CODEN: INJABN 19(1) i-viii, 1-118 (1984)
ISSN: 0020-773X

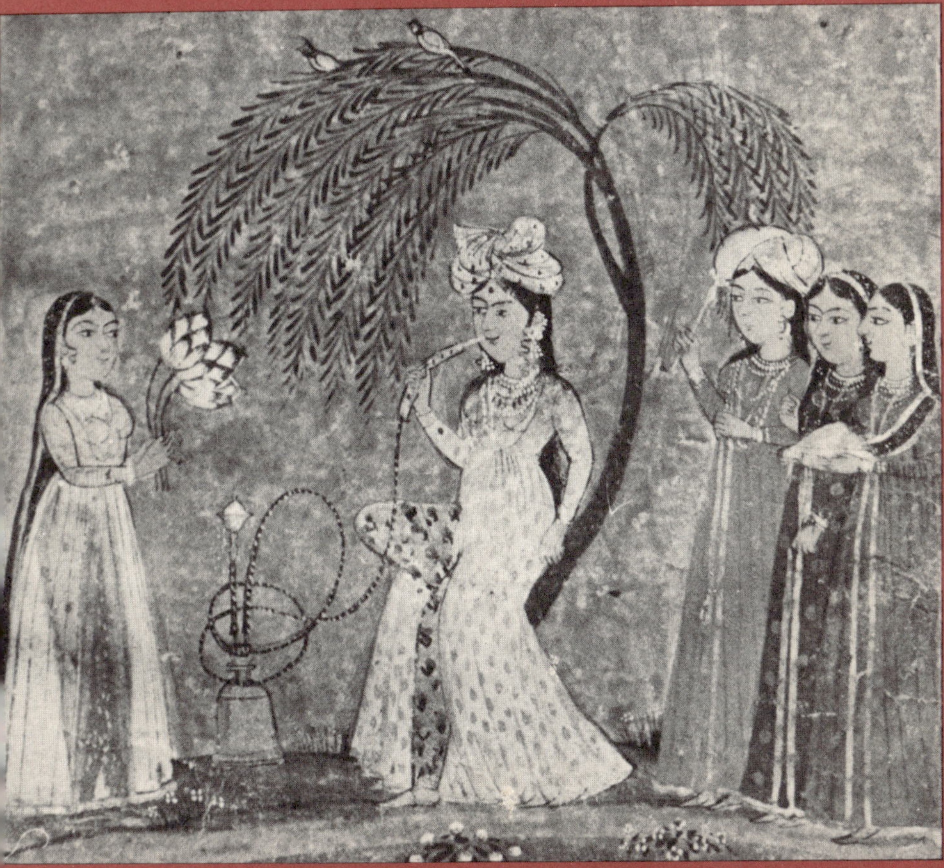

THE INTERNATIONAL JOURNAL OF THE Addictions

Volume 19 Number 1 1984

THE INTERNATIONAL JOURNAL OF THE ADDICTIONS

February 1984

Aims and Scope. This journal is a comprehensive medium for worldwide communication among both concerned laymen and professionals in research, training, and treatment in the field of addiction and substance misuse.

Indexing and Abstracting Services. Articles published in *The International Journal of the Addictions* are selectively indexed or abstracted in:

• Adolescent Mental Health Abstracts • ASCA • Bibliographic Index of Health Education Periodicals (BIHEP) • BioSciences Information Service of Biological Abstracts (BIOSIS) • Classified Abstract Archive of the Alcohol Literature • Current Contents/Clinical Practice • Excerpta Medica • Index Medicus • International Pharmaceutical Abstracts • ISI/BIOMED • Journal of Abstracts of the All-Union Institute of Scientific and Technical Information of the USSR • Psychological Abstracts • Science Citation Index • Selected List of Tables of Contents of Psychiatric Periodicals • Social Sciences Citation Index • State Central Scientific Medical Library/International Book Exchange–USSR

Articles published in *The International Journal of the Addictions* are listed in Selected List of Tables of Contents of Psychiatric Periodicals.

Manuscript Preparation and Submission. See inside back cover of this issue.

Subscription Information. *The International Journal of the Addictions* is published eight times annually in February, April, May, July, August, September, November, and December by Marcel Dekker, Inc., 270 Madison Avenue, New York, New York 10016. The subscription rate for Volume 19 (1984), containing eight numbers, is $225.00 per volume (prepaid). The special discounted rate for individual professionals and students is $112.50 per volume. To secure this special rate, your order must be prepaid by personal check. Add $20.00 for surface postage outside the United States. For airmail to Europe, add $32.48; to Asia, add $40.48.

Mailing Address. *Please mail payment with order to:* Marcel Dekker Journals, P. O. Box 11305, Church Street Station, New York, New York 10249.

Contributions to this journal are published free of charge. Second-class postage paid at New York, New York and at additional mailing offices.

Library of Congress Catalog Card Number 66-9896

Cover illustration courtesy of the Picture Collection, The Branch Libraries, New York Public Library.

Cover Illustration: Women using a hookah, probably to smoke a form of hashish (14--). Painting miniature, illustrating a Persian manuscript by Koka, *Kama Sastri*. Courtesy of the National Library of Medicine, Bethesda, Maryland 20014.

THE INTERNATIONAL JOURNAL OF THE Addictions

The International Journal of the Addictions, 19(1), iii–vii, 1984

Editorial

Coping and Drug Misuse Intervention

In the attempt to understand drug use/misuse and do something about it (as well as to minimize our own sense of failure and impotence in the face of its very existence and apparent increase), a number of critical concepts have been introduced to aid in intervention efforts and plans. *Coping* is one of these concepts. The term's use has become so common, by treatment agents and policymakers as well as by drug users, that we:

1. All too often attribute meaning to it which may be lacking
2. Limit the scope of its potential meaning(s)
3. Tend to overlook its varied implications
4. Confuse our ability to name the strategy and/or process of coping with our ability to understand and effectively utilize it

Coping has become yet another one of the shibboleths in the ongoing ritual of drug use intervention. We all too often attribute magical qualities to the drugs which are misused by categorizing them as *chemical coping mechanisms*. We continue to dehumanize the drug user by imputing limited abilities to him/her for successful functioning (coping, adaptation, life-styles) both without the help of his/her drug choice and because of the drug's chemical action(s). In essence the *concept of coping* permits us to conclude, without knowing the individual drug user or group of drug users, why the drug user began his/her socially unacceptable behavior, how he/she continues to misuse drugs, and why it is quite unlikely that drug misuse will ever change—for the better. Last, coping as a strategy, process, and life-style continues to be limited to only one segment, albeit a small segment, of those participating in drug intervention—the drug user.

Rarely, if ever, has this concept been explored with regard to:

1. The family of the drug user
2. The drug user's social network, which may (and often does) facilitate and reinforce drug use and the drug user's behavior
3. The intervention agents who have the responsibility to effect personal change
4. The policymakers who have the mandate to effect institutional and societal change

5. The institutional support sytem, which rarely is—but which should be—an integral component for effective intervention, planning, and delivery of needed appropriate services
6. The various communities within which drug use occurs, which are almost entirely responsible for funding intervention efforts, which on the surface do not tolerate drug use or the drug user, and which are ultimately responsible for the integration/reintegration of the treated drug users

In a sense, over time we have come to believe that *coping* is a problem only for the drug user—the identified drug user. The rest of us—individuals, systems, and institutions—are somehow immunized against the problems of chemical coping and chemical copers—other than being affected by "*them.*" The focus, for coping, from this perspective is "*them*" and not "*us.*" How realistic is this world view of drug use? In order to explore this question, it makes sense to briefly examine what coping is (and isn't) and what are some of the options in a given society, culture, or community.

No doubt you, the reader, have your own definition of coping. For the purpose of this brief note, *coping* is defined as a *style of or a stylized way of existing and/or functioning, for individuals and for systems.* There is nothing magical about coping. If the term, and the concept, didn't exist we would surely have to create another one in its place in order to describe patterns of existence, behavior, and functioning. Since *coping* is our term for describing complex patterns of behavior, it is obvious—or it should be obvious—that it cannot be a unitary concept. It covers a broad range of foci which are constantly in flux because of individual, systemic, institutional, and institutionalized factors (social, legal, political, economic, religious, educational, cultural, etc.). These foci cope with these various factors—both within and because of the factors—at various levels, at any given time.

For heuristic reasons we can categorize coping styles in terms of *primary focus* if we remember that every individual and/or system is in a sense a multicoper. Table 1 lists a number of coping options. The reader can add to this list or delete some of the options in terms of his/her own theoretical and/or existential perspective. Central to the utilization of this table is our having to reasonably understand those factors which permit a specific individual and/or system to experience the option as being available, utilizable, and meaningful in order to achieve specific goals; and those factors underlying the rejection of the coping option or its postponement.

Drug use intervention continues to:

1. Present itself as an organized, systematic, systemic effort designed to negate the seductiveness and power of certain chemicals which result (somehow) in maladaptive behavior/functioning
2. Prevent non-drug users from becoming *chemical copers*

Table 1
Some Categories of Coping Styles: A Beginning[a]

Selected coping options	Examples	Facilitating/inhibiting factors
Self	Own resources	Must be able to organize one's environment (internal and external)
Other people	Help from others	Availability of others; making oneself available to others
Systems	Family Networks Organizations Neighborhoods Communities Cultures	Membership, identification, participation (active/passive)
Things/ substances	Drugs Social substances Medicines	
Activities	Work Leisure Hobbies	
Beliefs	Religions Ideologies	
Other (specify)		

[a]Two other critical factors are not included in this schematic tool so as not to complicate it. These are *strategy* and *process*. The interested reader may choose to explore the needed strategies and processes by which selected coping options are achieved, postponed, maintained, or totally rejected.

3. Integrate/reintegrate active chemical copers into a world of multiple satisfying non-chemical-coping options

Reports continue to be issued noting that our successes are minimal and our failures are massive. Why is this so—if indeed it is so? A brief analysis of the lack of use, or inappropriate use, of the concept of *coping* in treatment planning may serve to help us to understand how we continue to build failure into our efforts.

If *healthier, socially acceptable coping* is a reasonable intervention goal, what prevents us from utilizing it more effectively with drug users? There are numerous possible answers to this loaded question! No doubt you, the reader, can add your own answer(s).

- One possibility is that we really don't want the drug user to cope in a healthier, more acceptable way. If drug users did, then they would be like us. And *we know* that they are different from us–intrinsically different!
- Second, many of us may not know how to go beyond the concept of coping in our own lives. In order that we can help others who are stigmatized, maladaptive copers, we would be forced to *join with them* in a mutual venture, rather than continue to treat them as we currently do at a *therapeutic distance.*
- A third possibility is that the concept of coping has yet to be effectively integrated into the process of treatment.

For example, the variety of screening processes and techniques currently in use do not seem to pay adequate attention to the scope of coping mechanisms or to potential coping typologies. An accurate diagnosis doesn't necessarily help us to understand the various coping mechanisms which the person and/or system has used, is currently using, has the ability to use, or is likely to use in the future. We are inundated with: levels of psychosexual development, defense mechanisms, traumas, deprivations, traits, personality types, histories of reinforcements and punishments, biochemical states, etc. But we have yet to develop typologies of copers from the material which has been gathered during screening and intake, material which is or should be usuable for the next major stage in treatment planning–appropriate goal selection. In simplistic terms, what treatment goals (short and long term, change related and maintenance related) are most appropriate for different types of *primary copers*? Were we able to answer this question, we would be challenged by yet another problem which has yet to be adequately solved to date. What therapeutic techniques are most appropriate for specific coping goals for different types of copers? The reader can obviously see where this line of thinking/questioning is likely to lead.

- What policies are needed to achieve selected types, levels, and qualities of coping as a function of treatment?
- What types of therapist-copers are needed in order to plan for and then achieve the desired coping on the part of the current chemical coper?
- Under what condition are the coping styles of systems and institutions that are (or should be) involved in the treatment-rehabilitation-intergration of the chemical coper detrimental or helpful in the intervention process?
- And, of course, we owe it to ourselves to ask what criteria should be used in order to reasonably conclude whether we–the drug user and the intervention system–have failed or succeeded. Is abstinence versus drug use to be the only major criterion?

These are but some of the issues and questions which are related to the continued use of the concept of *coping*. No doubt the term will continue to be used to answer questions which are rarely if ever asked. It is unfortunate that the term has become a mechanism of closure rather than a stimulus for further needed efforts. It is unfortunate that we have limited its meaning (s) and implications to selected chemicals, as well as to stigmatized segments of the visible drug-using population, rather than extending its potential outcome to all of us who are involved in and/or affected by drug use intervention. The latter option still exists for those of us who can be turned on by an exciting and relatively unexplored process after years of being turned off by a semantic cul-de-sac.

S. Einstein, PhD
Jerusalem, Israel

The International Journal of the Addictions, 19(1),1-23, 1984

Human Garbage and Physical Garbage: A Sociological Case Example of Institutional Violence

Nachman Ben-Yehuda, PhD

Department of Sociology, Hebrew University, Jerusalem 91905, Israel

Stanley Einstein,* PhD

Institute for the Study of Drug Misuse

Abstract

Since 1981 hundreds of drug addicts have been "treated" with methadone in the midst of the largest garbage dump in Israel. This paper details how this "treatment" program came into being and suggests the term "institutional violence" as the appropriate analytical concept to interpret this phenomenon.

INTRODUCTION

Historically speaking, *deviance* has almost always been thought of and analyzed as an act of an individual or individuals. Rarely, if ever, was deviance thought of as a product of institutions.

There are at least two glaring exceptions to this observation. The first is the labeling approach in deviance (e.g., Goode, 1978; Rubington and Weinberg, 1971; Schur, 1971, 1979). The labeling approach conceptualizes deviance in the following manner:

*To whom requests for reprints should be sent at 113/41 East Talpiot, Jerusalem, Israel.

0020-773X/84/1901-0001$3.50/0

> . . . social groups create deviance by making the rules whose infraction constitutes deviance, and by applying those rules to particular people and labeling them as outsiders. . . . Deviance is not a quality of the act a person commits, but rather a consequence of the application by others of rules and sanctions to an "offender". The deviant is one to whom that label has successfully been applied: deviant behavior is behavior that people so label. . . . (Becker, 1963, p. 9)

The labeling approach thus shifted the focus of attention from the deviant-actor to the environment in which he/she functions, drawing attention to the *societal reaction* to a presumed act of deviance. Within this theoretical framework, emphasis is being put on the role of society at large and social control agencies in particular in the amplification and actual manufacture of deviance. Thus Garfinkel (1980) analyzed the degradation ceremonies that deviants go through, and Goffman (1963) showed how deviants become stigmatized.

The second exception is a continuation partly of the labeling approach and partly of the Marxist approach to deviance research (see, e.g., Taylor, Walton, and Young, 1973). However, this approach can also be viewed independently of the labeling process. In this approach scholars again shifted attention from the deviant to his/her environment, but instead of asking how this environment helped crystallize deviance, the approach examined the question How much is this environment, totally or partially, deviant?

At least since the mid-1970s, and especially after the Watergate affair in the United States, researchers have been alerted to the fact that social institutions themselves are–more than once–involved in perpetrating various deviant and violent acts. This idea is, relatively speaking, new for social science research.

One of the first scholars to write from this perspective was Liazos (1972). Criticizing contemporary deviance research, Liazos suggested that both law enforcement and deviance researchers concentrated their efforts on small-scale deviances, neglecting the institutional form of deviance. Liazos stated that:

> The powerful "deviants" are . . . left untouched. . . . Because [deviance researchers] . . . concentrate their attention on those who have been *successfully labelled as "deviant"* and not on those who break laws, fix laws, violate ethical and moral standards, harm individuals and groups, etc. . . . (pp. 100–109)

Liazos continued by suggesting that:

> . . . violence is presented as the exclusive property of the poor in the slum, the minorities, street gangs, and motor cycle beasts. But if we take the concept *violence* seriously, we see that much of our own

> political and economic system thrives on it. In violence, a person is *violated*—there is harm done to his person, his psyche, his body, his dignity, his ability to govern himself. . . . We must see that *current institutional violence* is much more destructive than overt individual violence. . . . Violence is committed daily by the government, very often by lack of action. . . . (pp. 111-112)

In the forthcoming analysis we use the concept of *covert institutional violence* to analyze and explain drug abuse treatment programs in Israel and particularly the largest drug abuse treatment program available in Israel since 1981. In this program drug addicts daily receive large amounts of a narcotic substance—methadone—plus a variety of barbiturates. This occurs in the midst of what is the largest garbage dump site in Israel and probably one of the largest in the Middle East. An understanding of the relationship between covert institutional violence and the treatment of Israeli drug abusers necessitates a brief historical background.

HISTORICAL AND SUBSTANTIVE BACKGROUND

Drug abuse as an acknowledged phenomenon and social problem in Israel is relatively new. The continued view is that drug abuse, and its problematic manifestations, occurred after the Six Day War, in 1967. The etiology of the drug use problem is associated with Western/Westernized Jewish students who brought drugs and drug use to Israel as a way of adaptation; with Christian volunteers who introduced drug use to kibbutz youth and young adults; and with the Bedouins, who smuggled drugs, primarily hashish, from the administered areas or over the borders of neighboring countries. From this perspective the drug use problem is a new phenomenon introduced by foreigners. This has resulted in the continued effort by the public at large and all government agencies (national, municipal, regional), as well as professional agencies, to distance themselves from the existence of drugs, their increasing availability and use, and the existence of a broad variety of drug users. The initial denial that drugs were available and used by many different types of Israelis has been transformed into a "homogenizing" process. Drugs are seen as unusual, unacceptable, dangerous, and illegal substances used by societal deviants. As a result of this active cognitive and emotional homogenizing, the drug user is stripped of all actual and potential roles and functions, other than that of being a drug user.

The vast majority of treatment programs in Israel, for most illnesses and conditions, utilize and/or are influenced by the traditional hierarchical medical model. Many, if not most, treatment policymakers and treatment agents have had little experience with the treatment of drug use and the drug user. Paralleling this reality are the extensive use of medications for primary, secondary, and tertiary prevention, and the lack of interest in, lack of use of, and resistance to a broad variety of other reasonably effective and available treatment techniques. Thus, the Israeli drug abuser has generally been diagnosed, prior to being personally examined and listened to, as an untreatable nonfunctioning personality who is dangerous and violent; who will not cooperate with treatment staff; who is either incapable or not desirous of complying to the demands of a treatment regimen; who is unmotivated; who is most likely to disrupt day-to-day functioning of a treatment facility.

Three types of treatment are available to Israeli addicts. The first is detoxification. Detoxification is legally and traditionally available (condoned) in closed wards in psychiatric hospitals. How many detoxifications are done annually is not known. Nor does any individual or agency seem to be interested in knowing. The second type of treatment is methadone maintenance. There are three such programs; all have been founded and funded by the Israeli Ministry of Health since 1975. Two are directly administered by the ministry (Acco, Jaffa/Tel Aviv); one is administered by Israel's largest sick fund, Chupat Cholim (Haifa). The third type of treatment was established in Jerusalem and is administered by a private psychiatric hospital. This latter clinic provides a variety of treatment techniques but does not provide methadone. There can hardly be a question that the creation of these four specialized programs (other than detoxification) has permitted the health care delivery system to isolate drug users. Furthermore, while the central region of Israel is well covered by programs, north of Haifa and Acco and south of Jerusalem, no programs are available for addicts. There are no therapeutic communities, hostels, or halfway houses for drug users in Israel. It is important to note that the total number of drug users treated monthly by all four programs averages between 300 and 350. From 1978 until 1982 all four outpatient programs treated a total of no more than 500 drug users. Government guesses estimate that the number of narcotic addicts in Israel ranges between 4,000 and 8,000. These numbers lack any type of validity and have never been used for treatment planning.

Services are limited or unavailable for so-called special populations. There are no long-term outpatient treatment services available for teenage drug users. There are no programs available for the pregnant drug user. The unique needs of the female deviant drug user are rarely, if ever, met in any of the specialized drug centers. This is of particular concern when one considers that the majority of the female drug users who are in treatment were born into and reared in a familial and neighborhood culture which attributes first-class status to males and a second-rate and a service-oriented role and status to females. One of the specialized treatment centers has a unit designed to meet the needs of Arabic-speaking patients. There are no treatment services available for the aged drug user. Family therapy, as an ongoing process for the entire family, for drug users and nonusers, is available as an integral part of treatment in only one center.

These limitations result in treatment being given to (and taken by) male, adult Jews primarily (Ben-Yehuda, 1979). It is interesting to note that all four specialized outpatient clinics are directed by nonphysicians, in a medical-model-oriented delivery of care system. The great majority of the interdisciplinary staffs working in each of these centers have had relatively little experience in treating patients generally, and even less experience treating drug users. The development of specialized drug user treatment centers is not associated with special knowledge, skills, or experience on the part of clinical and/or policy-making staff. Rather it has been associated with the physical isolation of the pathologically laden and tainted—the labeled, visible drug users. This is further reinforced by the selected sites of treatment. Many of the approved treatment sites for drug users are either inappropriate, dehumanizing, or both. For a number of years the Acco Center was in a bomb shelter; the Haifa Center is situated in a respectable clinic building with a special entrance for drug users which does not permit them to enter onto other floors or mingle with other types of medical patients. The Jaffa program is in a physically isolated, dreary, dilapidated building, with barred windows, close to the seashore. The Jerusalem program was not permitted to enter a building designated and refurbished for its activities and was put into a relatively uninhabited part of town bordered on one side by a train terminal.

Thus, it is evident that the institutionalized treatment, in Israel, of drug users since 1975 has been, and remains, control oriented, and not change oriented. Furthermore, the drug users' access to a broad variety of needed psychological, social welfare, vocational-remedial, and existential services—which do exist in Israel—is virtually blocked. Social disability benefits are not given to known addicts, and the National Insurance Institute (Bituach Leumi), the primary governmental agency responsible for granting and monitoring social welfare payments, has formally disallowed health insurance to known drug users; clearly this is a strange decision in a country where alcoholism is acknowledged to be a disease and drug abuse is not.

In summary, failure is built into inappropriately based and dehumanizing detoxification efforts; a limited number of relatively newly developed government-funded specialized drug user outpatient treatment centers offer a limited number of treatment techniques to a small percentage of Israel's "estimated" active drug users; the needs of special populations of drug users are rarely, if ever, met; the needed and available services from the existing treatment and service support system are generally unavailable to active, as well as former, multiproblem multiple-drug users. These events and their implications and consequences exist within a country and culture which continues to deny the incidence and prevalence of drug use; which chooses to "blame" the existence of visible drug users upon personal and/or specified environmental pathology as well as foreign elements; which "homogenizes" the drug user into a visible, unacceptable entity and therein dehumanizes him/her; which offers treatment to those who are willing and able to fit into the role and status demands of a medical-model-oriented care delivery system.

The foregoing description provides a basis for understanding how a private treatment program, situated in Israel's largest garbage dump (and probably one of the largest in the Middle East), in the Tel Aviv region, came into being.

THE GARBAGE DUMP TREATMENT OF DRUG USERS

For a number of years a substantial group of drug users in Israel had not been in treatment in any of the four specialized centers for a number of reasons which are not the primary focus of this paper. They consisted of both Tel Aviv residents and those living in other parts of the country. A number of these drug users managed to receive prescriptions from physicians for methadone, as well as other medications. The Israeli police have contended that there were a group of "script" doctors who sold prescriptions. Israeli law, and the backing of the Israeli Medical Association regarding the right of the physician to prescribe as s/he sees fit, had effectively prevented police intervention. There were those who claimed that implicit and explicit threats by drug users–in the privacy of the physician's office, clinic, or even home–served to ease the receipt of such prescriptions. Few Israeli professionals presume that the majority of such prescriptions, for a broad variety of "medications," were issued to ill drug users who had been examined.

Over time a local pharmacy situated in Tel Aviv's famous Dizengoff Street became the place for honoring these prescriptions. Dizengoff Street is a hub of activity for Israelis and tourists alike, filled with shops and coffee houses. Indeed, Hebrew slang has made a verb of Dizengoff which expresses window shopping, walking, relaxing, sipping coffee–doing what is done by fun-loving conventional people on other famous streets in the main cities of the world. And within this ecology of conviviality the dreaded drug user arrived. Initially their numbers were small, so that the mechanism of denial on the part of shop-owners, residents, and the municipal powers was sufficient. In 1980 the numbers grew; complaints were made; pressure mounted. The pharmacist, who had emigrated from England, claimed he was simply carrying out his duties in both a professional and humane manner.

The pharmacist, not withstanding his humane professionalism, chose not to focus upon the factor of economic gain from a growing captive audience which was not being served by other pharmacies. As the pressure mounted, Israel's only informally structured private methadone program was transferred by the pharmacist to a shack in Jaffa. The shack was soon mysteriously burned down. While perhaps the Tel Aviv pharmacist could have removed himself from the program and the pressure–he chose not to. Tel Aviv's mayor, ostensibly bowing to community pressure—in a city in which Dizengoff Street is neither a neighborhood nor a community—offered a most clever solution. The sale of legal methadone and other medications to addicts holding valid prescriptions was moved by municipal order to Israel's largest garbage dump, on the outskirts of the Tel Aviv municipality, and was retained as a private venture. This occurred in August 1981, and at the time of writing this paper it is still continuing (see Figs. 1 and 2). During 1982 the number of drug users serviced by this organized chemotherapy happening has been acknowledged to be between 800 and 900 self-declared drug users. There are other estimates which approach 1,200. This program serves at least four times more drug users than all of the official Israeli programs combined. On any given day, from Sunday to Thursday, from 1 P.M. to 3 P.M., approximately 120 prescription holders are served. The vast majority of them are males, generally ranging in age from 20 to 30; approximately 5% are females. The vast majority of these self-declared addict prescription holders are

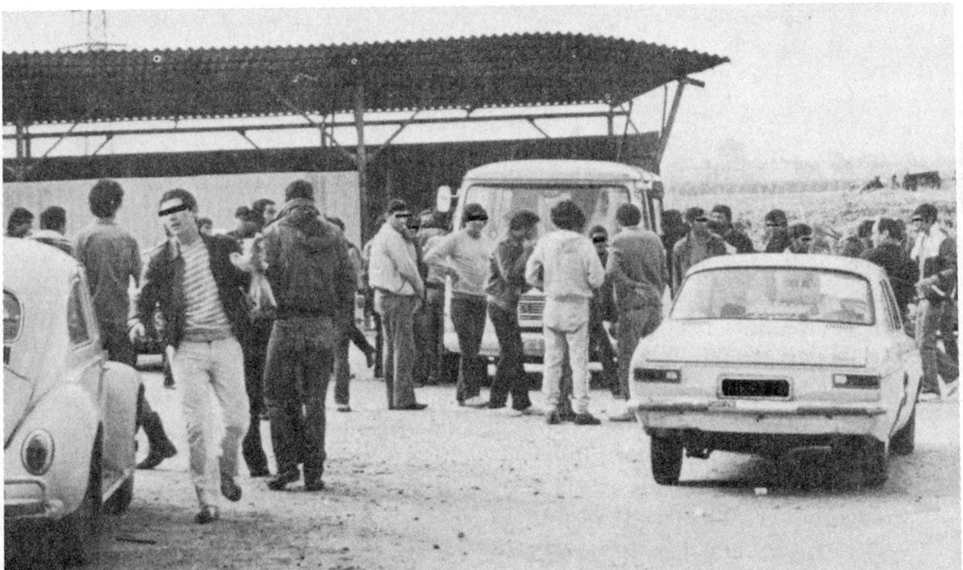

Fig. 1. Drug users waiting to purchase their "chemotherapy from a mobile pharmacy in the garbage dump.

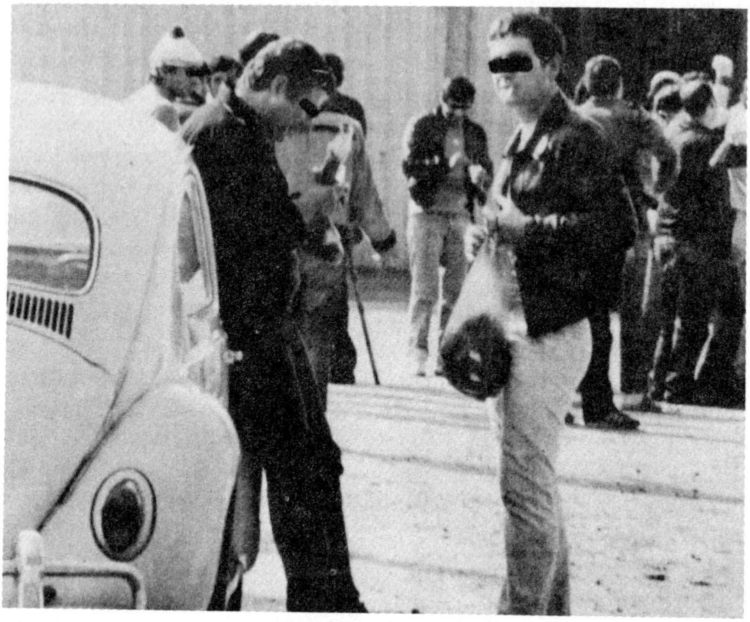

Fig. 2. A completed purchase.

of Sephardic or North African ethnic background, the same group which is primarily treated in the four specialized centers. This is the very same ethnic group which has been associated with the concept of *social deprivation*, which necessitates individual, group, and neighborhood intervention and rehabilitation. The 2-hour private, mobile chemical supermarket offers bottles of methadone (100 mg/bottle), barbiturates, and amphetamines. It is guarded by two border policemen, who do not interfere when these legal medicines are exchanged or sold to others (with no prescriptions).

The "happening" site is off a major highway to which there is no public transportation. Since many, if not most, of these "social garbage entities" don't own cars, they hire cabs to take them there and then back home to Tel Aviv, or to a bus stop to go back to their own town or city. "The Garbage Dump Program" is one of the few nonregionalized programs in Israel. Residency is not a criteria. The reality is that there are no criteria other than getting there physically with a valid prescription and money to pay for the legal drugs. One does not have to appear every day. This "program" permits participants to receive a methadone supply for up to 14 days (1,400 mg) at one time. There are no age criteria. Since there is no valid evidence that physical examinations occur, there are no medical contraindications to methadone use. In this light, pregnant women addicted to methadone in that "program" are essentially on their own regarding prenatal care, giving birth, and postnatal care for themselves and their infants. Since there are no mental health examinations, there are no psychiatric contraindications to methadone, barbiturates, or amphetamines. Since there is no anamnesis available, there are no adaptational contraindications to any of these drugs, the amount used, how they are mixed, and their frequency of use. Since the parental role of the participant, at the garbage dump, is unknown, there is no way of preventing young children from mistakenly using their parents' "medicines," or older children from commencing drug use in the bosom of their family. Since there is no ongoing follow-up, which is believable, the medical tradition of titration is nonexistent. These are only a selected number of the issues involved in the "garbage program."

The economic facts of this protected and condoned chemotherapy happening are an issue unto themselves but are not the primary focus of this paper. Suffice it to say that a microeconomic system has been developed by an entrepreneurial pharmacist with a growing captive audience in collusion with government and municipal officials and agencies against a backdrop of public disinterest.

Assuming that a drug user made an appearance only once every two weeks, the immediate costs would be 966 IS* per 14 bottles of methadone (a bottle a day), 100 IS payment for the biweekly prescription, and approximately 200 IS for the cab fare—a total of 1,266 IS. The payments for barbiturates and amphetamines are purposely not included in this "budgetary" example. The annual cost to each drug user is 32,916 IS. This cost is certainly not an insurmountable one for the average street drug user, particularly when one considers that at the same time a bottle of methadone in the black market costs about IS 110 (compared to 69 IS in the licit market). One must also remember that from a pharmacological point of view many, if not most, drug users can satisfy their theoretical biochemical need with half a bottle, leaving the other half for sale (7 bottles for use and 7 for sale). In this sense, after the initial layout during the first few trips to the garbage dump, the venture becomes a self-funded one, if not a profitable one. When one moves from the individual to the group, using an estimate of 1,000 participants, the economic value increases to 3,291,600 IS ($126,600) annually.

From the pharmacist's perspective this program is a windfall occurring in a land of secular miracles. His overhead is minimal. Indeed, the program's hours

*IS = Israeli shekel. The exchange rate in August 1982 was $1 = 26 IS.

do not interfere with his pharmacy; stores are traditionally closed in Israel from 1 to 4 P.M. The estimated profit made by the pharmacist on each bottle of methadone he sells is very close to 50% (based on the manufacturer's price for a bottle vs the price to the individual customer). Even if we accept the low figure of 800 drug users in the program, 800 bottles a day for 365 days a year still result in a considerable profit. This is a tidy sum for 2 hours daily of dehumanizing isolation among human rubble and physical garbage. On the surface it would seem that the "program" meets the needs of the participating applicants—the satisfied customers. It surely meets the needs of the pharmacist. This garbage dump program also meets the needs of a number of other critical vested interest groups. It meets the needs of the *police*. They can monitor a large number of drug users at a given time and place. Indeed, the police over the last few years have become advocates of methadone treatment rather than other available treatment techniques. It meets the needs of the *Tel Aviv Municipality* in removing an undesirable human blight from one of Tel Aviv's show places. In this sense, it also meets the needs of the *Ministry of Tourism*; Dizengoff Street is a tourist haven. It meets the needs of the *Treasury* in a number of ways. At a relatively insignificant level, the microeconomic system which has been created results in available tax money (e.g., manufacture of methadone, the pharmacist, and cab drivers). It saves the Treasury public funds which theoretically would/might be expended to treat these 800 drug users. It meets the needs of the *Ministry of Health* is a variety of ways. They have used (misused?) this program to demonstrate how bad things can get in an attempt to get more money from the Treasury. The goal has not been achieved. In a theoretical sense this example of institutionally fostered inhumanity and malpractice has also served the *professional treatment community*: Treatable citizens don't behave this way; they don't permit themselves to be engaged by inexpensive medical seduction. The stereotype of addicts who are obviously unmotivated to change is thus reinforced.

This program was not hidden. Almost as soon as the program began, the media reported it. Newspapers, electronic images, and radio broadcasts were unable to stop the program. The Interministerial Committee on drug abuse, mandated to develop a national program and given executive powers to initiate new programs and monitor ongoing programs, was not effective in stopping the profit-making chemotherapy maltreatment. Indeed, the deputy attorney general, who represented the Ministry of Justice within the Interministerial Committee, pointed out to relevant ministers and government officials that the program was illegal. And yet it continued. Apparently, a major reason for the continuation of the "program" is the fact that the interests of both the pharmacist and the municipality of Tel Aviv match almost perfectly on this matter. Thus, in the summer of 1983, when the deputy attorney general attempted to force the municipality of Tel Aviv to let other pharmacists in Tel Aviv provide methadone–the attempt failed. Pharmacies which advertised in the local newspaper that they would sell methadone were visited by city inspectors falsely threatening them that this was illegal and that their business licenses would be revoked.

One has to add that, in a sense, the visible drug users are passive but willing participants in an activity designed to anihilate their sense of worth and being, maintain their malfunctioning, and isolate them from society at large and the very agencies and institutions which are mandated by law and tradition to be responsible for the comprehensive welfare, present and future, of the constituency of man. It is these agencies, individually and collectively, which have choreographed a societal-professional tragedy (see Table 1).

AN EXPERIMENT

The authors of this article were naive enough to believe that this pseudo-treatment program was created simply because of temporary pressure and was

Table 1

Passive and Active Participants Associated with the Institutionalized Violence of Drug User Treatment[a]

The Knesset	Professional organizations
Ministry of Health	Physicians
Ministry of the Interior (Police)	Psychiatrists
Ministry of Justice	Psychologists
Ministry of Labor and Social Welfare	Social workers
Ministry of Tourism	Nurses
Interministerial Committee on a Comprehensive Drug Strategy	Pharmacists
	Lawyers
Tel Aviv Municipality	General hospitals
The pharmacist (selling the "drugs")	Psychiatric hospitals
	Specialized clinics treating drug users
Physicians (providing prescriptions)	Religious institutions
	Rabbinate
Cab drivers	Churches
Chupat Cholim (Sick Fund)	Kaddis
	WAQF
Al-Sam (National Organization of Citizens Against Drug Use)	Israeli citizens
	Media

[a]Two years after the initiation of a privately developed program which formalized the institutionalized violence of the treatment of drug users in Israel, the program was ended by threat of legal intervention instituted by the Ministry of Justice. A number of "script" doctors were arrested and a number of pharmacies in the Tel Aviv area undertook to fill legitimate prescriptions.

due to some basic misunderstandings about treatment. As members of the Interministerial Committee on drug abuse they urged members of the committee, as well as a multiplicity of institutional contacts, to close down this form of maltreatment and offer reasonable treatment, including methadone maintenance, in a dignified, humane, and professional manner to fellow citizens.

Representatives of the police and Ministry of Health (responsible for all psychiatric-mental health treatment in Israel) who served on the Interministerial Committee were disinterested or unwilling to close the program. The chairman of the committee, who was director-general of a large and prestigious medical center, chose not to use his executive powers, his professional and personal status in the community, and his government connections to effectively intervene. The vast majority of committee members chose not to get involved. Al-Sam, the only national citizens organization committed to drug use prevention and the stimulation of community interest and action, carried out its lip service intervention by sending telegrams, making a number of phone calls, and having a limited number of meetings with governmental officials. Its national office is housed in Tel Aviv. The chairman of the board is a well-known journalist with many contacts.

The government-mandated committee, responsible to a committee of ministers, was clearly unable to stop the shameful maltreatment of drug addicts.

A second attempt to intervene in this shameful "garbage program" was undertaken by the second author, the founder and director of the center treating drug users and their families in Jerusalem. This attempt/experiment can be thought of as an attempt at both giving the facts and their potential implications and at moral persuasion of actual or potential power brokers. A letter was sent to key political and religious leaders on March 8, 1982, as well as to heads of national organizations representing the treatment professions of Israel. A follow-up letter was sent to those individuals/organizations who did not respond to the first letter. (A copy of the original, long letter can be obtained by writing to the second author.) The letters were standard and focused on two points: First, the dreary facts about the "garbage program" were given, and, second, the "selected power broker" was asked to do whatever he/she could to solve the problem of the "garbage treatment." With the exception of two organizations, all those who received the letter answered. No response was received from the National Association of Israeli Social Workers. The Israeli Criminological Association also did not respond. At the urging of the first author, during the annual Israeli Criminological Association convention in Jerusalem, the presidential address mentioned the shameful "garbage treatment" and urged attenders to sign a petition against its existence. While a few hundred signatures were collected–nothing was actually done with them.

Table 2 briefly summarizes the essence of each response by quoting, from the authors' perspective, the key message. The differential answers reveal a clear

Table 2

In Their Own Words: Responses by National Political/Governmental, Moral, Religious, and Professional Leaders to a Request for Intervention

Prime Minister Menachem Begin

"It is difficult for me to understand why you turn to me with your complaint. . . . I never heard of this program that you write about in your letter of March 14, 1982. Now I know. Therefore I am forwarding your letter to the Minister of Health and am asking him to take care of this immediately. This is the responsibility of the Minister of Health and his task." [No response from the Ministry of Health was ever received.]

President Yitzhak Navon

"I acknowledge receipt of your letter of April 12, 1982 as well as a copy of your letter of March 9. We never saw your letter of March 9, and in my opinion the second letter was totally unnecessary. I will put the copy of your letter on the President's desk." [Signed by the personal assistant to the president. There was never a response from the president or from his office.]

Chief Rabbi Shlomo Goren

"Because the Chief Rabbi of Israel is not sufficiently knowledgeable about the drug issue, he was unable to fully understand your opinions in your letter, he does not understand the meaning of your letter or what you are requesting him to do about this issue. The Chief Rabbi requests that you explain the intentions of your letter."

Minister of the Interior Dr. Joseph Burg

[Printed form letter] "This is to acknowledge receipt of your letter of March 12, 1982 to the Minister of the Interior. [It] has been forwarded for action to those individuals who are involved with it at the National Police Headquarters, who will investigate the issue and will communicate the outcome of their actions as quickly as possible." [A letter was sent to the author by superintendent Zvi Ariel from the Israeli police. His response is given later.]

Labor and Social Affairs Committee, The Knesset: Chairman Mr. Menachem Porush

"I acknowledge the receipt of your letter regarding the issue of the legal use of the drug methadone. Unfortunately the pressure under which the Labor and Social Affairs Committee has operated prevented us until today to give our opinion about the problem which you raised. I don't know what the committee can do practically; I only wish we were able to contribute."

Israel Medical Association: Chairman Dr. R. Ishai

"I read your letter of March 4 with much interest. I am as sorry as you are about the matter of the distribution of the drug and on the basis of the treatment. . . . However I must acknowledge that perhaps this activity is intrinsically less serious than what it looks like when focusing on it from the outside. But even if things are as you have described them I don't see what the Medical Association can do about this issue. Surely we can not take a position.

Do we have a treatment suggestion as to how to handle this problem? I thought about it and didn't find a suggestion. Therefore I am sure that you should apply your sharp arrow to the Minister of Health, which is supposed to be responsible for [handling] these problems."

The Israeli Bar: Director of Central Committee Micha Yinon

"I was sorry to read the content of your letter regarding the use of drugs and their sale in the garbage dump near Tel Aviv. I don't see in what way the Central Committee of

(continued)

Table 2 (continued)

Lawyers can be involved. Nevertheless I will see to it that the contents of your letter is printed in our newsletter in order to make our members and their institutions aware [of the problem]."

Israel Nurses Association, Jerusalem Branch of Nurses: Secretary Sima Winter

"I am forwarding [your letter] to the National Secretary of the Nurses Association, for a decision regarding a response to this issue.

I hope that a solution will be found to the important problem that you raised in order to help these patients." [No further response was ever received.]

Israeli Psychiatric Association: President Elect Dr. M. Neuman

"In response to your letter of April 27, 1982, I wish to inform you that the chairman of the Psychiatric Association currently and for the next two years is Prof. ——. I was elected President Elect and will enter into my role in two years.

The same day that I received your letter I forwarded it to Prof. —— and requested that he respond to you. Enclosed is a copy of my letter to Prof. —— dated April 11, 1982. As you can see I behaved properly although I may have erred in not sending you a copy of the letter which I sent to Prof. ——. I apologize for that.

Permit me to make you aware that your critical letters will not contribute towards cooperation. I hope that you will get a letter from Prof. ——.

I value your important activities very much and strengthen your hand in your humanitarian battle." [No additional answer was ever received.]

Attorney General's Office (Ministry of Justice): Deputy Attorney General Yudith Karp

"The Attorney General is able to be active only in his own area of jurisdiction with his own tools. With the creation of the Interministerial Committee a direction has been selected to cope with the complex question of drug use in Israel. A representative of the Attorney General is a member of this Committee and the Attorney General expresses his position through this representative. It would not be appropriate for the Attorney General to interfere at this point by taking a position regarding subjects which are basically social [and in which] their legal expression is a side issue. . . . The authority [regarding the program] is, after all, not in the hands of the Attorney General and as long as the Interministerial Committee hasn't issued its final report, there is no place for the Attorney General's intervention."

Israel Police (Chief, Dept. of Intelligence and Detectives–Drugs): Superintendent Inspector Zvi Ariel

"Treatment of drug users is the sole responsibility of the Ministry of Health . . . [as is] the issuing of medical prescriptions of dangerous medical drugs and their distribution."

Prof. Elchanan Mair, Chairman, Israeli Psychological Association

5/4/82: "Thank you for your letter of 7/3/82. I don't feel that I understand the issue sufficiently and therefore it is my intention to forward this to colleagues who are more informed."

11/5/82: "I received your first letter of 7/3/82 and also the current one. The question was not neglected (honestly!). Rather up until now we have not been prepared for activities such as these. We are just beginning now. Your contribution [letter] has served as a catalyst. We have spoken for some time about a 'think tank' and a 'responding group' which will be active in regard to suitable/[professional] questions. At the last meeting of the Central Committee I presented your first letter. We decided

(continued)

Table 2 (continued)

upon a small staff which will check out the possibilities for responding to the issue which you raised, as well as to other issues. We decided that we will attempt to respond to and relate to issues which have public significance as well as to those which contribute to psychological knowledge. Therefore there is a need for teams of experts which will weigh what to do as well as how to do it. The staff decided to ask you to select 2 other psychologists as a 'think tank' team which will suggest what to do and how, in regard to the general issue of drugs and addiction [in Israel]."

We, the Central Committee, will be able to contribute: a formal and legitimizing backing [to the suggested activities], resources, i.e. press conferences, study days, contacts with the media, etc. . . .

How does this seem to you?"

A. Bass, Chairman, and A. Regev, Secretary, Pharmaceutical Association of Israel

3/24/82: "In response to your letter of 3/8/82, I am enclosing a letter [see Appendix A] which was sent by us to Prof. Modan, Director General of the Ministry of Health, in which we suggested a solution to the problem of the drug users. In addition we have met, because of this issue, with Dr. Philosoph, Director of Mental Health Services, Ministry of Health. We have requested her to help to get a place in Donolo B Hospital in order to distribute medications to drug users.

We are thankful to you for helping us to promote this issue."

5/12/82: "I received your letter of 4/29/82 and am sorry that you didn't receive my answer which was sent to you 3/24/82. I am enclosing a copy of my letter for your interest. I wrote to the Mayor of Tel Aviv, Mr. Shlomo Lahat, and requested that we be given a place in Donolo B Hospital for the purpose of legally distributing narcotics to patients in an organized place.

I received an answer that by the end of this month there will be a meeting including a representative of the Tel Aviv Municipality as well as the Chief of Police of Tel Aviv. A final decision will be made whether or not we will receive a place to open a pharmacy for this purpose.

If we are not successful in convincing the Mayor of Tel Aviv, and the Chief Police, that it is forbidden to distribute methadone to drug addicts in the garbage dump we will appeal to the High Court and demand that the Ministry of Health be forced, as well as the Israeli Police, to regulate this issue for the benefit of the patients."

---

and consistent pattern of avoiding the issue, throwing responsibility to other agencies/people, evasion, etc. This pattern seems to strongly support Liazos's (1972) definition of institutional violence as that "committed . . . by the government, very often by lack of action . . ." (p. 112).

DISCUSSION

The discussion is divided along two main axes: first, an analysis of the background of how the "garbage dump" methadone program could come into being, and second, a theoretical framework.

Background Factors

The first issue we have to address ourselves to involves two questions: How did the "garbage dump" program start? What enables its continued existence? To understand the answers to these questions, one has to familiarize oneself with a few relevant background factors. First, Israel is a small developing country which does not easily accept or understand the unusual or different phenomena, styles, individuals, or groups—in either the secular or the religious sphere. Drug use and the publically visible/identified drug user continue to be rejected and isolated, as being incompatible with Israel's past, present, and future existence and life-style. This has resulted in the continued effort by the public at large and all government agencies (national, municipal, and regional), as well as the professional ones, to distance themselves from the existence of drugs and their increasing availability/use, as well as the existence of a broad variety of drug users. The initial denial that drugs were available and used by different types of Israelis has been transformed into a "homogenizing" process. Drugs are unusual, unacceptable, dangerous, and illegal substances used by *them*: societal deviants.

As previously noted, one result of this active cognitive and emotional homogenizing process is that the drug user has been stripped of all actual and potential roles and functions, other than that of being a drug user—now and forever. Having gone outside Israel's conventional society—actual, as well as aspired, normative borders, values, and behavior—and having been caught and "tagged," the visible drug user has almost always not been permitted or helped to be integrated into conventional society again. Under the best of circumstances a minority of drug users have been given the option of partaking in a limited number of therapies, but never as a planned and evaluated treatment process designed to effectively meet their coping, adaptational, and existential needs.

Second, drug use is perceived by professionals and the community at large as being either symtomatic of personal pathology or, more recently, a side effect of environmental distress. Within the context of environmental distress it is presumed that only the weak, or sick, choose drug use as their means of escape. One must note that this view does not permit the acknowledgment of *self-medication* as a meaningful description or explanation; to admit this possibility is somehow to acknowledge that the drug user is suffering from a disease, condition, or problem with which he/she is attempting to cope, albeit in a socially unacceptable way. If a drug user is a "sick person" rather than a pathological entity or deviant, s/he would be entitled to all of the benefits of a patient role. These include the rights, responsibilities and obligations, and status of an acute or chronically ill citizen. The Israeli drug user, as a pathology-ladden deviant, is generally permitted to partake of various forms of social-behavioral control, but not in treatment designed for patients.

Third, the vast majority of treatment programs in Israel, for most illnesses and conditions, utilize and/or are influenced by the traditional hierarchical medical model. Many, if not most, treatment policymakers and treatment agents have had little experience with the treatment of drug use and drug users. Paralleling this reality are the extensive use of medications for primary, secondary, and tertiary prevention; and the lack of use, interest in, and resistance to learning about a broad variety of other reasonably effective treatment techniques. A number of serious consequences have resulted from this medical model orientation by treatment agents of all disciplines when faced with a drug user seeking detoxification or help. Having little firsthand experience regarding the drug user as a functioning person, average treatment professionals, and their agencies, will make their immediate, as well as ongoing, response(s) on thirdhand "information." This information, which most often stereotypes the drug user and attributes magical qualities to drugs and their actions, is based upon mythology, rather than upon facts which are, or can be, verified. The drug user has generally been diagnosed, prior to being personally examined and listened to, as having an untreatable nonfunctioning personality disorder; as a person who is dangerous and violent, who will not cooperate with treatment staff, who is either incapable or not desirous of complying to the demands of a treatment regimen, who is unmotivated, who is most likely to disrupt the day-to-day functioning of a treatment facility, and who is most likely to "infect" non-drug users in the same general treatment facility. When the drug user (who is perceived to be a pathology-laden entity, solely responsible for his/her current situation) requests help/treatment from a blaming and frightened medical model institution, a number of institutionally self-fulfilling options have been developed in Israel. For example, detoxification is legally condoned in closed wards in psychiatric hospitals. No general hospitals accept citizens only for detoxification. Addicts who need treatment for medical illness or surgery will be admitted (but not easily). Very often a staff psychiatrist or a consulting psychiatrist will be called in. No referrals will be made for posthospital treatment if it is wanted, or needed, by the patient. With the exception of the few government centers mentioned earlier, there are no therapeutic communities, hostels, or halfway houses for drug users in Israel. As a result the Israeli drug user can leave his/her immediate environment for short periods of time for hospitalized detoxification or treatment of medical conditions, go to prison for longer periods of time, or be forced to cope with either a rejecting community or one which may have a blatant vested interest in maintaining his/her drug user status and role.

Services are limited or unavailable for so-called special populations. As previously mentioned, institution-based detoxification, primarily a physical process with time-limited symptoms, is condoned and condemned to closed wards in psychiatric hospitals—environments which have been questioned in recent times as to their suitability and applicability for even the treatment of psychological processes and symptoms. Among the various conclusions that can be reached regarding the planned-for outcome of the treatment of the Israeli drug user, is ongoing visible isolation of a drug user, rather than a change in status from sick to healthy and a change in functioning from unacceptable to acceptable. In this sense institutionalized treatment in Israel of drug users since 1975 has been and remains control oriented, and not change oriented.

Fourth, a broad variety of psychological, social welfare, vocational, and remedial services exist in Israel for all her citizens including noncitizens living in the administered territories. Since 1976 the vast majority of these services have been regionalized. Newly developed, as well as long-established, neighborhoods offer local community mental health centers, health clinics, prenatal and post-natal mother-child care centers, welfare offices, community centers, etc. The encatchment area for inpatient psychiatric and medical services, while broader, is still well defined. Certain services—such as vocational testing, vocational training, disability insurance, unemployment insurance, and remedial education—are generally regionally centralized rather than being neighborhood oriented. Many of these services are either unavailable for the drug user or are available contingent upon the drug user's entrance into treatment, active participation in treatment, and a recommendation from the treatment program. The irony, if not the injustice, of this is so obvious as not to need further analysis. What does merit further attention is that this form of *institutional violence* is a mixture of formal policies and increasingly inflexible traditions engaged in by the service agency support system. Thus, whereas conventional work is an institutionally aspired to and designated criteria for successful treatment outcome, either in the open work arena or in a sheltered environment, vocational testing and vocational rehabilitation are rarely available for the drug user. Sheltered workshops, which are rare to begin with, very rarely accept drug users; governmental, municipal, and defense employers are loath to hire drug users (particularly those with prison records or those who have never served their mandatory army service because they were known drug users); and the private employment sector, in a country blessed with full employment, has not often felt the need, or been forced, to hire the known active drug user or even the known former user. Under these conditions, the drug user in treatment or posttreatment is helped to be supported, as an adult, by dependency-producing public support and/or familial support, or by illegal and/or deviant activities. In this sense the myth and stereotype of the nonconventionally functioning drug user becomes verified as a self-fulfilling myth.

Disability in Israel is limited by law and policy to two major categories: physical and psychological. Alcoholism is acknowledged to be a disease; drug use is not.

Social disability—the inability to fit into acceptable conventional roles and functions—as a concept and as an acceptable criterion, is legally alien to Israel. In reality, the situation is even worse than the obvious implications of the current policies regarding public support for acknowledged disabilities. A drug user temporarily or permanently impaired by medical or psychiatric illness/conditions (drug use or non-drug use related) may still not be categorized as disabled. The status of disability is the outcome of examinations and the perusal, trust, and acceptance of the veracity of available written reports about the drug user, including those from the specialized centers. Psychiatrically disturbed drug users, including those who have been or are currently blatantly psychotic, are rarely given a disabled status. The National Insurance Institute (Bituach Leumi), the primary government agency responsible for granting and monitoring social welfare payments, has formally disallowed health insurance to known drug users at the request of the national sick fund (Chupat Cholim), which administers the nation's largest network of outpatient health clinics and guarantees payment for inpatient hospitalization. Medical health care is made difficult to attain for a drug user who by public and professional tradition is preconceived to be dysfunctional or malfunctioning but not disabled. Outpatient mental health care is also generally denied the active or former drug user. Drug use becomes the general diagnosis, necessitating treatment in the four available specialized treatment centers. Drug users not living in these four encatchment areas are left to the pity of God (Jewish, Muslim, or Christian) or to the continued concern of their pusher, ongoing self-medication, or self-care. It is as if the drug user cannot possibly be a psychotic or neurotic who can benefit, as all other citizens theoretically can, from available outpatient psychological treatment. In a country with three-digit inflation, public housing is a significant service to disadvantaged populations. Drug users, because of who they are and/or who they are thought to be, all too often encounter serious problems with their need for such a basic need as reasonable living conditions.

The previous discussion makes it clear that drug addicts in Israel have not received proper care and that many of their rights—enjoyed by non-drug-abusing citizens—have been violated. This background helps explain how such a dehumanizing methadone "program" in the central "garbage dump" in Israel could have come into existence. The continued existence of this program is possible because the same background which enabled the creation of such a program does not do anything to stop its existence. The letters quoted in Table 2 only verify this point.

Theoretical Considerations

Morality is the process through which any object/process in the world is defined as being good or bad. Obviously, what is regarded as good or bad, desired or not, not only varies among societies but could very well change within one society during different time periods. Furthermore, in pluralistic societies, definitions of morality and deviance are not the same even within the same society in a specific time period. While there is an argument on this point between those who characterize society as conflictual and those who characterize it as consensual, there can hardly be a question that in modern, complex society morality is simply negotiated. Laws and punishments, therefore, reflect not only hierarchies of morals and values but also outcomes of complex value and morality negotiations.

Morality, one has to see, has a deeper meaning than just the "technical" or "definitional" aspect of it. Becker (1963) developed the concept of "hierarchies of credibility," which in essence means a stratification principle in the hierarchy of morals and credibility. Rock (1973) stated too that "In complex societies, the distribution of deviant phenomena is closely linked to the distribution of power and life-chances. . . . A stratification system can also be viewed as a moral system: major organization of beliefs about the rights, duties and moral properties of the members of a society. . . . A system of control based on authority rests, in part, on a recognition of the *moral* right of the authoritative to make decisions. . . . Thus, in a stable, but unequal society class position is often identified with moral position–the higher one's position in a stratification order, the greater is one's moral worth . . ." (p. 47).

Rock's and Becker's theoretical formulations suggest that some members in society are more protected than others. Likewise, the social-moral system of societies increases the probability that some people–and not others–will develop a deviant career.

While the Marxist-oriented criminology brought attention to, focused on, and sharpened the perception of deviance as a moral-political threat, the modern approach to deviance as a "threat" was formally developed by Horowitz and Liebovitz (1968) and Lofland (1969). The first two authors stated (p. 282) that deviance should be thought of as a conflict between at least two parties: superordinates who make and enforce rules, and subordinates whose actual behavior violates these rules. When Becker (1963) wrote that deviance was created by society because social groups made rules whose infractions constituted deviance (p. 9), it only gave a good theoretical antecedent to Horowitz and Liebovitz's approach. In 1969 Lofland continued this line, when he suggested that deviance was a name of a conflict game where individuals (or loosely organized small groups) with little power were strongly feared by a well-organized, sizable minority (or majority) who had a large amount of power (p. 14). Turk's (1979) views also strongly supported this "threat" perspective. Turk stated explicitly that "deviations are whatever is felt, consciously or not, to be threatening . . ." (p. 466).

That addicts somehow threatened the Dizengoff area is clear. As Dizengoff Street is a showwindow of Israel, these addicts presented a moral threat in, and to, what is considered by many Israelis to be a symbolically very important area in Israel. These addicts were considered as "not belonging" to Dizengoff, as not representing the "true" Israel. Thus, they found themselves in the midst of a far-away large garbage dump–again with a clear symbolic message.

From the perspective of the general background of the treatment of drug addicts in Israel, the "garbage dump" treatment program near Tel Aviv constitutes a clear case of *institutional violence*, as defined by Liazos (1972). There, the senses and sight–indeed, the human image–of a large number of addicts/drug users are being violated daily, with clear harm done to the addicts' psyches, bodies, dignity, and ability to govern themselves. The covert institutional violence is done with the actual approval of a large variety of agencies and people in Israel. These agencies, usually ranking high in the hierarchy of credibility and enjoying a high position in the societal moral hierarchy, enable–even by their silence–the continued existence of the garbage program. In that program, powerless, stigmatized, and feared people receive "treatment" which in fact is no treatment at all. Furthermore, the institutional violence against the addicts also becomes possible because the addicts have never organized themselves as a group acting collectively to achieve their needs.

APPENDIX A: LETTER FROM THE PHARMACEUTICAL ASSOCIATION TO THE MINISTRY OF HEALTH

Prof. Baruch Modan, Director General
Ministry of Health
Jerusalem

2/8/82

Dear Prof. Modan:

Angry voices have been heard in the media regarding the distribution of proscribed medicines to "Narkomanim" at the garbage dump (in Tel Aviv), which adds to the suffering and humiliation of the drug user and injures their self respect as humans.

Our professional society has decided to help to solve this painful problem by distributing methadone–which is currently distributed at the garbage dump from a car, and not from a pharmacy–at a pharmacy which is agreed upon by the Ministry of Health. [It is suggested that it be] at the Donolo B Hospital, which we were told has a place for distribution, or at any other hospital which will be accredited (for this project) by the Ministry of Health. The drug user will receive methadone from a pharmacist (in the agreed upon pharmacy).

As you know the sum total of methadone sold to drug users in the garbage dump has reached 24,000 bottles (100 mg/bottle). The bottle is purchased by the pharmacist at the price IS 49.80/bottle and is sold to the drug user at the price of IS 74.30/bottle. Gross monthly sales are 1,783,200.00 IS. There is a gross profit of 25%. The gross monthly profit for the pharmacist is 445,800 IS.

If methadone were to be marketed by the Ministry of Health, the profits would not be taxed. We suggest to transfer the profits earned by the selling of the drug to drug users to LIBI.* This would bring in a permanent monthly profit to the LIBI fund, after subtracting the essential expenses which are part of methadone distribution–salary for the dispensing pharmacist (the place would be donated by the Ministry of Health).

Our Society will fund the purchase of the initial supply of methadone and pay ABIC Pharmaceuticals the total of IS 1,195,200 (24,000 × 49.80) and will receive this amount back from the sale of methadone by the Ministry of Health.

Our Society will supply the LIBI Fund with a pharmacist who will be needed during the initial stages of the development of this project.

We are requesting to meet with you to discuss this issue in order to solve this painful problem.

Sincerely yours,
A. Bass, Pharmacist, Chairman

A. Regev, Secretary

The Pharmaceutical Association of Israel

c.c. General R. Eitan, Chief of Staff, LIBI Foundation
Prof. Menczel, Pharmacist, Ministry of Health, Jerusalem
Dalia Cohn, Regional Pharmacist
A. Turneau, Pharmacist, Ministry of Health, Tel Aviv

REFERENCES

BECKER, H.S. *Outsiders*. New York: Free Press, 1963.

BEN-YEHUDA, N. *Drug Abuse in Israel–A Survey*. Jerusalem: Ministry of Welfare and Social Affairs, 1979 (in Hebrew).

GARFINKEL, H. Condition of successful degradation ceremonies. *Am. J. Sociol.* 1:720-724, 1980.

GOFFMAN, E. *Stigma*. Englewood Cliffs, NJ: Prentice-Hall, 1963.

GOODE, E. *Deviant Behavior*. Englewood Cliffs, NJ: Prentice-Hall, 1978.

HOROWITZ, I.L., and LIEBOVITZ, M. Social deviance and political marginality: Towards a redefinition of the relation between sociology and politics. *Soc. Probl.* 15(3): 280-297, 1968.

*LIBI is a voluntary fund established to help soldiers who are lacking in basic educational skills to study during their army service.

LIAZOS, A. The poverty of the sociology of deviance: Nuts, sluts and perverts. *Soc. Probl.* 20: 103–120, 1972.

LOFLAND, J. *Deviance and Identity*. Englewood Cliffs, NJ: Prentice-Hall, 1969.

ROCK, P. *Deviant Behavior*. London: Hutchinson University Press, 1973.

RUBINGTON, E., and WEINBERG, M.S. (eds.). *The Study of Social Problems*. New York: Oxford University Press, 1971.

SCHUR, E.M. *Labeling Deviant Behavior*. New York: Harper and Row, 1971.

SCHUR, E.M. *Interpreting Deviance*. New York: Harper and Row, 1979.

TAYLOR, I., WALTON, P., and YOUNG, J. *The New Criminology*. London: Routledge and Kegan Paul, 1973.

TURK, A. Analyzing official deviance: For nonpartisan conflict analysis. *Criminology* 16(4): 459–476, 1979.

The International Journal of the Addictions, 19(1), 25–44, 1984

A Diagnostic Tool with Important Implications for Treatment of Addiction: Identification of Factors Underlying Relapse and Remission Time Distributions

Nancy R. Mann,* PhD

V. Charles Charuvastra, MD

V. K. Murthy, PhD

Abstract

The results of analysis of successive relapse and remission times of many opiate addicts were examined. It is discovered that motivation is the preeminent factor that governs the distribution of lengths of remission times (periods of abstinence), differences in types of motivation leading to an underlying mixture of three or fewer Weibull distributions. On the other hand, two distinct factors–namely wear-out (dysfunction resulting from exhaustion or tiring out brought on by the addict's enforced life-style) and precipitation of events that may not be beyond the control of the addict–govern the distribution of lengths of relapse times (periods of using opiates), leading, typically, to an underlying competing-risk distribution. Methods for using this information to aid in treatment and in research are described.

*To whom correspondence should be addressed at BM–82, Department of Biomathematics, School of Medicine, University of California, Los Angeles, California 90024.

0020-773X/84/1901-0025$3.50/0

INTRODUCTION

The present study, as well as previous research (Brill, 1972; Waldorf, 1973; Waldorf and Biernacki, 1979), suggests that feelings of dysfunction regarding heroin and the related life-style, "rock bottoms" that precipitate "surrender," existential crises, and other events that change the way in which the addict views his or her use of the drug are among the major contributing factors leading addicts to quit the use of heroin for extended periods of time. Dysfunction is expressed usually in terms of being tired: tired of the life, the "changes," the "hassles"; tired of the junkies and being in and out of jails (Waldorf and Biernacki, 1979). One might view this as a type of "wearing out." "Rock bottom" is a subjective state wherein the individual reaches some low point in his or her life and is sometimes motivated to surrender and make a radical change in behavior. On the other hand, existential crisis (Kierkegaard, 1941a, 1941b) is a more profound emotional and psychological state in which the addict questions the very nature and meaning of his or her whole life and being. Other precipitating events may take the form of falling in love, becoming a parent, having a "eureka" (sudden insightful) experience, etc.

The present authors are thus led to the hypothesis that these different types of factors, as well as factors precipitating shorter periods of abstinence, "compete" during periods of use of heroin to motivate the patient to quit the use of the drug. In statistical terminology, the hypothesis states that the distribution of successive intervals of use of heroin by an individual behaves as a random sample from an underlying distribution corresponding to a competing-risk model.

The question now arises: How does the addict stay successful in maintaining abstinence? For help in answering this question and in validating our hypothesis concerning the distribution of intervals of use, an analysis was made of histories of successive intervals of remission and relapse in addicts from several populations.

DESCRIPTION OF DATA SOURCES AND METHODS

The data for this study were obtained from three different institutions. They are the Maryland Psychiatric Research Center (MPRC), the Brentwood Veterans Administration Hospital Methadone Maintenance Program, and the New Jersey Medical School. The data from the MPRC pertain to a community-wide study, made in Baltimore beginning in 1965 and continuing throughout the decade of the '70s, in which detailed use histories of 405 male narcotic abusers were obtained by intensive interviews and validated by follow-up investigations. The initial study involving part of the data is described by Nurco et al. (1975).

The Brentwood Methadone Program, under the direction of Dr. V. C. Charuvastra (Ling and Charuvastra, 1976), began in 1974 as part of the Brentwood Hospital drug treatment program. The recidivism data from this program were obtained for this study in early 1980 from 88 randomly selected patient records, about a third of the patient population (all males) who were active at the time of selection. Additional data from the methadone clients were obtained by means of an interview program. Informed consent was obtained after the purpose of the research was fully explained. All recidivism data were extracted from the patient records and resulted from randomly performed weekly urinalyses made to determine presence or absence of various drugs, including both heroin and methadone.

Information from the New Jersey Medical School (NJMS) was provided in 1980 by Dr. A. Sheffet (Lavenhar et al., 1975). The data used from the NJMS study pertain to periods of both inpatient and outpatient residency that were terminated prematurely, by Newark residents only among over 5,000 narcotics abusers in the various Newark community treatment programs from 1969 to 1980.

The sequence of consecutive remission times and the sequence of consecutive durations of relapse, along with demographic and background profiles of the addict, were available for all of these populations. The methods used in this paper are directed toward characterizing the basic underlying distributions of remission and relapse times.

Earlier analyses (Mann, 1979; Mann and Rothberg, 1980) of the type performed in this study were made by one of the authors on data stored at the Walter Reed Research Center, concerning U.S. Army personnel who were repeatedly hospitalized for alcoholism.

ANALYSIS

In the present context it has been found that detoxification provides a time that one may fruitfully define as the initiation of a life test which ends in "failure" if and when the subject returns to use of heroin. Thus, a single patient beginning with detoxification may generate successive times to failure, first, second, third, . . ., etc., just as would light bulbs successively tested until failure (burnout) in a single electrical outlet.

"Detoxification" is used in this analysis rather loosely as the time an addict abstains from ingestion of the substance to which he or she is addicted long enough to eliminate the drug and its immediate toxic effects from his or her body and brain. Detoxification in this sense may result from inpatient or outpatient treatment at a hospital or a treatment center, or it may be self-induced. It may be a result of legal pressure or of social pressure brought to bear by family members, a friend, or an employer, or by temporary unavailability of the substance. Or it may result simply from a decision on the part of the addict or drug abuser to give up the habit because of its deleterious effects on his or her life and the lives of others.

Also, we define "remission time" (number of days to relapse, or failure) as the number of days from detoxification until resumption of use, leading (hopefully) to a subsequent detoxification. A "relapse time" is defined as the time following resumption of use until a subsequent remission. In utilizing historical hospitalization data (treatment program data), one may define "time to relapse" as the number of days between hospitalizations resulting from drug use (number of days from entry until premature termination). However, such measures of time to failure are biased since they often include time of using and, indeed, may be affected by various extraneous factors, including strength of drug.

The methods used in this paper for the analysis of remission and relapse times are survival analysis techniques (Mann, Schafer, and Singpurwalla, 1974). Essentially, this methodology provides a means of characterizing the underlying distributions governing the histories of consecutive relapse and remission times of a patient. Characterization of the distributions gives insight into the mechanics of the phenomena of relapse and remission, and provides an objective tool to aid in prediction of treatment outcome and for detecting treatment effects, spontaneous or otherwise. The tool provided is one that is much more sensitive than the usual procedures based solely on an arbitrary time threshold. Also, one can use this type of methodology with "time to first relapse" or "extent of longest period of abstinence" of patients in a treatment program for comparing different treatment modalities. These various issues of prediction and comparison will be, for the most part, addressed in a subsequent paper.

Statistical Models

The three statistical models that have emerged from the analysis are a single Weibull distribution, a mixture of two or more Weibull distributions, and a competing-risk distribution. The Weibull distribution is one in which, for an addict in remission, the logarithm of conditional probability of a relapse is proportional to the logarithm of the duration of remission. When the constant of proportionality is 0, the distribution becomes the well-known exponential distribution governing relapsed times between Poisson (or purely random) events. The Weibull mixture model is one in which the distribution is a linear combination of two or more Weibull distributions.

Suppose "time to failure" in a random sample of hardware such as, for example, razor blades, exhibits a frequency distribution that suggests a single Weibull population. Then one would be justified in inferring that failure is precipitated by a single cause (wear-out, e.g.), and that the razor blades are from a single population. If two (three) distinct distributions are indicated, suggestive of perhaps a bimodal (trimodal) frequency distribution, then one would again hypothesize a single cause of failure, but in this case with two (three) different types of razor blades with very different average failure times.

Finally, the competing-risk distribution is the distribution of "time to event" (relapse, remission) in which two or more forces are competing throughout the time until the event (relapse, remission) to pressure the addict to give up.

A convenient hardware analogy for competing risk is given by the two processes of wear-out and destruction by vandals of light bulbs in a street lamp post. Each bulb will eventually wear out unless it is prematurely destroyed by a vandal. In this model the vandalism may occur at any time throughout the life of each bulb. In an alternative light bulb model that is seen to be clearly a mixture, one would observe a single cause of failure in a sample from two or more populations of light bulbs with very different average failure times.

Graphical Plotting of the Data

Based on a random sample of N times to an event (relapse or remission) from a single individual or a single population, the underlying distribution of duration of a remission or relapse can be estimated as follows: The data are first ordered according to increasing size. Let $T(i)$ be the ith smallest time to the event in a sample history of N observed times. The quantity $1-(i-.5)/N$ is calculated for each i as an estimate of the probability that the event does not occur before time $T(i)$. The graph of $(i-.5)/N$ plotted against $T(i)$ is a graph of the underlying cumulative distribution of time to the event.

To capture any pattern of the type we are after, we plot $\ln(-\ln[1-(i-.5)/N])$ versus $\ln[T(i)]$. A straight-line plot (Kao, 1959) suggests that the original (unordered) observations are independent events and that the underlying distribution belongs to the Weibull family. A pattern of two (or three) distinct consecutive straight lines suggests that the underlying distribution is a mixture of two (or three) Weibull distributions. A corresponding frequency distribution for time to failure would be bimodal (or trimodal), unless one or more of the Weibull distributions has no mode.

If, on the other hand, the plot is a curve with several twists and turns, then it indicates an underlying competing-risk model. The competing-risk plot for a large sample of successive intervals of use of heroin looks like a sample randomly selected from two or more different (possibly Weibull or mixture of Weibull) distributions which completely overlap. A corresponding frequency function would be the result of two or more unimodal or multimodal frequency distributions (with possibly one or more frequency distributions among these devoid of a mode). As opposed to a unimodal, bimodal, or trimodal mixture model, the competing-risk frequency function could be characterized as a lumpy mass formed by the two or more overlapping modes and/or masses of density.

Computerized graphical (Versatec) plots of time to relapse were made for each of the subjects who exhibited three or more failure times among all of the methadone clients, all of the Baltimore addicts, and a sample of 200 of the Newark residents with premature terminations. Plots of periods of use (time to remission) were made for eight of the methadone clients who exhibited 20 or more such periods.

DISCUSSION

The authors found, from analysis of the data, that the type of motivation (or "intention") appears to be the preeminent factor determining length of remission times of addicts. From the many sets of longitudinal time-to-relapse data, they identified three different levels (or strengths) of intention, corresponding to a mixture of three different failure patterns with different average failure times. These three patterns appeared randomly distributed over time in individual histories and over individual subjects in "time to chronologically first (or kth, $1 \leqslant k \leqslant N$, or most recent) failure" in samples of N cohorts. (It is interesting that a study of prison recidivism by Carr-Hill and Carr-Hill [1972], which investigates time to first failure, also finds a mixture of three distributions.) The three levels appear, on the basis of interview results, to be associated with, respectively, uninternalized motivation (such as compliance arising in response to coercion), ordinary internalized motivation (somewhat akin to that leading to New Year's resolutions, going on a diet, and the like), and very profound motivation (such as provided by falling in love, having a spiritual experience, or by an extremely strong feeling of dysfunction).

Thus, an intention (or resolve) to abstain and to make changes in behavior and/or life-style that facilitate abstinence is formed and may or may not be strengthened or changed after the original formation. Meanwhile, the stresses and traumas that the addict experiences, or time itself, will tend to erode away this intention. Making behavior modifications and changes in one's environment is for an addict analogous to using a beard softener that can to some extent prolong the life of a razor blade. Only in cases in which there is an ingredient in the beard softener that profoundly strengthens the blade can it be changed from an ordinary one to one designed to last for years.

Thus, the type of intention alone determines whether the period of remission will be, for the individual in any particular instance during his or her history of use, of more or less average length, unusually short or unusually long. This leads one to the hypothesis that successive periods of abstinence in an individual addict behave like a random sample from an underlying distribution corresponding to a mixture of three or fewer distributions, each individual distribution corresponding to one of the three possible degrees of motivation.

Previous research (Simpson et al., 1977) has shown that background family responsibility and background socioeconomic status are predictors of performance following narcotic treatment programs. What is suggested here is that these background variables give a measure of the ability of a subject to be motivated.

CONCLUSIONS

Identification of Failure Patterns

The slopes of the Weibull plots estimate the Weibull shape parameter. If the slope of the true plotted line is greater than unity, then the corresponding distribution has a (single) mode, and the implication is that the hardware is wearing out and that the failure rate is increasing. By "failure rate" we mean the probability of failure in the next instant, given survival until that instant. We therefore conclude or hypothesize that in applications to recidivism in which the Weibull shape parameter is greater than 1, the subject's intention to abstain (involving both physiological and psychological factors) is wearing out. Thus, as time goes on, the impact required to destroy the intention to abstain becomes less and less.

When the Weibull shape parameter is less than 1 (decreasing failure rate), one sees failure times ranging from very early to average combined with extremely long ones. Samples of electronic equipment often exhibit this kind of failure pattern. In a random sample of a dozen television sets, for example, a few may fail early because of loose connections, faulty components, etc., but most will operate for hundreds of hours before exhibiting any kind of failure. This is a type of mixture involving some pieces of equipment with parts that wear out very early, mixed with sample elements that are devoid of such quality defects.

This kind of behavior in an addict sometimes appears to be manifested as a result of a treatment program that occasionally makes a strong impact but sometimes fails completely. And, if a subject whose failure data are of this type abstains for a rather moderate period of time, one might predict that there is a high probability that he or she will abstain for an extended period.

When the Weibull shape parameter is unity, then failure is purely catastrophic or random. In this special case, the distribution is exponential and the failure rate is constant. Some electronic systems that have been "burnt in" (i.e., operated long enough to eliminate the early failure modalities) exhibit this type of failure behavior. Exponential failure data for an addict might imply a lack of commitment to abstain. In this case the addict apparently responds without resistance to random stresses and traumas that occur as a homogeneous Poisson process.

Table 1

Sources of Data

Types of data	Methadone patients	Baltimore community	Newark residents
Periods of abstinence from opiates	Urinalysis records	Records from intensive interview combined with police reports, peer and family follow-up	Patient records indicating treatment periods prematurely terminated
Periods of using opiates	Urinalysis records	Same as above	Patient records indicating periods out of treatment following premature termination–before return for new treatment
Background and demographic information	Patient records	Same as above	Patient records
Information related to motivational levels	Intensive interviews	–	–

The three different samples are representative of completely different diverse populations engaging in three different types of recidivism activities and would ordinarily not be compared (see Table 1). The Brentwood and Baltimore samples include only males, while the Newark patients are of both sexes. Each Brentwood patient is exposed to a single type of treatment (methadone), but for each of a large number of the Baltimore and Newark clients, there are several treatment modalities. Still, all of the various patterns that have been discussed—that is, single distributions, mixtures, and increasing, constant, and decreasing failure rate—were exhibited in all three of the plotted individual time-to-relapse data sets. There is no outstanding feature of the individual failure patterns that characterizes the different populations except that the number of relapse and remission periods exhibited per individual tends to be larger for the methadone clients than for the other subjects. The principal cause for this may be the ease with which the methadone client may terminate periods of using, so that fears ordinarily associated with detoxifying do not aid in deterring reinitiation of use.

Figures 1 and 2 give the times to relapse and the associated graphical plots for two methadone patients. One sees for each, two different wear-out distributions with distinctly different average failure times. In Fig. 2 there is a single observation significantly longer than the others (suggesting a very much stronger motivation associated with this remission period). Analytical methodologies

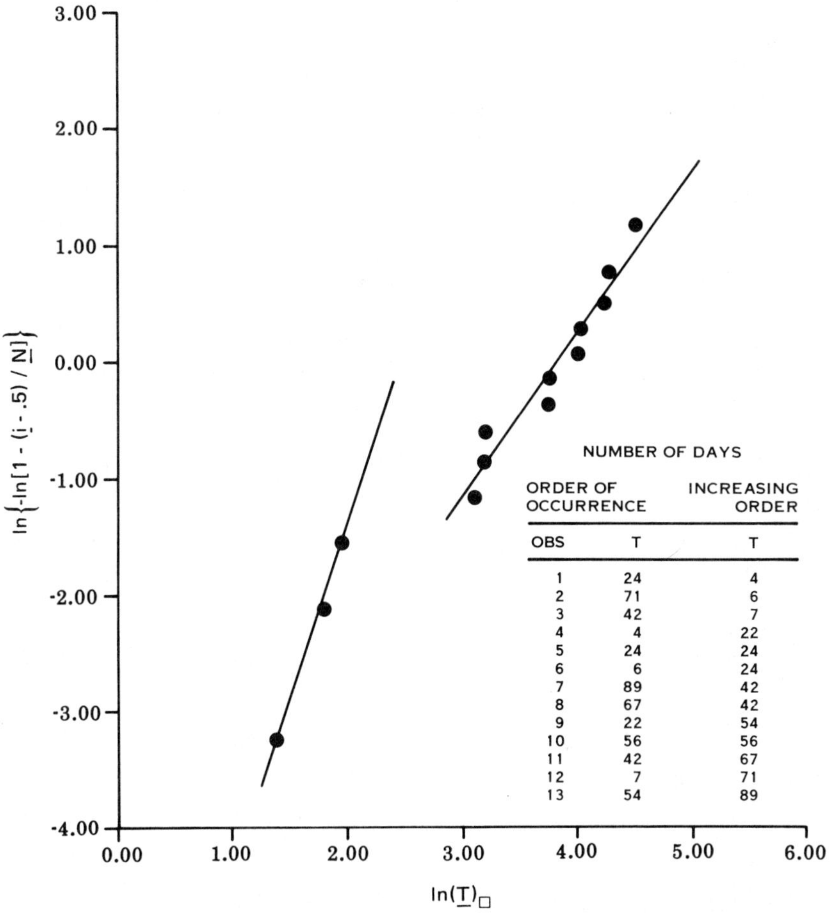

ORDER OF OCCURRENCE		INCREASING ORDER
OBS	T	T
1	24	4
2	71	6
3	42	7
4	4	22
5	24	24
6	6	24
7	89	42
8	67	42
9	22	54
10	56	56
11	42	67
12	7	71
13	54	89

Fig. 1. Subject ME 6: Weibull probability plot of time until drug relapse.

(Fertig et al., 1980; Mann, 1982) have recently been developed for testing for statistical significance of suspected outliers, such as this single large observation, and for testing whether a next period of remission (after initiation of a new treatment program) is significantly longer than to be expected. Typically, as shown in Figs. 1 and 2, the slope of a second line is smaller than the first when the first is associated with very early failure.

The time-to-failure data from the Baltimore study were stored as numbers of months, so that it is impossible to tell, for these subjects, the type of behavior exhibited for the period extending less than 1 month after detoxification.

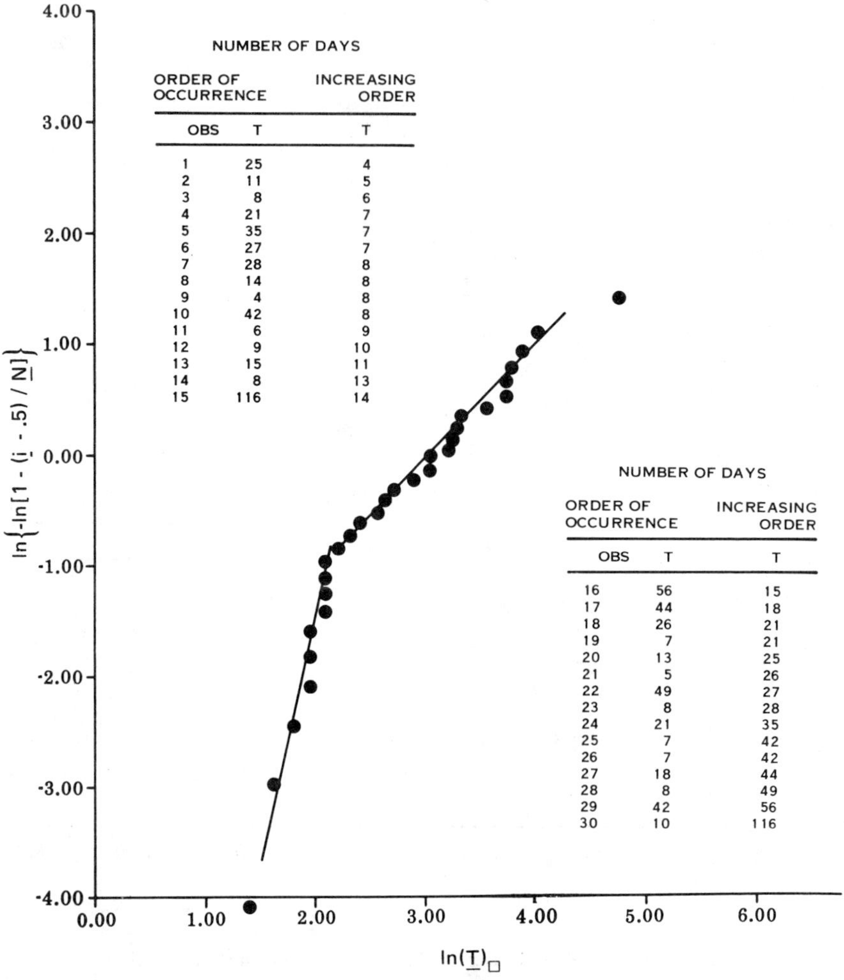

NUMBER OF DAYS

ORDER OF OCCURRENCE OBS	T	INCREASING ORDER T
1	25	4
2	11	5
3	8	6
4	21	7
5	35	7
6	27	7
7	28	8
8	14	8
9	4	8
10	42	8
11	6	9
12	9	10
13	15	11
14	8	13
15	116	14

NUMBER OF DAYS

ORDER OF OCCURRENCE OBS	T	INCREASING ORDER T
16	56	15
17	44	18
18	26	21
19	7	21
20	13	25
21	5	26
22	49	27
23	8	28
24	21	35
25	7	42
26	7	42
27	18	44
28	8	49
29	42	56
30	10	116

Fig. 2. Subject ME 18: Weibull probability plot of time until drug relapse.

Figures 3 and 4 give the time-to-relapse data and the associated probability plots of two Baltimore heroin addicts. The subject of Fig. 3 exhibits a decreasing failure rate pattern. For this individual there is a strong probability of a very long current period of remission when the current period has exceeded 2 months. The subject whose data are plotted in Fig. 4 exhibits two inordinately long periods of abstinence.

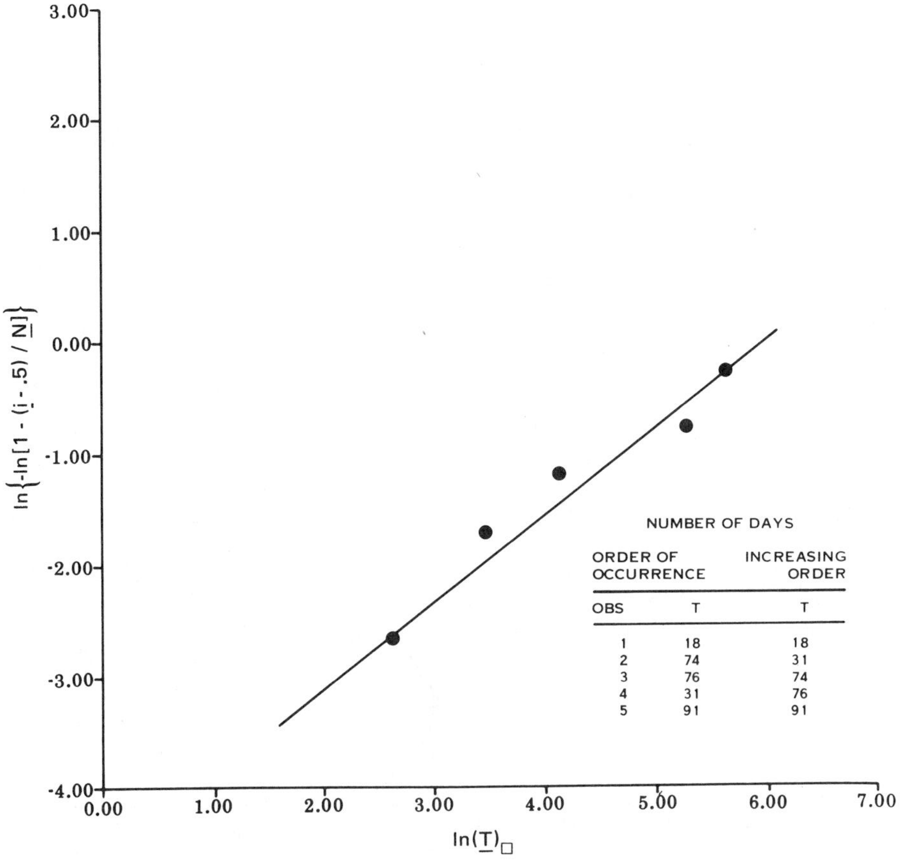

Fig. 3. Baltimore, subject 27: Weibull probability plot of time until drug relapse.

The successive premature treatment termination times for subject 2870 of the New Jersey Medical School study are shown in Fig. 5. The probability plot indicates that the patient tends to wear out after a treatment period has lasted about 1 to 3 months.

Figure 6 gives data pertaining to periods of relapse (periods of use of heroin) and the resulting plot for a typical methadone client among those who exhibited sufficient recidivism so that the time-to-remission patterns could be identified. Note the several twists and turns.

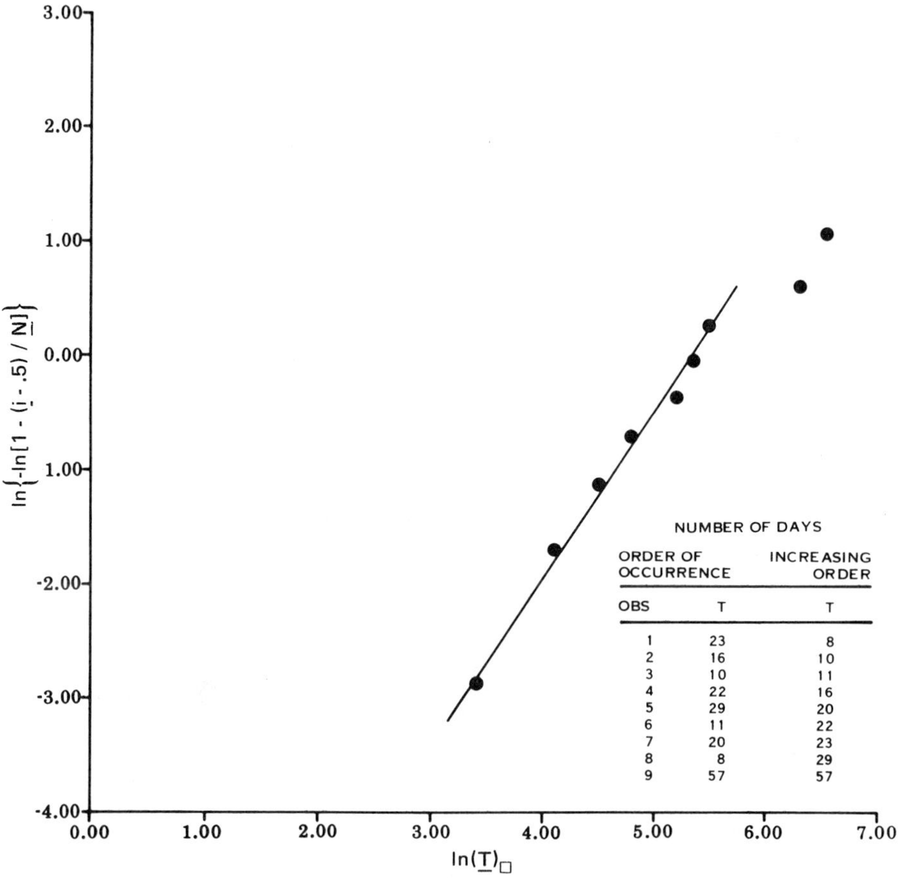

ORDER OF OCCURRENCE		INCREASING ORDER
OBS	T	T
1	23	8
2	16	10
3	10	11
4	22	16
5	29	20
6	11	22
7	20	23
8	8	29
9	57	57

Fig. 4. Baltimore, subject 104: Weibull probability plot of time until drug relapse.

Characterization of the Recidivism Process

Probably the most important implication of this study results from the fact that when different failure mechanisms operate within a single individual, the time-to-relapse data plot as mixtures of distributions, rather than as competing-risk distributions. The fact that a competing-risk model does not apply to this kind of data suggests that if an addict exhibits, for example, two distinct types of failure patterns with very different average failure times, the resulting patterns are exhibited only because there are two completely different types of motivation, like two different types of hardware. In other words, the intention that is

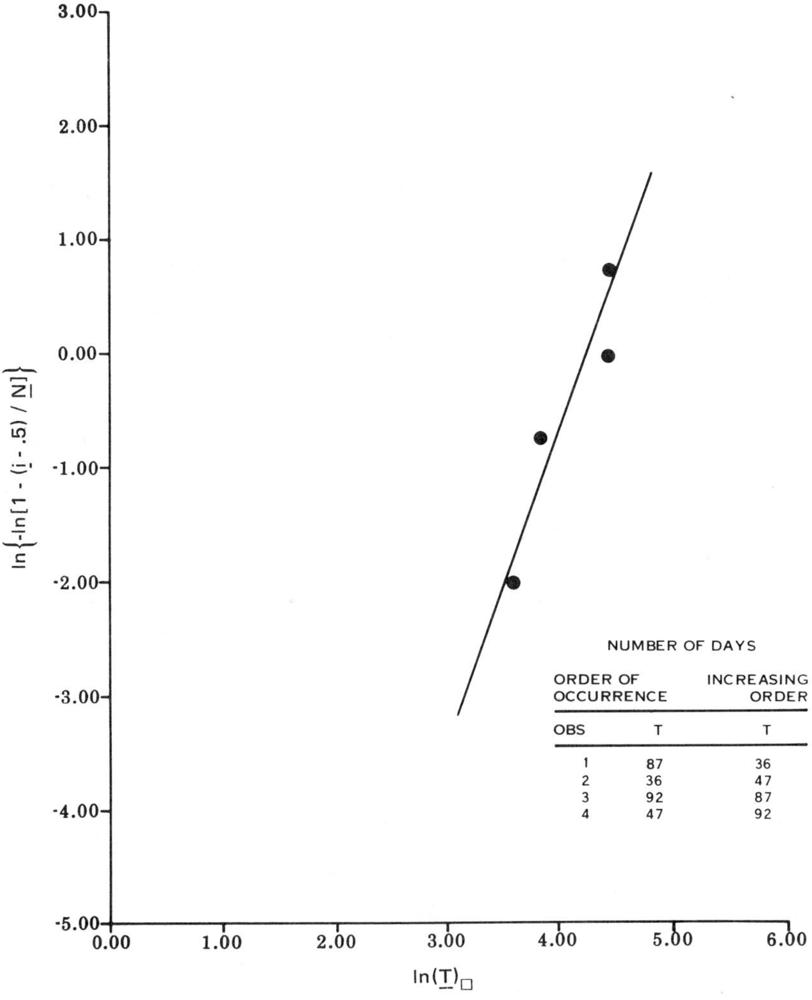

Fig. 5. Newark, subject 2870: Weibull probability plot of time until drug relapse.

creating the abstinence is associated with one of the two patterns of failure: one that is early, on the average, and one that is late, on the average. It is this fact that demonstrates that the most important factor in determining expected length of abstinence of a subject is the type of motivation that is operating.

In the case of wear-out, we draw an analogy between the razor blades, which a subject selects repeatedly and randomly from one or more prescribed

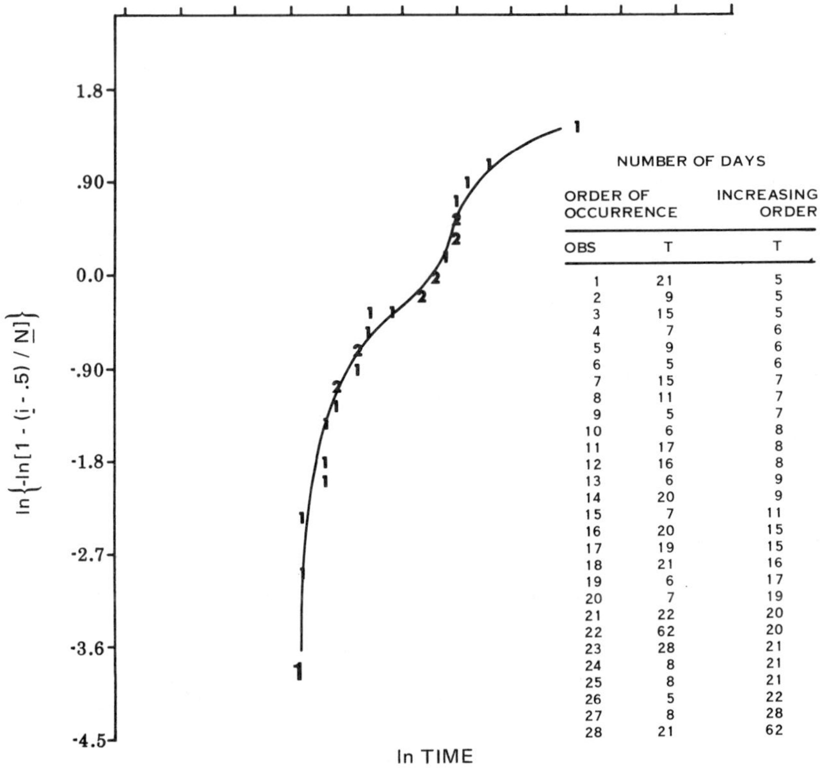

NUMBER OF DAYS

ORDER OF OCCURRENCE		INCREASING ORDER
OBS	T	T
1	21	5
2	9	5
3	15	5
4	7	6
5	9	6
6	5	6
7	15	7
8	11	7
9	5	7
10	6	8
11	17	8
12	16	8
13	6	9
14	20	9
15	7	11
16	20	15
17	19	15
18	21	16
19	6	17
20	7	19
21	22	20
22	62	20
23	28	21
24	8	21
25	8	21
26	5	22
27	8	28
28	21	62

Fig. 6. Extent of time using heroin: plot of methadone patient 53. Numbers on curve indicate the number of observations at the given intersection.

populations after wear-out of a blade used previously, and the intentions of an addict to abstain from use of heroin. (For failure patterns characterized by other than wear-out, another hardware analogy may be more appropriate.) The intentions are very often formed repeatedly after extinction of a previous intention and appear, from the data, to be independent of previous responses, long and short periods being apparently randomly intermixed with those of more or less average length. One never sees a clear-cut trend toward either longer or shorter duration of remission periods. (See, e.g., the data in Figs. 1-5.) The fact that data for individual addicts plot as would failure data from random samples from three or fewer specific types of hardware corroborates an assumption of independence of events.

Thus, what is observed here is not a nonhomogeneous Poisson process indicating a tendency toward gradual increase or decrease in time to failure throughout the history of the addiction. Such a process would suggest that the recidivism phenomenon involves something like "repair" of the addict before returning to using and continuation of a trend (Crow, 1974). In fact, only in the special case of exponential data resulting from a homogeneous Poisson process (for which we hypothesize a lack of intention) might one interpret the recidivism phenomenon as one involving repair before return to use. For exponential data, even when conceptualized as resulting from a failure and repair process, there is no trend in either direction. Hence, in general, one cannot use a single most recent failure time to predict a next failure time for an individual, except in a special situation in which an individual exhibits extreme wear-out. (In such a case the addict might always terminate periods of abstinence after some fixed period of time, plus or minus a very small percentage of that period, as long as his or her motivational level was not dramatically changed.)

On the other hand, if one examines results of analysis of the methadone program data set (which has received the most thorough scrutiny in this study to date), one sees that some individuals do improve with respect to length of period of abstinence in an unexpected and subtle way. As noted earlier, failure times for each methadone patient moved more or less randomly within each of the patterns (as many as three) that he or she exhibited, as well as between patterns. Nevertheless, there appeared to be a tendency over calendar time for the patient population to experience fewer of the short-term failure times (9 most recent failure times vs 23 times to first failure out of each total sample of 88 that were less than 21 days—significant at the .006 level) and more of the extremely long-term failure times (16 most recent failure times vs 5 first failure times greater than 665 days—significant at the .03 level).

The overall mean time to failure increased from 196 days to 366 days, but the proportion of the sample that experienced failure times that were of moderate average length stayed relatively constant. For the razor blade analogy, one can assume that later deliveries to a retail outlet contain fewer blades with extremely short lives and more that last an extremely long time.

Lengths of periods of using heroin by the methadone patients exhibited the same sort of random variation as did lengths of periods of abstinence. However, the sample median for both time of first use and time of most recent use was 8 days, and the mean times of using were 11.3 and 11.7 days, respectively. That is, improvement in the recidivism behavior reflected in the increase in number of longer periods of abstinence was not reciprocated by a corresponding improvement (decrease) in the duration of periods of use. This gives corroboration to intuitive feelings that lengths of periods of using drugs are not useful in measuring performance since they are often terminated by random events completely out of the control of the addict.

Uninternalized Motivation

Further corroboration (in addition to the interview data) of the interpretation, stated earlier, concerning uninternalized motivation is given by the following. Probation and other legal restraints on the methadone patients upon entering the program were highly predictive of a time to first failure in the early range, that is, less than 21 days (15 patients out of 39 on probation vs 8 out of 49 not on probation–significant at the .02 level). Presence or absence of these early legal restraints, however, had essentially no effect on the graphical plots (number of early failures, slopes of the three lines, mean, etc.) of time to longest failure or time to most recent failure, both of which sometimes occurred several years after the patient entered the methadone program. For example, the probation and nonprobation data sets for time to most recent failure both exhibited approximately 10% failure times less than 21 days and had a mean time to failure of 367 and 365 days, respectively.

The implication of legal restraint being often associated with uninternalized motivation is not in conflict with that of earlier research (Desmond and Maddux, 1977; Vaillant and Rasor, 1966) which compared addicts on probation with those that appeared to be unmotivated. What is suggested here is that although law enforcement agencies exacerbate the difficulties of the addict in coping with his or her habit, and thus add pressure for at least temporary wear-out of drug use, their coercion is ineffective in producing internalized motivation for maintaining abstinence (except perhaps in their cumulative effect on feelings of dysfunction).

This phenomenon is in agreement with results of previous research (Zander and Curtis, 1962) which found that, in an experiment, high school boys evidenced a weaker motivation to do well on a group task when they were subjected to the threat of being expelled from the group than when no threats were employed. It has been demonstrated by recent research in the field of personality (Carver and Scheifer, 1981) that excessive coercion may lead to aversion, movement away from the communicator's idea, while gentle persuasion may move one into closer agreement with the communicator. It seems that attempted influence causes psychological reactance, a motivational state which occurs when an individual's freedom is threatened. Reactance, hence, causes an attempt to reassert the threatened freedom.

RECOMMENDATIONS

Motivating the Patient

A rather clear implication of this analysis is that a necessary ingredient of any really successful drug treatment program is a method of strongly motivating the patient to want to abstain and to want to maintain any modifications of behavior or changes in environment and life-style that help him or her to abstain. It also suggests that the use of willpower alone (i.e., simply "trying hard") in fighting return to use of a drug dooms the subject to eventual failure unless he or she is profoundly motivated during the period of abstinence in which the willpower is being exerted.

Obviously, a treatment facility has no control over most of the motivating factors mentioned earlier, such as, for example, parenting. There are some such factors, however, that treatment personnel can conceivably influence. For example, it may be possible to intensify the patient's awareness of the dysfunction caused by use of heroin and/or his or her awareness of other behavior options available to him or her besides use of drugs and to demonstrate the incongruence between a patient's behavior and his or her goals and values. Also, it may be possible to initiate insightful experiences so that use of heroin is then seen to be an undesirable, or at least a less desirable, activity.

Given these goals, one may ask how to go about achieving them. Results of the present study, combined with previous research (Brill, 1977; Simmell, 1948), give us several valuable clues. Interview responses demonstrate that instances in which addicts have had eureka experiences, spiritual experiences, or any other kinds of experiences that have turned their lives around have often been times of withdrawal from drugs. The time of withdrawal and detoxification is usually one during which the addict experiences feelings of hitting bottom and has the potential for surrender and a commitment to abstinence. Altered states of consciousness and the physical trauma caused by the chemical detoxification can intensify this potential. This suggests that treatment effects can be enhanced if a significant part of treatment resources are allocated to very early stages of treatment, beginning with detox.

Using the Methodology to Predict Behavior

Most recidivism studies measure only time to first failure (e.g., relapse, return to prison) or number of subjects who have failed after some specified period following "treatment." On the basis of such measurement, some investigators have characterized subjects in terms of their levels of responsiveness. This study makes clear that length of time before relapse to undesirable habitual behavior does not characterize an individual, but rather temporarily characterizes the motivational level of an individual.

Thus, neither the most recent period of relapse nor, as stated earlier, any other one single previous period of relapse can be used to predict how an individual will tend to respond following detoxification. An individual's history of time to relapse, however, will allow one to determine (1) how long a next period of remission must be before it can be considered significantly different from previous ordinary behavior and (2) if and under what conditions treatment effects were experienced in the past. The latter can be used to direct treatment.

To facilitate this sort of analysis, the senior author (N.R.M.) has developed special graphical plotting papers (each one appropriate for a specified number of times to relapse) for plotting the individual historical time-to-relapse data. Using these plots, one can identify failure patterns, identify instances of treatment effects, and predict future recidivism behavior. The recidivism data can be solicited by means of a questionnaire (which is also available from the senior author, along with suggestions for its administration). The two publications (Fertig et al., 1980; Mann, 1982) give procedures for detecting, respectively, past and present potential treatment effects by means of the probability plots. Use of this methodology requires staff training and/or a good understanding of survival analysis techniques.

Using the Methodology in Selecting Experimental Samples

One important byproduct of this study is the identification of a method for selecting two experimental groups who are to receive treatment for elimination or alleviation of their addictive behavior. This has been a problem in the past because of difficulties involved in making sure that one of the populations does not exhibit an imbalance with respect to some concomitant variable that could possibly influence outcome.

Although extent of "time to most recent relapse" cannot be used to characterize an individual, the distribution of such relapse times and the parameters of this distribution can be used to characterize the current motivational level of a population at any given time, such as before treatment. Thus, we saw earlier that the two groups who were identified as being with or without legal restraints upon entry into the methadone program exhibited sample distributions of time to first failure that were significantly different and distributions of time to most recent failure (occurring in general after elimination of the legal restraints) that were without discernible differences. It seems appropriate to conclude (on the basis of comparison of probability plots and sample parameters) that after some initial period of exposure to the program, the distributions of motivational levels of the two groups were identical for all practical purposes. If such a near equivalence can be established for two experimental groups in terms of their most recent relapse experience before entry into an experimental program, then it is only necessary to ensure that, aside from experimental parameters that are to be varied, there are no systematic differences in dealing with the two groups by treatment personnel or legal authorities. If the two groups are large enough, external motivational factors will tend to balance out within and between the two populations. Thus, a question relating to "length of most recent period of abstinence" should be added to patient intake forms, even when more extensive abstinence histories are not solicited.

ACKNOWLEDGMENT

Financial support was given by grants 1H81DA02118-01 and -02 from the National Institute on Drug Abuse.

REFERENCES

BRILL, L. *The De-Addiction Process*. Springfield, IL: C. C. Thomas, 1972.

BRILL, L. The treatment of drug abuse: Evolution of a perspective. *Am. J. Psychiatry* 134(2): 157–160, 1977.

CARR-HILL, G.A., and CARR-HILL, R.A. Reconviction as a process. *Br. J. Criminol.* 12: 35–43, 1972.

CARVER, C.S., and SCHEIFER, M.F. Self-consciousness and reactance. *J. Res. Pers.* 15: 16–29, 1981.

CROW, L.H. Reliability analysis for complex repairable systems. In F. Proschan and R.J. Serfling (eds.), *Reliability and Biometry*. Philadelphia: Society for Industrial and Applied Mathematics, 1974.

DESMOND, D.P., and MADDUX, J.F. The effect of probation on behavior of chronic opioid drug users. *Contemp. Drug Probl.* Spring 1977, pp. 41–58.

FERTIG, K.W., MEYER, M.E., and MANN, N.R. On constructing prediction intervals for samples from a Weibull or extreme-value distribution. *Technometrics* 22: 567–573, 1980.

KAO, J.H.K. A graphical estimation of mixed Weibull parameters in life testing of electron tubes. *Technometrics* 1:389–407, 1959.

KIERKEGAARD, S. *Fear and Trembling*. Princeton, NJ: Princeton University Press, 1941a.

KIERKEGAARD, S. *The Sickness unto Death*. Princeton, NJ: Princeton University Press, 1941b.

LAVENHAR, M., SHEFFET, A., DUVAL, H., and LOURIA, D. The New Jersey Medical School narcotics case register: Methodology and summary of first four years of operation. *Addict. Dis.* 1(4): 513–527, 1975.

LING, W., and CHARUVASTRA, C. Methadyl acetate and methadone as maintenance treatments for heroin addicts. *Arch. Gen. Psychiatry* 33: 709–720, 1976.

MANN, N.R. *Use of life-test data analysis methodology for analyzing undesirable habitual behavior*. George Washington University School of Engineering and Applied Science Institute for Management Science and Engineering, Serial T-406, July 1979.

MANN, N.R. Optimal outlier tests for a Weibull model–To identify process changes or to predict failure times. In J.S. Rustagi and S. Zanakis (eds.), *Optimization in Statistics*. North-Holland, 1982.

MANN, N.R., and ROTHBERG, J. *Using life-test data analysis methodology to think about human behavior*. Presented at TIMS/ORSA Annual Meeting, Washington, DC, May 5–7, 1980.

MANN, N.R., SCHAFER, R., and SINGPURWALLA, N. *Methods for Statistical Analysis of Reliability and Life Data*. New York: Wiley, 1974.

NURCO, D.N., BONITO, A.J., LERNER, M., and BALTER, M.B. Studying addicts over time: Methodology and preliminary findings. *Am. J. Drug Alcohol Abuse* 2(2): 183–196, 1975.

SIMMEL, E. Alcoholism and addiction. *Psychoanal. Q.* 17: 6–31, 1948.

SIMPSON, D.D., SAVAGE, L.J., LLOYD, N.R., and SILLS, S.B. *Evaluation of drug abuse treatments based on the first year after DARP: National followup study of admissions to drug abuse treatments in DARP during 1969–1972.* Institute of Behavioral Research Report No. 77-10, Texas Christian University, 1977.

VAILLANT, G.E., and RASOR, R.W. The role of compulsory supervision in the treatment of addiction. *Fed. Probation* 30: 53, June 1966.

WALDORF, D. *Careers in Dope*. Englewood Cliffs, NJ: Prentice-Hall, 1973.

WALDORF, D., and BIERNACKI, P. Natural recovery from heroin addiction: A review of the incidence literature. *J. Drug Issues* 9(2), 1979.

ZANDER, A., and CURTIS, T. Effects of social power on aspiration setting and striving. *J. Abnorm. Soc. Psychol.* 64: 63–67, 1962.

The International Journal of the Addictions, 19(1), 45–56, 1984

Impression Management and Testing for Control Locus in an Alcoholic Sample

Raymond M. Costello,* PhD

The University of Texas Health Science Center at San Antonio
San Antonio, Texas 78284

Kathleen A. Wicoff, BS

The University of Texas at San Antonio
San Antonio, Texas 78284

Abstract

In response to a debate as to whether alcoholics as a group score in an internal or an external direction on Rotter's I-E Scale, a projective, TAT measure of locus of control was proposed. In this pilot study a multivariate storytelling measure was used to test the hypothesis that alcoholics may resort to "impression management" when responding to questionnaires and that a "projective" device may yield different results regarding personality variables like locus of control. An internal score on the I-E was observed for 30 alcoholic subjects to shift to an external score on the Thematic Locus of Control (TLC). Spearman's rho for I-E and TLC was .47 ($p < .001$). Six subjects had markedly incongruent ranks across instruments; three of these were extreme I-E "internals" who shifted to extreme TLC "externals."

Research into generalized beliefs or subjectively held probabilities of the "real" nature of the control of valued events has resulted in an objective

*To whom correspondence should be sent at P.O. Box 3, Helotes, Texas 78023.

 0020-773X/84/1901-0045$3.50/0

questionnaire measure–Rotter's (1966) Internal-External Locus of Control Scale (I-E). The measure is conceptualized as representing a generalized expectancy regarding behavior reinforcement sequences prominent in predicting behavior in social contexts in which there is no clear and uniform labeling of reinforcement contingencies as dependent on skill versus luck. Clear and uniform labeling of reinforcement contingencies defines the situation with regard to the skill versus luck dimension, and generalized beliefs give way to specific expectancies for control appropriate to the situation.

In the alcohol literature a finding on the I-E contrary to expectation was reported by Goss and Morosko (1970), replicated by Costello and Manders (1974) and others, and subsequently challenged by still others. The puzzling finding was that alcoholics in treatment scored more in the "internal" direction than was expected. It had been expected that alcoholics would perform as had other mixed psychiatric patients and reveal an I-E pattern consistent with maladjustment (i.e., externality). In the manner of an explanation, Rotter (1975) suggested that all questionnaires are subject to error under particular testing conditions, that questionnaires are limited by their dependence on conscious awareness, and that questionnaire responses are subject to the bias of impression management and conformity. Specifically, he suggested that as alcoholics are often told that "cure" is "up to them," this could lead to a questionnaire presentation which conforms to treatment staff expectations (i.e., internality). Thus, a more subtle form of examination might be more appropriate for this population.

Adams-Webber (1969), a student of Rotter's, developed a projective measure of internal-external control which correlated positively with the I-E Scale. This measure involved a story-completion test in which a central actor initiates an immoral course of action. The examinee then projects an ending to the story. Story endings are scored for an expectancy for punishment for moral transgression as imposed externally.

Dies (1968) also developed a projective measure of internal-external control using the Thematic Apperception Test (TAT). Dies suggested that the TAT format allows the introduction of a broader spectrum of situations and possible responses, and includes significant interpersonal and intrapersonal concerns not tapped by Rotter's questionnaire. His measure involves a single externality score summed and averaged over any number of TAT stimulus cards. Scores of 5 were given for stories in which there was a "relative absence of self-initiated, responsible action or personal mastery . . . the central figure is viewed as almost powerless in the face of favorable and /or unfavorable events or as unable to overcome life's dilemmas. There may be some attempts to use fantasy to escape from intolerable situations, but few efforts to solve problems realistically are shown" (p. 488). Scores are graded down to 1, which suggests the relatively greatest demonstration of competence of figures central to the story. Principal figures are depicted as "coping with problems and conflicts in a competent, self-determined fashion." This scoring scheme reduces highly complicated stories, with regard to the I-E construct, to a single numerical summary.

PROBLEM

The present report is an exploratory study to determine if a multiaspect scoring system can be devised to score TAT stories to correlate modestly with the 23-item I-E Scale. It was expected that such a system could be devised, that correlations would be much less than unity but statistically significant, and that marked deviations of TAT-predicted scores on the control dimension might provide important clues for biased responding (i.e., impression management or conformity) or differentiation of "defensive externals" from true externals (Rotter, 1975).

METHOD

TAT

In the ordinary TAT procedure, the respondent is asked to weave a story to answer a number of questions about a particular scene. Each scene is ambiguous with regard to the identity of the actor or actors, ambiguous with regard to the emotional state of the actors, ambiguous with regard to the antecedent conditions which led up to the present scene, and ambiguous with regard to future events implied by the scene. The respondent may be asked to consider any of these dimensions and others as well. To capitalize on the complex nature of TAT storytelling, an alternative scoring system for TAT stories is proposed. Rather than a single numerical summary, the (1) projected social transactions, (2) identity of the actor, (3) emotional state of actor, (4) antecedent conditions, and (5) potential outcome can each be rated as independent contributions to a score of generalized expectancy about the nature of the control of valued events. Presumably, this multivariate method of scoring could improve reliability of measures in a fashion analogous to that observed in other psychometric instances involving tests of increased length.

Hypothetically, in the completely "internal" story the projected action statement reveals that the actor is the "origin" of the action, that the actor holds a social identity characteristic of a person who must assume personal initiative and responsibility for actions in order to acquire the identity, that the feeling state of the actor reflects self-satisfaction, that antecedents to the action reflect freedom from external constraints, and that the story's outcome reflects a "reinforcement" contingent upon the actor's self-initiated behavior sequence. The completely "external" story would depict the obverse. Any story receiving the lowest or highest possible score would represent a stereotypic internal or external presentation, respectively.

An example of the proposed Thematic Locus of Control (TLC) scoring method is provided for TAT Card 17BM. This card depicts an apparently naked man holding onto a rope. He appears to be in the act of climbing up or down and is facing forward.

The first question is asked to determine the "action" of the scene as perceived by the respondent: *1. What is happening in this scene*? The objective description of the card involves a man in relationship to a rope. He is either climbing up or descending the rope, or is clinging in a static fashion. No internal-external control value is implied when the respondent sticks to an objective description of the scene. Many respondents, however, project an action statement scorable for its implication of internal-external control. On this card, at least for alcoholic subjects, stories seem to vary on a thematic continuum, suggesting, on one end, an "escape" from the control of powerful others or from highly complex forces surrounding the actor, including the actor's own emotions or physiological drive states. When the respondent projects a social transaction (even if and perhaps especially when only one actor is depicted in the card) which describes the central actor as "finding himself" in a situation in which he must cope with, defend against, or escape from powerful external or internal forces, the implication is that the actor is in some way a victim of forces (including character "defects") which have rendered him in a devalued position. It is this implication of having been put-upon which is scored 2 for externality. On the other end, however, is a story of a self-initiated action free of external constraints, with no hint of having been put-upon. This action statement is scored 0 for internality. Between these extremes lies the noncommittal, objective card description and/or a negotiated social transaction suggesting that the actor acts because of the recognition of a socially determined behavior reinforcement sequence (e.g., It's a requirement of the job). In this case, specific reinforcement contingencies are operative, rendering general expectancies irrelevant with regard to the "psychological" control issue. These latter descriptions are scored 1, neither external (2) nor internal (0).

The second question is asked to determine the perceived identity of the actor: *2. Who is the person in the scene*? The objective description of the card indicates simply that the person in the scene is a naked man. No internal-external control value is implied in this description. Many respondents, however, project an elaborated identity or social role for the actor. On Card 17BM, the thematic continuum considered most relevant for internal-external control involves projection of a role of social prominence, attainable only as a result of an investment of much personal effort. A score of 2 is given to projected identities of a social role of "no prominence or influence" when the actor is the unwilling, incompetent, or passive subjugate of powerful others or of personal ego-dystonic forces or obvious character "defects," or is clearly labeled a child. A score of 0 is given to projected identities of "social prominence or influence" when the actor is an internally motivated achiever. Between these extremes (scored 1) lies the noncommittal card description (e.g., apartment tenant), identification of the actor as "me" (when there is no other description of control value), identification of the actor as a cartoon character or other figment such as Tarzan, and/or identification of the actor as occupying a negotiated social role involving a socially determined behavior reinforcement sequence (e.g., employee).

The third question asks for a description of the actor's emotional state: *3. What is this person thinking or feeling*? The objective description of the card does not suggest any emotional state; the naked man simply holds onto a rope. The thematic continuum considered most relevant for internal-external control involves a projected emotional state suggesting turmoil, distress, tension, or painful indecision, on the one end (scored 2), as the actor is unable to resolve or is painfully attempting to resolve whatever social predicament he might be in. At the other end is a sense of euphoria or excitement as the actor realizes the fruits of personal effort (scored 0). Between these extremes lies the noncommittal card description and/or a detached emotional attitude suggesting a ritualized conformance to a socially determined behavior reinforcement sequence (e.g., He's wondering how much he will be paid), or an emotional state consistent with or required by the action statement (e.g., He feels the strain of the climb).

The fourth question is asked to determine the degree to which the actor played a part in the development of the scene: *4. What led up to this situation (that is, what has happened in the past)*? The objective description of the card suggests no clues in this regard. The thematic continuum considered most relevant for internal-external control involves projected antecedents ranging from an actor who is basically unconscious (i.e., behavior is a predictable result of character "defect") or unaware (e.g., careless, irresponsible, impulsive, or an unwitting victim of some sort) (scored as 2); to one who is fully conscious and aware, who prepares and plans ahead, and who "willfully" and with full awareness initiates a course of action (scored 0). Between these extremes (scored 1) lies the noncommittal card description and/or a highly predictable consequence of a socially determined behavior reinforcement sequence (e.g., job demands).

The scoring difficulty encountered here involves two distinctions. The first distinction to be drawn is that between acceptance of culpability post hoc and the decision to initiate a course of action a priori with "full awareness" of personal motivation and ramifications of whatever consequences might be encountered by the actor. The second distinction to be drawn is between actors who appear to be making a "responsible" decision to initiate an action; but one is the victim of unwitting self-deception and the other is not. Although this adjustment to what otherwise might be a fairly objective scoring scheme introduces an element of subjectivity, and therefore increases the risk of error, it is recommended in order to take advantage of the "projective" nature of the instrument. This adjustment is necessary to avoid the problem of impression management which has been proposed as undermining the validity of the questionnaire method of examination.

The final question asks the respondent to project a future scenario for the present scene: *5. What will happen (what will be done)*? The objective description of the card suggests no terminal scenario. The thematic continuum considered most relevant for internal-external control involves projected scenarios ranging from the vanquishing of the actor by powerful forces beyond personal control, including emotions (scored 2); to self-determined achievement of personal success or gain (scored 0). Between these extremes (scored 1) lies the noncommittal card description and/or a routine performance of a socially determined behavior reinforcement sequence (e.g., He'll do his job).

The following story, produced by one of the subjects for this study, illustrates the concepts and the scoring system. This individual scored 2 on the I-E Scale, suggesting a very strong generalized expectancy for personal (i.e., internal) control of valued events. His score on the Marlow-Crowne Social Desirability Scale was 7, suggesting no particular need to produce socially desirable responses.

Illustrative Protocol

1. What is happening in this scene?

> The man is trying to get down to the ground, because the construction lift on the building is out of order. He needs a drink of water and must come to the ground to get some.

This response was given a score of 2. This respondent perceives the actor to be the victim of a broken construction lift and of a physiological drive—thirst. The attempt to get to the ground is necessitated by these forces.

2. Who is the person in this scene?

> His name is Joe Brown, a married man with a wife and three children. He doesn't like his job, but circumstances make it necessary for him to work to support his family.

This response was given a score of 2. The respondent identifies the actor as an employee (usually scored 1) who apparently has been victimized by circumstances beyond his control which dictate his behavior.

3. What is this person thinking or feeling?

> Joe is thinking, "My God, how the hell did I get myself into this fix?" Upon thinking somewhat deeper, he realizes that he is responsible, himself. He thinks, "If I hadn't done this and if I hadn't done that, I wouldn't be in this fix."

This response was given a score of 2. The projected emotional state is one of turmoil and distress as the actor realizes that he is "in a fix." This recognition of personal responsibility for the predicament does not modify the score, as this is recognition of behavior determined by character "defect."

4. What has led up to this situation? What has happened in the past?

> Joe likes to be one of the boys and, in doing so, spends more than he should. Consequently, he is not able to pay his bills that are required in order to take care of his family. Under these existing conditions he has to take any kind or type of work that he can get. He has been getting gradually deeper and deeper into debt and is providing less care for his family.

This response was given a score of 2. Despite the present recognition of personal culpability, we must assume that the actor was basically unconscious or unaware as he got himself deeper into trouble. He was the victim of a wish to be "one of the boys" and consequently acted immaturely, impulsively, and without restraint.

5. What will happen? What will be done?

> He resolves to stop being one of the boys, and really provide better care for his family. Joe makes an effort to straighten up and fly right, but he feels somewhat confined when he spends all of his time with his family. His attitude and manner towards his family has become bitter and aggressive. His wife has told him that he must change his attitude toward them or leave. He goes to a psychiatrist for counseling and finds out what is wrong. He has therapy and becomes well. His family and he live happily from then on.

This response was scored 1. Although the story has a happy ending involving an effortful initiation of a course of action on the part of the actor, 0 cannot be scored. The outcome is a stereotyped product of a socially determined behavior reinforcement sequence (i.e., Psychotherapy changes people), and the motivation for the actor's effort was, in part, imposed from without (i.e., the ultimatum from his wife). An argument could be raised that a score of 2 is appropriate in that the actor acted under duress from the wife, experienced internal turmoil throughout, and was simply the lucky recipient of the good work of a therapist. The initial statement of personal resolve to change, however, seems to balance out the marital duress and results in a score of 1, neither internal nor external in control value.

The final externality score for this card was 9 of a possible 10. This individual scores nearly as external as possible, in marked contrast with his I-E score of 2. If a significant positive correlation were found for the study sample between I-E scores and the TAT-derived score, this individual would be labeled a TLC miss, and further examination would be indicated to determine reasons for the incongruity. It is also possible that this individual represents an I-E miss, as he may have been conforming his questionnaire behavior to what he may have perceived to be the expectations of the investigators or treatment staff. Whichever might be the case, further evaluation would be recommended.

Subjects

Volunteers were solicited late in 1974 from the resident membership of a rehabilitation center for alcoholics in the southwestern United States. The sample of 30 included both men and women. No identifying information whatever was requested, both as it was not essential for the project and as an attempt to decrease the potential confounding of bias associated with impression management. The facility is known to treat chronic alcoholics who are primarily unemployed and maritally distressed. The average age at admission is in the 40s, and many have police records and prior treatment experiences for alcoholism (Costello, Bechtel, and Giffen, 1973; Costello and Hodde, 1981; Costello and Manders, 1974).

The subjects were examined in a single session with group instructions. Subjects worked at their own desks, first to complete the I-E and then to write stories to TAT Cards 17BM and 14. As only 15 TAT sets were available, one-half of the group worked on Card 17BM while the other half worked on Card 14. These cards were chosen because only one actor is depicted, so that social transactions reported are entirely the product of projection, and thus there is no labeling whatever of social reinforcement contingencies as dependent on skill versus luck. There are, of course, no apparent clues as to identity or feeling state of the actor, and no clues regarding antecedent conditions or possible outcome.

Scoring and Analysis

The I-E questionnaire was scored after Rotter (1966). The TLC score was a sum of externality scores for the two cards. Spearman's rho was calculated for

I-E versus each TAT card, for I-E versus TLC, and for Card 17BM versus Card 14.

RESULTS

Ranks assigned on the basis of performance on Card 17BM were statistically unrelated to ranks assigned on the basis of performance on Card 14 (ρ = .04). A marginal relationship was discovered for I-E ranks and 17BM ranks (ρ = .22, $t(28) = 1.32$, $p < .10$). Statistically significant relationships were found between I-E ranks and 14 ranks (ρ = .46, $t(28) = 3.31$, $p < .001$), and between I-E ranks and TLC ranks (ρ = .47, $t(28) = 3.36$, $p < .001$). Table 1 displays raw scores and associated subject ranks for I-E and TLC.

Table 1

I-E and TLC Raw Scores and Subject Ranks for 30 Chronic Alcoholics

I-E		TLC		I-E vs TLC
Score	Rank	Score	Rank	rank difference
1	1.0	15	21.0	20.0
2	2.5	15	21.0	18.5
2	2.5	10	4.0	1.5
3	6.0	9	1.5	4.5
3	6.0	10	4.0	2.0
3	6.0	12	12.5	6.5
3	6.0	11	8.5	2.5
3	6.0	16	24.0	18.0
4	10.5	10	4.0	6.5
4	10.5	11	8.5	2.0
4	10.5	12	12.5	2.0
4	10.5	14	18.5	8.0
5	14.5	13	15.5	1.0
5	14.5	13	15.5	1.0
5	14.5	13	15.5	1.0
5	14.5	13	15.5	1.0
6	19.0	16	24.0	5.0
6	19.0	11	8.5	10.5
6	19.0	14	18.5	0.5
6	19.0	11	8.5	10.5
6	19.0	9	1.5	17.5
7	23.5	11	8.5	15.0
7	23.5	18	27.5	4.0
7	23.5	15	21.0	2.5
7	23.5	16	24.0	0.5
8	26.5	11	8.5	18.0
8	26.5	19	29.0	2.5
9	28.0	18	27.5	0.5
10	29.0	20	30.0	1.0
11	30.0	17	26.0	4.0

The average I-E score was 5.33, classifying the group as "internal." Range restriction was also evident in that no I-E score greater than 11 was obtained. The distribution of I-E scores appears quite platykurtic over the observed range.

The average TLC score was 13.5. The distribution appeared normal with a mode of 11, but with obvious range restriction (no score lower than 9 was observed). Thus, the group tended to score in an "external" TLC direction, as contrasted with their "internal" I-E performance.

The average I-E versus TLC difference in ranks was 3.3 for 24 of the 30 subjects. The difference for the six subjects remaining, however, was 16.5. The most "external" I-E scorers had concordant TLC scores, but three very "internal" I-E scorers had markedly incongruent TLC scores.

DISCUSSION

The TLC results provided both an intriguing similarity and an intriguing contrast to the I-E results and suggested some support for Rotter's impression management hypothesis for samples of alcoholics. A modest positive correlation between the instruments suggested that, indeed, they were measuring the same or a highly similar construct. The positive correlation, in fact, increased from .47 to .85 after removal of the six cases of marked test incongruence. Thus, 80% of the subjects generally maintained their relative ranks across test modalities, whereas 20% gave very unpredictable performances across measures. This finding of essential concurrent test validities, however, does not presage the additional finding that the group as a whole appeared to have an "internal" locus of control as measured by the I-E method, yet shifted to an "external" locus on the projective method. This finding may be peculiar to alcoholic samples, it may be a more general finding, or it may be a function of TLC scoring peculiarities. No conclusion can be drawn without further testing.

The incongruity, however, does point to the need for multimethod measurement when attempting to validate instruments or theories. The Goss and Morosko (1970) conclusion that alcoholics are an internal I-E group because they "control" the most important reinforcer in their lives is a post hoc argument against which many alternative arguments can be drawn. Heretofore, alternative explanations for the phenomenon have emphasized subject characteristics such as age and social class (e.g., Bowen and Twemlow, 1978) or incomparability of control/comparison groups (e.g., Butts and Chotlos, 1973). The most parsimonious alternative explanation may be that of impression management (Rotter, 1975). If so, serial testing under various apparent demand characteristics might be an important experimental research design to explicate the conditions under which some alcoholics (approximately 20%?) modify their questionnaire behavior to reflect a perceived external reality rather than a genuine internal one.

An additional finding of heuristic value is that of no correlation across TAT cards. This is an excellent situation from a psychometric vantage point, as the cards appear to provide unique rather than redundant information, yet both cards provide information which correlates positively with an external criterion. Scores from the sum of the two cards should prove to have greater reliability and, thus, greater predictive validity when exposed to further validation than would the score from either card taken alone. Further, it is of interest to determine the pattern of intercorrelations across the many TAT cards. Some cards may pull more for "internal" stories than others. If so, not only would this have methodological significance in designing future studies, but it may have clinical significance, for both psychodiagnostic and treatment design purposes, to discover which social/interpersonal/psychological situations provoke an attitude of expectancy for power versus impotence, internal versus external control, or optimism versus pessimism for alcoholics or any other clinical group.

Further research is needed to develop and standardize the psychometric properties of the TLC instrument on a normal population. This is presently underway with protocols obtained from students at the University of Texas at San Antonio, and a scoring manual is being compiled. Another question in need of consideration involves the nature of such a projective device. Should the emphasis be mainly on the story's characteristics or on the choices (projections) made by the storyteller? This question raises the possibility of an altogether different concept in the interpretation of this instrument.

REFERENCES

ADAMS-WEBBER, J.R. Generalized expectancies concerning the locus of control of reinforcements and the perception of moral sanctions. *Br. J. Clin. Psychol.* 8: 340–343, 1969.

BOWEN, W.T., and TWEMLOW, S.W. Locus of control and treatment dropout in an alcoholic population. *Br. J. Addict.* 73: 51–54, 1978.

BUTTS, S.V., and CHOTLOS, J. A comparison of alcoholics and nonalcoholics on perceived locus of control. *Q. J. Stud. Alcohol* 34: 1327-1332, 1973.

COSTELLO, R.M., BECHTEL, J.E., and GIFFEN, M.B. A community's efforts to attack the problem of alcoholism. II. Base rate data for future program evaluation. *Int. J. Addict.* 8(6): 875-888, 1973.

COSTELLO, R.M., and HODDE, J.E. Cost of comprehensive alcoholism care for 100 cases over four years. *J. Stud. Alcohol*, 1981.

COSTELLO, R.M., and MANDERS, K.R. Locus of control and alcoholism. *Br. J. Addict.* 69: 11–17, 1974.

DIES, R.R. Development of a projective measure of perceived locus of control. *J. Project. Tech. Pers. Assess.* 32: 487–490, 1968.

GOSS, A., and MOROSKO, T.E. Relation between a dimension of internal-external control and the MMPI with an alcoholic population. *J. Consult. Clin. Psychol.* 34(2): 189–192, 1970.

ROTTER, J.B. Generalized expectancies for internal vs. external control of reinforcement. *Psychol. Monogr.* 80, 1966 (1, whole No. 609).
ROTTER, J.B. Some problems and misconceptions related to the construct of internal vs. external control of reinforcement. *J. Consult. Clin. Psychol.* 43: 56–67, 1975.

The International Journal of the Addictions, 19(1), 57–77, 1984

A Review of the Reliability and Validity of the Drug Abuse Warning Network

John D. Swisher

Teh-wei Hu

Center for Research on Human Resources
Institute for Policy Research and Evaluation
The Pennsylvania State University
University Park, Pennsylvania 16802

Abstract

The Drug Abuse Warning Network (DAWN) is a government-funded drug abuse data gathering system used extensively at the federal, state, and local levels in policy formulation and program evaluation, and as an indicator of changing trends in substance abuse. This paper (1) briefly describes the DAWN data, (2) examines reviews of the DAWN system, (3) assesses the strengths and limitations of the DAWN data, and (4) illustrates some possible further uses of these data for research and policy purposes.

INTRODUCTION

The Drug Abuse Warning Network (DAWN) is a government-funded drug abuse data gathering system frequently used in federal-level policy formulation and program evaluation.

In addition to federal activities, many state drug prevention and enforcement agencies use DAWN data to formulate state plans. Cost-benefit analysis of drug abuse treatment programs and estimates of the cost of drug abuse (Rufener, Rachel, and Cruze, 1977) have relied heavily on the DAWN data. DAWN is also recommended as a data source in the NIDA drug abuse prevention evaluation guidelines (French and Kaufman, 1979). Since important policy decisions are in

 0020-773X/84/1901-0057$3.50/0

part based on DAWN data, DAWN has also been reviewed in terms of its data collection procedures, response quality, accuracy, and completeness of its information on drug abuse by a number of authors (Barton, 1975; Franklin Research Center, 1979; Lasagna, 1976; Person, 1976; Ungerleider, Lundberg, Sunshine, and Walberg, 1980a). The purposes of this paper are: (1) to provide a brief description of the nature of DAWN data, (2) to examine the reviews on the DAWN system, (3) to assess the strengths and limitations of DAWN data, and (4) to illustrate the possible further use of the DAWN data for research and policy purposes.

THE NATURE OF DAWN DATA

The DAWN system started its annual collection in 1972, at the initiative of the Drug Enforcement Administration (DEA). In 1975 the National Institute on Drug Abuse (NIDA) became a cosponsor of the project. DEA uses DAWN data for its enforcement, compliance, scheduling, and research activities. NIDA uses the data primarily for policy formulation regarding research, prevention, and treatment programs.

DAWN presently collects reports of drug abuse episodes from hospital emergency rooms and county medical examiners/coroners located in 26 Standard Metropolitan Statistical Areas (SMSAs) throughout the United States. SMSAs are integrated economic and social units with a large population nucleus composed of a relatively large core city, or cities, plus the adjacent contiguous counties. In addition, data from a random sample of hospital emergency rooms outside the 26 SMSA areas are used in conjunction with the SMSA data for projecting nationwide estimates of drug abuse.

DAWN SMSAs were originally selected in 1972 so that all former 13 DEA regional areas (formerly BNDD) would be represented and so that no fewer than two SMSAs would be included from each DEA region. Population criteria were also employed to identify the number of SMSAs within a given region. The initial coverage of 38 SMSAs was reduced in April 1973 to the 24 SMSAs which coincided with those drug abuse areas designated by the Special Action Office for Drug Abuse Prevention as part of a data coordination effort with other federal information systems. (The Baltimore, Maryland, and St. Louis, Missouri, SMSAs entered the DAWN system in May 1979.) Therefore, the final sample of SMSAs was never intended to represent a sociological cross-section of America; rather, the system was intentionally designed to focus on areas which would most likely provide early warning indicators of new drug abuse patterns.

The sample set of hospital emergency rooms eligible for DAWN reporting is limited to those nonfederal, short-term general hospitals which have at least 1,000 emergency room visits of all kinds per year. They must be open 24 hours a day, 7 days a week. Not every eligible hospital within the 24 SMSAs is included in the system due to the lack of adequate recordkeeping systems or sufficient available staff to report the data (Franklin Research Center, 1979, Table 12, Sec. 4, p. 6).

The reporting facilities are individually recruited and each DAWN reporter is individually trained and tested according to standardized procedures by members of the contractor's professional field staff. In addition, each facility's data are analyzed by computerized statistical procedures each month to identify any reporting idiosyncracies. The objective in standardized reporter training is for all DAWN reporters to use the same definitions and procedures for completing the DAWN data forms. Diagnostic information relative to the data elements on the forms is expected to be provided by appropriate medical staff. In addition, emergency room data reported to DAWN are transcribed directly by these trained reporters from available hospital medical records, in many cases after consultation with the doctor and/or nurses attending the episode. In a variety of audits, carried out on an almost continuous basis from the beginnings of the DAWN system and ranging in sponsorship from the General Accounting Office to the Franklin Research Center, the reliability of these data has been tested and they have proven to be highly accurate.

The DAWN reporters identify only those episodes which meet the following definitions adopted for the project:

1. *Drug Abuse Episode*—The nonmedical use of a substance for any of the following reasons: psychic effects, dependence, and attempted or successful self-destruction. Within this definition, the major items were also defined:
   a. *Nonmedical use*—The use of
      (1) Prescription drugs in a manner inconsistent with accepted medical practice.
      (2) Over-the-counter (OTC) drugs contrary to approved labeling.
      (3) Any other substance (heroin, marijuana, peyote, glue, aerosols, etc.) considered nonmedical with the exception of alcohol, caustics, household poisons, and other hazardous material. Alcohol, caustics, etc., should be reported only if used in conjunction with another drug; for example, alcohol-diazepam, Clorox-barbiturates.
   b. *Psychic effects*—Euphoria, high, kicks, mood alteration, alleviation of unhappiness, sexual enhancement, trips, and drug experiences. Drug experiences include experimental use for pleasure, fulfillment, social or recreational purposes, and for peer acceptance.
   c. *Dependence*—A psychological or physical state characterized by behavior that always includes a compulsion to take the drug on a continuous or periodic basis in order to experience its effects or to avoid the discomfort of its absence.

d. *Suicide attempt or gesture*—Successful or unsuccessful suicide attempt or gesture verified by a witness, a note left by patient, physician's medical record, or other evidence.

2. *Drug-Involved Death*—Any death which is drug induced or drug related:
   a. *Drug induced*—Caused by a drug "overdose" where a toxic level is found or suspected, or caused by a synergistic effect of the drug with another drug.
   b. *Drug related*—Drug or drugs are present and a contributing factor to the death but not the sole cause of death.

The DAWN report forms contain 18 data elements relating to the reporting facility information, patient information, and drug substance information. The emergency room patient information includes age, race, sex, employment status, drug program participation status, reason for taking substance, reason for contact, patient disposition, and clinical status. The medical examiner report forms differ in patient information from the emergency room forms because the main items of interest in a drug-related or drug-induced death are the cause and manner of death. The drug substance information requested on both forms, however, is almost identical; the major exception is that the source of substance is peculiar to the emergency room forms. Only the medical examiner forms provide for a listing of the toxicological testing methods and concentration of drug(s) found.

As many as six drugs or substances can be mentioned on each report form. The episode reports are completed and sent to the contractor's processing facility. Data editors then review each report, resolve any problems with missing data or data anomalies, and maintain regular written and telephone contact with each assigned facility to ensure data quality and timeliness. The reports are coded and processed following these extensive quality control procedures. Throughout the remainder of the data processing a high degree of error control is further achieved by numerous computer edit programs.

For the purpose of illustration, the data in *Project DAWN Annual Report 1979* revealed that 121,575 drug abuse episodes were reported to the DAWN system. Approximately 97% came from hospital emergency rooms, and the rest from medical examiners (IMS America, 1979, p. 16). (Crisis Centers no longer participate in DAWN.) The distributions of drug abuse episodes from the two facility types vary only slightly in a given year.

The DAWN system has reported over 6,700 different substances in the incidents of abuse during the past 8 years. In 1979 approximately 30 of these substances accounted for 67% of all drugs mentioned from emergency rooms. Data on alcohol used in combination with other drugs are also collected in the system, but medical emergencies and deaths caused only from alcohol ingestion are not collected. Collection of all other alcohol-alone data is currently the sole responsibility of NIAAA.

At the present time, the DAWN data system is the single most comprehensive source of drug abuse information which has accumulated data on an individual patient/client basis for more than 8 years. These data are available in aggregate statistical reports and/or monthly, quarterly, and annual reports. These reports are available to the public upon request from the Drug Enforcement Administration, Washington, DC. Unidentified episode records are also contained in computer tapes and have been provided by DAWN to individual researchers upon review of an appropriate request. Data collection, processing, limited analysis, and reporting are presently performed by the DAWN contractor, IMS America Ltd., of Ambler, Pennsylvania, at the request of the Drug Enforcement Administration.

RELIABILITY AND VALIDITY OF DAWN DATA

There has been considerable discussion regarding the nature and quality of the DAWN data system. This can be attributed to the fact that the data have significant impact on government drug and scientific research policies. There are five major critiques which address these aspects of the system: Barton (1975); Lasagna (1976); Person (1976); Franklin Research Center (1979); and Ungerleider, Lundberg, Sunshine, Walberg (1980b). This section presents a brief review of these publications and provides a synthesis of the comments.

Among these reviews varying degrees of accurate, objective, and constructive suggestions and/or cautions for DAWN data collectors and users are found. The exception is Lasagna's review (1976), in which comments appear to be based more on personal bias than professional evidence.

Reliability of DAWN Data

Barton's (1975) nonstatistical review suggested several possible limitations of the early DAWN system. First, DAWN covered only 24 SMSAs and a small portion of hospitals in "other cities"; thus Barton felt DAWN was not nationally representative. As indicated earlier in this paper, DAWN was not designed to be a nationally representative survey. Second, he pointed out that the hospitals are not compelled to report their drug abuse information to the DAWN system. To the contrary, it is a voluntary decision on the hospital's part to become part of the DAWN system and report drug abuse episodes. Although facilities are paid a small monetary incentive (which in most cases does not pay for the amount of work effort required for the reporting), this cannot be considered an incentive to the facility to report. Facilities choose to report to DAWN because they believe DAWN contributes to solving a significant social problem. DAWN reports could also be used to document a community's need for treatment and prevention programs. Barton's third apprehension was that even if hospitals were willing to supply the information, the emergency rooms may not have adequate record files. He suggested that this condition would be responsible for causing reporting errors. The contractor now maintains an external field staff of professional health administrative personnel to minimize any such reporting errors, and for training and awareness programs for medical and nursing staff who are familiar with hospital emergency room record filing systems. To assist with potential problems in this area, they provide on-site advice and thorough training to facility reporters on how best to accomplish their reporting responsibilities under all types of filing systems.

Lasagna (1976) stated that DAWN data could not be used to assess changes or trends in drug abuse. Several examples reported later in this paper prove that DAWN data are very useful as indicators of substance abuse. Lasagna expressed concern about the possibility of double counting a crisis center episode and hospital emergency room episode which could theoretically involve the same person on the same day. He also contended that DAWN understated alcohol and that the reported overall drug rankings are misleading. Lasagna neglected, however, to provide supportive data for the last three accusations.

Since rebuttals are based on questioning the evidence used to state a hypothesis, the absence of Lasagna's supportive data casts a shadow of doubt in the authors' minds as to the veracity of Lasagna's accusations and prevents the present authors from presenting any rebuttals for the accusations. However, the alcohol statement can easily be refuted because DAWN does not collect data on alcohol-alone episodes. The "double counting" observation represents a further misunderstanding by the author. The DAWN system contains no patient identifiers and therefore makes no claims regarding the tracking of a particular abuser.

Person's review (1976) contended that raw drug-mention data cannot be used for comparisons among different SMSAs because the data are not adjusted for population size. He felt the data should be limited only to a given SMSA and not used for national indicators. This limitation identified by Person has since been rectified. Since June 1977 specific drug problems as reported by hospital emergency rooms can be compared between SMSAs due to the development of statistical criteria to compensate for late reporting, non-DAWN facilities, and differing SMSA populations. A statistical model has also been developed by DEA which permits estimation of specific drug problems to be made for the universe of eligible hospital emergency rooms throughout the United States.

Person further indicated that the level of reporting contributed by the participating facilities influenced the underreporting aspect of the whole system. The level of hospital emergency room (ER) reporting among the various SMSAs refers to the criteria which the government directed the contractor to follow in soliciting ER participation in the DAWN network, commonly referred to as "saturation." The goal of "saturation" was to enlist as near to 100% of all qualified hospital ERs within 20 DAWN SMSAs and a 50% sample of ERs from

New York, Chicago, and Los Angeles. In 1976, for various reasons, ER coverage was less than 100%, with an overall average of 89% for the 20 SMSAs.

In May 1977 the selection process was changed to reflect the total hospital emergency room visits occurring within a given SMSA. In the current DAWN program, the contractor is required to solicit ER participation in 22 SMSAs such that at least 80% of the total number of hospital ER visits in the entire SMSA is regularly screened for DAWN episodes. Adequate ER distribution of these facilities must also be reflective of the central city and surrounding counties of the SMSA. In New York, Chicago, and Los Angeles, at least 50% coverage is required. Currently, the average ER visit coverage in 20 SMSAs (excluding the recent recruitment of St. Louis and Baltimore SMSAs) is 86%; and New York, Chicago, and Los Angeles contribute 46%, 51% and 51%, respectively. (Only seven hospitals in San Francisco County currently report to DAWN.)

DEA statisticians indicate that the identification of drug abuse episodes from a given population is more complete and cost efficient when based upon total hospital ER visits rather than when based upon an absolute number of hospitals.

Person concluded with a recommendation for more careful training for the reporters, using standardized definitions and procedures and instituting quality control procedures to ensure the reliability of DAWN data. He also pointed out that DAWN validity, as tested via the biochemical identification of the purported drug of abuse, is a much more difficult issue to resolve. However, Person did indicate that "validity" of the DAWN data, in a somewhat different sense, might be established by correlating the DAWN drug picture with ancillary sources of drug abuse information.

Person's overall opinion was that if necessary caveats are mentioned, DAWN information is a helpful data source for decision makers.

It should be pointed out that a number of Person's comments or suggestions concerning the reliability of the DAWN data have been addressed by the DEA. During the last 3½ years, revised procedures have been instituted concerning (1) clarification of definitions, (2) development of reporting and training manuals, and (3) quality control of input data; and (4) revised computer edits and checks have been implemented by the contractor throughout the DAWN system. All trended data presently used from DAWN have been generated by this revised, upgraded DAWN system.

The 1979 Franklin Research Center Study was an extensive study of the reliability of the hospital data reported to the DAWN system. This independent study was supported by DEA and NIDA and focused on the major source of DAWN data, the hospital emergency room drug abuse episodes.

A random sampling of 134 DAWN hospitals was visited by FRC evaluators. The FRC staff reviewed 4,484 records and found that DAWN drug abuse episodes were underreported by approximately one-third. Stated another way,

DAWN reported about two-thirds of the actual drug abuse episodes treated in the emergency rooms.

The problem of underreporting is perhaps the greatest weakness in the system, and major efforts are being made to reduce the problem. Although data are being underreported, use of DAWN data and their reliability are not significantly impacted. Nor does the underreporting appear to significantly affect in any way the distribution of cases which are reported to DAWN. The government is fully aware that the important scheduling, enforcement, and treatment policy decisions using DAWN data result from a conservative data base.

The FRC Study also did error analyses on the individual data cells of the report forms. The average error was about 2.5% for factual information and about 15% on drug substance information. FRC attributed most of these errors to the turnover rates in the emergency room personnel, the pressures of working in the emergency rooms, and the hospital staff's lack of understanding of the DAWN instruction booklets.

The appropriate recommendations from this study are currently being implemented into the system. For example, hospital emergency room personnel training materials have been revised and standardized testing executed at the end of training. DAWN field personnel are making more frequent facility visits to ascertain the accuracy and completeness of reporting and to assist with facility problems.

The integrity of the emergency room record (from which DAWN reports are derived), when used as a source of drug abuse information, was recently evaluated by Anglin et al. (1980). This study involved the evaluation of a sample of 494 sedative-hypnotic overdose patients selected from the records of four hospital emergency room facilities (three of them DAWN-reporting hospitals) in New York City. Miami. Houston, and Boston, respectively. This study clearly indicated that emergency room reports were reliable indicators of drug abuse.

Validity of DAWN Data

This section of the paper presents information indicating that DAWN statistics are related to and can be validated by external sources of data. It is particularly evident in several examples involving PCP and methaqualone trends. These examples, reflecting other data sources of information, represent a traditional form of validating a data collection procedure.

The best form of external validation would involve confirmation of the purported drugs of abuse by laboratory analysis. Ungerleider, Lundberg, Sunshine, and Walberg published two articles, one in the January 1980 issue of the *Archives of General Psychiatry* and the other in the November/December 1980 issue of *Journal of Analytical Toxicology*. Both articles use data collected in 1977 which attempted to correlate DAWN abuse mentions with toxicological analysis. While the overall study was of very questionable design, one interpretation of the data did substantiate 89% partial laboratory confirmation of specific drug substances cited in abuse episodes. A more in-depth evaluation of this study is found later in this section.

DAWN hospital emergency room data provide regular, ongoing information which correlates the purported drug of abuse with the episode. A 1978 analysis of 117,023 emergency room episodes revealed that 61% of the drugs mentioned were voluntarily identified by the patient, 22% by the physician, 7% by possession of the actual dosage form, and 7% by laboratory analysis of blood, urine, or tissue specimens; from January 1976 through September 1979, medical examiner data indicated 99% laboratory validation involving 2,082 drug-abuse-related death mentions.

Anglin et al. (1980), in the previously mentioned sedative-hypnotics study, investigated the correlation between purported drugs of abuse in four hospital emergency room facilities and the biochemical verification of those substances through independent toxicological analysis of specimens taken from emergency room patients. For five specific drug substances—diazepam, secobarbital/amobarbital, ethchlorvynol, methaqualone, and phenobarbital—the authors found an average of 75.2% agreement between the medical records and the laboratory reports. The results of this limited study provide definitive, although indirect, credence to the validity of DAWN hospital emergency room data, since three of the four hospitals studied were DAWN-reporting hospitals which generated DAWN reports from the same emergency room records evaluated in the Anglin study.

Moreover, the Anglin study provides valuable insight into the reasons why some drugs which are identified in the toxicological analysis are not reported by the patient when seeking emergency medical attention. The Anglin study found that drug substances reported when the patient first sought treatment were commonly found at high levels in the patient's serum toxicology, indicating that the level of the drug probably was related to the medical emergency (DAWN reportable). In those cases in which the patient did not report the drug substance when seeking treatment, the level of the substance in the patient's serum toxicology was far less, indicating less likelihood that the substance was of any relevance in causing the medical emergency (not reportable to DAWN). These results clarify the misleading conclusions of the earlier Ungerleider et al. study (1980a, 1980b), which made no such distinction and simply defined all disagreement with any toxicological positive as a "DAWN error."

Anglin et al. (1980) summarized their finding that the medical record, from which DAWN data are derived, is both a valid and reliable source of information:

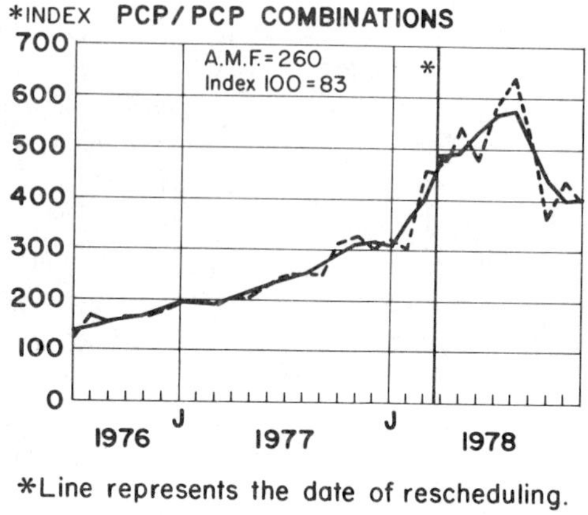

Fig. 1. Trends for PCP. From consistently reporting emergency rooms in TCDS, July 1976-December 1978.

An example of external validation is presented in Fig. 1, which reflects a significant increase in the mentions for PCP from midyear 1978 (*DAWN Quarterly Report*–IMS America, 1978). DEA officials, noting the PCP problem as indicated by DAWN data and other sources of information, initiated rescheduling procedures in December 1977 to move PCP from Schedule III to Schedule II. The rescheduling action was effected on February 24, 1978. At about this same time DEA initiated a concentrated enforcement effort against PCP clandestine laboratory activity. Three to four months after the effective date of these actions, the upward abuse trend made a significant shift downward. Figure 2 reveals a continuing downward trend for PCP to a 1977 level of activity.

In addition to the rescheduling of PCP, there was widespread concern for PCP abuse expressed in the media and at special conferences (White House, 1977). While one could speculate as to the weight of various factors that contributed to this downward trend, there is a reasonable probability that the pattern change was effected by a combination of (1) rescheduling actions, (2) media publicity, (3) appropriate medical warnings, and (4) enforcement efforts directed at clandestine laboratories. In this case, it can be reasonably surmised that the DAWN data reflected the true PCP abuse picture both before and after the rescheduling action.

The case of methaqualone is a particularly clear-cut example of the validity of DAWN data. Florida government officials became concerned when a 1975–

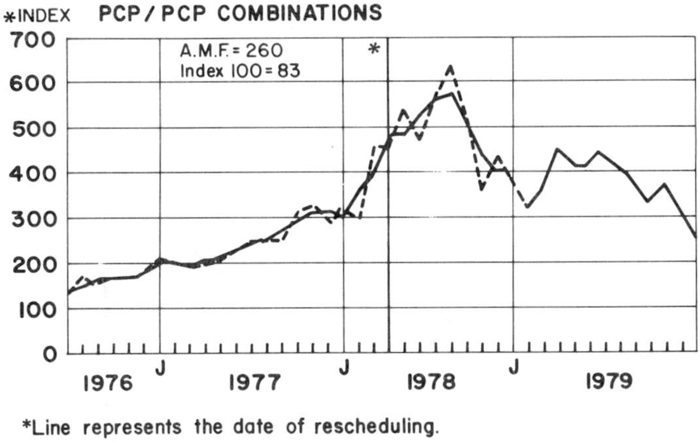

Fig. 2. Trends for PCP. From consistently reporting emergency rooms in TCDS, July 1976-December 1979.

1977 DAWN trend indicated a continuously increasing pattern of methaqualone abuse in Miami (see Fig. 3). A check of the commercial distribution of methaqualone (see Fig. 4) in Florida revealed a high level of sales to one particular physician. Based on this information, enforcement agents successfully intervened. The lines in Figs. 3 and 4 represent the approximate time when the physician's indiscriminate activity was curtailed. There was an immediate downward shift in Miami methaqualone emergency room mentions (see Fig. 5).

However, in comparison with all methaqualone data (see Fig. 3), Miami DAWN incidents did not decline as much as would have been expected. It was subsequently hypothesized that either DAWN was not accurate or there were other sources of methaqualone in the Miami area. Further investigation revealed a relatively new and extensive illicit importation of the substance in question from Colombia. This touched off a widespread effort by government officials to find the illegal importation source. Once again, DAWN data accurately reflected both licit and illicit substance abuse activity and was extremely helpful in alerting the Miami community to the problem.

Another example of the validity of DAWN data is associated with a series of articles which appeared in the *Chicago Tribune* during June 1979. The articles described the excessive prescribing of stimulants and depressants by a local "weight and stress" clinic. The *Tribune* initiated its investigations based on DAWN reports which indicated extensive emergency room abuse mentions of the prescribed substances. In this instance, DAWN data displayed the existence of a particular local community abuse pattern. A questionable "clinic" was

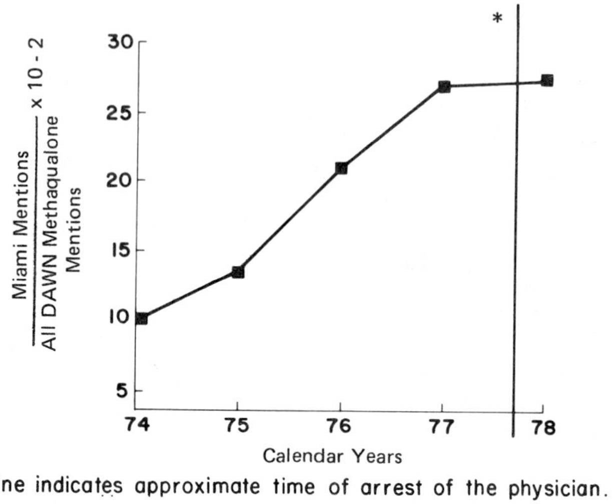

Fig. 3. Methaqualone abuse. From DAWN hospital emergency rooms.

implicated as a major contributor to the abuse problem through further solid investigative newspaper reporting and efforts of concerned local groups. After 4 days of adverse publicity, the "clinic's" physicians resigned and the clinic closed.

The toxicological verification study published by Ungerleider, Lundberg, Sunshine, and Walberg (1980a, 1980b) attempted to validate DAWN drug mentions from only one emergency room by reviewing toxicology reports for the same patients during a period of time in 1977. The authors used about 1,000 emergency room patient drug abuse episodes from the Los Angeles County/ University of Southern California Medical Center to compare retrospectively the drug substances mentioned in the DAWN reports with chemical analysis of biological specimens. Their research approach, however, contained several questionable methodological procedures which significantly erode the veracity of their findings:

1. Specimen samples for analysis were taken from only 52% of the total number of patient drug abuse episodes. No reason was given for sampling only half of the subjects. This selection bias may well have affected the magnitude of the test results.
2. The laboratory analyses ordered for the clients had no connection with the drugs reported by the patients. The analyses were ordered by physicians in the course of basic medical treatment rather than being specific analyses to

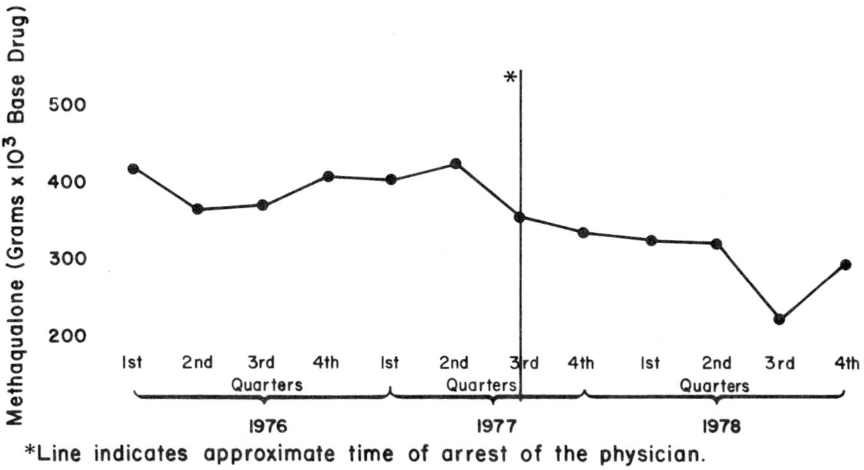

Fig. 4. Methaqualone distribution in Florida.

check for the drugs reported by the patients. The authors specifically stated this on page 108 of their article: "The toxicology laboratory assays were based on those specific laboratory tests the physician requested, not on the DAWN mention or the diagnosis." Thus, another bias was probably introduced because physicians were not instructed to run tests for the drugs reported by the patients. A comparison of results between the tests requested and the DAWN mentions could hardly be valid under this set of circumstances.

Several statements by Dr. Ungerleider and his colleagues regarding the study results need clarification. The article abstract states that the DAWN reports were "verified in 20 percent of the tested samples, found to be incorrect in 11 percent and partially correct in 69 percent." The terms "partially correct" and "partially incorrect" were never defined in the article. Both terms could mean that all drugs mentioned by the patient were found, plus some drugs that the patient did not mention. On page 108 of the article, the authors seem to be defining the terms in question as we have surmised when they state: ". . . 103 reports (20 percent of those for which analyses were done) were consistent with the DAWN reports; 56 (11 percent) indicated the DAWN reports were incorrect; and 369 (60 percent) [Note: The percentage as printed in the body of the article was in error. It should have been 70% (369/528), which was correctly stated in the abstract] indicated the DAWN reports contained some correct information but also were incomplete and omitted some drugs that were involved but not re-

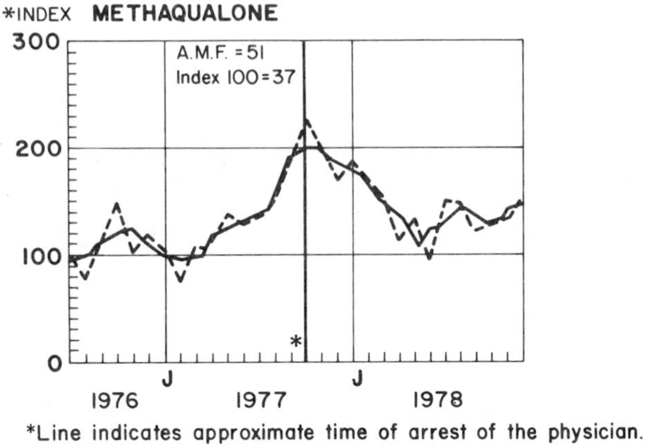

Fig. 5. Miami trends for methaqualone. From consistently reporting emergency rooms in SMSA, July 1976-December 1978.

ported." Thus, it can be stated that as much as 89% of the records could be correct if laboratory verification was based on the drugs reported by the emergency room patient instead of the drug analyses requested by the physician.

The authors also inaccurately state that nonacute "recreational use" of drugs (i.e., friends calling a hospital to report their pleasant reactions) are reported to DAWN and quote the DEA project officer as the source. Only acute medical emergencies consistent with the DAWN criteria for reportable drug abuse cases, which are treated in person at hospital emergency rooms, are entered into the DAWN system, and the DAWN project officer at DEA indicates that the authors' interpretation is erroneous (Murphy, 1981).

It is confusing that the authors initially stated that their retrospective DAWN study contained considerable limitations but yet in a subsequently published February 1980 article in *The Journal*, a Canadian alcohol and drug publication, the authors disregarded these limitations and branded the DAWN data as "worthless." The inaccuracies and problems associated with the Ungerleider et al. research as reported by them in both articles were recently pointed out by Hinkley (1980), who stated that "the statements made by Thomas Ungerleider regarding the results of a recent reliability study of DAWN data at the Los Angeles County University of Southern California Medical Center are essentially misleading." Contrary to the opinions of Ungerleider et al., the present authors consider the current DAWN system with its quality control features as a reliable and valid drug abuse indicator.

Greenburg and Roberson (1978) performed a sophisticated research study using the DAWN emergency room heroin-related cases as one of the dependent variables to examine drug abuse correlates. They also employed a Heroin Problem Index (HPI) based on four drug use indicators (treatment admissions, emergency room cases, heroin-related deaths, and serum hepatitis cases) using the principal component factor analysis. Among these four indicators, only emergency room data are obtained from the DAWN system.

The correlation analysis among 24 of the DAWN SMSAs shows that there are simple correlations of approximately .80 between the DAWN emergency room variable and the heroin-related death variable, which is a relatively high degree of correlation. (The Baltimore and St. Louis SMSAs are excluded because of late entry into the system.) The extensive analysis of five SMSAs (Detroit, Chicago, Washington, D.C., Dallas, and Phoenix) indicates that among the composite index (HPI), the DAWN emergency room variable contributed the highest proportion of variance in explaining the magnitude of the HPI. In a separate regression analysis, both the DAWN emergency room variable and the drug treatment admission variable provide equally good predictions of the heroin use indicators. These empirical analyses have shown that the DAWN data have been a consistent and adequate indicator for drug use status in these SMSA areas.

Expected Levels of Reliability and Validity

The reliability and validity reviews can be summarized into two categories: One is concerned with the data collection procedures while the other is concerned with the implications of collected results.

The initial design of the DAWN hospital emergency room (ER) reporting network was to collect abuse statistics primarily from selected SMSAs. In addition to the ERs from selected SMSAs, statistics were also collected from a random sample of hospital ERs outside the existing DAWN SMSAs. This smaller data base was to be used later to develop a nationwide hospital ER estimating procedure. DEA statisticians have developed and satisfactorily tested such an estimating procedure which will provide national drug abuse estimates. Details of the method and results were published by DEA officials recently.

Prior to the development of this estimating procedure, it was generally recognized that since the source of the data was primarily generated from the SMSAs, it would be inappropriate to interpret the results as statistically representing the entire United States. This is clearly recognized by the DAWN Project (IMS, 1978, p. 3), and such statistical coverage has never been claimed by the government as a capability of DAWN. This data limitation should not, however, be considered a major problem for using or interpreting the DAWN SMSA data. One must simply recognize this limitation and consider the DAWN SMSA data as primarily reflecting urban drug abuse information throughout various sections around the country.

With the advent of the national estimating procedure, the present DAWN system can reflect the abuse problem from 26 selected areas and estimate the specific abuse problem on a nationwide basis, to the total universe of eligible hospital ERs. This is a significant accomplishment of the DAWN system.

The present authors know of no other drug abuse reporting system, with a continuously reporting hospital ER data base since July 1973, which can provide nationwide specific drug abuse estimates. With the addition of a national hospital ER estimating procedure, the capability of the present DAWN system has now been enhanced to provide nationwide profiles for types of drug abuse and the abusers themselves.

Second, as pointed out by the Franklin Research Center (1979), the DAWN system presently underreports actual drug abuse cases by about 30% and also contains about 5-8% incorrect information. While underreporting may be due to lack of hospital staff or other sources (such as only screening the emergency room log book for primary diagnoses), the incorrect information may also be due to misunderstanding on the part of either patients or recorders (i.e., nurse, clerk, etc.). Further revisions in the data collection procedures could improve underreporting; however, the present reporting error rate of only 5-8% is certainly within a very acceptable research range as compared to other social and health statistics systems. For example, the Health Interview Survey conducted by the National Center for Health Statistics has accounted for more than 10% nonrespondent bias (Kovar and Wright, 1973). Most national opinion surveys allow for errors of plus or minus 3% and even clinical/toxicological laboratories generally allow for a normal variation range of plus or minus 10% (a factor not considered by Ungerleider et al).

Further Validation Needs

The studies reviewed in this section have indicated that DAWN data are both reliable and valid. The major problem with DAWN data appears to be that they underestimate the extent of the problem. An adequate validity study using laboratory analyses to confirm drug mentions has not been conducted, and it is recommended that a study of this nature be considered by DEA and NIDA through a separate evaluation effort.

Since important legal and program decisions are presently being made in part on the basis of DAWN data, it would be appropriate to establish a periodic or continuous reliability and validity analysis of DAWN. Obviously, this effort should be conducted as objectively as possible and, as such, should be the role of a third party. In spite of expected limitations typical of similar data systems, the DAWN system is by far the most valuable source of information on the status of drug abuse among large segments of urban populations. It provides very accurate information on the relative frequency (ranking) of drug abuse in the targeted SMSAs. Obviously, further improvements as suggested by the Franklin Research Center would be desirable, together with periodic monitoring of the data system.

DATA UTILITY

DAWN data have been used extensively within federal agencies, such as the Drug Enforcement Administration, the National Institute on Drug Abuse, the Department of Defense, and the Food and Drug Administration for planning, monitoring, and evaluation purposes. While national aggregate DAWN data are very useful for the stated purposes, another attractive aspect of the DAWN data is their availability for research analyses of individual data from the past 8 years. Furthermore, in a given area or time period, the DAWN data can be used by DEA and NIDA in conjunction with other drug prevention or enforcement information including state and local laboratory reports.

Many single-state authorities, county, and municipal authorities also use DAWN data for needs assessment and monitoring substance abuse patterns within a specific area. New York, Pennsylvania, New Jersey, and other states regularly use the DAWN data for their annual planning based on monthly or quarterly statistical DAWN reports.

The State of New Hampshire has established a statewide DAWN-type system for its specific needs (Rhodes, 1979, 1980), using the federal DAWN system as a model. Barry Rhodes, deputy director for drug abuse services in New Hampshire, reported in 1979 that "One of the more significant impacts that Mini-DAWN data has had has been in the area of sensitizing physicians to the prescription drug abuse problem" (Rhodes, 1979, p. 5). The majority of New Hampshire emergency room mentions of substance abuse were for drugs primarily acquired through prescriptions. In fact, New Hampshire Mini-DAWN data revealed that a large number of women between the ages of 20 and 39 were abusing alcohol in combination with valium. A series of meetings held with physicians ended in a recommendation by the New Hampshire Medical Society that physicians consider counseling as an option in the treatment of depression, stress, and anxiety for women.

Fourteen other states have requested and are presently considering formal proposals to implement statewide DAWN systems in order to track the pattern and extent of alcohol and drug abuse in their states. Approximately 20 single-state (drug abuse) agencies have requested DAWN briefings. The United States Department of Defense recently participated in a 6-month pilot test (November 1979 to April 1980) for gathering drug abuse statistics from 30 military hospitals and is now considering adopting a similar system throughout military medical installations worldwide. In addition, the Pan American Health Organization has initiated programs to develop national drug abuse and other health data systems in Mexico, Peru, and Argentina patterned after the DAWN program and has received information requests relative to DAWN from five other member countries. DAWN data were used extensively in preparing the barbiturate study requested by the Office of Drug Abuse Planning and by the Food and Drug Administration for the amphetamine hearings conducted in December 1977. DAWN data have been used in the Senate hearings on d-propoxyphene.

Obviously, care should be exercised in targeting specific trade name substances which would unnecessarily harm the pharmaceutical industry. However, the pharmaceutical industry could also use DAWN-type data to encourage responsible medical practice and responsible individual decisions regarding specific substances which show a high potential for abuse. One pharmaceutical firm (Lemmon Pharmacal Company) has urged greater prevention and enforcement efforts to reduce the abuse of methaqualone, but emphasized the need to take actions which do not prohibit its use as a responsible medical agent.

In addition to social policy formation, DAWN data may also be used for basic research and program evaluation. For example, if one were interested in examining the factors that affect the extent of drug use and different types of substances being taken by users, a statistical relationship could be formulated using the type of substance as a dependent variable in an analytical model. There are many factors affecting the use of these drugs, such as age, race, sex, employment status, and location of users, and this information is self-contained in the DAWN data file. Additional information such as income level, price of the substance, and the degree of enforcement of prevention activities in the SMSA, all of which are available from the U.S. Census, DEA, and/or NIDA statistics, are data which may be used in conjunction with DAWN data.

Such a study using the type of substance as a dependent variable would not have to use the entire DAWN sample. For example, one could use the hospital emergency room records alone, and the data could also be limited to a particular age group (e.g., 20–29). Further limitations could focus on a particular SMSA and examine the time trend by grouping the entire 7-year data and incorporating time dummy variables in the equation. Yearly differences could then be compared by controlling for the possible differences of sociodemographic changes over time within an SMSA.

The DAWN data files also have information regarding treatment and the outcome of the treatment. For instance, it is possible to examine the relationships between the substances used, the reasons for treatment, the disposition of the patient, and the related sociodemographic factors among drug users. Statistical relations could be studied by considering the reasons for treatment or disposition status as dependent variables. Identifying the major factors that affect the extent of use and type of substances used could provide important insights for prevention, enforcement, intervention, and treatment activities.

The incorporation of drug program and policy information together with the DAWN system is another important type of program evaluation. For example, if one SMSA has implemented a large-scale drug prevention program, the effect of the prevention program on drug abuse behavior could be partially studied by comparing the data collected by the DAWN system for this given geographical area before and after implementing the prevention program, provided other sociodemographic factors remain the same. If the sociodemographic factors have been changed, multivariate regression analysis can again help to isolate the program effects (e.g., if a large-scale television media drug prevention campaign is carried out in certain eastern SMSAs while the western SMSAs are not exposed to the campaign). A comparison of these cross-sectional differences among eastern and western SMSAs may provide some information on the impact of the television campaign. By introducing multivariate regression analysis, a possible difference in sociodemographic factors may be controlled.

Another comparison of DAWN data with policy and program resource data is illustrated by the City of Baltimore, which studied the geographical, age, and sex distribution of various types of drug abuse emergencies. As a result, the city concluded that the populations at risk and the locations of treatment services which could effectively assist the at-risk populations did not match. In some cases, treatment programs designed originally for clients with hard-drug problems were located in areas where almost no such problem existed, while programs serving young, less chronic polydrug users were located in the areas characterized by hard-drug use by older clients.

These illustrations are only small examples of how the DAWN data system can and is being used for purposes of program planning and evaluation as well as social policy research. The data can be used at the national, state, local, and individual levels over a period of 8 years. As stated previously, it is important to note that DAWN data are interpretive and should not be used alone.

CONCLUDING REMARKS

The DAWN system is a well-known and useful data source which has been used extensively at the federal level and more recently at the state and local levels to evaluate the changing trends of drug and alcohol abuse by various client populations. This paper provides a review of the DAWN data and illustrates further usefulness of the data system. Several facts stand out:

The DAWN data base has been subjected to external review and, while no human-behavior data are without some error, the point at issue is the nature and degree of error in the DAWN system. Errors in DAWN can be attributed to respondents, instrument design, records, and data processors. As a result of previous reviews, the early DAWN system (1972–1976) was extensively modified, and the data collection system and internal quality control mechanisms were improved significantly 4 years ago.

If the rural aspect of drug use is not sufficiently represented in the data, a further expansion of the non-SMSA random sample of facilities across the United States could be considered.

DAWN data serve important purposes in their present form. Recent reviews have assured that recording errors are only 5-8% on substances and 2-3% on sociodemographic information. The ranking and relative distribution of drug use have been found to be generally accurate and consistent. Therefore, for the purpose of formulating drug program, enforcement, prevention, and treatment policies, the DAWN data provide quite accurate information. Extreme caution should be used not to generalize the criticisms of antiquated and/or misleading studies to this valuable system, since such criticisms focus on system problems which do not characterize the system since its reorganization in 1976–1977. Rather, the illustration of the potential uses of DAWN in this paper indicates that a much broader use of the data system could efficiently be achieved by the drug inforcement, prevention, and academic research communities, especially since the DAWN system now provides a high-quality national reporting network of hospitals from which extensive new health data could be retrieved at minimal cost.

ACKNOWLEDGMENT

This review was supported by DEA contract number 80-10.

REFERENCES

ANGLIN, C.L., SANTO, Y., HARMATZ, J.S., and SHADER, R.I. *An Evaluation of Sedative Hypnotic Patients in DAWN Reporting Hospitals*. Final Report by Macro Systems, Inc., for Services Research Branch, National Institute on Drug Abuse, Contract 271-77-4524, November 30, 1980.

BARTON, W.A. *DAWN: An Operational Analysis and Evaluation*. Rockville, MD: National Institute on Drug Abuse, 1975.

CHICAGO TRIBUNE. The pill peddlers: Our No. 1 drug abuse dilemma. June 17-21, 1979.

FRANKLIN RESEARCH CENTER. *DAWN Quality Assurance Study*. Prepared for the Drug Enforcement Administration, Washington, DC, 1979.

FRENCH, J., and KAUFMAN, N. (eds.). *Prevention Evaluation Guidelines* (National Institute on Drug Abuse). Washington, DC: U.S. Government Printing Office, 1979.

GREENBERG, S.W., and ROBERSON, C.B. *Analysis of Drug Abuse Correlates*. Final report by Research Triangle Institute for the Drug Enforcement Administration, 1978.

HINKLEY, S.W. Statistician casts "clarifying light" on DAWN. *The Journal* (Toronto: Addiction Research Foundation), May 1980.

IMS AMERICA LTD. *DAWN Quarterly Report* (October-December, 1978). Ambler, PA: The Author, 1978.

IMS AMERICA LTD. *Project DAWN Annual Report 1979*. Ambler, PA: The Author, 1979.

KOVAR, M.B., and WRIGHT, R. An experiment with alternative respondent rules in the National Health Interview Survey. In *Proceedings of the American Statistical Association, Social Statistics Section*, Washington, DC, 1973.

LASAGNA, L. The DAWN's early light: A flickering flame. *The Sciences*, 1976.

MC CONNELL, H. Data about worthless numbers. *The Journal* (Toronto: Addiction Research Foundation), February 1, 1980, p. 6.

MURPHY, J.B. Chief, Information Systems Section, Drug Enforcement Administration, personal communication, January 1981.

PERSON, P.H. The Drug Abuse Warning Network: A statistical perspective. *Public Health Rep.* 91: 395–401, 1976.

RHODES, B. *The New Hampshire Mini-DAWN: The nation's first statewide saturation drug abuse warning network: The data and its uses.* Unpublished report, Governor's Office of Alcohol and Drug Abuse Prevention, State of New Hampshire, 1979.

RHODES, B. *Mini-DAWN: New Hampshire's experience.* Paper presented at the National Alcohol and Drug Coalition Conference, Washington, DC, September 17, 1980.

RUFENER, B., RACHAL, J., and CRUZE, A. *Management Effectiveness Measures for NIDA Drug Abuse Treatment Programs*, Vol. 1: *Cost-Benefit Analysis* (National Institute on Drug Abuse Technical Paper). Washington, DC: U.S. Government Printing Office, 1976.

RUFENER, B., RACHAL, J., and CRUZE, A. *Management Effectiveness Measures for NIDA Drug Abuse Treatment Programs*, Vol. 2: *Costs to Society of Drug Abuse* (National Institute on Drug Abuse Technical Paper). Washington, DC: U.S. Government Printing Office, 1977.

UNGERLEIDER, J.T., LUNDBERG, G.D., SUNSHINE, I., and WALBERG, C.B. The Drug Abuse Warning Network (DAWN) program. *Arch. Gen. Psychiatry*, 1980a.

UNGERLEIDER, J.T., LUNDBERG, G.D., SUNSHINE, I., and WALBERG, C.B. DAWN: Drug Abuse Warning Network or data about worthless numbers? *J. Anal. Toxicol.* Vol. 4, November-December, 1980b.

UNGERLEIDER, LUNDBERG, SUNSHINE, and WALBERG, *The Journal*, February 1980c.

U.S. DEPARTMENT OF JUSTICE. *CSA Drug Activities Since October 27, 1970.* Washington, DC: Drug Enforcement Administration, 1978.

WHITE HOUSE. Seminar on Primary Prevention. Meeting held at the White House, December 1977.

The International Journal of the Addictions, 19(1), 79–92, 1984

Substance Abuse: Assessment of the Outcomes of Activities and Activity Clusters in School-Based Prevention

Jay Sexter,* PhD
Arthur P. Sullivan, PhD
Stephen F. Wepner, PhD
Robert Denmark, PhD

Office of Research Services
Fordham University
Bronx, New York 10458

Abstract

The purpose of the research reported herein was to associate prevention activities in the schools with abusing behaviors of the students, after statistically controlling relevant variables. Discrete activities and clusters of activities ("programs" or "models") were studied with a randomly assigned control group design. This approach was selected so that effective activities could be identified even against an overall background of increasing abuse during and after the prevention experience.

Research on prevention activities over the years has focused on certain outcomes. One of these is increase in knowledge about drugs and their effects on users. This was shown to be like other educational content areas, and the prevention programs were easily shown to be achieving this goal (e.g., Swisher and Crawford, 1971; Swisher, Warner, and Herr, 1972). Improvement in attitude toward drugs was the next target outcome. Initially this goal was, perhaps, somewhat more elusive than knowledge, as reflected in some early studies (e.g.,

*To whom requests for reprints should be addressed.

 0020-773X/84/1901-0079$3.50/0

Swisher and Crawford, 1971; Swisher et al., 1972), but shortly thereafter a breakthrough in either program effectiveness or measurement sensitivity began yielding research results indicating that the technology needed to improve student attitudes toward drugs now existed and was in use (e.g., Warner, Swisher, and Horan, 1973).

A third objective for prevention programs became the cluster of behaviors which researchers indicated was associated with abuse and abusers. Investigators pointed to patterns of relationships with parents, schools, peers, and societal institutions which systematically differentiated abusers from nonabusers (e.g., Gossett, Lewis, and Phillips, 1972; Smith, n.d.; Streit, Halsted, and Pascale, 1974), and some of these patterns involved variables which fall within the educational bailiwick. Thus, student grades, attendance at school, disciplinary problems, and low self-esteem were identified as trouble signs and used programmatically either to identify potential abusers or as actual prevention outcomes. The intent of this latter style of prevention program was apparently indirect. Educators were found capable of correcting these trouble signs (Bry, 1978; Visco and Finotti, 1974), but the causal link by which these corrections would eventually reduce drug abuse was never established.

A fourth prevention outcome was reduction in actual substance abuse. While this seems a more salient outcome than knowledge, attitude, or associated behaviors which are expected to impact abuse only indirectly, it poses significant research design problems. First, since prevention of abuse is in question, not treatment of abusers, little abusing behavior is expected in the prevention population. Second, since prevention is often considered an emergency measure for students seen as likely abusers, true experimental designs erode as control group members seek alternative services in the community. Third, all difficulties attending field research in a health-related investigation apply, including problems associated with obtaining fully informed consent, maintenance of strict confidentiality, etc. And yet the need for experimental designs to identify prevention activities which are directly effective (i.e., impact abusing behavior itself) is clear (Bry, 1978).

The singular lack of success of researchers in obtaining positive findings in this fourth area, abusing behavior, either underlines the difficulties inherent in this type of research noted in the previous paragraph or reflects less than positively upon prevention efforts. For, while the casual observer would expect effective prevention efforts to extinguish any abusing behaviors among participants, researchers have had to accept increases in abuse as normal even during the prevention process itself, and they have had to test prevention effectiveness against the yardstick of "preventing large increases in drug abuse" (Blum, 1975; Kleber, Berberian, Gould, and Kase, 1975).

The research reported herein seeks to link prevention activities directly to substance abuse: Specific prevention efforts are associated with self-reported abuse of a broad variety of substances. Thus, it was hypothesized that there exist singular prevention activities and clusters of activities which predict to desirable abusing outcomes (lower level of abuse than control group), when interfering variables are controlled.

PROCEDURE

Prevention Models

Directors of substance abuse prevention programs were surveyed during 1978-1979 (Board of Education, 1980) to determine the degree to which they engaged in each of 28 molecular prevention activities. The behaviors are listed in Table 1. The resulting data were factor analyzed to show similarities in prevention procedure in five broad categories of programs. The first category consisted of prevention programs using activities designed to clarify values and stimulate thought, opinion making, and decision making. This is called the *humanistic education model*. A second category focused on group formation, and when group dynamics indicated, this moved to an agenda of problem solving and risk taking. This was named the *peer group model*. A third category of program devoted major resources to teaching parents more effective parenting styles and to improving communication between parents and children, both their own and those of others. This was named the *parent effectiveness model*. A fourth model was named *network*. Programs in this fourth category built prevention groups around shared common problems and drew upon members' resources to support each other (psychologically); these programs frequently grouped children in pairs. The fifth model was named *advocacy*, and programs of this type focused on providing information to aid in solutions of problems. It differed from problem-solving work in other models chiefly in that the educator or leader was a primary resource and engaged in seeking solutions with the youngsters. Expansion of response alternatives was encouraged in these programs, as were students' responding to challenges and their taking of each others' parts to aid expression and mutual supportiveness. The five models are summarized in Table 2.

Subjects

One program was selected of each model type. Each selected program followed its standard intake procedure on 20% more students than it could accommodate. One-sixth of the students were then assigned at random to the control group in each program. Control students from all programs were combined in analysis, to form one cross-model control group. This procedure resulted in random assignment to prevention and control conditions within each model but

Table 1

Molecular Behaviors Used to Cluster Prevention Program Models

1. Peer-run drop-in centers
2. Unstructured rap groups
3. Students meet individually with a staff member
4. "Buddy" system so that each student has a buddy to talk to at any time
5. Discussions with ex-addicts
6. Discussions led by the students themselves, with the staff member facilitating
7. Providing the individual with information to make him/her aware of alternative responses to a situation
8. Presentation of alternatives to drug use
9. Parent workshops
10. Support group of peers
11. Dealing with a situation or problem through information provided by the staff member
12. "Hot line"—telephone number to call at anytime to discuss a problem
13. Student involvement in program planning
14. Providing the student with information which will make it possible for him/her to understand the ramifications of her/his actions
15. Discussions directed by the staff member
16. Role playing, where the student is himself/herself, another student, an adult, etc.
17. Dialogue between parents and their own children
18. Risk taking in a group situation
19. Group of individuals sharing common problems meeting regularly
20. Direct class/group instruction
21. Teaching of effective parenting styles
22. Dialogues between children and parents other than their own
23. Another student speaks for an individual who is having trouble expressing his/her feelings
24. Problem solving in a group
25. Stress on developing a value system of one's own
26. Parent dialogues, without children present
27. Staff members follow same scope and sequence of prevention activities
28. Staff members follow same scope and sequence of intervention activities

not across models. Distributional irregularities on important variables, therefore, may have distorted results, but random assignment to program is not an option open to researchers in this area. While effects of nonrandom assignment cannot be corrected, replication of findings using different programs to represent the prevention models may ameliorate the problem. This replication is underway as part of the present research project.

After students from whom informed parental consent had not been received were excused, and students from whom properly completed instruments could not be obtained were deleted, subjects were distributed across prevention and control conditions as shown in Table 3. Students were enrolled in grades five

Table 2

Five Models for Prevention of Substance Abuse

Name	Activities	Immediate goal
Advocacy	1. Information provided 2. Alternatives suggested	Students more self-sufficient
Parent Effectiveness	1. Teach parents to listen and counsel their own and others' children	Parents improve parenting skills
Peer Group	1. Sharing 2. Problem solving 3. Risk taking	Students experience psychological support of peers
Network	1. Buddy system 2. Group work on shared problems	Students develop insight into their presenting problem; have a "buddy" to aid and rely on for aid
Humanistic Education	1. Value clarification 2. Opinion formation 3. Decision making	Students improve self-knowledge and self-esteem

Table 3

Distribution of Subjects between Experimental and Control Conditions Across Prevention Models

	Experimental	Control	Total
Advocacy	44	31	75
Parent Effectiveness	162	21	183
Peer Group	377	81	458
Network	433	100	533
Humanistic Education	260	66	326
Total	1,276	299	1,575

through nine and their mean age was 12.72; 53.9% were female. Data were collected from September 1980 to June 1981.

Materials

A modified version of the New York State survey of substance abuse, the *Periodic Assessment of Drug Abuse among Youth*, was used to assess abusing behaviors. Responses were grouped into seven scales of abused substances: alcohol, marijuana, psychedelics, stimulants, depressants, opiates, and a composite scale including glues, solvents, and sprays. The number of items in each scale is shown in Table 4 along with the associated coefficient alpha, which is reported as a summary indicator of measurement error. The posttest, or outcome scale, consisted of a subset of the pretest scale, namely those items which do not ask about abuse from before the beginning of the program. Alphas for this scale have been corrected to full pretest length.

Table 4

Measurement Error of Scales

	Pretest		Posttest	
Scale	Item *N*	Alpha	Item *N*	Alpha (corrected)
Alcohol	9	.75	5	.71
Marijuana	9	.87	5	.82
Psychedelics	8	.84	4	.80
Stimulants	8	.83	4	.79
Depressants	13	.86	6	.87
Opiates	12	.71	4	.85
Glues, etc.	8	.76	5	.68

Table 5

Measurement Error of SYMLOG Scales

Scale	Item *N*	Alpha
Nurturance (P)	9	.89
Unfriendliness (N)	9	.81
Task orientation (F)	9	.72
Expressiveness (B)	9	.55
Dominance (U)	9	.92
Submissiveness (D)	9	.69

The Systematic Multiple Level Observation of Groups (SYMLOG) developed by Bales (1979) was used to determine whether the prevention programs maintained the distinctiveness in operation that was suggested by their membership in different model categories (Board of Education, 1980). Scale lengths and coefficient alpha for each scale are shown in Table 5.

Methods

The modified drug abuse survey was administered to prevention participants at the beginning and the end of each program, corresponding to the school semester. Trained observers collected SYMLOG observations from a subsample consisting of all groups directed by any two of the staff members from each program. The observers visited the sampled groups, in pairs, six times during the semester.

RESULTS

Hierarchical multiple regressions were used to associate prevention models with outcomes. Each abuse category was regressed upon a stock of carriers consisting of the prevention models (entry level 1), presenting abuse level as measured by pretest, sex, age, and self-esteem of the subject at pretest time (entry level 2).

Each regression was respecified and reestimated as nonsignificant coefficients were adjusted to zero. Final regression estimates for the seven scales of substance abuse are shown in Table 6.

These analyses investigated prevention efforts of the five procedural clusters observed elsewhere (Board of Education, 1980) but defined and labeled by the present authors. Evidence was sought regarding the integrity and differentiability of the models in operation, both to replicate previous research and to establish a basis for the meaningfulness of findings of prevention effectiveness.

Table 6

Summary of Regression of Substance Abuse Levels on Prevention Models with Control Variables

	Advocacy	Parent eff.	Peer group	Network	Humanistic educ.	Presenting level	Age	*sc*	r^2	*K*
Alcohol	−.08	−.13*	−.13**	−.05	.15**	.35***	.03**	.00	.35	−.19
Marijuana	−.03	−.08	−.11**	−.07	.06	.52***	.03**	.00	.53	−.22
Psychedelics	−.03	−.04	−.03	−.03	.11**	.34***	.02**	.00	.31	−.21
Stimulants	−.01	−.04	−.01	.00	.03**	.41***	.00	.00	.38	.04
Depressants	−.04	−.03	−.04	−.03	−.04	.42***	.01**	.00	.29	−.13
Glues, etc.	.12	−.07	−.09*	−.02	.08	.36***	.00	.003**	.23	.27
Opiates	−.03	−.01	.00	−.01	.03	.18**	.00	.00	.04	.03

*$p < .05$.
**$p < .01$.
***$p < .001$.

Table 7

SYMLOG Half-Scales on Which Row and Column Prevention Models Differ Significantly

	Model		
	Peer Group	Network	Humanistic Education
Advocacy	Submissiveness Nurturance Task orientation	Submissiveness Nurturance Expressiveness	Nurturance Task orientation
Peer Group		Submissiveness Nurturance Task orientation Expressiveness	Submissiveness Nurturance Task orientation
Network			Submissiveness

Two analyses bear on this point. First, using the SYMLOG, six half-scales were constructed from the observers' ratings by summing appropriate items (Bales, 1979). Two observations were included for each student in each occasion, one from each observer in the assigned pair. These were treated as separate data points to help correct for systematic differences in observer rating remaining even after training. Observations of the same students on different occasions were also treated as separate data points so that changes on the SYMLOG half-scales attributable to ordinary group development would accrue to the error term: Only differences attributable to the students' relationships to the leader, parents, and each other because of the uniqueness of the program style were being sought. Analysis of variance showed that the four models represented differed on four of the six half-scales. These discriminating scales were the negative half of the dominance scale (submissiveness), both halves of the task-orientation scale (task orientation and emotional expressiveness), and the positive half of the nurturance scale (supportiveness). The post hoc comparisons are summarized in Table 7.

In addition to regressing the scales of substance abuse on the stock of carriers consisting of prevention program models and control variables, these scales were also regressed on the discrete, molecular behaviors used originally to cluster and define the prevention models (see Table 1). These analyses are summarized in Table 8, which shows, irrespective of program cluster, which molecular behaviors are associated with lower (−) or higher (+) abuse or difference in other categories, relative to the control group. Significance levels are indicated. Note that the full results are summarized both with and without presenting levels (pretest measurement) controlled. Refer to Table 1 to decode significant molecular behaviors by number.

Table 8

Summary of Molecular Prevention Behaviors Significantly Related to Prevention Outcomes[a,b]

Outcome variable	Molecular behavioral predictor	Molecular behavioral predictor with pre-test level controlled
Alcohol abuse	Behav. 1 +**	
	Behav. 3 –**	Behav. 3 –*
	Behav. 28 –**	
Marijuana abuse	Behav. 1 +**	
	Behav. 3 –**	Behav. 3 –*
	Behav. 4 –**	Behav. 4 –*
Psychedelics abuse	Behav. 1 +**	
	Behav. 3 –**	Behav. 3 –**
	Behav. 4 –**	Behav. 4 –*
CNS stimulant abuse	Behav. 1 +**	
	Behav. 3 –**	Behav. 3 –*
	Behav. 4 –	Behav. 4 –*
CNS depressant abuse	Behav. 1 +*	
	Behav. 3 –**	Behav. 3 –*
	Behav. 4 –*	
Glue, solvent, spray abuse	Behav. 1 +*	
	Behav. 3 –*	None
	Behav. 28 –**	
Opiate abuse	None	None

[a]Behavior numbers 1-28 are identified in Table 1.
[b]+, behavior associated with increase in outcome variable; –, behavior associated with decrease in outcome variable.
*$p < .05$.
**$p < .01$.

CONCLUSIONS

From the foregoing results it was concluded, first, that discrete, differentiable program strategies exist in the studied population. This was evidenced both by differences in students' reported perceptions of significant persons and the differences in group dynamics as measured by the SYMLOG scales with between-observer and between-observation error collapsed.

Second, it was concluded with extreme caution, because of nonrandom assignment to prevention program, that certain programs systematically encounter less abusing behavior after prevention than found for students in the control condition. In addition to these positive findings, there are a few analyses showing abuse after prevention significantly worse than the control condition; it is particularly with respect to these occurrences that the reader is reminded that regression procedures undercorrect for baseline differences among non-randomly assigned groups. Replication of these findings, which (as already noted) is presently underway, is essential to reduce the liklihood of results attributable more to distributional oddities than to prevention realities. Specifically, it was concluded that parent effectiveness and peer group models significantly surpassed control group performance in prevention of abuse of alcohol; advocacy and network models were indistinguishable from control, and humanistic education performed significantly worse. These relations are diagrammed in Fig. 1. Figure 2 shows the peer group model as the only one outperforming the control group in limiting marijuana abuse, and it is the only model surpassing control in preventing abuse of glues, solvents, and sprays (Fig. 3). Note that the control variables sex, age, presenting abuse level, and presenting self-esteem were entered in each analysis; only those with significantly nonzero coefficients in the final regression estimate are listed as controlled variables in the figures displaying these results. These control variables are held constant at the mean or other frequently occurring value to permit the graphic presentation.

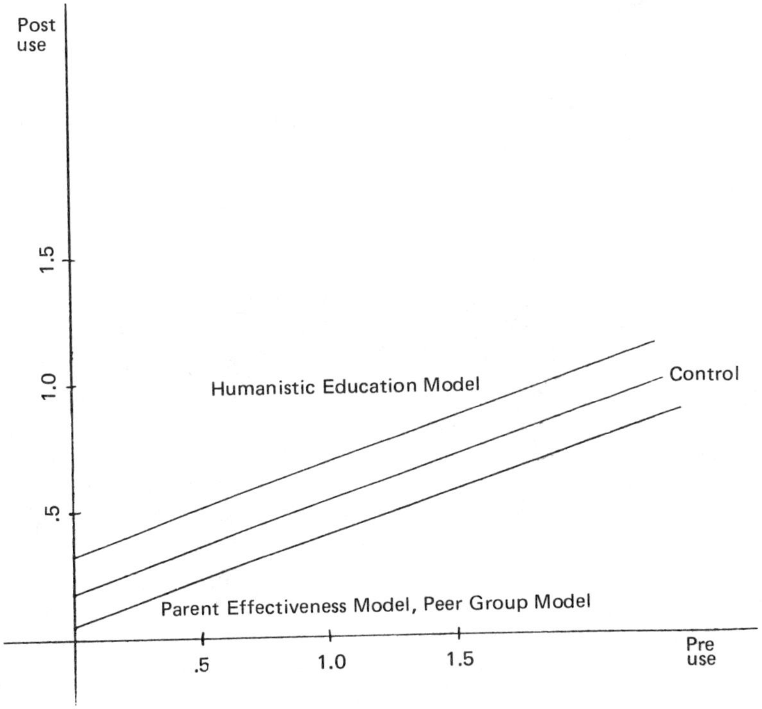

Fig. 1. Models differing significantly from control in preventing alcohol abuse. Age and race controlled; age = 13.

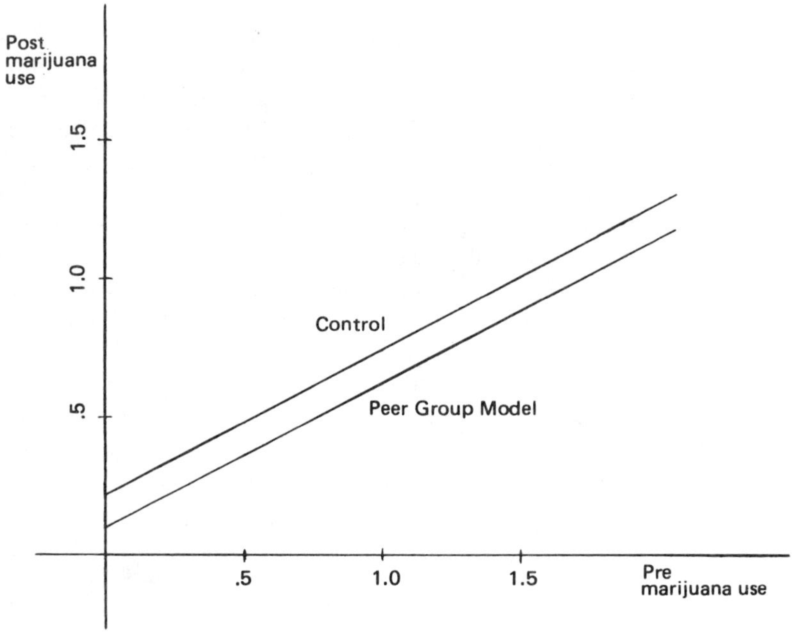

Fig. 2. Model differing significantly from control in preventing abuse of marijuana. Age controlled.

Third, it was concluded that age functions prominently as an interfering variable in abuse prevention research. Age is significantly, positively related to increase of abuse in virtually all categories of substances and undesirable behaviors. Thus, age must be experimentally and/or statistically controlled to investigate impact of prevention upon abuse.

Fourth, it was concluded that certain prevention activities are associated with lower drug abuse than encountered in the control group, across prevention program models, with outset abuse levels held constant. Use of one-on-one sessions where students meet individually with staff members and use of the "buddy" system, where each student has another student available to talk to, were both associated with better results than control in almost all substance abuse categories.

Future research must be relied upon to establish the stability of regression coefficients observed here and the extent to which prevention outcomes are attributable to nonrandom inclusion of students in the various programs.

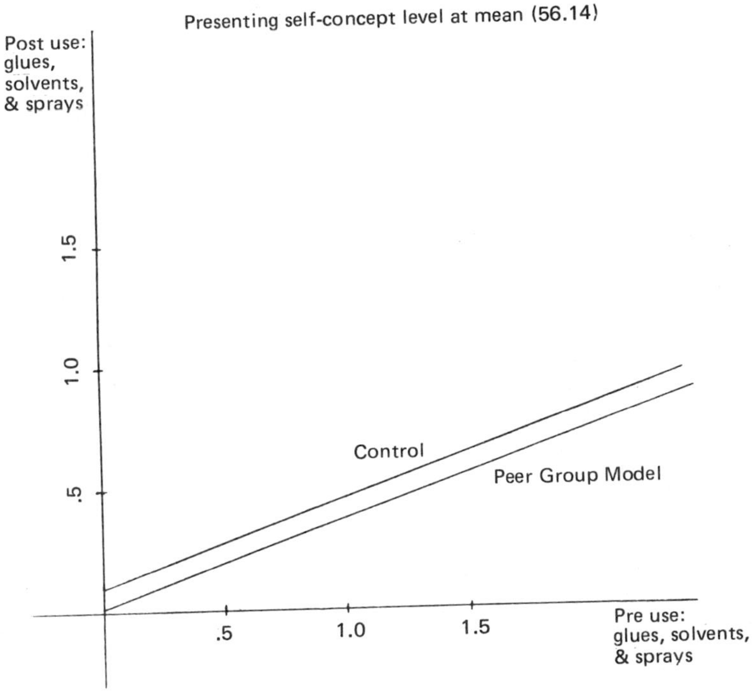

Fig. 3. Model differing significantly from control in preventing abuse of glues, solvents, and sprays. Self-esteem controlled.

ACKNOWLEDGMENT

The research reported herein was supported by National Institute on Drug Abuse grant number 5 R01 DA02316-03.

REFERENCES

BALES, R.F., and COHEN, S.P. *Symlog: A System for the Multiple Level Observation of Groups.* New York: Free Press, 1979.

BLUM, R.H. *Drug Education: Impact and Outlook.* Rockville, MD: National Institute on Drug Abuse, 1975.

BOARD OF EDUCATION OF THE CITY OF NEW YORK. Office of Educational Evaluation. *Alcohol and Substance Abuse Education Program.* New York: The Author, 1980.

BRY, B.H. Research design in drug abuse prevention: Review and recommendations. *Int. J. Addict.* 13(7): 1157–1168, 1978.

GOSSETT, J.T., LEWIS, M.J., and PHILLIPS, V.A. Psychological characteristics of adolescent drug users and abstainers. *Bull. Menninger Clinic* 36: 425–435, 1972.

KLEBER, H.D., BERBERIAN, R.M., GOULD, L.C., and KASE, S.V. *Evaluation of an Adolescent Drug Education Program.* Rockville, MD: National Institute in Drug Abuse, 1975.

OSGOOD, C., SUCI, G.J., and TANNEBAUM, P.H. *The Measurement of Meaning.* Urbana: University of Illinois Press, 1957.

SMITH, G.M. *Antecedents of teenage drug use.* Unpublished manuscript (available from the Department of Psychiatry, Massachusetts General Hospital, Boston, MA 02114), n.d.

STREIT, F., HALSTED, D.L., and PASCALE, P.J. Differences among youthful users and nonusers of drugs based on their perceptions of parental behavior. *Int. J. Addict.* 9(5): 749–755, 1974.

SWISHER, J.D., and CRAWFORD, J.L. An evaluation of a short-term drug education program. *School Counselor*, March 1971, pp. 265–272.

SWISHER, J., WARNER, R., and HERR, E. An experimental comparison of four approaches to drug education. *J. Counsel. Psychol.* 18: 328–332, 1972.

VISCO, E.P., and FINOTTI, J.F. *Spark Program Analysis.* Washington, DC: Geomet, 1974.

WARNER, R.W., SWISHER, J.D., and HORAN, J.J. Drug abuse prevention: A behavioral approach. *Natl. Assoc. Secondary School Principals Bull.* 57(372): 49–54, 1973.

The International Journal of the Addictions, 19(1), 93–117, 1984

Construct Validity of Heroin Abuse Estimators

J. Arthur Woodward

University of California, Los Angeles
Los Angeles, California 90024

Robert L. Retka

Bureau of International Narcotics Matters
U.S. Department of State
Washington, DC 20520

Lin Ng

University of California, Los Angeles
Los Angeles, California 90024

Abstract

The construct validity of two methodologically unrelated procedures for estimating the prevalence of heroin abuse was studied using a covariance structure model-fitting approach. A factor analytic estimation procedure and a log-linear-based capture-recapture method of estimation were simultaneously applied to 24 major metropolitan areas of the nation. A test of the construct validity of these procedures for estimating the prevalence of heroin abuse was carried out in the context of structural equation models where the results of the two methods were compared directly.

INTRODUCTION

The purpose of this research is to test the construct validity of two methodologically unrelated procedures for estimating the prevalence of heroin abuse. The factor analytic approach of Person, Retka, and Woodward (1976) is expanded conceptually to include hypothesized influences of both heroin abuse

 0020-773X/84/1901-0093$3.50/0

prevalence and heroin availability. Concurrently, a log-linear-based application of the capture-recapture method of estimation is developed for use in the Client Oriented Data Acquisition Process (CODAP). A test of the construct validity of these procedures for estimating the prevalence of heroin abuse is carried out in the context of structural equation models where the results of the two methods are compared directly.

BACKGROUND

During the last decade the federal government has attempted to monitor trends in drug abuse prevalence in order to appropriate treatment rehabilitation resources, develop drug abuse prevention and control activities, and determine research and training priorities. In this context, the epidemiology of drug abuse has assumed great importance, and a variety of extensive, nationally based reporting systems and indicator networks have been devised to aid in the study of changing patterns of drug abuse (Greene and Nightingale, 1975).

Today this network of data collection systems is operated at the federal level to yield, at regular time intervals, drug abuse relevant information for metropolitan areas in every region of the nation (for a description, see Greene, 1974; Hunt, 1974). Among the most extensive are the Drug Abuse Warning Network (DAWN), jointly operated by the Drug Enforcement Administration (DEA) and the National Institute on Drug Abuse (NIDA); the Client Oriented Data Acquisition Process (CODAP), operated by the National Institute on Drug Abuse; and the Drug Enforcement Administration's extensive data files: the Defendent Statistical System, the Drug Theft System, and the computerized system STRIDE.

Because the drug abuse indicators contained in these reporting networks are the major sources of drug abuse specific information available at regular time intervals on a substantial, cross-national sample of communities, researchers have studied the indicators for a variety of theoretical and practical reasons. Efforts to chart changing trends in illicit drug use were undertaken by DuPont and Greene (1973), Greene and DuPont (1974), Greene and Nightingale (1975), and more recently by the Forecasting Branch, NIDA (O'Donnell et al., 1976; Richards and Blevens, 1977). Variations in supply were studied nationally using heroin abuse indicators from a variety of sources (Greene and Nightingale, 1975).

Incidence and prevalence estimation based on indicators has received considerable attention. Incidence analysis has been based on hepatitis indicators (Minichiello, 1974), treatment admissions (Greenwood, 1974), and on a variety of different indicators (Hunt, 1974). Estimation of prevalence has progressed from single-indicator studies (e.g., Greenwood, 1971; Greenwood and Crider,

1978) to multiple-indicator approaches at the level of the SMSA (Person, Retka, and Woodward, 1977; Riley, Wagenfeld, and Sonnad, 1981) and at the level of the county (French, 1977). Recently, intermetropolitan correlates of drug use have been investigated by testing a variety of demographic models of inter-SMSA variation in indicator-derived prevalence (Schlenger and Greenberg, 1978). Similarly, demographic models of census tract variation in drug abuse prevalence recently were tested by Demaree (1978). Excellent reviews have appeared (e.g., Greene, 1974) and the recent report of a major conference on the epidemiology of drug use has surveyed the entire spectrum of epidemiologic issues (Richards and Blevens, 1977).

As the number of applied research projects using drug abuse indicators has increased, so has the emphasis on basic scientific issues of reliability and validity of indicators as measures of drug abuse prevalence. Person, Retka, and Woodward (1976) addressed the conceptual problems of estimating heroin abuse prevalence from indicators. Because of difficult problems of definition (as well as measurement), they concluded that the terms "heroin problem index" and "relative prevalence" better describe that which is estimated from the indicators than does the traditional term "prevalence." In this paper we will adopt the Person et al. convention and use the term "heroin abuse," rather than "prevalence." In addition, Person et al. (1976) studied the internal consistency of a set of heroin abuse indicators drawn from medical, treatment, and law enforcement sources for the 24 DAWN SMSAs. Each of the three sources represents a different method of measurement; thus, the research used a "multimethod-single trait" design to study the internal consistency of the indicators. An explicit measurement model was developed in which it was hypothesized that each indicator (regardless of the method of measurement) was a monotone function of heroin abuse and an error term unique to the indicator. Tests of the measurement model using nonmetric statistics revealed an adequate fit of the model to data collected at four different time periods (i.e., the model was accepted as plausible). Based on these analyses it is possible to compute the reliability of the indicator-based estimates of heroin abuse. For the four quarters of 1974, the estimates of reliability (coefficient α) were .69, .76, .76, and .82. Considering that the prevalence estimates are formed from only six measures, these reliabilities are adequately high. Certainly they are consistent in magnitude with typical psychological measures used in drug abuse research. The fact that their magnitude ranges from .7 to .8 does not support the claim that the indicators are unacceptedly "messy" or "noisy."

Since the reliability estimates are based on only 24 observations (i.e., SMSAs), a statistical correction is necessary to avoid overestimating the population reliability. Using the statistical lower-bound estimator of reliability developed by Woodward and Bentler (1978), we can be highly confident (probability $\geqslant .95$) that the population reliabilities of the indicator-based estimates are at least .51, .61, .62, and .72. Thus, even with a stringent correction for sampling error, the reliabilities of the indicators are encouragingly high.

Subsequently, Woodward (1978) applied linear structural equation models to test statistically a variety of measurement models of the heroin abuse indicators drawn from medical, treatment, and law enforcement domains. Three reliability-validity issues were addressed. First, within a given quarter of the year, two alternative measurement models were contrasted. The first model allowed for so-called method factors (i.e., factors defined by variables having a common method of measurement), and the second model postulated a single heroin abuse construct underlying all indicators. The single-construct model could be accepted as plausible while the method factor models could not. Second, the single-factor model was fitted simultaneously at two time periods separated by a single quarter (3 months). Not only could the longitudinal model be accepted as plausible, but the correlation between the heroin abuse constructs across time was estimated to be .946, indicating the expected high degree of stability across the 3-month time period. In addition, cross-lag relationships among the indicators in the longitudinal model revealed that for a 3-month lag there was a significant negative relationship between purity at quarter 2 and subsequent treatment admissions at quarter 4. Similar relationships were found by Stoloff, Levine, and Spruill (1975) in a longitudinal study carried out within a single SMSA. Third, the two-point longitudinal model was fitted in the context of two drug abuse related demographic characteristics of the communities–urbanicity and employment. Again, the model showed adequate fit, and the significant coefficients of the model were in a direction consistent with the interpretation that the single factor underlying the indicators is a measure of the intensity of heroin abuse. That is, the heroin abuse construct was positively related to urbanicity and negatively related to employment (cf. O'Donnell et al., 1976, p. 111).

While these recent studies of the reliability and validity of indicator-based estimates of heroin abuse are important, they can be considered to be only an initial step in the right direction (cf. Richard and Blevens, 1977, p. 5). Because the two major indirect methods (i.e., factor analysis and capture-recapture) involve so many untenable assumptions, so many inaccuracies and influences beyond the control of the researcher, their practical utility remains in serious doubt. In theory, the factor analytic method works well (for a simulation, see Person et al., 1976), but application to SMSA aggregate data remains a problem because of potentially shifting reporting bases underlying the indicators, distributional problems of the data, and other practical violations of assumptions. The same can be concluded of the other major indirect estimation procedure, the capture-recapture method. In theory, the capture-recapture method is ideal, but in practice its validity can be doubted because of inaccuracies of data and obvious violations of assumptions of random sampling, independence among samples, and constant population size.

Even though the problem of validity arises from practical issues, the force of circumstance appears beyond the control of the researcher at this time. Thus each method, applied in isolation, contains a lack of demonstrated validity. Before the continued practical use of the indirect estimation methods can be condoned on scientific grounds, a construct validation study must be carried out in which the two methods of measuring prevalence are compared *directly*. This direct comparison of the factor analytic and capture-recapture method is a major purpose of the research reported here.

METHOD

Observational Units

Twenty-four metropolitan statistical areas currently covered by the Drug Abuse Warning Network (DAWN) were studied. This level of aggregation was necessitated by the data collection networks and was not regarded as optimal on other methodological grounds. These communities are representative of every geographical region of the country and account for more than 30% of the total national population. The SMSAs are:

Atlanta	Indianapolis	Oklahoma City
Boston	Kansas City	Philadelphia
Buffalo	Los Angeles	Phoenix
Chicago	Miami	San Antonio
Cleveland	Minneapolis	San Diego
Dallas	New Orleans	San Francisco
Denver	New York	Seattle
Detroit	Norfolk	Washington, DC

Drug Abuse Indicators

The drug abuse indicators used in the present study are drawn from three data collection networks, as shown in Table 1.

The source of the medical indicators is the DEA-NIDA Drug Abuse Warning Network (DAWN). The treatment program data (number of admissions to federally funded programs) were obtained from NIDA's Client Oriented Data Acquisition Process (CODAP). The law enforcement information was obtained from the DEA.

Expansion of the Factor Analysis Model

The factor analytic model originally proposed by Person, Retka, and Woodward (1976) hypothesized a single common heroin abuse influence underlying a

Table 1

Heroin Abuse Indicators

Indicator		Source	No. SMSAs
Er:	All narcotic analgesic emergency room episodes	DAWN	24
D:	All narcotic analgesic medical examiner episodes	DAWN	24
T:	All CODAP admissions where opiate was primary drug	CODAP	24
Arr:	All arrests where opiate consumption was involved	DEA	24
Ph.T:	All pharmacy thefts where opioid was stolen	DEA	24
Pr:	Retail price of heroin	DEA	24
Pur:	Retail purity of heroin	DEA	24

set of five heroin abuse indicators. In the current research, the indicator base was expanded to include "pharmacy thefts" and "heroin-related arrests" so as to define a second hypothetical influence that we will call "availability," or supply. The supply construct is conceptualized as the number of dosage units of heroin per user within a given SMSA. The expanded factor analysis model of the indicators is shown in Fig. 1.

Figure 1 represents an improvement over other previously published factor analytic models in that it now contains both heroin abuse and availability constructs as hypothesized explanations of SMSA variation and covariation in the heroin abuse indicators. The inclusion of arrests and pharmacy thefts is important in conceptualizing the new model. For example, in SMSAs where heroin has become unavailable, the number of treatment admissions is hypothesized to be greater than in SMSAs with highly available heroin—hence the negative sign relating availability and treatment admissions (T). The hypothesized relationships between availability (Avail) and price (Pr) and purity (Pur) are self-explanatory.

The absence of an arrow connecting availability and arrests (Arr) represents the hypothesis that variation across SMSAs in availability is not related to variation in arrests. This zero relation is hypothesized because the indicator represents only opiate-related crimes and will not reflect, for example, increases in property crime that might accompany increased price of heroin.

Development of a Capture-Recapture Method for the CODAP Admission Files

In order to use a methodologically unrelated estimation technique concurrently with the factor analytic model of the previous section, we have developed

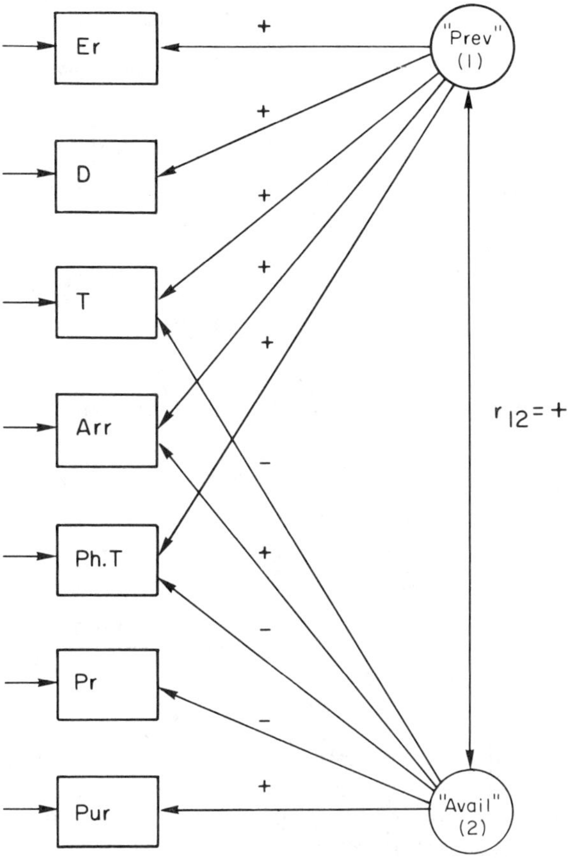

Fig. 1. Hypothesized measurement model of SMSA variation and covariation on seven heroin abuse indicators.

a way to apply the capture-recapture technique to the national CODAP files. The two-sample capture-recapture method is easily illustrated by the two-way contingency table presented in Table 2. The dimensions of the two-way table represent two independent samples of heroin abusers. It is assumed, among other things, that the length of time between samples is sufficient for all persons captured in Sample 1 to be returned to the general population so that they potentially can be captured in the second sample. Three of the cell frequencies can be observed directly, while one cell frequency, two marginals, and the total population size are not observed. These missing numbers, specifically $f_{22}, f_{.2}, f_{2.}$, and N, are enclosed in parentheses to indicate that they are unknown and must be estimated from the observed frequencies.

Table 2

Illustration of the Two-Sample Capture-Recapture Method

		Sample 2 Captured	Sample 2 Not captured	
Sample 1	Captured	f_{11}	f_{12}	$f_{1.}$
	Not captured	f_{21}	(f_{22})	$(f_{2.})$
		$f_{.1}$	$(f_{.2})$	(N)

As is well known, the maximum likelihood estimator of N is given by

$$\hat{N} = \frac{f_{.1}\, f_{1.}}{f_{11}}$$

with variance

$$\mathrm{VAR}(\hat{N}) = \frac{f_{1.}\, f_{.1}\, f_{12}\, f_{21}}{(f_{11})^3}$$

The three-sample capture-recapture method represents an important advance over the two-sample procedures. The three-way table is shown in Table 3. The missing cell frequency, f_{222}, and the missing marginal frequencies are enclosed in parentheses as in Table 2.

The maximum likelihood estimator for N, the total population, can be derived for a variety of models that do not assume independence among successive

Table 3

Illustration of the Three-Sample Capture-Recapture Method

	Sample 3 Captured: Sample 2 Captured	Sample 3 Captured: Sample 2 Not captured		Sample 3 Not captured: Sample 2 Captured	Sample 3 Not captured: Sample 2 Not captured	
Captured	f_{111}	f_{121}	Captured	f_{112}	f_{122}	
Not captured	f_{211}	f_{221}	Not captured	f_{212}	(f_{222})	
						(N)

samples in the three-sample versions of the capture-recapture method. This fact represents a very important advance in capture-recapture methodology as it is applied in the area of drug abuse, since an assumption of independence among successive samples is almost certainly false (see Greene, 1974, for a discussion).

The reader will be spared the details of the log-linear models on which this fact is based; the end result is that in the case that each sample is dependent on each of the other samples (in the sense of two-way interactions in a log-linear model), the maximum likelihood estimator of N is

$$\hat{N} = \eta + \frac{f_{111}\, f_{221}\, f_{122}\, f_{221}}{f_{121}\, f_{211}\, f_{112}}$$

with variance

$$\mathrm{VAR}(\hat{N}) = \hat{M}_{222}\left(\frac{1}{f_{111}} + \frac{1}{f_{121}} + \frac{1}{f_{211}} + \frac{1}{f_{221}} + \frac{1}{f_{112}} + \frac{1}{f_{122}} + \frac{1}{f_{212}} + \frac{1}{\hat{M}_{222}}\right)$$

This result, as well as closed-form estimators for other models, can be found in Bishop, Feinberg, and Holland (1975).

Conceptually, the adaptation of the three-sample capture-recapture method to the CODAP admission files is straightforward. Within a given SMSA, all heroin-related admissions of unique clients to federally funded treatment programs during a specified time interval can be considered a (nonrandom) sample drawn from the population of heroin users. The second and third samples can be defined in an identical manner, but separated by 3-month periods. By recognizing readmissions of clients, the intersections of Table 3 could be filled in, with the exception of f_{222}. Obviously, only clients that have been discharged prior to the end of the closest subsequent sample would be eligible for recapture. Thus, only clients with such discharge dates would be considered to constitute each sample. An exact description of two temporally nonoverlapping replications of a three-sample strategy is shown in Table 4. In order to create two nonoverlapping replications, 2 months from 1978 were used, even though this complicates the interpretation of the resulting estimate.

With subjects selected in the manner described in Table 4, the cells of Table 3 could be filled in and an estimate of the total population size computed from one of the log-linear model estimators. Prior to actually carrying out such a strategy, however, it was necessary to develop an admission report matching procedure whereby the anonymous records belonging to the same client could be identified. This posed the most serious practical problem of the research.

The matching procedure described here is based simply on the logical relationships inherent in the CODAP admission and discharge reports. A two-stage

Table 4

Parameters of a Three-Sample Capture-Recapture Application in 1977

Time period	Sample 1	Sample 2	Sample 3
Replication 1	(March-April)	(July-August)	(November-December)
Replication 2	(May-June)	(September-October)	(March-April)

Admission record selection
1. All nonduplicate records of admissions within one of the above time periods; and
2. All such admission records with discharge dates prior to end of adjacent (later) sample.

[a]These months were taken from records with admission dates in March-April 1978.

procedure was developed in the form of a computer program that utilized certain information about each admission and discharge record. The easiest way to conceptualize the procedure is to think of two admission records being compared to determine if they belong to the same client. The admission record with the earlier admission date is indicated by the subscript E, and the record with the later date is indicated by the subscript L. In the first stage, the records would be sorted into the cells formed by the crossing (cross-tabulation) of four variables, as shown in Table 5. The cartesian product of the four variables defines a four-dimensional structure containing 81,216 cells. If an admission record falls into a cell by itself, then it is considered to be unique and not matched with any other admission record. If several records fall into the same cell, they are considered potential matches, and then we proceed to the second stage of the matching procedure, as described in Table 6. The logical tests in Table 6 are recognized to be fallible, since the accuracy of the admission report may not be perfect; thus, an empirical study was carried out to determine the accuracy of the last six tests in Table 6. The study used the subsample of clients who were readmitted to the same clinic and who thus had the same client number. By comparing the matching procedures of Tables 5 and 6 with the

Table 5

Rules for Profile Matching: Stage 1

Stage 1: Admission records are located in the cells formed by the cross-tabulation of the following four variables:

Variable name	No. levels
1. Month and year of birth	564
2. Ethnicity	4
3. Sex	2
4. Level of education ($\text{Ed}_L - \text{Ed}_E \leqslant 2$)	18

Table 6

Logical Rules for Capture-Recapture Method: Stage 2

Stage 2: Pairs of records located in same cell of Stage 1 are compared on seven tests. If the test is passed, then the records are judged to be from different clients.[a]

1. Client number, within clinic and within year (*CNW*):

   If $CNW_E \neq CNW_L$

2. Form type (*FT*):

   If $FT_E = FT_L = C$

3. Admission date (*AD*):Discharge date (*DD*):

   If $DD_E > AD_L$

4. Marital status at admission (*AMS*) and discharge (*DMS*):

   a. If $[(AMS_E =$ ever mar.) and $(AMS_L =$ never mar.)$]$
   b. If $[(DMS_E =$ ever mar.) and $(DMS_L =$ never mar.)$]$

5. Number of prior admissions (*PA*)

   If $PA_L \leqslant PA_E$

6. Reason for discharge (*RD*):

   If $RD_E =$ Death

7. Drug abuse code (*DA*), year of first use (*YFU*):

   If $[(DA_E = DA_L = 1)$ and $(YFU_E - YFU > 2)]$

[a]The subscripts *E* and *L* refer to the earlier and later admission dates, respectively. Thus CNW_E means the client number of the admission record with the earlier admission date.

correct information, as represented in the client numbers for this special subsample, the accuracy of the procedure was estimated. The results of the validation of the matching procedure are described in detail in the results section.

Structural Equation Model of Heroin Abuse and Supply

The purpose of the structural equation model of this section is to test the hypothesis that the factor analytic approach and the capture-recapture approach measure the same construct—namely, the intensity of heroin abuse at the SMSA

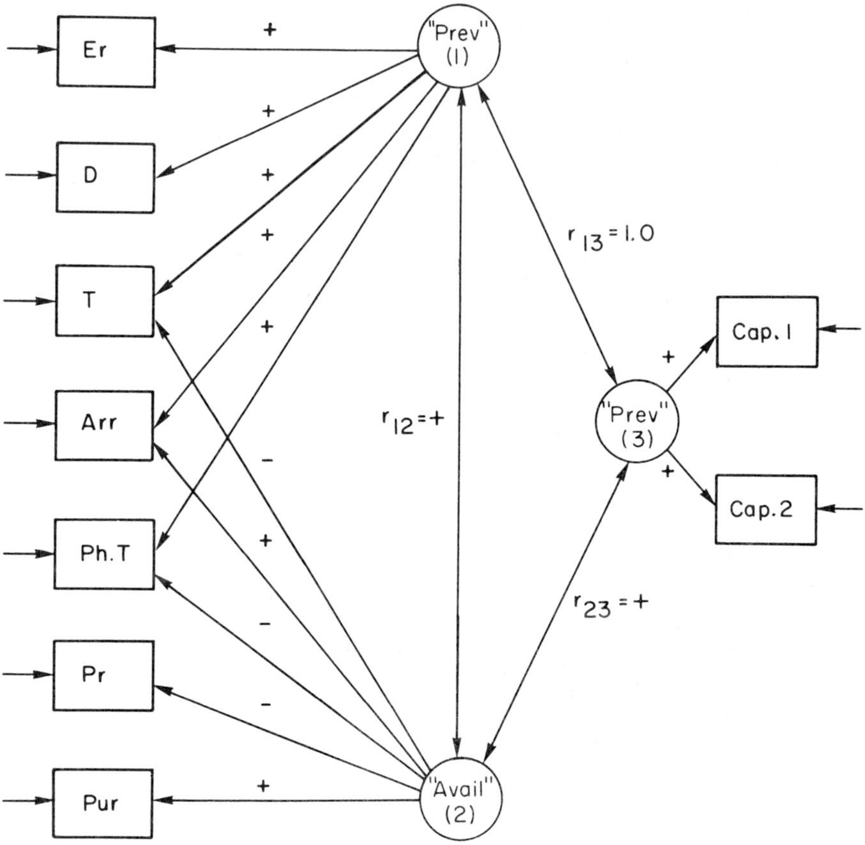

Fig. 2. Hypothesized measurement models and correlations among constructs of indicator-based prevalence, availability, and capture-recapture prevalence.

level of aggregation. The model is presented schematically in Fig. 2. At the left is the heroin abuse construct expressed in the confirmatory factor analysis model in terms of the seven heroin abuse indicators. At the right of the figure is the heroin abuse construct expressed in terms of the two capture-recapture estimates. If the two approaches to estimating heroin abuse do indeed measure the same thing, then the correlation r_{13} should be high and the correlations r_{12} and r_{23} should be equal. Such a comprehensive test based on structural equation models has the advantage that the correlations (e.g., r_{12}, r_{23}) are not biased (or attenuated) by the effects of arbitrary levels of measurement error. In addition, it will be informative to obtain estimates of the reliabilities of the estimation procedures.

The statistical methodology used to estimate the parameters of the structural equation models and to test the goodness-of-fit is a standard application of covariance structure modeling using maximum likelihood estimation (e.g., Jöreskog, 1978).

RESULTS AND DISCUSSION

Results of the Capture-Recapture Method

The results of the capture-recapture method are described first, since the testing of the expanded factor analytic model is carried out and presented in the context of the general construct validation model of Fig. 2.

Accuracy of the Matching Procedure

The accuracy of the profile matching procedure is of importance in the application of the capture-recapture method. In order to assess its accuracy, a special subsample of admission records was selected as a calibration sample. These were pairs of admission records known to be matched because the clients were readmitted to the same clinics and thus received the same client numbers. When the matching procedure (omitting the use of within-clinic client number information, Test 1 in Table 6) was run on these 10,450 admission records (5,225 matched pairs) the accuracy information of Table 7 was obtained. Because of the relative balance between the number of false positives and the number of false negatives, the obtained number of matched records in many cases is very close to the true number of matched records. The least favorable error rate is 31%, for Buffalo and Denver, and the average percent error is 12.04. While not perfect, these results were deemed sufficiently accurate for use in the capture-recapture method; however, two replications were obtained to help reduce the effects of possible inaccuracies and to generalize results across different combinations of months that have different treatment admission patterns.

Capture-Recapture Results

Two temporally nonoverlapping replications of the three-sample capture-recapture method were carried out using the setup described in Table 4. The procedure was carried out separately within each of the 24 SMSAs, and the basic data produced were of the form of Tables 2 and 3. An example of such a table is presented in Table 8. For this contingency table a variety of log-linear models were tested, each model corresponding to different combinations of dependencies among the successive samples. For the case of the Detroit data presented in Table 8, only the model including dependency among all three

Table 7

Results of Accuracy Study of Matching Procedure Using Within-Clinic Admissions

	True *N* matched pairs	Obtained *N* matched pairs	False positives	False negatives	% error
Atlanta	103	100	12	15	03
Boston	117	98	7	26	16
Buffalo	29	20	0	9	31
Chicago	216	187	17	46	13
Cleveland	94	84	7	17	11
Dallas	104	91	8	21	13
Denver	16	11	0	5	31
Detroit	349	359	15	5	03
Indianapolis	27	24	0	3	09
Kansas City	34	27	0	7	21
Los Angeles	844	816	91	119	03
Miami	97	86	5	16	11
New Orleans	92	81	4	15	12
New York	1,305	1,470	481	316	13
Norfolk	11	9	0	2	18
Oklahoma City	71	60	4	15	15
Philadelphia	526	514	77	89	02
Phoenix	138	132	22	28	04
San Antonio	51	48	2	5	06
San Diego	81	72	0	9	11
San Francisco	746	740	109	115	01
Seattle	33	29	2	6	12
Washington	130	115	9	24	12
Total *N* matched pairs	5,225				
Average % error					12.04

samples fitted the data. Consequently, the estimate of the total population size was based upon the equation derived for that model as shown at the bottom of Table 8. The data from each of the 24 SMSAs were analyzed in precisely this manner; in each case, the simplest log-linear model (i.e., the model with the fewest parameters) that fitted the data was chosen as the basis for calculating the estimate of heroin abuse population size. As it turned out, only two log-linear models were selected on this basis—the independence model (all three samples independent) and the dependence model (all three samples dependent). A summary of the results of both replications is shown in Table 9. As can be seen, in about half the SMSAs, the hypothesis of independent sampling was rejected.

Table 8

Example of Three-Sample Capture-Recapture Method Applied to Detroit for the Months (May-June), (September-October), and (March-April)

		Sample 3 (3,4)					
		Captured Sample 2 (9,10)			Not captured Sample 2 (9,10)		
		Captured	Not captured		Captured	Not captured	
Sample 1 (5,6)	Captured	107	140	247	107	926	1,033
	Not captured	109	680	789	1,014	–	1,014
		216	820		1,121	926	

$$\hat{N} = \eta + \frac{f_{111} f_{221} f_{122} f_{212}}{f_{121} f_{211} f_{112}}$$

$$\hat{N} = 3{,}083 + 41{,}841 = 44{,}924$$

The estimates yielded by the estimators appropriate to the fitted model are also shown in Table 9. The two replications differ somewhat in the average magnitude, but the linear correlation between the two estimates is .97.

Construct Validation Model of the Two Estimation Procedures Based on Raw Indicators

In order to compare the results of the capture-recapture method with the factor analysis model, the structural equation model shown in Fig. 2 was fitted to the correlation matrix among the seven indicators, the two capture-recapture estimates, and total SMSA population. These correlations are shown in Table 10. Since the "raw" indicators were studied in this initial analysis, it can be seen that each variable is related to the SMSA population. In order to remove the linear effects of differing population base, the model of Fig. 2 was fitted again, but this time with the effects of population partialled out. This treatment of population was important in verifying that the measures of raw prevalence contain useful information that is independent of population size.

The results of the first analysis are shown in Fig. 3. The goodness-of-fit chi-square test statistic yielded a value of 38.45 on 28 degrees of freedom. Since the critical value of 50.89 ($\alpha = .01$) was not exceeded, the model is not rejected. The

Table 9

Results of Capture-Recapture Applications to 24 SMSAs[a]

SMSA	Replication 1		Replication 2	
	Best-fitting model	Estimate of N	Best-fitting model	Estimate of N
Atlanta	D	3,841	I	3,848
Boston	I	8,606	I	7,280
Buffalo	I	5,788	D	11,871
Chicago	D	47,042	D	28,890
Cleveland	I	2,176	D	3,827
Dallas	I	5,808	I	5,723
Denver	I	2,482	I	3,896
Detroit	D	63,533	D	44,924
Indianapolis	I	1,861	I	3,439
Kansas City	I	8,580	I	4,929
Los Angeles	D	92,978	D	55,786
Miami	I	6,151	I	6,212
Minneapolis	I	8,268	I	14,818
New Orleans	I	5,375	I	6,567
New York	D	132,154	D	71,671
Norfolk	I	6,552	I	8,937
Oklahoma City	I	7,141	I	12,527
Philadelphia	D	31,344	D	32,785
Phoenix	I	10,176	I	8,567
San Antonio	I	16,986	I	11,084
San Diego	I	4,792	I	4,896
San Francisco	D	42,812	D	34,583
Seattle	I	7,217	I	4,808
Washington	I	6,523	D	14,292

[a]I = independence model; D = dependence model.

numbers attached to the arrows indicate the magnitudes of the linear relationships. As can be seen, the pattern of significant paths relating the latent variables and manifest indicators is not exactly as hypothesized in Fig. 2. There are two differences. First, the weight (i.e., loading) relating treatment and the availability construct is not significant. Thus, during a given time period, one does not observe the tradeoff between treatment admissions and availability that can be seen in longitudinal models (e.g., Woodward et al., 1978). Second, the relationship between raw pharmacy thefts and availability is positive. This is difficult to understand since it suggests that with greater availability, there would be greater pharmacy thefts.

All of the remaining parameter estimates, including the correlations among the constructs, are consistent with the hypotheses of Fig. 2. It is important to note that the correlation between the two prevalence constructs is 1.00, a value

Table 10

Correlations among Seven Heroin Abuse Indicators, Two Capture-Recapture Estimates, and Total Population for 24 SMSAs

	1	2	3	4	5	6	7	8	9	10
1. Er	1.000									
2. D	0.690	1.000								
3. TR	0.861	0.822	1.000							
4. Ph.T	0.724	0.671	0.810	1.000						
5. Arr	0.738	0.543	0.648	0.604	1.000					
6. Pr	-0.148	0.032	0.032	0.019	-0.190	1,000				
7. Pur	0.253	0.250	0.205	0.307	0.496	-0.382	1.000			
8. CRC 1	0.904	0.805	0.967	0.822	0.691	0.030	0.209	1.000		
9. CRC 2	0.866	0.806	0.967	0.764	0.606	0.054	0.142	0.973	1.000	
10. Pop	0.861	0.786	0.901	0.885	0.738	0.002	0.248	0.931	0.902	1.000

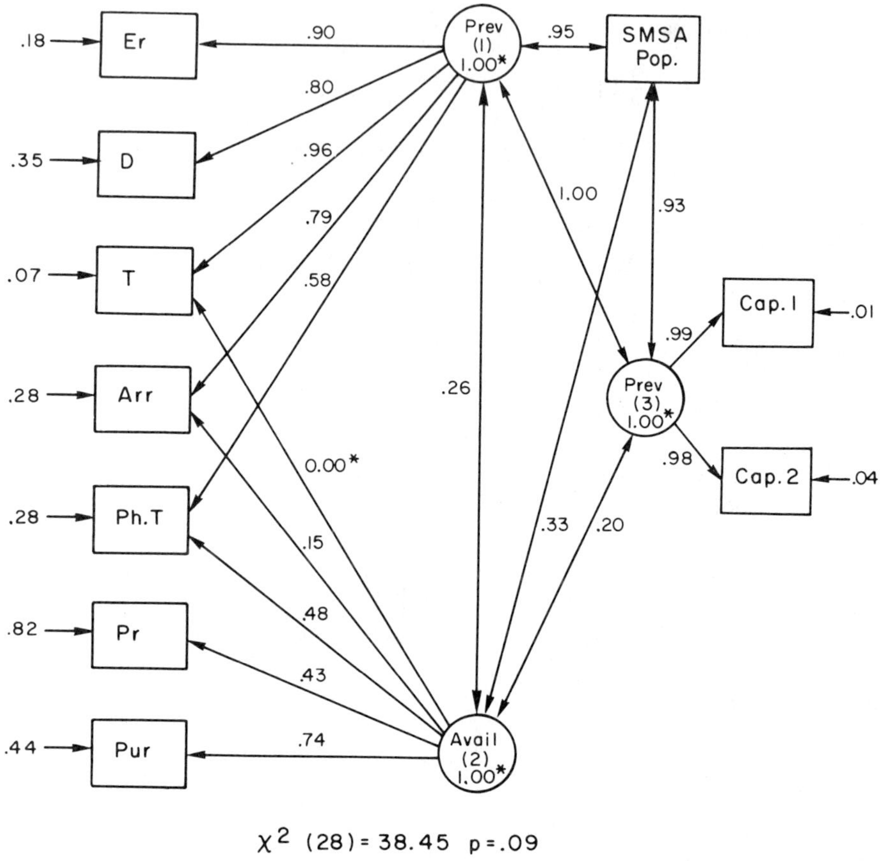

Fig. 3. Standardized maximum likelihood estimates and goodness-of-fit test for the three-construct model, including SMSA population. Asterisks indicate parameters constrained to values shown.

certainly within two standard errors of 1.00. Thus, we accept the hypothesis that in the population, the correlation between these two constructs is unity.

The model in Fig. 4 is identical to that in Fig. 3, but with the linear effects of population partialled out. As can be seen, the correlation between the prevalence constructs is still 1.00 (i.e., $.115/\sqrt{(.08)(.13)} \doteq 1.00$). Thus, even those portions of the latent constructs that are linearly independent of population are correlated at unity.

From this we conclude that there are two latent constructs underlying the raw indicators and capture-recapture estimates of prevalence. These we interpret

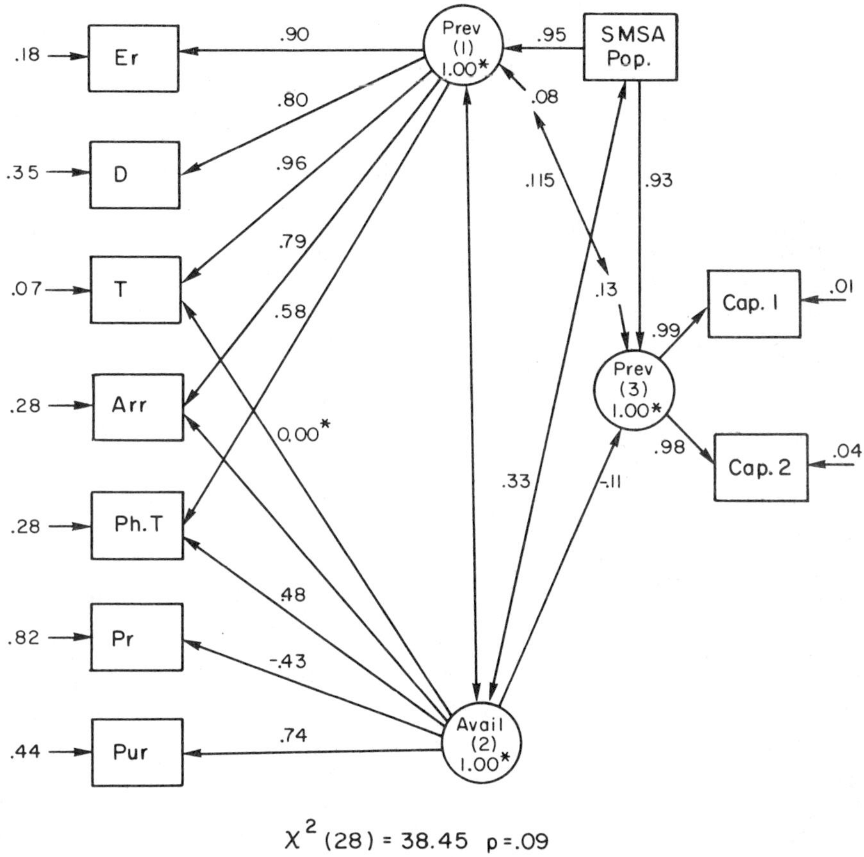

Fig. 4. Standardized maximum likelihood estimates and goodness-of-fit test for the three-construct model with SMSA population partialled out. Asterisks indicate parameters constrained to values shown.

to be prevalence and availability. The fact that there are not two prevalence constructs corresponding to the two different methods of measuring prevalence provides evidence of the construct validity of the methods.

In order to examine the availability latent variable more closely, we have estimated the scores of the 24 SMSAs on the latent variable using a standard approximation (Harman, 1975). In Table 11 the 24 SMSAs are listed in rank order of availability. The estimated scores on the latent variable are also shown, but these scores are on an arbitrary scale and cannot be interpreted directly. The rank orderings appear quite reasonable, in that the greatest heroin availability

Table 11

Estimated Scores of 24 SMSAs on the Availability Factor

SMSA	Estimated score on availability construct
Detroit	2.748
Chicago	1.053
New York	0.929
San Francisco	0.355
San Diego	0.295
Los Angeles	0.130
Boston	0.104
Washington, DC	0.095
Phoenix	0.035
Philadelphia	0.024
Indianapolis	−0.182
Seattle	−0.183
Buffalo	−0.204
Denver	−0.214
Miami	−0.216
Cleveland	−0.226
Atlanta	−0.248
Minneapolis	−0.250
Kansas City	−0.260
San Antonio	−0.260
Dallas	−0.261
New Orleans	−0.285
Oklahoma City	−0.288
Norfolk	−0.295

during 1977 would appear to be in Detroit, Chicago, New York, San Francisco, San Diego, and Los Angeles.

Construct Validation Model of the Two Estimation Procedures Based on Per Capita Indicators

Because of the differing SMSA populations, the raw indicators are difficult to interpret in terms of the seriousness or intensity of drug use differences across communities. Following common practice, we now present a study of the per capita occurrence of the drug abuse indicators. Each indicator that reflects a frequency (namely, Er, D, TR, Arr, Ph.T, and Cap. 1, Cap. 2) can be transformed into a sample proportion by dividing by the SMSA population. Thus, these ratios express, on a common scale, the "probability" of each occurrence in a community. These estimated probabilities, or proportions, are of interest in epidemiologic investigations where questions are addressed such as "Why is heroin abuse a more serious problem in region x than in region y?"

In spite of the interpretational importance of such ratios, their use is frequently criticized on a variety of methodological grounds (e.g., Freeman and Kronenfeld, 1973). In a recent review of the controversy, Long (1980) concludes that the traditional objections of confounding and bias when analyzing ratio variables are not entirely justified. Assuming that the ratio variables are of interest in and of themselves, and assuming that the components are free from measurement error, then the use of ratios appears quite acceptable, in spite of the numerous expressions to the contrary.

In this paper we are interested in demonstrating that the two methods of measuring the prevalence rates are in agreement. The major problems with the current analysis of the rates are that the distribution of these ratios is highly nonnormal and that the presence of measurement error in the common component of the ratios cannot be assessed. The sample univariate kurtosis values ranged from 4.00 to 12.00, and the bivariate scatterplots among the ratio variables suggested nonlinear relationships. Considering the extreme departures from univariate normality, and the presence of nonlinearities, we must reject the assumption of multivariate normality. Since it is now known (e.g., Browne, 1980) that the test statistic used in the analysis of the previous models of Fig. 3 is not valid under conditions of excess kurtosis, the corresponding model does not fit the indicator rates. Analysis of such a model appears particularly inappropriate in this case because of the nonlinearities present in the bivariate relationships.

With complex data such as these ratio variables, it is necessary to formulate a more complex model that does not assume simple linear relationships in multivariate normal data. In psychophysics, simple power functions frequently are used (Stevens, 1951). In econometrics, nonlinear models identical in form to those used in psychophysics are referred to as the Cobb-Douglas production function (e.g., Barten, 1964; Douglas, 1948). For the current ratio variables, the Cobb-Douglas function is attractive since it is an intrinsically linear model, a transformation of which can be analyzed using the covariance structure approach used in the previous model.

The version of the Cobb-Douglas function hypothesized here is a simple form of nonlinear (but intrinsically linear) factor analysis (e.g., MacDonald, 1967). In equation form, for the typical indicator ratio such as number of deaths (D), we hypothesize

$$(D/\text{pop}) = (\text{no. users/pop})^{\lambda} \cdot e^{\epsilon}$$

In the logarithm this equation is linear, and parameter estimates (λs) and variances of errors ($\sigma_{\epsilon}{}^2$) can be estimated using the covariance structure approach employed in Figs. 3 and 4. An advantage of such a model is that a compressive transformation such as the logarithm will tend to normalize the platykurtic distributions observed for the rates. In addition, when such a model fits

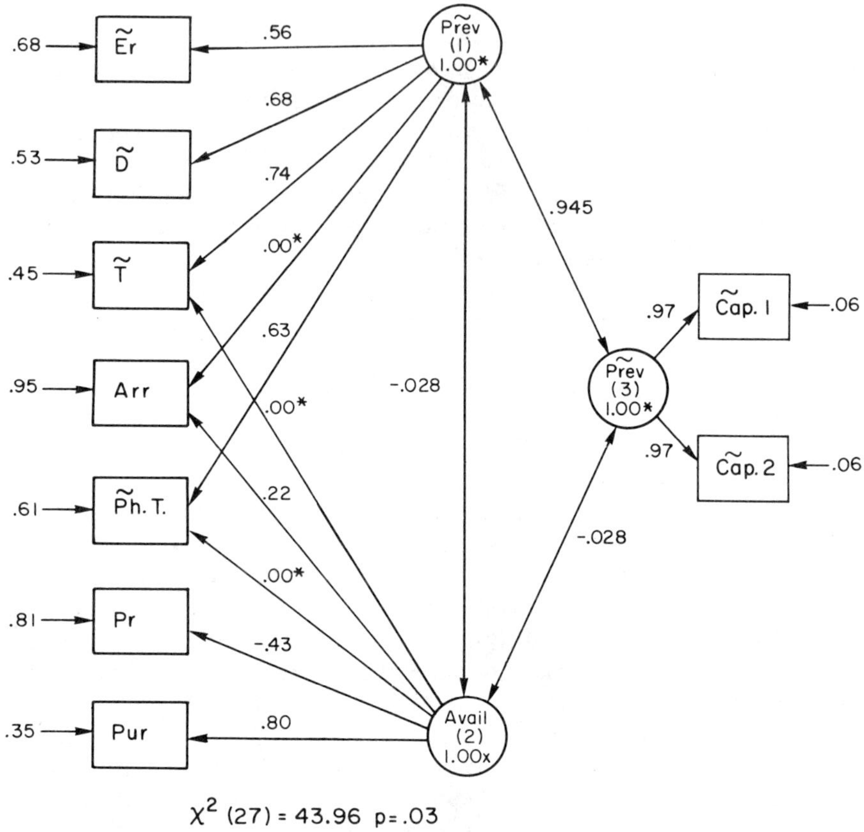

Fig. 5. Standardized maximum likelihood estimates and goodness-of-fit test for the log rate three-construct model.

the data, then the estimates of the weights (the λs) are in fact the elasticities, which for the Cobb-Douglas model are known to be constant.

The model in Fig. 2 was fitted to the logarithm of the indicator rates, yielding the results shown in Fig. 5. In the figure, the log rates are indicated by the tilde (~). Price and purity are entered as the logarithms of the raw values used in the previous model. It should be noted that for the log rates, the sample univariate kurtosis values range from -1.00 to 1.00, and the bivariate scatter plots appear linear.

As can be seen in the figure, the obtained chi-square test statistic does not exceed the critical value, and thus the model is not rejected. The weights relating the latent variables and the log rate indicators are almost identical to the previous results using the raw frequencies. In one respect, the results are more consistent with the hypotheses in that the relationship between pharmacy thefts and the latent availability construct no longer takes a paradoxical positive value. In other respects, except for the treatment-availability relationship and the arrest-prevalence relationship, the model is consistent with the hypotheses of Fig. 2. The correlation between the two prevalence constructs is still within sampling error of unity. As in the case of the raw frequencies where population was partialled out, the relationships between the prevalence construct and the availability construct are negative.

Thus, we conclude again that the two methods of measuring prevalence indeed measure the same underlying construct. Thus, for Fig. 5 we accept a two-construct model where a single prevalence construct is manifested in the indicator rates and in the capture-recapture rates, and where availability is manifested in price, purity, and arrests.

In conclusion, the results of this study reveal a convergence of two methodologically unrelated techniques for estimating the intensity of heroin abuse at the SMSA level of aggregation. For both the raw indicators expressed as frequencies and for the logarithms of the indicator rates, the factor analytic and capture-recapture approaches do indeed appear to measure the same underlying construct. Because of the importance of the epidemiology of heroin abuse, this demonstration of the construct validity of these indirect estimation procedures is a crucial step in building a scientific substrate for indicator-based heroin abuse estimation. Had such validation not been possible, then continued use of the heroin abuse indicators for such estimation could not have been condoned on scientific grounds. Additional work will be required, of course, to develop further methods for extracting useful information from the heroin abuse indicators. Such research is important, since the indicators represent a unique accessibility to that large subpopulation of heroin users who have encountered legal, medical, or social complications as a result of heroin use.

ACKNOWLEDGMENT

This research was supported in part by grant number DA 01070 from the U.S. Public Health Service.

REFERENCES

BARTEN, A.P. Consumer demand functions under conditions of almost additive preferences. *Econometrica* 32: 1–38, 1964.

BISHOP, Y.M.M., FEINBERG, S.E., and HOLLAND, P.W. *Discrete Multivariate Analysis: Theory and Practice*. Cambridge, MA: MIT Press, 1975.

BROWN, M.W. Covariance structures. In D.M. Hawkins (ed.), *Topics in Applied Multivariate Analysis.* Cambridge University Press, 1982.

DEMAREE, R.G. *Demographic models of census tract variation in drug abuse prevalence.* Paper presented at the 1978 meeting of the Society for Multivariate Experimental Psychology, Cincinnati, Ohio, 1978.

DOUGLAS, P.H. Are there laws of production? *Am. Econ. Rev.* 38: 1–49. 1948.

DU PONT, R.L., and GREENE, M.H. The dynamics of a heroin addiction epidemic. *Science* 181: 716–722, 1973.

FREEMAN, J.H., and KRONENFELD, J.E. Problems of definitional dependency: The case of administration intensity. *Soc. Forces* 52: 108–121, 1973.

FRENCH, J.F. *Prevalence of heroin use in New Jersey*. Unpublished report of Department of Health, Alcohol, Narcotic and Drug Abuse Unit, State of New Jersey, October 1977.

GREENE, M.H. *Estimating the prevalence of heroin use in a community*. Special Action Office for Drug Abuse Prevention Report, August 1974.

GREENE, M.H., and DU PONT, R.L. The epidemiology of drug abuse. *Am. J. Public Health* (Suppl.) 64: 1973.

GREENE, M.H., and NIGHTINGALE, L. Evolving patterns of drug abuse. *Ann. Int. Med.* 83: 402–411, 1975.

GREENWOOD, J.A. *Estimating number of narcotic addicts*. Bureau of Narcotics and Dangerous Drugs Report SCID-TR-3, October 1971.

GREENWOOD, J.A. *Estimating relative incidence of narcotic addiction using treatment facility admissions*. DEA Report RTP-TR11, June 1974.

GREENWOOD, J.A., and CRIDER, R. *Estimated number of heroin addicts 1977*. NIDA Administrative Report, 1978.

HARMAN, H.H. *Modern Factor Analysis*. Chicago: University of Chicago Press, 1975.

HUNT, L.G. *Drug Incidence Analysis*. Special Action Office Monograph, Ser. A, No. 3, August 1974.

JÖRESKOG, K.G., and SÖRBOM, D. *LISREL IV*. Chicago: National Educational Resources, 1978.

LONG, S.B. The continuing debate over the use of ratio variables: Fact and fiction. In K.F. Schuessler (ed.), *Sociological Methodology*. San Francisco: Jossey-Bass, 1980.

MC DONALD, R.P. *Nonlinear Factor Analysis*. Psychometrika Monograph 15. Chicago: University of Chicago Press, 1967.

MINICHIELLO, L. *Indicators of intravenous drug use in the United States 1966–1973*. IDA Paper P-1068, October 1974.

O'DONNELL, J.A., VOSS, H.L., CLAYTON, R.R., SLATIN, G.T., and ROOM, R.G.W. *Young Men and Drugs–A Nationwide Survey*. NIDA Research Monograph 5, February 1976.

PERSON, P., RETKA, R., and WOODWARD, J.A. *Toward a heroin problem index–An analytic model for drug abuse indicators*. NIDA Technical Paper, DHEW Publ. No. (ADM)76-367, 1976.

PERSON, P., RETKA, R.L., and WOODWARD, J.A. *A method of estimating heroin use prevalence*. NIDA Technical Paper, 1977.

RICHARDS, L.G., and BLEVENS, L.B. *The epidemiology of drug abuse: Current issues*. NIDA Research Monograph 10, March 1977.

RILEY, W.J., WAGENFELD, M.O., and SONNAD, S. Triangulated investigating: An approach to the estimating of the extent of heroin use. *Int. J. Addict.* 16: 97–108, 1981.

SCHLENGER, W.E., and GREENBERG, S.W. *Final Report: Analysis of intermetropolitan correlates of heroin use*. NIDA, January 1, 1978.

STEVENS, S.S. *Handbook of Experimental Psychology*. New York: Wiley, 1951.

STOLOFF, P., LEVINE, D.B., and SPRUILL, N. *Public drug treatment and addict crime*. Public Research Institute Study, October 1975.

TORGERSON, W.S. *Theory and Methods of Scaling*. New York: Wiley, 1958.

UNDERWOOD, B.J. Individual differences as a crucible in theory construction. *Am. Psychol.* 30: 128–134, 1975.

WEEKS, D.G. *Structural equation systems in latent variables within a second-order measurement model*. Unpublished doctoral dissertation, UCLA, 1978.

WOODWARD, J.A. *Structural equation models of drug abuse indicators*. Paper presented at the National Drug Abuse Conference, Seattle, WA, April 3, 1978.

WOODWARD, J.A., and BENTLER, P.M. Statistical lower bounds to population reliability. *Psychol. Bull.* 85: 1323–1326, 1978.

THE AMERICAN JOURNAL OF DRUG AND ALCOHOL ABUSE

Volume 9, Number 4, 1982-83

CONTENTS

Recidivism among Opioid Addicts after Drug Treatment: An Analysis by Race and Tenure in Treatment. 371
G. W. Joe, M. R. Lloyd, D. D. Simpson, and B. K. Singh

Fetal Outcome in Narcotic-Dependent Women: The Importance of the Type of Maternal Narcotic Used 383
B. Stimmel, J. Goldberg, A. Reisman, R. J. Murphy, and K. Teets

Families and Drugs: A Life-Span Research Approach. 397
T. J. Glynn

A Quantitative Inventory of Alcohol Disorders (QIAD): A Severity Scale for Alcohol Abuse 413
J. L. Stinnett and J. O. Schechter

Prodromal Syndromes in Delirium Tremens 431
F. Miller

Grief and Alcohol 435
A. Blankfield

Cognitive Impairment and Other Psychological Scores Derived from the Content Analysis of Speech in Detoxified Male Chronic Alcoholics 447
L. A. Gottschalk, J. C. Hoigaard-Martin, M. J. Eckardt, R. L. Gilbert, and R. J. Wolf

Medical-Behavioral Treatment of the Older Alcoholic Patient. 461
A. N. Wiens, C. E. Menustik, S. I. Miller, and R. E. Schmitz

Book Reviews. 477

Books Received. 485

Announcement 487

Erratum. 489

Index to Volume 9 491

Collective Contents to Volume 9 497

MARCEL DEKKER, INC. New York and Basel

Contributions to this journal are published free of charge

INFORMATION FOR AUTHORS SUBMITTING MANUSCRIPTS

Send a clear double-spaced typewritten original and one duplicate to Ms. Nancy Reid-Rappolt, Editorial Assistant, *International Journal of the Addictions,* c/o Winch, Smith, Ostermann and Mates, MD's, 4141 Geary, Suite 326, San Francisco, California 94118. Also send one duplicate to the Chief Editor, Dr. Stanley Einstein, Building 113/41, East Talpiot, Jerusalem, Israel. DOUBLE-SPACE the entire manuscript; do not use single spacing anywhere, including references.

Include authors' academic degrees and present affiliation. If applicable, cite auspices under which work being reported was done. Specify address to which requests for reprints should be sent.

Begin your TITLE with a word useful in indexing. A 75- to 100-word ABSTRACT should be provided, which precedes each article. A summary is then not necessary. Major and minor headings may be used in the text; indicate major headings by typing in capitals.

Use METRIC UNITS of measure. If measurements were made in English units, give metric equivalents.

Cite all TABLES and FIGURES in the text. Tables should have titles, and figures should have brief legends. In tables, give each column a heading. Indicate units of measure in parentheses in the heading for each column. Do not use vertical rules. Do not use horizontal rules other than those in the heading and at the bottom. Submit PHOTOGRAPHS as glossy prints, untrimmed and unmounted; identify each with pencil lightly on the back and indicate top.

ARTWORK will not be returned unless specifically requested, and will be disposed of three months after publication.

REFERENCES in the text should be enclosed in parentheses and include the author's surname and the date of the item cited. Keep footnotes to a minimum. Footnotes should be collected at the end of the manuscript in their numerical order of appearance.

The BIBLIOGRAPHY (double-spaced) should be given at the end of the article in alphabetical order. Journal references should include authors, title, name of journal abbreviated according to *Chemical Abstracts List of Periodicals*, inclusive page numbers, and date. Book references should include authors, title, place of publication, publisher, and date.

AUTHOR RESPONSIBILITY: It is the sole responsibility of the author(s) to obtain written permission from the author(s), publisher(s), etc. for figures, tables, or any other information excerpted from previously published works which are used in the manuscript(s) considered for publication. It is understood that the manuscript(s) considered for publication in the *International Journal of the Addictions* have not been previously published nor are they under simultaneous publication consideration elsewhere.

Statements and opinions expressed in the articles and communications herein are those of the author(s) and do not necessarily express those of the Editor or publisher.

THE INTERNATIONAL JOURNAL OF THE ADDICTIONS

Volume 19 Number 1 1984

CONTENTS

Editorial: Coping and Drug Misuse Intervention: S. Einstein iii

Human Garbage and Physical Garbage: A Sociological Case Example of Institutional Violence: N. Ben-Yehuda and S. Einstein 1

A Diagnostic Tool with Important Implications for Treatment of Addiction: Identification of Factors Underlying Relapse and Remission Time Distributions: N. R. Mann, V. C. Charuvastra, and V. K. Murthy 25

Impression Management and Testing for Control Locus in an Alcoholic Sample: R. M. Costello and K. A. Wicoff 45

A Review of the Reliability and Validity of the Drug Abuse Warning Network: J. D. Swisher and T.-W. Hu 57

Substance Abuse: Assessment of the Outcomes of Activities and Activity Clusters in School-Based Prevention: J. Sexter, A. P. Sullivan, S. F. Wepner, and R. Denmark 79

Construct Validity of Heroin Abuse Estimators: J. A. Woodward, R. L. Retka, and L. Ng 93

MARCEL DEKKER, INC., New York and Basel

CODEN: INJABN 19(2) i-vi, 119-232 (1984)
ISSN: 0020-773X

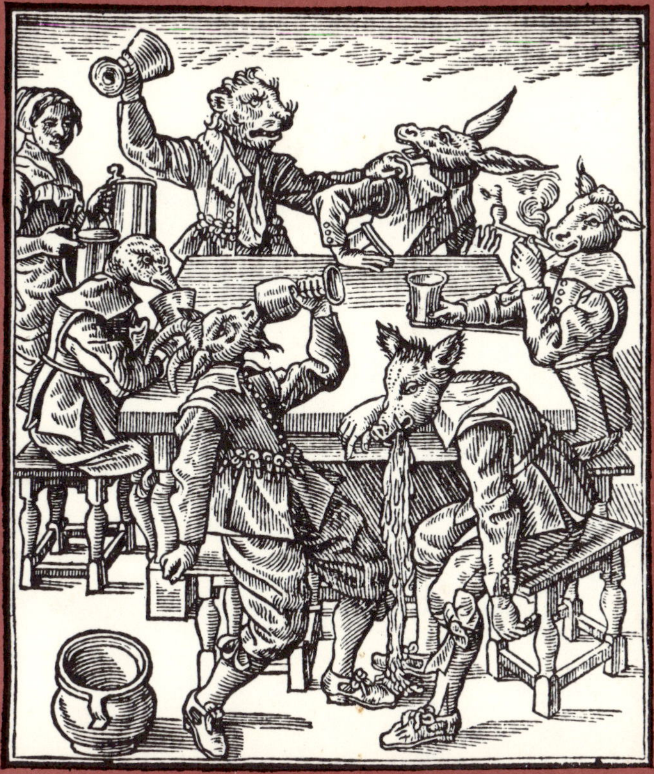

THE INTERNATIONAL JOURNAL OF THE Addictions

Volume 19 Number 2 1984

THE INTERNATIONAL JOURNAL
OF THE ADDICTIONS

April 1984

Aims and Scope. This journal is a comprehensive medium for worldwide communication among both concerned laymen and professionals in research, training, and treatment in the field of addiction and substance misuse.

Indexing and Abstracting Services. Articles published in *The International Journal of the Addictions* are selectively indexed or abstracted in:

• Adolescent Mental Health Abstracts • ASCA • Bibliographic Index of Health Education Periodicals (BIHEP) • BioSciences Information Service of Biological Abstracts (BIOSIS) • Classified Abstract Archive of the Alcohol Literature • Current Contents/Clinical Practice • Excerpta Medica • Index Medicus • International Pharmaceutical Abstracts • ISI/BIOMED • Journal of Abstracts of the All-Union Institute of Scientific and Technical Information of the USSR • Psychological Abstracts • Science Citation Index • Selected List of Tables of Contents of Psychiatric Periodicals • Social Sciences Citation Index • State Central Scientific Medical Library/International Book Exchange–USSR

Articles published in *The International Journal of the Addictions* are listed in Selected List of Tables of Contents of Psychiatric Periodicals.

Manuscript Preparation and Submission. See inside back cover of this issue.

Subscription Information. *The International Journal of the Addictions* is published eight times annually in February, April, May, July, August, September, November, and December by Marcel Dekker, Inc., 270 Madison Avenue, New York, New York 10016. The subscription rate for Volume 19 (1984), containing eight numbers, is $225.00 per volume (prepaid). The special discounted rate for individual professionals and students is $112.50 per volume. To secure this special rate, your order must be prepaid by personal check. Add $20.00 for surface postage outside the United States. For airmail to Europe, add $32.48; to Asia, add $40.48.

Mailing Address. *Please mail payment with order to:* Marcel Dekker Journals, P. O. Box 11305, Church Street Station, New York, New York 10249.

Contributions to this journal are published free of charge. Second-class postage paid at New York, New York and at additional mailing offices.

Library of Congress Catalog Card Number 66-9896

Cover illustration courtesy of the Picture Collection, The Branch Libraries, New York Public Library.

THE INTERNATIONAL JOURNAL OF THE Addictions

The International Journal of the Addictions, 19(2), iii–vi, 1984

Editorial

Considering the Risks of "Populations at Risk"

The special qualities of the active drug user (personality, traits, dysfuntional behavior, etc.) or the drug user in remission (the infamous ex-drug addict) have over time been significantly broadened. Apparently individuals working actively in the field of drug use intervention—those actively demanding that *others* solve the drug use problem (or at the very least, demanding that it be kept at a safe distance from them) and those funding a vast number of intervention efforts and programs (many of which cannot be learned from)—somehow feel that there is not enough to do.

As a result, the foci of plans and efforts have been conceptually enlarged over time, from both visible and hidden drug users to include *populations at risk*. Depending upon one's semantic perverseness and one's vested-interest commitments, one is at liberty to arbitrarily limit the meaning of *populations at risk* or to presume that the term includes the living and the yet to be born, but excludes the dead.

Before continuing upon this semantic trip there is an additional semantic issue which deserves our attention. *At risk* seems to carry with it a pejorative or negative valence. As a result it has been suggested that this concept be replaced with the concept *susceptibility*. Unfortunately the use of more than twice as many letters does not diminish the implications. Nor does it diminish the implicit and explicit dangers to those without status and/or power who are about to be tagged and "saved" by others with status, power, a mandate, or a "personal calling."

In a sense, use of *populations at risk* may be little more than a continuation of the dehumanizing process of stigmatizing a unique individual to that of encompassing and stigmatizing a unique cohort, group, social network, subculture, or even a community.

It could prove useful to consider some of the implications of this concept, since it has so readily entered the semantics of drug use intervention. So many are expecting so much from what may ultimately prove so little! One way of exploring the utility of *populations at risk* is to consider it in terms of *personal and social integration.* The presumption would be that differential degrees of integration are somehow related to differential degrees of susceptibility to drug use. Obviously integrated individuals/groups don't/won't seek out disintegrative behavior, experiences, life-styles, etc. And drug use is obviously initially and/or ultimately disintegrative—in the eyes of almost everyone.

From such a perspective, high degrees of personal and social integration lead to or are related to *secure populations.* Low levels of integration can be considered to be associated with populations at risk. The in-betweens, depending upon their cultural and environmental options, may be *coping* (another mystical term) with the aid of acceptable social substances or legalized psychotropics, or with an endless variety of available non-substance options.

Table 1 schematically presents the presumed outcome of interfacing levels of personal and societal integration with risk potential for unacceptable behavior such as drug use.

At first glance, and with initial efforts (including free if not loose associations), one could easily agree that the lowest risk, for drug use, is for those who are highly integrated themselves as well as with a variety of others (individuals and systems). It would be intriguing to investigate the extent to which such people, whoever and whatever they are, use and misuse a variety of chemically active substances.

A further analysis could lead to the consensual agreement that those whose ties are weak to themselves and within themselves, as well as to others and to the society in which they exist and reside but are not engaged in, are at the highest risk for disapproved *chemical coping*. It would be most useful to gather empirical data about the numbers of nonintegrated, as well as the disintegrated, who are or have been drug users. Paralleling such as effort one could search within this population for the nonchemical copers in the hope of understanding their behavioral arrogance in challenging our theoretical wisdom.

Table 1

Levels of Risk and Selected Types of Integration

	Societal integration (family, friends, peers, society, etc.)	
	High	Low
Personal integration	Lowest risk	
	Highest risk	
	Low	

But these two groups—*high- and low-risk populations*—are predefined, and therefore need not concern us. We remain confronted with two empty cells, which for the sake of closure demand our attention.

- There are those, many or few in number and/or potential impact, who are so highly integrated personally that they march to their own drummer, alone or with a selected few, instead of to the tunes of others. What is their need for the drug experience? What is their need for ongoing social experiences? What is their role and place in society, with peers, and within their own family—as well as the family of man? Do their current life-style and quality of coping and adapting immunize them from the magic, mystique, and seductiveness of drugs, so that we need not intervene with them in order to forestall future disintegration?
- And then there are those who live in, with, and through a variety of groups, highly integrated within them, who have distanced themselves from themselves or perhaps were never sufficiently personally integrated. What is their need for personal experiences—drug or non-drug related? Are the drugs of chemistry an option for them when the drugs of "others" are a readily available and continuing option? What should be the realistic and legitimate concern of drug use prevention agents with respect to the increasing number of young and old who lose themselves ecstatically in group roles, activities, and rituals in what may be arbitrarily termed the "social psychology of the pseudoindividual"? This latter term is used descriptively and not pejoratively.

It would appear upon further perusal that concepts such as *risk, susceptibility*, and *integration*, while semantically wholesome and satisfying, are not necessarily very helpful or usable as we seek to immunize the masses because of the interests, concerns, and fears of the few.

This arrogant assertion may be even further substantiated when we explore the implications and relationships of *risk* to a number of drug user parameters. Table 2 is designed to permit the reader to enunciate his/her own views, feelings,

Table 2

Risk/Susceptibility and Drug Use

Drug use	Level of risk/susceptibility
Never/currently abstaining	
Initial use	
Experimental/recreational use	
Acute/self-medication	
Chronic use	

and private collection of facts regarding both the actual and the potential interface of risk/susceptibility and drug use. Is risk regarding the potential for the phenomenon of drug use a predictable or quasi-predictable gradient of the many variations of drug use? Is it a unique happening? Are the necessary parameters for "chronic" or even "acute" abstinence substantially different from other arbitrary categories of drug users in regard to the substance(s) and meaning of risk/susceptibility?

Indeed, what are the implications of considering the notion of a *population at risk* with regard to abstinence, utilizing a negative term in regard to a positive value? The possibilities may be awesome once we break away from the limiting barriers of pejorative controls.

Last, it would be useful to consider the relationship between the *at risk* concept and the *quality of the drug experience.* Upon taking a drug one can have any one of a variety of experiences which are generally unpredictable. They can arbitrarily be categorized as being:

- Positive +
- Mixed ±
- Negative –
- No experience

No doubt the same can be said about the abstinence state.

Are different qualities of the drug experience differentially and predictably associated with or "caused by" specific types and/or levels of risk/susceptibility? The implications of such a question are potentially mind boggling. If, for example, the highest of the high-risk populations are or may be doomed to drug use, can we (should we) intervene in order to effect a positive drug experience? After all, their being *at risk* is enough of a burden without adding to it with untoward reactions. On the other hand, we may be provoked to create intervention models which induce negative drug experiences (short term, long term, or even chronic) for those on the outskirts of personal and societal integration in order to challenge them into self-integration.

The end may justify the means, as it currently apparently does, regarding the use and misuse of a concept which has the virtues of a slogan. It is amazing how easily so many permit themselves to become drugged by concepts and convinced of their merit in this field, and amazing that so few have made the effort to integrate and accept the drug user—as a person—and find merit in who s/he is and who s/he can be.

S. Einstein, PhD
Jerusalem, Israel

The International Journal of the Addictions, 19(2), 119-151, 1984

Drug-Induced Ego States. I. Cocaine: Phenomenology and Implications

James V. Spotts,* PhD

Greater Kansas City Mental Health Foundation
Kansas City, Missouri 64108

Franklin C. Shontz, PhD

Department of Psychology
University of Kansas
Lawrence, Kansas 66045

Abstract

The ego state experienced by chronic users of cocaine is described in terms of sensorimotor functioning, cognitive functioning, emotionality, spatiality, temporality, causality, and materiality. At low use levels the state is pleasurable, but at high levels fear, anxiety, and paranoia increase, and ultimately reality contact breaks down. Q-sort, Semantic Differential, and other data suggest that low-level users take cocaine to overcome personal insecurities and relieve boredom. Heavy users take it to support overvaulting ambitions and intense strivings for self-sufficiency. Psychotherapy with such persons must deal with their counterdependency, anger, and despair, and with their underlying sense of betrayal. These persons have unacknowledged needs for spiritual experience that must be dealt with openly. A description of persons most vulnerable to heavy use of cocaine is provided, and recommendations for research and social policy are presented.

*To whom correspondence should be addressed: Assistant Director, Greater Kansas City Mental Health Foundation, 600 East 22nd Street, Kansas City, Missouri 64108.

 0020-773X/84/1902-0119$3.50/0

INTRODUCTION

In the last two decades a number of Western countries have experienced a resurgence in illicit use of cocaine; at present, this resurgence is most evident in the United States. Although cocaine was not a serious problem in America in the 1960s, its use increased slowly but steadily through the mid-1970s with explosive increases in use in the latter part of the decade. By 1980, 14-17 million Americans had tried the drug and 4-5 million were using it with some regularity (Gwynne, 1982; Kozel, Crider, and Adams, 1982). Cocaine use continues to increase despite the fact that *heavy* consumption can induce severe dependence, produce devasting physical and psychological effects, and even kill. Efforts to cope with this social problem have been hampered because, until the mid-1970s, there was no up-to-date information regarding the lethality, hazards, or sequelae of cocaine use in man (Byck, 1974).

Patterns of drug abuse that appear in one industrial country often emerge later in others. If trends for cocaine follow those of amphetamine (Brill and Hirose, 1969; Ellinwood, 1974; Inge, 1969) illicit use of cocaine could soon become a matter of international concern (Bewley, 1965; Connell, 1969; Jeri, Sanches, del Pozo, and Fernandez, 1978; Ling and del Prado, 1978; Noya, 1978). From 1977 to 1981 the number of cocaine seizures in the European nations increased almost fourfold (U.S. Department of Justice, Drug Enforcement Administration, 1982). These trends, if unchecked, would suggest that by the mid to late 1980s, cocaine could become as serious a drug problem in Europe as it is in the United States today. Consequently, experts in all nations should learn as much as they can about the drug and the effects associated with its heavy use.

This report describes some important psychological factors associated with heavy, chronic use of cocaine. Earlier reports have presented in-depth analyses of the developmental characteristics of male, heavy, chronic cocaine users and have described how these men perform on several personality tests (Spotts and Shontz, 1980a, 1982, 1983). This article presents an analysis of the phenomenological structure of the ego state induced by chronic use of cocaine. The analysis is derived from interviews and Q-sort data; findings from the Semantic Differential are also summarized. These findings are integrated with other facts to produce a theory of why some persons are drawn to heavy, chronic use of cocaine; to describe persons most at risk for heavy use of the drug; and to provide recommendations for treatment, research, and social policy.

The term *ego* is defined here as the point or focus of consciousness (Jung, 1958); *ego state* refers to the properties of the field of consciousness within which the ego is located at a given time. Heavy use of cocaine propels the ego into a state with definable characteristics that distinguish it from those produced by all other major drugs of abuse.

Cocaine

Cocaine is known colloquially as *snow, flake, girl, coke, heaven dust, she, happy dust, Bernice, happy trails, her, lady,* etc. (Spotts and Shontz, 1980a). It is an alkaloid derived from the leaves of *Erythroxylon coca,* a shrub cultivated on the mountain slopes of Peru, Chile, and Bolivia. Pure cocaine is a colorless to white crystal or crystalline powder that is odorless, decomposes on standing in air, and has a melting point of 98°C. Cocaine hydrochloride (USP) dissolves in half its weight in water; its saturated solution is alkaline (Clark, 1973). The drug has two distinctive pharmacologic actions: (1) as a topical or local anesthetic of high efficacy and toxicity, and (2) as a powerful central nervous system stimulant (Eiswirth, Smith and Wesson, 1972).

Cocaine is absorbed at all sites of application. After application to mucous membranes it may be detected in the blood within 3 minutes, reaches a peak in plasma concentration in 15-60 minutes, and may be detectable for as long as 6 hours. Most cocaine is hydrolized in the body to benzoylecgonine and is eliminated in the urine within 24-36 hours (Van Dyke, Barash, Jatlow, and Byck, 1976; Van Dyke, 1981; Woods, 1977). For many years it was thought that cocaine was metabolized by the liver, but recent research suggests that serum cholinesterase may play a major role in metabolizing the drug (Inaba, Stewart, and Kalow, 1978; Van Dyke, 1981).

Detoxification of cocaine is estimated to be at a rate of 30-40 mg/hour and in incremental doses the body may be able to detoxify 10 g/day (Eisworth et al., 1972; Gay, Sheppard, Inaba, and Newmeyer, 1973). Absorption can easily exceed the rate of detoxification; hence the high toxicity of the drug. Ritchie, Cohen, and Dripps (1970) estimate the *fatal dose* (causing death 100% of the time) to be 1,200 mg after oral ingestion. Eiswirth et al. (1972) estimate the *lethal dose* (causing death 50% of the time) with intravenous injection at approximately 500 mg in a 150-pound person, but upon application to mucous membranes as little as 20-30 mg may be fatal (Ritchie et al., 1970). With incremental consumption, users can often absorb amounts cumulatively larger than lethal dose limits.

Cocaine is the most potent of all sympathomimetic agents and can induce *rapid elevation of heart and respiration rates,* and *blood pressure* (Fischman, Schuster, Resnekov, Schick, Krasnegor, Fennell, and Freedman, 1976; Post, Kotin, and Goodwin, 1974). Heavy use can produce *euphoria; anorexia and insomnia; anxiety; agitation and confusion; depression; visual, auditory, and tactile hallucinations;* and an *acute psychosis, with paranoia and delusions,* similar in some respects to the amphetamine psychosis (Chopra and Chopra, 1930/1931; Cohen, 1981; Gay et al., 1973; Grinspoon and Bakalar, 1976; Jeri et al., 1978; Noya, 1978; Post, 1975; Spotts and Shontz, 1980a, 1981; Wesson and Smith, 1977).

Cocaine is not believed to induce physical dependence. However, *intense psychic dependence* often does occur. Most investigators report that no long-term tolerance develops. Cocaine is widely used in clinical medicine as a local and regional anesthetic and is particularly valuable for anesthetizing the mucous membrane in oral-pharyngeal surgery and in other otolaryngological procedures (Barash, 1977; Barash, Kopriva, Langou, Van Dyke, Jatlow, Stahl and Byck, 1980; Van Dyke, 1981).

Contrary to popular belief, cocaine is not a safe recreational drug. Although its lethality is thought to be low, it is known to kill (Finkle and McClosky, 1977; Wetli and Wright, 1979). In deaths associated with intravenous injection, users collapse and die within a few minutes. Following oral or intranasal administration, users typically display a symptom-free period for up to an hour, after which they go into grand mal seizures and die shortly thereafter. The mechanism of death is usually respiratory collapse, mediated by the effects of cocaine on the central nervous system. Postmortem data indicate that the highest blood concentrations of cocaine occur with oral use and the lowest with intravenous use, with intermediate concentrations among those practicing nasal insufflation (Wetli, 1980).

During the last decade the predominant method of administration of cocaine in the United States has been nasal insufflation (snorting), although a considerable number of users practice intravenous injection. Recently a riskier practice of "free basing" cocaine (smoking a chemically treated and purer form of the drug) has become popular (Siegel, 1979, 1980; Van Dyke, 1981).

Research Context

The men whose experiences are described in this report participated in a program of research on carefully matched groups of heavy, chronic users of cocaine, amphetamine, opiates, and barbiturate/sedative-hypnotics, as well as a comparable group of men committed to the nonuse of drugs. The research employs the Representative Case Method (Shontz, 1965, 1977) and is based on intensive studies of carefully selected persons who epitomize patterns of heavy, chronic drug use. This method provides a unique perspective on specific drugs, their effects, dynamics and determinants of use, antecedents, consequences, and social correlates. It focuses upon heavy, chronic users who possess knowledge about drug effects that can be obtained from no other sources (Spotts and Shontz, 1980a).

METHODS

The Experts

Using paid intermediaries and users as finders, nine expert consultants (participants) were selected from more than 800 men who were reported to be knowledgeable about cocaine (Spotts and Shontz, 1980a). The men selected were not experimental, occasional, or social-recreational users. All had experimented with numerous drugs, but each was intensely committed to cocaine, preferred it over all others, and had used it long enough to be fully acquainted with its effects. Each participant was examined individually for 14 or more full days over a period of 4-6 months: Data collection for all nine men took approximately 1.5 years. These men were studied in 1974-1975, before cocaine use had become pandemic in the United States. Our research, therefore, may represent the first in-depth study of heavy cocaine users in the industrial West.

The participants were from 21 to 44 years of age and of above average intelligence, with from 10 to 13 years of formal education. Most were White, single, and came from small, intact, middle-class families (Table 1). Although four were married at the time of these studies, two men left or divorced their wives during the project; another divorced his wife shortly afterward. Only one marital relationship produced a child.

As in all studies in the research program, participants were drawn from many sectors of society and included: a millionaire's son, a blue-collar worker, a musician or entertainer, a manager of performers, a thief, an entrepeneur, an ambitious, achievement-oriented individual, a social misfit, and a two-worlder (who maintained full-time legal employment to cover another illegal occupation [Brotman and Freedman, 1969]). Heterogeneity in life-styles ensured that findings were not due to selection of a single psychological type.

None of the men in these studies had completed college or other formalized programs designed to provide specialized employment skills. Although their work histories varied considerably, whatever specialized skills they had acquired were of the on-the-job training variety. Despite this fact, one man, a highly successful salesman, was earning an annual salary of $65,000-$70,000 per year (in estimated 1982 dollar equivalents), and those in illegal occupations (i.e., cocaine dealers) were earning considerably more. During their involvement with the research project, five men maintained full-time employment and were working in legitimate occupations as a fry cook, service station manager, musician, maître d' and salesman. Three were pursuing what were essentially illegal occupations as gamblers, procurers, or cocaine dealers, and one had enrolled in college and was working fitfully toward a college degree.

On the average, participants had used cocaine (Table 2) for 11 years (range 2-18 years) and on a daily basis (estimated number of years of daily use) for an average of 4.6 years (range 1.0-12.0 years). Typically daily doses ranged from 20 to 3,000 mg (median 1,000 mg). All but one man used cocaine intravenously; most had practiced nasal insufflation previously and therefore knew the effects produced by both methods of administration.

Six men reported a history of five overdoses on heroin and four on cocaine. Cocaine overdoses were described as producing stabbing precordial chest pain or

Table 1

Personal and Family Characteristics of Participants

	Chronic cocaine users (N = 9)
1. Personal characteristics	
Age	
Median	28
Range	21-44
Intelligence (revised beta)	
Mean IQ	105.8
SD	11.21
Educational achievement	
Median	12.0
Range	10-13
Marital status	
Single	3
Married	4
Divorced	2
Socioeconomic background	
Median	Middle class
Range	Upper-lower class[a]
Race	
Black	3
White	6
2. Family characteristics	
Parents' marital status	
Intact[b]	6
Divorced	1
One parent deceased	2
Parents' educational achievement (yr)	
Father	
Median	12
Range	4-20
Mother	
Median	13
Range	6-16
Siblings	
Brothers	
Median	1
Range	0-3
Sisters	
Median	2
Range	1-5
Birth Order	
Median	3
Range	1-9

[a] A five-class typology (upper, upper-middle, middle, lower-middle, lower) based on the father's occupation and income, using a modification of status assessment procedures developed by Hollingshead (1965).

[b] An intact marital relationship does not necessarily mean a healthy one, but only one in which the parents remained together until the participant was age 15 or older.

Table 2

Participant Drug Use Characteristics

	Chronic cocaine users ($N = 9$)
1. Presenting characteristics	
Primary method of administration	
Nasal insufflation	1
Intravenous	8
Chronicity of use (yr)[a]	
Median	11
Range	2-18
Estimated years daily use of drug of commitment[b]	
Median	4.6
Range	1.0- 12.0
Estimated typical daily dosages (mg)	
Median	1,000
Range	20-3,000[c]
Number of drug overdoses reported	9
Median	1
Range	0-2
Number in treatment at time of investigation	4
Longest voluntary termination of use of drug of commitment (mo)	
Median	1.0
Range	1.0-3.0
2. Historical background of use	
Age first-ever use of illegal substance[d]	
Median	15
Range	13-19
Age first-ever use of drug of personal commitment	
Median	18
Range	14-26
Number of different drugs ever used	
Median	15
Range	8-22
Abuse of drugs by parents	
Alcoholic mother	1
Abuse of drugs by siblings	
Alcoholic sister	1
Introduced to drug of personal commitment by	
Friends	7
Acquaintances	2

[a] Age of last use of drug of personal commitment minus age of first use.
[b] Total days lifetime use converted to years.
[c] Relatively low dosages appear at the bottom of the drug use range because participants were selected to depict the entire drug use continuum, from low to high. The man with the lowest use level practiced nasal insufflation and was deliberately selected to anchor the low end of the dose-use continuum.
[d] Defined as the use of illicit substance(s) or illicit use of licit substances other than alcohol.

severe respiratory distress. All were terminated by injection of opiates, in one instance by a friend and in the others by the users themselves. Four men were in treatment at the time of our studies; three of these were in methadone maintenance programs, having become addicted to opiates in efforts to control adverse reactions to cocaine.

These men were relatively free of the medical complications that can accompany intravenous drug use. None ever had hepatitis or had received emergency treatment for drug-related medical conditions. However, two had been hospitalized for a pneumothorax (collapsed lung) which they thought was related to cocaine use, and one had suffered damage to a heart valve, apparently due to use of unsanitary paraphernalia.

First-ever use of drugs was at about age 15 (range 13-19); first-ever use of cocaine was at about age 18 (range 14-26). Most men were introduced to cocaine by close friends. Although these men had experimented with a number of drugs (median 15, range 8-22), they had tried only half as many substances as heavy, chronic users of amphetamine, opiates, and barbiturate/sedative-hypnotics (Spotts and Shontz, 1983).

Abuse of licit of illicit substances by parents or siblings was minimal. One user reported his mother to be an alcoholic; another described a sister as an alcoholic.

Certain findings presented in this report were extended and substantiated in 1982 by searching out and interviewing five additional heavy cocaine users. The additional interviews became necessary partly because the practice of free basing was not popular at the time data were first collected, and it was necessary to determine the extent to which the effects of free basing could be considered comparable to those of intravenous injection. Also, in the original interviews, questioning about some aspects of the phenomenology of the cocaine state (temporality, in particular) was incomplete. It was therefore felt to be desirable to obtain direct confirmation of inferences drawn from data collected earlier (see footnote to Table 3).

Instruments and Procedures

Subsequent descriptions of the cocaine ego state reconstruct the experience from many kinds of data. These data came from intensive and extensive interviews concerning drug use history, use patterns, social context of use, reasons for selecting drug of choice, and drug preferences (Spotts and Shontz, 1980a). In addition, each participant responded to two checklists: one described physical/physiological effects of cocaine; the second described psychological effects. Checklist items were drawn from the research literature (Table 3). Each participant was read each item and asked whether he had experienced that effect and if so what percentage of the time. He was then requested to add comments to

Table 3

Drug Effect Items[a]

Physical/Physiological Effects	
Dizziness	Yawning
Tremors, muscle spasms	Fainting
Sweating	Abscesses
Gooseflesh	Diarrhea
Tightness in chest or chest pains	Headaches
Elevation of pulse rate	Cellulitis (inflammation following administration)
Infection of nasal mucous membrane	Increased or decreased urination
Weight loss	Tolerance
Increased sensitivity to allergies	Insomnia
Loss of fatigue	Nausea
Feeling of insects being on or under the skin	Rhinorrhea
Visual hallucinations	Mydriasis
Auditory hallucinations	Reactive hyperemia
Tactile hallucinations	Increased heart rate
Olfactory hallucinations	Local anesthesia, numbness
Itching	Increased respiration rate
Lacrimation or tearing	Respiratory difficulties or distress
Emesis or vomiting	Hyperphrenia (excessive mental activity)
Dryness of mouth and throat	Hepatitis or liver infections
Nosebleed	Convulsions, seizures
Ringing in the ears	Coma
Anorexia, loss of appetite	Visual difficulties or anomalies
Psychological Effects	
Increased or decreased feelings of self-control	Increased optimism, courage
Increased restlessness, excitement	Feeling of increased physical strength or ability to do work
Intensified feelings of well-being	Feeling that everything is perfect
Euphoria	A physical orgasm in the "rush"
An exquisite "don't care about the world" attitude	Increased thinking power and imagination
Increased self-confidence, aggressivity	Increased garrulousness
Feeling that the mind is quicker than normal, the feeling that one is smarter than everyone else	Acceleration of mental activity
Reduced sensitivity or indifference to pain	Decreased interest in work, failure of ambition, loss of ambition for useful work
Depression	An aphrodisiac or sexual stimulant
Prolonged sexual performance	Irrational fears
Better or more spectacular orgasm	Paranoia or paranoid ideas
Terror or panic	Increased anxiety
Changes in reality or the way a room or objects look	Causes one to carry a gun or run from imaginary enemies
A trigger for violence	Delusions

[a]The following questions were posed to heavy users interviewed in 1982 to confirm hypotheses from the 1974-1975 studies: alterations of experienced time, increased or decreased dreaming, more pleasant or unpleasant dreams, direction of cocaine experience, increased feelings of personal unity or completeness, and color(s) of drug experiences.

explain, clarify, or elaborate his answer. Complete drug use interviews required 2-3 days per person.

Each participant used Q-sorts to describe his usual, ideal, and worst self; and himself when wanting cocaine, when under its influence, and after its use, as well as several other aspects of his personal identity. Q-sorts were obtained 14 times, at each of three testing sessions approximately 2 months apart. Each person also rated nine substances (amphetamine, beer, barbiturates, cocaine, hard liquor, heroin, LSD, marijuana, and speedball combinations of cocaine and heroin) on 26 scales of a Semantic Differential. The Q-sort and Semantic Differential procedures are described in Spotts and Shontz (1980a).

RESULTS

Descriptive Framework

Nearly all the men studied epitomize the heavy, chronic user. Consequently, dosage levels are higher in this research than in most investigations. *Low-level users* are persons who consume no more than 50 mg of cocaine (of variable quality) per day for extended periods. *Moderate users* practice intravenous use of up to approximately 1,000 mg per day (ranging from an estimated 45% purity to pharmaceutical grade cocaine) for prolonged periods, and *heavy users* practice intravenous use of more than 1,000 mg of high-grade cocaine per day for extended periods.

The following descriptions cover seven aspects of the ego state induced by the chronic use of cocaine: *sensorimotor functioning, cognitive functioning, emotionality, spatiality, temporality, causality,* and *materiality* (Ellenberger, 1958).

Phenomenological Structure of the Cocaine Ego State

Sensorimotor Functioning

The sensorimotor effects of cocaine are intense and diverse. After injection, the user feels an immediate "rush" (often compared to sexual orgasm) so powerful it takes his breath away. His heart pounds, his pulse races, and he breathes deeply and heavily. He sweats profusely but simultaneously experiences chills and gooseflesh, ringing in the ears, tightness of the chest, dizziness, and vertigo. His mouth and throat are dry, and he may be overcome by nausea of the kind some people report with sexual orgasm. Lights seem to dim, the room darkens, and the user fears he may faint. Within minutes the rush subsides.

During the rush, the user enters an ecstatic state characterized by feelings of exaltation, as if he were being lifted upward. At the same time, he feels strong and energetic. His reflexes seem quicker, more accurate and precise. His body feels lighter and more bouyant; movements seem more agile and graceful. Although bright lights hurt his eyes, vision seems sharper; sounds are clearer; odors are more distinctive and colors seem warmer, richer, and more intense. Fatigue and pain are abolished; hunger vanishes. Users frequently have bowel movements immediately after the rush and urinate more frequently than normal. These reactions (along with loss of fatigue and sensations of hunger) occur because this powerful sympathomimetic activates the body for emergency fight-flight reactions.

Except for vertigo with the rush, no serious disturbances in gait, balance, or coordination were reported. Cocaine users related no difficulties operating cars or other vehicles while using the drug, though some said they drove faster. None reported seizures or convulsions, but three men said they had witnessed them in other users. In the cocaine ego state, restlessness, excitement, and need for activity increase. Some individuals are able to harness these energies for constructive activities. In most cases, however, motivation for any activity other than the drug experience is gone.

Since most men terminated the cocaine experience with drugs that reduce REM sleep (opiates, sedative-hypnotics, and alcohol), little can be said about the effect of heavy use of cocaine on dreaming. Low-level users reported that cocaine produced more active and unusual (but not necessarily frightening) dreams.

Continued heavy use of cocaine produces striking alterations of sensorimotor functioning. Binocular vision becomes difficult; vision begins to blur; the world appears misty, milky, and hazy; and the individual may see bright pinpoints of light ("snow lights") flashing like swarms of tiny, blinking electronic insects. The room begins to look like it was being seen through a fog or snowstorm. The user begins to feel numb, and tremors and involuntory spasms may begin in his extremities. His skin may itch as if insects are crawling on it.

As use continues, the individual becomes hyperalert and overreacts to sounds that are normally ignored. He thinks he hears people whispering and talking about him outside his apartment; he believes he sees persons hiding behind trees or scurrying about in the shadows. He may now be vomiting with every injection, as his body tries to reject the drug. However, since it continues to produce ecstatic effects, he persists in its use. By this time he is toxic. He becomes fearful that his enemies (or the police) will break in at any moment. In panic, he may flush the drug down the stool or drive into the countryside at great speed, where he hides for hours furtively watching for an enemy that never appears.

Even if the user never reaches toxicity, he cannot rest or sleep. After prolonged use he is physically and mentally exhausted, tense, and nervous; but if he lies down he cannot relax. His body is mobilized and his mind reels from the rapidly changing ideas tumbling through consciousness. At this point, he may turn to other drugs to terminate what is now a distinctly unpleasant experience.

Cognitive Functioning

Cocaine is a powerful organizer of mental activity. Therefore, some users take it for instrumental purposes (e.g., to perform at peak levels or to work long hours without rest) as well as for pleasure. With low to moderate use, ego functions (thinking, memory, concentration, judgment, etc.) seem to be enhanced. The user feels that his mind is clear, quicker, alert and more effective in managing transactions with the environment. Rumination ceases; extraneous ideas are quickly discarded and decisions are made effortlessly. The ego expands; the user feels he has risen above the problems of existence and is in firm control of his destiny.

With further use, mental activities continue to accelerate; thoughts pile on top of one another, and control becomes difficult. Previously pleasant stimulation is transformed to anxiety, which disrupts cognitive functioning. Cocaine now begins to crowd out other thoughts and becomes the organizing principle of mental life: a Grail, or symbol of transcendence that dominates thinking and around which everything is now organized. A point is reached where nothing matters except cocaine and the experience it produces. Reality testing weakens, and the user begins to misperceive and mininterpret events. Ultimately, the overinflated ego implodes and the person becomes delusional. He believes he can trust no one; he thinks others can read his mind and are plotting his destruction. In the cocaine psychosis, he is exposed to the full fury of the "Bitch Goddess," the Dark Side of the cocaine experience.

Typically, the person in the cocaine psychosis does not act against the object(s) of his delusions. He may flee in panic, he may simply try to endure until delusions abate, or he may inject another drug (often an opiate) to reestablish control. The third strategy is quickest but makes the person vulnerable to addiction, a not uncommon price paid for heavy, chronic use of cocaine.

Emotionality

Low-level users experience an enhancement of personal well-being. Depression and dysphoria fade and fears diminish. They feel more competent, optimistic, and self-assured. Being less inhibited, they reach out to others more easily. The low-level users we studied took cocaine in small groups or at parties with 8-10 people and reported that the drug enhances social relationships. They also reported that cocaine increases sexual desire, prolongs intercourse, and produces more intense and satisfying orgasms. No low- or moderate-level users experienced severe or disabling emotional disturbances, none had gone through the cocaine psychosis, and several were angered by the suggestion that "their drug" could produce such effects.

Heavy users reported the same pleasurable experiences as low- and moderate-level users but with greater intensity. However, their joy is mixed with a dysphoria that low-level users never encounter. Unlike low-level users, these individuals consume cocaine in isolation or with a trusted friend and go to considerable effort to ensure their privacy (locking or barricading doors, closing windows and shades, turning out lights, etc.).

Heavy users tend to dominate women and evidence little desire for close or equalitarian relationships with them. These men are phallic and sexually active during abstinence but report that their sexual interests decline in the cocaine state. They agree that the drug may prolong intercourse (if the user can acheive erection) but not that it produces more spectacular orgasms ("I don't know how you can have a more spectacular orgasm when you're so numb.").

With intravenous injection, the depression, malaise, and ruminative worries that normally plague the heavy user's life vanish, and his suffering melts away. He experiences pleasurable ego expansion, increased feelings of dominance and control over self and environment, and a sense of ethereal wholeness that some people occasionally report with sexual intercourse. Huddled in his darkened room, he feels an ecstatic satisfaction of desires. For a time he feels almost complete unto himself; captured by a quintessential experience so ripe and fulfilling that he believes he needs no one ("You don't need *anyone.* It's just you and your best girlfriend, coke.").

The intense emotion induced by heavy intravenous use of cocaine is ephemeral, a quick up and a quick down lasting about 10 minutes, but so compelling that the user feels he must possess it repeatedly. Therefore, when the effects of the first injection abate, the heavy user injects again. He may continue injecting every 15-20 minutes for a day or more, around the clock. He continues to experience euphoria and exaltation, but fear, anxiety, and apprehension increase as well.

As dosage and chronicity of use increase, the drug ceases to be seductive and becomes coercive. Even moderate doses produce intense cravings to continue its use. ("You get this crazy compulsion that you have to have more and more of it." "It's impossible to control cocaine. It controls you." "Cocaine is evil . . . its so easy to abuse. If I only do one hit I can probably walk away from it, but if I get beyond two hits I can't stop.") Persons who have not used the drug for a year or more may still fear to discuss their experiences. Some say they can taste the drug just talking about it. Others terminate the discussion because talking about cocaine threatens to arouse the desire to use it again.

With continued use, ego functions crumple and the user becomes frightened and apprehensive; he is afraid to be on the streets or in cars. He begins to experience delusions and hallucinations. He becomes terrified and paranoid, believing people are watching his house and will break in at any moment to take the drug, his money, and his life.

For low-level users, termination of the cocaine state brings fatigue and regret that a pleasurable experience is past; for moderate users it brings fatigue and mild depression. For heavy users termination is associated with insomnia, physical and mental exhaustion, and depression, occasionally accompanied by suicidal ideation; an experience so unpleasant some users inject others drugs and fall into a dreamless sleep.

Spatiality

Spatiality is described here in terms of a *vertical* and a *horizontal vector.* Movement upward indicates elevation toward ethereal or spiritual states, and movement downward indicates depression and dejection (Ellenberger, 1958). The horizontal plane is the mundane world of everyday activities. Movement outward indicates involvement with the environment, the world of action, and movement inward indicates withdrawal.

The men we studied are not spiritual people during abstinence but stubborn and pragmatic individuals who live in the world of everyday affairs. Consciously, at least, they are interested only in conquering and expanding their personal worlds. At some point in their lives all had entertained dreams of conquest, glory, and the achievement of godlike status. When we studied them, some were just entering the struggle, some had already given up their dreams and had accepted a limited space, while others were still striving to overcome a complex and hostile world.

Despite their desires to transcend through conquest, these men live in restricted spaces, isolated, alone, and without allies. They evaluate the world in terms of what it can do for them; they wrest what they can from it and react with anger or despair when it resists. It is these men's acute recognition that their life is confined to a narrow space that produces much of the anger, bitterness, and resentment they display.

Cocaine can produce a brief transcendence that carries the user upward toward ethereal realms. For low and moderate users who have resigned themselves to living in a limited space, the drug warms and enlightens the day, takes the rough edges off life, and makes confinement more tolerable. Like the Brompton Cocktail (Carruthers, 1980), which contains cocaine and is prescribed for terminal cancer patients, the drug dulls pain and lightens the user's mood.

Despite intense and stubborn efforts, heavy users are unable to expand their spatial worlds. They find themselves sinking below the horizontal plane; they become depressed and turn to cocaine for salvation. Cocaine does not change their worlds, but it does expand the ego, lifting it up and out of confinement and creating a brief illusion that the expansion could be continued indefinitely.

Temporality

Temporality refers to the directional orientation (future, past) of life and to personal tempo, or the experience of time. The long-range temporal orientations of the men we studied were mixed. Two were living in the past. The first was locked in a life-long struggle with his father that should have ended years ago. The second had been a successful pimp but had a future only to the extent that he could restore the past. Three men (a crippled street hustler, a thief, and a cocaine dealer) lived in a protracted present. The other men (mostly heavy users) were future oriented to varying degrees. One was working toward becoming a studio musician; a second was striving for middle-class acceptability; while a third experienced religious conversion, stopped using cocaine, married, and began rebuilding his life. The last man lived in despair at the years he had wasted in the violent world of a ghetto cocaine dealer but was trying to create a future with some peace and serenity.

Tempo was not dominant in the lives of low- and moderate-level users. Time was generally experienced as slow, even sluggish. Since most of these men were going nowhere in particular, they seemed to move unhurriedly through life. All were able to stop, enjoy the moment, and take pleasure in an interesting experience without feeling that anything had been lost. In the ego state induced by low to moderate cocaine use, temporal events move more slowly than during abstinence but are tinged with a sensuous quality that enriches and enlivens them. The world seems brighter; the user feels bouyed up, more animated and carefree; music sounds better; people seem friendlier and more accessible; etc. Time flows slowly, but someone who takes pleasure in momentary experiences could hardly ask for more.

Time and events are experienced quite differently by heavy users. When not using cocaine these impatient men live in quick-paced, linear time, but only two were able to sustain efforts toward long-range goals. One was constantly attempting to slow time down and fill it with more and more activities. The other had learned (painfully) to pace his actions and was working toward a promised promotion. The rest were restless and impetuous individuals who seemed unable to direct their energies toward anything beyond immediate goals.

Heavy, intravenous use of cocaine produces striking alteration of experienced time. In the rush that follows injection, the user feels lifted beyond temporal existence to a point where time not only seems to slow down, it stops or freezes. ("You're above the world, out of time." "Time stops. It's irrelevant, meaningless." "When the coke's all gone you come back into time.") Because the passage of time seems to cease, the troublesome processes of mundane existence seem to cease also and therefore become completely unimportant to the user. He stops ruminating about the disappointments of his past, the frustrations of his present life, and his despair over prospects for the future. During the cocaine rush he believes, or wants to believe, that he has entered a permanent state of ecstasy. He feels he is in the Winner's Circle, and he wants to stay there eternally. Despite his wants, however, the state of ecstasy is transitory.

Afterward, like Tannhauser (Barto, 1916), the user may feel he has been touched by a goddess. As a result, temporal existence no longer holds any appeal for him. He is willing to struggle with day-to-day life only because he must do so to acquire money to buy cocaine: his return-trip ticket to the ethereal realm. For the heavy, chronic user, everyday life may become an alternating movement between linear time and apparent timelessness, but only the latter has any significant meaning.

Causality

Causality refers to the degree to which the person regards his world as ordered and lawful, and the extent to which he feels capable of influencing events in his life.

Though constantly struggling to control their own destinies, the cocaine users we studied live in a disorganized, unpredictable, and even paranoid world of primitive psychological causality or *participation mystique* (Levy-Bruhl, 1923, 1928). Cocaine users are men of the 20th century. Yet they live like the primordial Hunter, for whom strength and cunning, guile and deception, power and intimidation are necessary skills; and ability to quickly identify potential dangers, accurately assess the intentions of others, and act boldly and decisively is essential to success of even survival. Such a world is vital and exciting, but it is not controllable, for in this world, Chance, Luck, and Fate are integral elements of life.

For low- and moderate-level users, cocaine temporarily makes this world seem less frightening and overwhelming. However, cocaine mobilizes the heavy user; sharpens his vision, reaction time, and thinking; and makes him feel stronger, more powerful, and better able to cope with a world where a man with a weakness can be a victim.

Materiality

Materiality refers to the way the person experiences the primary and secondary qualities of his phenomenal world, the number and variety of objects it contains, and its textural quality (rough, sharp, smooth, jagged, etc.) as well as the properties of the medium through which psychological movement takes place (Ellenberger, 1958).

The chronic cocaine user lives in a richly furnished environment that seems ripe with possibilities. Yet, metaphorically speaking, it is a jungle: vital and alive; beautiful yet hazardous; frightening yet fascinating. As a jungle, this world is not clearly structured, and dangers may be hidden anywhere. Movement is difficult and energy draining, for the path is always treacherous. One must not lose his way and must be constantly alert, for an apparently tranquil scene can suddenly erupt into quick violence (one man we studied was slain during the research and another shortly thereafter).

The rules governing life in this civilized jungle are simple; only the fit, clever, and strong prevail. Low-level users are frightened by this dangerous environment and do not venture far from well-traveled trails. Heavy users are stimulated by the challenges and opportunities it offers and believe they can succeed in a world where every man is alone. For low and moderate cocaine users, cocaine makes the world seems brighter, more attractive and desirable, and less frightening. For the heavy user, it relieves depression, reassures him of his power and potency, and silently tells him he could rule it all, if he would but try.

Findings from Q-Sorts

Q-sort data fill out the picture of the ego state induced by cocaine and bring into focus some of the psychodynamic factors associated with its heavy, chronic use.

During *abstinence,* most cocaine users we studied appear (at first glance) to be satisfied with themselves. They approximate their own ideals, are the opposite of their worst selves, and see their ideal selves as polar opposites to their worst selves (usual self vs ideal self, r = .784; usual self vs worst self, r = −.570; ideal self vs worst self, r = −1.000; these and all subsequent values are median correlation coefficients, corrected for attenuation due to temporal instability of sequential sortings; values beyond ±1.000 are reported as ±1.000). However, the negative correlation between the ideal and worst self is too high and too rigid for healthy adjustment. It suggests that these men have not integrated the dark and potentially destructive components of their personalities into consciousness. Thus excluded or repressed, these elements (the Shadow: Jung, 1958) threaten to overwhelm the ego whenever the opportunity appears.

Low-level users see themselves as being like nonusers (usual self vs nonusers, r = .966). However, moderate and heavy users are ambivalent about people who do not use drugs. On one hand, they see nonusers as happy, friendly, and successful persons who can lean on others and are at peace with themselves. On the other hand, they look down upon nonusers as being clinging, dependent, and weak. They feel little in common with nonusers yet envy their successes and tend to idealize them for that reason (usual self vs nonusers, r = .203; ideal self vs nonusers, r = .703).

Two heavy users displayed patterns of relationships opposite to those one normally finds in Q-sort data. Both of these men expressed extreme dissatisfaction with themselves (usual self vs ideal self, r = −.712 and −.870, respectively).

Both had been successful cocaine dealers, both were experiencing extreme guilt, and both were strongly identified with their worst selves (usual self vs worst self, r = 1.000 and .951, respectively). For the first man (Tom P.), use of cocaine brought about a profound change, making him unlike his worst self and more like his ideal (cocaine self vs worst self, r = –.847; cocaine self vs ideal self, r = .771). The pattern reversed with the second (Willie M.). Cocaine made him less like his ideal and more like his worst self (cocaine self vs ideal self, r = –.949; cocaine self vs worst self, r = 1.000). One other person (Fred S.) became less like his ideal in the drug state. This individual, also a heavy user, was a seriously disturbed young man who used cocaine as a weapon in an ongoing struggle with his wealthy father. When using cocaine, this man's identity shifted to that of his worst self (usual self vs worst self, r = –.461; cocaine self vs worst self, r = .669), thus producing something akin to a transformation from a Dr. Jekyl to Mr. Hyde.

Two patterns were evident in the psychological state that precedes drug use. Low and moderate users described themselves in the *predrug state* as being happy, in charge, feeling good, friendly, mellow, and adventurous. Heavy users, however, experienced massive losses in self-regard in the period preceding drug use. These men entered a state characterized by erosion of self-control, inability to sustain the usual self, increased depression and despair, and flooding of consciousness with violent, hostile impulses; a state that could be described as the Arousal or Unchaining of the Worst Self. In the predrug state, these men became less like their usual or ideal selves and more like their Shadows (usual vs wanting cocaine self, r = .524; ideal self vs wanting cocaine self, r = –.279; and worst self vs wanting cocaine self, r = .451). When wanting cocaine, heavy users described themselves as depressed, uptight, lonely, weak, anxious, dependent, aggressive, ready to explode, sociopathic, cruel, violent, selfish, and vicious.

For most men, cocaine blocks emergence of the Worst Self and lifts the user out of depression or malaise. The drug not only restores the congruence between usual and ideal selves that existed during abstinence but elevates the user beyond this to a point where he feels even more complete than before. Most of the men described themselves in the *drug state* as being more like their usual and ideal selves, and more unlike their worst selves (usual self vs cocaine self, r = .905; ideal self vs cocaine self, r = .942; worst self vs cocaine self, r = –.871). In the cocaine ego state, they drop the negative and undesirable parts of themselves and briefly approximate their ideal.

Q-sort descriptions of the cocaine experience depict a state of exhilaration, elevation of mood, and a heightened sense of well-being and mastery. In this state, users say they are happy, satisfied, on top of things, successful, excited, intelligent, carefree, friendly, attractive, sensuous, charming, self-assured, romantic, open, easygoing, independent, relaxed, and mellow. One heavy user, a successful salesman, reported that in the drug state he was "on top of the world–

successful, rushing, high, strong, powerful, energetic, free, independent, and happy with what I am doing!"

Intravenous cocaine is equally powerful in temporarily eradicating negative feelings and emotions. In this ego state, most users report themselves as not being sad, hurting, depressed, lonely, laughed at, sexually impotent, wishy-washy, stupid, slow, afraid of women, inept, inadequate, weak, cruel, foolish, vicious, anxious, or dependent.

For low- and most moderate-level users, the *postdrug state* is a positive one in which users feel weak, but relaxed, easygoing, lazy, happy, successful, and self-controlled. They are not troubled by concerns over sexual adequacy, aggression, or even success and achievement; they are more at peace with themselves than during abstinence (usual self vs after-cocaine self, $r = .975$; ideal self vs after-cocaine self, $r = .706$; and worst self vs after-cocaine self, $r = -.748$). For heavy users, however, the state following drug use in one of anxiety, sadness, depression, loneliness, and even victimization (the user may feel like a clown or fool). Inner peace is gone, as are self-control, willpower, happiness, independence, and personal honor. In the postdrug state, these men are unlike their usual selves, are opposite to their ideals, and for all practical purposes are their Shadows (usual self vs after-cocaine self, $r = -.480$; ideal self vs after-cocaine self, $r = -.814$; and worst self vs after-cocaine self, $r = 1.000$). The depression and despair described in the postdrug state may be traced to the fact that while these intensely self-sufficient men were able to ward off their Shadows, they were able to do so only by reliance upon cocaine.

The cocaine experience is described as being similar, in some respects, to that induced by heavy use of amphetamine (cocaine self vs amphetamine self, median $r = .910$). However, none of the men who had tried amphetamine enjoyed it; most stated in interviews that it was too harsh and made them feel edgy and uncomfortable (Spotts and Shontz, 1980a).

Semantic Differential

Data from the Semantic Differential support observations from other sources. The men described cocaine as: *mighty, beautiful, bright, strong, exciting, fast, refreshing, pleasant, clean, active, successful, good, heathy*, and *secure*. Even Willie M., the man who hated (and feared) cocaine most, described it as *good, soft, bright, beautiful, fast, active, valuable,* and *vigorous.*

When asked to describe the color of the cocaine experience (not the drug but the experience), most heavy users interviewed in 1982 described it as a white experience (bright white, pure white, blue or clear white). They described the opiates experience as dark and heavy (dark blue to black), the amphetamine experience as yellow to bright orange, the barbiturate and sedative-hypnotic experience as black to gray, marijuana as blue to yellow, and psychedelics as multicolored.

DISCUSSION

Summary

With low to moderate intravenous use, cocaine mobilizes bodily processes and increases the user's sense of physical well-being. It reduces anxiety and heightens the distinctiveness of the ego, making the user feel more aggressive, optimistic, and self-assured. Heavy, chronic users experience similar effects but more intensely. The drug also helps the heavy user manage depression and dysphoria, and control anger, bitterness, and impulses to violence. It inflates his ego and produces exceptional feelings of exhaltation and power. The heavy, chronic user pays a price for these benefits, however, for what begins as a bright and exhilarating experience becomes transformed into a dark, tumultuous condition: Visual-motor functions become impaired, ego functions fail, emotionality careens out of control, and reality testing collapses. A toxic state follows, with paranoia; insomnia; delusions of persecution; and visual, auditory, and even tactile hallucinations.

Phenomenologically, the trajectory of heavy, intravenous use of cocaine is steeply upward, an *ascension* toward the upper rim of the Sphere of Life. Injection instantly catapults the user to ethereal realms where he experiences ecstatic feelings of Power, Dominion, and Superiority. For a moment, the opposites of the Universe seem to come together in a *hieros gamos,* or divine union of the masculine and feminine that produces an intoxicating illusion of unity and completion. Heavy intravenous use of cocaine produces an experience best described as spiritual; however, it is *counterfeit* (Spotts and Shontz, 1980b) and is by no means religious in the ordinary sense of the word. It propels the user toward a paradisical Dionysian state depicted in age-old myths of mortal man becoming a god.

Theoretical Integrations

In a structural model of drug-induced ego states, the present authors (Spotts and Shontz, 1980b) described the cocaine state as being similar to the amphetamine state, in being associated with aggressive action and tendencies toward paranoia, but as being different from the amphetamine state in being ecstatic rather than violent. Because ego expansion characterizes the cocaine state, it is the opposite of the states induced by opiates or barbiturate/sedative-hypnotics. Like psychedelic drugs, cocaine produces transcendence, but the cocaine-induced transcendence is predominantly emotional, while that induced by psychedelics is predominantly cognitive and perceptual.

To explain *why* users seek the cocaine state requires a developmental or motivational schema. The following discussion describes how cocaine fits the need systems of persons who practice low and heavy, chronic use of the drug.

Needs for social support, status, and peer influence appear to be primary reasons for low-level cocaine use (Spotts and Shontz, 1980a). The low-level users we studied are insecure persons, troubled by self-doubts and feelings of inadequacy; they are easygoing people who avoid conflict and intense emotionality. Cocaine helps them feel more self-assured, enhances social ralationships, warms and enlightens a dreary day, or provides brief escape from an otherwise dull existence. It these individuals could find more effective ways to obtain social support and affirmation, they could probably do quite well without the drug.

For heavy users, however, cocaine provides *direct support* to topologically central psychological needs (Lewin, 1935). These people are intense, achievement-oriented men who are determined to be completely self-sufficient; they are strong but isolated loners who equate dependence with submission, intimacy with vulnerability, and expressions of weakness as setting the stage for defeat at the hands of others (Spotts and Shontz, 1982). They are stubborn and willful men who are willing to struggle, overcome obstacles, and compete with others to achieve their goals. Most are economically successful; all resent authority and seek out occupations where supervision is minimal.

Heavy cocaine users attempt to live a Yang existence and avoid the passive, receptive Yin. Therefore, they never achieve unity or wholeness. They do not recognize that the energies of the active principle (Yang) require the support of the passive one (Yin) to give the active force its direction and form (Albertson, 1973; Whitmont, 1969). These men attempt to live a pure *Animus* existence (Jung, 1958); strive for perfection but sacrifice completeness; avoid dependence upon anyone, live in confinement, and find victory denied them. They struggle stubbornly to break free, conquer their worlds, and achieve the glory they feel they deserve, but they fail to recognize that they have themselves set the conditions that restrict their worlds and make victory impossible.

Cocaine serves diverse purposes in the lives of heavy users. It provides them the energy, drive, and optimism they need to continue their struggle to overcome a hostile world; it rewards their efforts and serves as a balm for injuries received. Cocaine seems almost perfect to them, for it reassures them that their decision to live in isolation is correct, and it reinforces their beliefs that they are powerful persons who need no one. The drug provides temporary escape from harsh reality, gives the user a taste of the Power and Dominion he might feel if he were able to fulfill his dreams of glory, and helps him believe that his struggle, though painful, is worthwhile. The heavy user tolerates the adverse effects of cocaine because the drug briefly lifts him out of depression, helps ward off the Shadow, and seems to promise fulfillment of a need for balance and unity (cf. Maslow's concept of meta-need, 1970). Given the illusions that it fosters for the heavy user, cocaine is a pharmacological substitute for, and impediment to, normal psychological growth and individuation (Spotts and Shontz, 1980b).

The lives of these men are dominated by a dream or personal myth, in which they are heroes engaged in a noble quest (Levinson, Darrow, Klein, Levinson, and McKee, 1978). Though some had difficulty persisting toward goals in the face of adversity, others were able to achieve a great deal. However, none could keep or enjoy success; their dreams of glory were either abandoned with bitterness and despair or led to the downfall, disgrace, or death of their perpetrator (Spotts and Shontz, 1982). The collapse of the dreams of these impatient and ambitious men has ready parallels in myths of mortals who attempted to be gods. One is reminded of Phaethon, the presumptuous son of Helios, who perished in a disastrous attempt to drive his father's Sun Chariot across the sky; or of Icarus, who, against his father's advice, flew too close to the sun and was destroyed. Another metaphor is the parallel between the cocaine psychosis and the casting down of Lucifer (the Shining One) who dared try to be the equal of God.

Low to moderate use of cocaine can be adequately explained by many theories including those based upon homeostasis, tension reduction, conditioning (Wikler, 1965, 1973, 1980), addiction to pleasure (Bejerot, 1972, 1980), learning (Frederick, 1972, 1980), self-esteem (Kaplan, 1980a, 1980b), or status strivings (Demarest, 1981). However, such theories are less useful in explaining heavy chronic use of cocaine, for at high use levels the steady state of the organism is deliberately disrupted; tension, fears, and anxieties increase rather than diminish, and the person becomes increasingly disorganized and confused.

Implications for Treatment

Van Dyke (1981) states that there is no effective method for treating cocaine dependence. We are more optimistic but feel that innovations in therapy are required. Heavy, chronic cocaine users are poor candidates for psychotherapy as long as they desire and have access to cocaine. It is unlikely these individuals will voluntarily seek treatment, and give up a drug that makes them feel good and wipes out depression and malaise, until they have undergone many painful experiences with the drug's Dark Side. However, some will accept psychotherapy after arrest, adjudication, and the offer of treatment as an alternative to imprisonment.

Our data suggest that older heavy users (those 37 years of age or more), men who have both achieved and suffered more, may be more amenable than younger ones. However, the heavy cocaine users of all ages are strong and resourceful men with intense desires to achieve. The problem is to deal with these needs in light of the peculiar psychological characteristics these individuals display.

Psychotherapy

The heavy cocaine users we studied are not anxious people, either consciously or unconsciously; their problems are more existential than adaptive. For this reason, a therapist who treats such individuals should not expect therapy to follow the same course it would in classical neurosis. Psychotherapy with heavy users of cocaine must deal with three main *manifest problems* and two *underlying themes.*

The most obvious manifest problem is the *counterdependence* of these men. Heavy cocaine users do not trust people; they strive to achieve complete independence through competitive success and domination. They have vowed to lean upon no one. They cannot be intimate with women, whom they only use and control, and they cannot be friends with men, whom they regard as competitors. A serious problem will be that of finding ways to hold these persons in therapy until some kind of effective transference can be established, for they are prone to bolt or terminate the relationship when they feel the slightest dependence upon the therapist.

The second problem is an *intense anger* that is externally oriented but not directed at any specific object. Anger serves a dual purpose in these men's lives. It supports their struggle against the world and justifies their antagonism toward other people. It is also a response to the frustration they feel when their attempts to achieve self-sufficiency fail. It recharges their energies and goads them to try even harder for success next time.

The third problem tends to appear only after the user begins to realize the futility of his efforts at conquest. This is the problem of *despair,* and it is reflected in feelings of defeat, helplessness, bitterness, and disappointment. Despair may manifest itself in depressive symptoms, but its cause is not self-blame or guilt but a sense of futility, helplessness, and failure, for which the world is usually held at fault.

These three problems result from and feed into the first underlying theme, which is *betrayal.* We believe the intense counterdependence of these men stems from their infantile belief in the divinity of the mother imago and their subsequent sense of betrayal when this belief was destroyed by bitter experience. When children, these men reached out for affection, nurturance, intimacy, or support, but were subjected to embarrassment, humiliation, or even rejection by a stern mother. They withdrew and vowed to become strong and self-sufficient Warriors who would need to lean upon no one. As adults, they avoid personal closeness with women, for they fear the tyrant mother in every women they see. Developmentally, they also feel betrayed by their fathers, who were too weak to prepare their sons adequately to deal with the world at large.

The psychodynamic appeal of the cocaine state derives largely from its archetypal spiritual quality. In suitably predisposed individuals, it has the power to attract deep-seated, preverbal fantasies and arouse infantile states of Oedipal longing. The drug, therefore, has a special attraction for heavy users who believe they see the end to their betrayal in the promise of ecstatic reunion with the Eternal Feminine (a spiritual Anima: Jung, 1956), and they pursue this with all the deadly persistence of a genuine *repetition compulsion* (Freud, 1929).

Heavy cocaine users are like knights errant who are on a Great Quest, but many are too poorly armed and lack the skills they need to slay the dragons they meet, and those who do succeed are dismayed when they eventually find that the Grail they seek in not a divine vessel but only a drug, or an ordinary mortal woman. Like the fatherless knight Parsefal, in Chrétien Troye's account of the Grail myth, they are unable to possess the Grail because they have not completely broken free from the coercive power of the mother of childhood (R.A. Johnson, 1974; Spotts and Shontz, 1982).

Yet they cannot give up the Quest, for they suffer an even more fundamental deficiency. These men are unable to distinguish between that which is divine and that which is mundane. They spend their lives trying to become gods and yearning for paradise in a world where gods do not exist and chemical pleasure is the best that they can find.

Heavy cocaine users, like all people, have deep spiritual needs that are as important as, sometimes more important than, physical or psychological needs. Because they vigorously deny these needs, these men are victimized by their own *spirituality*. This is the second experiential theme. These men vainly attempt to take onto themselves attributes reserved for deities and to convert a chemical substance into an object of worship. The only therapeutic way out of their despair is for them to recognize the reality of their spiritual needs and to turn them toward more appropriate goals. To facilitate this, the therapist must help the person recognize and give up his equation of the cocaine state with divine ecstasy and his adoration of the drug as if it were a goddess. In addition, the patient needs to learn how, and discover what, to worship: to find something that is truly divine for him and that will satisfy his need for dependence on spiritual power.

Another major task will be to help the heavy cocaine user integrate important elements of his Shadow into consciousness so that it can become an ally instead of a demonic force that threatens to destroy. The Gordian Knot linking dependence to domination must also be severed. In addition, the therapist must help the user free the Anima from the subverting influence of the maternal figure so that he can come to see women as persons in their own rights and not just as faded daguerreotypes of the mother of childhood. Finally, the client must acknowledge and accept the limitations and frailties of all human beings, himself included. All in all, the therapist must help the heavy cocaine user come to recognize and accept his own humanity (warts, Shadow, and all) for only then will he have a chance of finding peace or contentment.

PRACTICAL AND SOCIAL IMPLICATIONS AND RECOMMENDATIONS

The practical and social implications of our findings are best considered following a preliminary consideration of some properties of cocaine and the persons who are most at risk for its heavy, chronic abuse.

Properties of Cocaine as a Substance of Abuse

Both users' reports and Q-sort data indicate that cocaine, at all use levels, is an *overcompensating drug* that carries the user to a pleasurable point well above his typical abstinence state. However, despite its reputation as the caviar of drugs, our findings indicate that cocaine is the *most unsatisfying drug* of all the major substances of abuse. It induces ecstatic experiences, but it does not and can never produce satisfaction, completion, or fulfillment. After a hungry person has eaten a meal, hunger is diminished and he feels contented; after the sexual act, people feel calm and the desire for sex recedes. However, use of cocaine produces no comparable sense of contentment or completion; its only residual is the desire for more. To bowdlerize a phrase from the soft-drink industry, "Coke is *not* it," for it *cannot* satisfy.

Cocaine is like a woman who leads her lover on with foreplay and then refuses consummation. Heavy, intravenous use of cocaine (and apparently free basing and heavy insufflation as well) produces an experience so close to completeness that the user feels compelled to return again and again, hoping that ultimate consummation will occur. It may be, however, that this sought-for union with the "divine goddess" is more like union with a black widow spider: attainable only with death.

Cocaine is a seductive and intensely coercive drug, one of the most powerful pharmacological reinforcers known. Animals conditioned to self-inject it will undergo prolonged bouts of intoxication, and when unlimited quantities of the drug are available it kills with amazing speed and regularity, sometimes in less than a week (Deneau, Yanigita, and Seevers, 1969; C.E. Johanson, Balster, and Bonese, 1976; Thompson and Pickens, 1970; Woods, 1977; Woods and Downs, 1973; Yanigita, 1973). Heavy use of cocaine by humans also produces an intense compulsion to continue its use (Eiswirth et al., 1972; Jeri et al., 1978; Noya, 1978; Spotts and Shontz, 1980a). Even among those who practice insufflation, any amount of cocaine set out at a social gathering gets used, and it is unheard of for any to be left over (Grinspoon and Bakalar, 1976). Although most recreational use is by insufflation, nasal ingestion of cocaine is sometimes associated with heavy consumption (up to 3 g/day). The effects of heavy use of this drug are equally debilitating, regardless of the mode of intake.

A number of investigators have commented on the similarity of the effects of cocaine and amphetamine (Bejerot, 1970; Fischman, Schuster, and Krasnegor,

1977; Jaffe, 1970; Kramer, Fischman, and Littlefield, 1967), and our studies confirm some of these similarities. However, careful analysis reveals that these two sympathomimetics produce ego states with distinctively different characteristics. A detailed discussion of some of these differences is presented elsewhere (Spotts and Shontz, 1980a).

Persons at Risk

The following discussion does not concern low-level, social-recreational users, who display diverse personality patterns, nor does it necessarily apply to the heavy cocaine users described in South American studies (Jeri et al., 1978; Noya, 1978).

To the extent that our data justify extrapolation, they suggest that the persons most at risk for heavy, chronic cocaine use in the United States are not the weak, emotionally disturbed, or deprived, but are strong and resourceful persons who epitomize many of the modal values of our society. Persons most at risk are typically White, aged 20-44 (the "years of achievement"), and well educated. Most have completed at least 1-2 years of college and some have advanced degrees. Those who come from minority groups may demonstrate somewhat lower academic achievement but are similar to heavy, chronic White users in most other regards. Individuals at risk come from intact (but conflicted) low- to upper-middle-class families which place emphasis upon striving, success, and achievement. They are strong, ambitious, intensely competitive persons who have difficulty with intimacy and whose lives are built upon opposition to dependencies of any kind. Many come to use of cocaine after previous experience with amphetamine or other sympathomimetics. A continuing struggle against underlying chronic depression increases vulnerability.

The at-risk individual, though sexually active, has difficulties with mutual relationships with members of the other sex and is probably single. Marriage, if undertaken, is most often short-lived and childless. Conversely, a stable marriage with children is a positive prognostic sign. In our opinion, men who have discovered satisfactory representatives of their Mother Imago, their Animas (Jung, 1958), in the real world and find intimacy with women gratifying are unlikely to become heavy, chronic users of cocaine.

At-risk individuals tend to be bright, hard working, and economically successful. They judge other people in terms of competence and self-sufficiency, and tend to be contemptuous of passive individuals or persons with strong affectional needs. They strive for perfection and are intolerant of weaknesses or frailties in themselves or others. They have problems functioning as "team players," have difficulties accepting authority, and gravitate to occupations where opportunities for independent action are maximal, supervision is minimal, and a person can attribute success to his/her own efforts. Typically, they are self-employed or in occupations such as sales, advertising, consulting, acting, or writing, or in professions such as law, dentistry, or medicine, which permit some autonomy of action.

Given this characterization, it is hardly surprising to find media reports of heavy cocaine abuse among actors and actresses, movie directors, dancers, professional athletes, business executives, and other persons in occupations where emphasis is placed upon competition, achievement, and success at almost any price (Demarest, 1981; Don Reese with John Underwood, 1982).

Not all such persons will become heavy users of cocaine. The traits described here are highly regarded in Western society and are present in many highly successful persons who never use illicit drugs. This description suggests only that, if provided the opportunity to experience the effects associated with heavy use of cocaine, individuals with the characteristics described will be more vulnerable than persons of other types.

Recommendations

Research

Research efforts must be intensified to identify the factors contributing to the lethality of cocaine. The conditions associated with fatal reactions to the drug are not known. Social planning would benefit greatly from thorough, case-by-case investigations of cocaine-related fatalities (Gottschalk, McGuire, Dinovo, Birch, and Heiser, 1977) which will permit investigators to tease out the factors contributing to deaths from use of this drug. For example, recent research suggests that serum cholinesterase may play a significant role in the metabolism of cocaine (Inaba et al., 1978). It would be important to know whether individuals deficient in this substance are overrepresented in cocaine-related fatalities.

Thorough and carefully designed naturalistic studies of humans who regularly use different dosages of cocaine (with different methods of administration) are needed to indentify the levels at which adverse physical or psychological effects appear. A number of investigators (Ashley, 1975; Sabbag, 1976; Waldorf, Murphy, Reinerman, and Bridget, 1977), who studied only low-dose, recreational cocaine users (snorters), found no evidence of serious adverse effects and concluded that such effects were "myths." However, Spotts and Shontz (1980a) found that cocaine produces diverse and even contradictory effects at differing dosage levels, with increasing psychopathology at higher levels. Noya (1978) also found that heavy, chronic use of relatively pure cocaine produces strikingly different effects than low-dose, episodic use. Recent studies in the United States, Boliva, and Peru demonstrate that heavy, chronic use of cocaine can produce anxiety; insomnia and anorexia; inability to maintain gainful employment; deep depression, with suicidal ideas and intentions; convulsions; hallucinations;

and a paranoid psychosis sufficiently debilitating to require hospitalization (Jeri et al., 1987; Noya, 1978; Spotts and Shontz, 1980a).

In 1975 only two men we studied knew anyone who had died a cocaine-related death. A much higher incidence of cocaine-related fatalities was reported by heavy intravenous users interviewed in 1982. Those who engage in the increasingly popular practice of free basing ingest cocaine of a higher purity and reportedly ingest more of it in shorter time spans than injectors. Free basing therefore may produce more adverse effects and increase the risk of lethality. The comparative hazards of these two methods of drug administration should be investigated.

Social Policy

To the extent that efforts of drug enforcement personnel keep the price of cocaine high and restrict its widespread availability, they reduce health hazards associated with its use. Byck (1980) and Grinspoon (1980) assert that occasional, low-level use of cocaine poses no serious health hazard; our position, however, is more conservative. Cocaine can kill, but the factors contributing to its lethality have not been identified. This is reason enough to argue that cocaine endangers those who use it. However, the most serious and debilitating effects associated with use of cocaine occur in persons who practice its heavy, chronic use. Cocaine is intensely coercive. If it were readily available at low prices the social costs would be enormous. It is generally believed that cocaine is not physically addictive, but it might as well be, for with heavy use, by any route of intake, psychological dependency develops very quickly. Even with the drug at current prices of $100-$130 or more per gram, clinics across the country are seeing increasing numbers of persons who have lost their jobs, marriages, and families as a direct or indirect result of their involvement with cocaine. Incidents of this sort would increase markedly were the drug more readily available.

Efforts to "decriminalize" cocaine would be inappropriate at this time. We restate the position we took in an earlier publication (Spotts and Shontz, 1980a). "First, cocaine in not benign; when used in excess it can produce paranoia, hallucinations, and psychosis. Second, while the current practice of 'snorting' small amounts may seem safe enough, even 'snorting' can kill. . . . Efforts should be made to better define the parameters of risk with cocaine prior to efforts to alter its legal status" (p. 461).

The media should be encouraged to use restraint and sound judgment in reports about cocaine. Media reports should be factual and evenhanded, and should provide the public with as much reliable information about the drug, its effects, and the hazards associated with its use as possible; otherwise, such reports will not serve the public interest. Some reports, though probably well intended, associate cocaine with the jet set, the "glitter people" and the successful, and only increase the drug's appeal to vulnerable individuals by linking use of cocaine to status strivings.

The most effective long-run strategy to reduce misuse and abuse of cocaine would be to rob the drug of its status. Successful advertising firms gross millions of dollars per year by attaching status to consumer products. If advertising techniques can augment the status of consumer products, they can also reduce it. Well-designed image-altering campaigns could go far to reduce cocaine's appeal, desirability, and attractiveness. At least six negative attributes of cocaine could be stressed to bring about its discountenance. First, the drug is extremely expensive. Second, the cocaine experience, though intense, is ephemeral. Third, the drug cannot produce any sense of satisfaction or completion. Fourth, cocaine's effects are counterfeit, for they produce no changes in personal structure that outlast the drug experience. Fifth, cocaine is a coercive substance that all but demands that the individual use more and more; and sixth, it can kill.

ACKNOWLEDGMENTS

This research program has been supported by contracts and grants from the Psychological Sciences Division of the National Institute on Drug Abuse. The authors wish to thank Dr. Daniel J. Lettieri for his encouragement and helpful suggestions.

REFERENCES

ALBERTSON, E. *Understanding the Kabbalah*. Los Angeles, CA: Sherbourne Press, 1973.

ASHLEY, R. *Cocaine: Its History, Uses, and Effects.* New York: St. Martin's Press, 1975.

BARASH, P.G. Cocaine in clinical medicine. In R.C. Peterson and R.C. Stillman (eds.), *Cocaine: 1977* (NIDA Research Monogr. No. 13, DHEW Publ. No. (ADM) 74-432). Washington, DC: U.S. Government Printing Office, 1977, pp. 193-200.

BARASH, P.G. KOPRIVA, C.J., LANGOU, R., VAN DYKE, C., JATLOW, P., STAHL, A., and BYCK, R. Is cocaine a sympathetic stimulant during general anesthesia? *J. Am. Med. Assoc.* 243: 1437, 1980.

BARTO, P.S. *Tannhauser and the Mountain of Venus.* New York: Oxford University Press, American Branch, 1916.

BEJEROT, N.A. A comparison of the effects of cocaine and synthetic central stimulants. *Br. J. Addict.* 65: 35-37, 1970.

BEJEROT, N. *Addiction: An Artificially Induced Drive*. Springfield, IL: C.C. Thomas, 1972.

BEJEROT, N. Addiction to pleasure: A biological and social-psychological theory of addiction. In D.J. Lettieri, M. Sayers, and H.W. Pearson (eds.), *Theories of Drug Abuse: Selected Contemporary Perspectives* (NIDA Research Monogr. No. 30, DHHS Publ. No. (ADM) 80-967). Washington, DC: U.S. Government Printing Office, 1980.

BEWLEY, T. Heroin and cocaine addiction. *Lancet* 738: 808-810, 1965.

BRILL, H., and HIROSE, T. The rise and fall of a methamphetamine epidemic: Japan 1945-1955. *Sem. Psychiatry* 1: 179-194, 1969.

BROTMAN, R., and FREEDMAN, A.M. *A Community Mental Health Approach to Drug Addiction* (Juv. Del. Publ. No. 9005). Washington, DC: U.S. Government Printing Office,1969.

BYCK, R. (ed.). *Cocaine Papers: Sigmund Freud.* New York: Stonehill, 1974.

BYCK, R. Cocaine: A major drug issue of the seventies. In *Testimony before Select Committee on Narcotic Abuse and Control, House of Representatives, Ninety-Sixth Congress, First Session, July 24-October 10, 1979* (SCNAC-96-1-9). Washington, DC: U.S. Government Printing Office, 1980, pp. 58-69.

CARRUTHERS, S.G. Clinical pharmacology of pain. In W.L. Smith, H. Mersky, and S.C. Gross (eds.), *Pain: Meaning and Management.* New York: Spectrum Publications, 1980, pp. 89-103.

CHOPRA, R.N., and CHOPRA, G.S. Cocaine habit in India. *Indian J. Med. Res.* 18: 1013-1046, 1930/1931.

CLARK, R. Cocaine. *Texas Med.* 69: 74-78, 1973.

COHEN, S. *The Substance Abuse Problem.* New York: Haworth Press, 1981, pp. 75-80.

CONNELL, P.H. Drug taking in Great Britian: A growing problem. *Roy. Soc. Prom. Health* 89: 92-96, 1969.

DEMAREST, M. Cocaine: Middle class high. *Time* 118: 56-63, 1981.

DENEAU, G.W., YANAGITA, T., SEEVERS, M.H. Self-administration of psychoactive substances by the monkey: A measure of psychological dependence. *Psychopharmacologia* 16: 30-48, 1969.

EISWIRTH, N.A., SMITH, D.E., and WESSON, D.R. Current perspectives on cocaine use. *Am. J. Psychedelic Drugs* 5: 153-157, 1972.

ELLENBERGER, H.F. A clinical introduction to psychiatric phenomenology and existential analysis. In R. May, E. Angel, and H. F. Ellenberger (eds.), *Existence.* New York: Basic Books, 1958.

ELLINWOOD, E.H. Jr. The epidemiology of stimulant abuse. In E. Josephson and E.E. Carroll (eds.), *Drug Abuse–Epidemiological and Sociological Approaches.* Washington, DC: Hemisphere, 1974, pp. 303-329.

FINKLE, B.S., and MC CLOSKY, K.L. The forensic toxicology of cocaine. In R.C. Peterson and R.C. Stillman (eds.), *Cocaine: 1977* (NIDA Research Monogr. No. 13, DHEW Publ. No. (ADM) 77-432). Washington, DC: U.S. Printing Office, 1977, pp. 153-192.

FISCHMAN, M.W., SCHUSTER, C.R., and KRASNEGOR, N.A. Physiological and behavioral effects of intravenous cocaine in man. In E.H. Ellinwood, Jr., and M.M. Kilbey (eds.), *Cocaine and Other Stimulants.* New York: Plenum Press, 1977, pp. 646-664.

FISCHMAN, M.W., SCHUSTER, C.R. RESNEKOV, L., SCHICK, J.F.E. KRASNEGOR, N.A. FENNELL, W., and FREEDMAN, D.X. Cardiovascular and subjective effects of intravenous cocaine administration in humans. *Arch. Gen. Psychiatry.* 33: 983-989, 1976.

FREDERICK, C.J. Drug abuse as self-destructive behavior. *Drug Therapy* 2: 49-68, 1972.

FREDERICK, C.J. Drug abuse as learned behavior. In D.J. Lettieri, M. Sayers, and H.W. Pearson (eds.), *Theories of Drug Abuse: Selected Contemporary Perspectives* (NIDA Research Monogr. No. 30, DHHS Publ. No. (ADM) 80-967). Washington, DC: U.S. Government Printing Office, 1980.

FREUD, S. *Beyond the Pleasure Principle* (J. Strachey, trans.). New York: Liveright, 1929.

GAY, G.R., SHEPPARD, C.W., INABA, D.S., and NEWMEYER, J.A. Cocaine perspective: Gift from the sun god to the rich man's drug. *Drug Forum* 2: 409-430, 1973.

GOTTSCHALK, L.A. MC GUIRE, F.L., DINOVO, E.C., BIRCH, H., and HEISER, J.F. (eds.). *Guide to the Investigation and Reporting of Drug Abuse Deaths: Problems and Methods* (National Institute on Drug Abuse, DHEW Publ. No. (ADM) 77-386). Washington, DC: U.S. Government Printing Office, 1977.

GRINSPOON, L. Cocaine: A major drug issue of the seventies. In *Testimony before Select Committee on Narcotic Abuse and Control, House of Representatives, Ninety-Sixth Congress, First Session, July 24-October 10, 1979* (SCNAC-96-1-9). Washington, DC: U.S. Government Printing Office, 1980, pp. 46-58.

GRINSPOON, L., and BAKALAR, J.B. *Cocaine: A Drug and Its Social Evolution.* New York: Basic Books, 1976.

GWYNNE, P. The cocaine high: Dangerous new drug of the 80s. *Glamour* 80(8): 280-312, 1982.

HOLLINGSHEAD, A.B. *The Two-Factor Index of Social Position.* New Haven, CN: Yale University Press, 1957/1965.

INABA, T., STEWART, J., and KALOW, W. Metabolism of cocaine in man. *Clin. Pharm. Ther.* 23: 547, 1978.

INGE, G. The present state of abuse and addiction to stimulant drugs in Sweden. In F. Sjoqvist and M. Tottie (eds.), *Abuse of Central Stimulants.* New York: Raven Press, 1969, pp. 187-214.

JAFFE. J.H. Drug addiction and drug abuse. In L.S. Goodman and A. Gilman (eds.), *The Pharmacological Basis of Therapeutics* (4th ed.). New York: Macmillan, 1970, pp. 276-313.

JERI, F.R., SANCHES, C., DEL POZO, L., and FERNANDEZ, M. El sindrome de la pasta de coca: Observaciones en un grupo de 158 pacientes del area del Lima. *Rev. Sanid. Minesterio Interior* (Peru), 39: 1, 1978.

JOHANSON, C.E., BALSTER, R.L., and BONESE, K. Self administration of psychomotor stimulant drugs: The effects of unlimited access. *Pharm. Biochem. Behav.* 4: 45-51, 1976.

JOHNSON, R.A. *He: Understanding Masculine Psychology.* New York: Harper and Row, 1974.

JUNG, C.G. *Symbols of Transformation* (Bolingen Series No. 20) Princeton, NJ: Princeton University Press, 1956.

JUNG, C.G. Aion. In V.S. deLaszlo (ed.), *Psyche and Symbol: A Selection from the Writings of C.G. Jung.* New York: Doubleday Anchor Books, 1958.

KAPLAN, H.B. Self-esteem and self-derogation theory of drug abuse. In D.J. Lettieri, M. Sayers, and H.W. Pearson (eds.), *Theories of Drug Abuse: Selected Theoretical Perspectives.* (NIDA Research Monogr. No. 30, DHHS Publ. No. (ADM) 80-967). Washington, DC: U.S. Government Printing Office, 1980a.

KAPLAN, H.B. *Deviant Behavior in Defense of Self.* New York: Academic Press, 1980b.

KOZEL, N.J., CRIDER, R.A., and ADAMS, E.H. National surveillance of cocaine use and related health consequences. In *Morbidity and Mortality Weekly Report* (MMWR), U.S. Department of Health and Human Services 31: 265-273, 1982.

KRAMER, J.C., FISCHMAN, V.A., and LITTLEFIELD, D.C. Amphetamine abuse: Patterns and effects of high doses taken intravenously. *J. Am. Med. Assoc.* 201: 89-93, 1967.

LEVINSON, D.J., DARROW, C.N., KLEIN, E.B., LEVINSON, M.H., and MC KEE, B. *The Seasons of a Man's Life.* New York: Ballantine Books, 1978.

LEVY-BRUHL, L. *Primitive Mentality.* London: G. Allen and Unwin, 1923.

LEVY-BRUHL, L. *The Soul of the Primitive.* New York: Macmillan, 1928.

LEWIN, K. *A Dynamic Theory of Personality: Selected Papers.* New York: McGraw-Hill, 1935.

LING, G.M., and DEL PRADO, J.G. International challenge of drug abuse: A perspective from the United Nations. In R.C. Peterson (ed.), *The International Challenge of Drug Abuse* (NIDA Research Monogr. No. 19, DHEW Publ. No. (ADM) 78-654). Washington, DC: U.S. Government Printing Office, 1978, pp. 60-68.

MASLOW, A.H. *Motivation and Personality* (2nd ed.). New York: Harper and Row, 1970.

NOYA, N.D. Coca and cocaine: A perspective from Bolivia. In R.C. Petersen (ed.), *The International Challenge of Drug Abuse* (NIDA Research Monogr. No. 19, DHEW Publ. No. (ADM) 78-654). Washington, DC: U.S. Government Printing Office, 1978, pp. 82-90.

POST, R.M. Cocaine psychosis: A continuum model. *Am. J. Psychiatry* 132: 225-231, 1975.

POST, R.M., KOTIN, J., and GOODWIN, R. The effects of cocaine on depressed patients. *Am. J. Psychiatry* 131: 511-517, 1974.

REESE, D., with UNDERWOOD, J. I'm not worth a damn. *Sports Illustrated* 56(24): 66-82, 1981.

RITCHIE, J.M., COHEN. D.J., and DRIPPS, R.D. Cocaine, procaine, and other synthetic local anesthetics. In L.S. Goodman and A. Gilman (eds.), *The Pharmacological Basis of Therapeutics.* New York: Macmillan, 1970, pp. 371-401.

SABBAG, R. *Snow blind.* New York: Avon Books, 1976.

SHONTZ, F.C. *Research Methods in Personality.* New York: Appleton-Century-Crofts, 1965.

SHONTZ, F.C. Single-organism designs. In P.M. Bentler, D.J. Lettieri, and G.A. Austin (eds.), *Data Analysis Strategies and Designs for Substance Abuse Research* (NIDA Research Issues No. 113, DHEW Publ. No. (ADM) 77-389). Washington, DC: U.S. Government Printing Office, 1977.

SIEGEL, R.K. Cocaine smoking [letter]. *New Engl. J. Med.* 1: 373, 1979.

SIEGEL, R.K. Freebase cocaine: Hazards and costly habit. *ADAMHA News* 7: 3, 1980.

SPOTTS, J.V., and SHONTZ, F.C. *Cocaine Users: A Representative Case Approach.* New York: Free Press, 1980a.

SPOTTS, J.V. and SHONTZ, F.C. A life-theme theory of chronic drug abuse. In D.J. Lettieri, M. Sayers, and H.W. Pearson (eds.), *Theories of Drug Abuse: Selected Contemporary Perspectives* (NIDA Research Monogr. No. 30, DHHS Publ. No. (ADM) 80-967). Washington, DC: U.S. Government Printing Office, 1980b, pp. 59-70.

SPOTTS, J.V. and SHONTZ, F.C. Research findings on cocaine use. In G. Volger (ed.), *Rapture and Reality: Drug Use in Cross-Cultural Perspective.* Cologne, West Germany: Museen der Stadt Koln, 1981.

SPOTTS, J.V. and SHONTZ, F.C. Ego development, dragon fights, and chronic drug abusers. *Int. J. Addict.* 17(6): 945-976, 1982.

SPOTTS, J.V. and SHONTZ, F.C. Psychopathology and chronic drug use: A methodological paradigm. *Int. J. Addict.* 18(8): 633-680, 1983.

THOMPSON, T., and PICKENS, R. Stimulating self-administration by animals: Some comparisons with opiate self-administration. *Fed. Proc.* 29: 6-12, 1970.

UNITED STATES DEPARTMENT OF JUSTICE. Drug Enforcement Administration. Cocaine trafficking trends in Europe. *Drug Enforcement* 9: 21-22, 1982.

VAN DYKE, C. Cocaine. In J.H. Lowinson and P. Ruiz (eds.), *Substance Abuse: Clinical Problems and Perspectives.* Baltimore, MD: Williams and Wilkins, 1981, pp. 158-166.

VAN DYKE, C., BARASH, P.G., JATLOW, P., and BYCK, R. Cocaine: Plasma concentrations after intranasal application in man. *Science* 191: 859, 1976.

WALDORF, D., MURPHY, S., REINERMAN, C., and BRIDGET, J. *Doing Coke: An Ethnography of Cocaine Users and Sellers.* Washington, DC: Drug Abuse Council, 1977, pp. 16-68.

WESSON, D.R., and SMITH, D.E. Cocaine: Its use for central nervous system stimulation inducing recreational and medical uses. In R.C. Petersen and R.C. Stillman (eds.), *Cocaine: 1977* (NIDA Research Monogr. No. 13, DHEW Publ. No. (ADM) 77-432). Washington, DC: U.S. Government Printing Office, 1977, pp. 137-152.

WETLI, C.V. Cocaine: A major drug issue of the seventies. In *Testimony before Select Committee on Narcotic Abuse and Control, House of Representatives, Ninety-Sixth Congress, First Session, July 24-October 10, 1979* (SCNAC-96-1-9). Washington, DC: U.S. Government Printing Office, 1980, pp. 69-81.

WETLI, C.V., and WRIGHT, R.K. Deaths caused by recreational cocaine use. *J. Am. Med. Assoc.* 241: 2519-2522, 1979.

WHITMONT, E.C. *The Symbolic Quest: Basic Concepts of Analytic Psychology.* Princeton, NJ: Princeton University Press, 1969.

WIKLER, A. Conditioning factors in opiate addiction and relapse. In D.M. Wilner and G.G. Kassenbaum (eds.), *Narcotics.* New York: McGraw-Hill, 1965.

WIKLER, A. Dynamics of drug dependence: Implications of a conditioning theory for research and treatment. *Arch. Gen. Psychiatry* 28: 611-616, 1973.

WIKLER, A. A theory of opioid dependence. In D.J. Lettieri, M. Sayers, and H.W. Pearson (eds.), *Theories of Drug Abuse: Selected Contemporary Perspectives* (NIDA Research Monogr. No. 30, DHHS Publ. No. (ADM) 80-967). Washington, DC: U.S. Government Printing Office, 1980.

WOODS, J. Behavioral effects of cocaine in animals. In R.C. Petersen and R.C. Stillman (eds.), *Cocaine: 1977* (NIDA Research Monogr. No. 13, DHEW Publ. No. (ADM) 77-432). Washington, DC: U.S. Government Printing Office, 1977, pp. 116-139.

WOODS, J.H., and DOWNS, D.A. The psychopharmacology of cocaine. In National Commission on Marihuana and Drug Abuse, *Drugs in America: Problems in Perspective. Appendix Vol. 1: Patterns and Consequences of Drug Use.* Washington, DC: U.S. Government Printing Office, 1973, pp. 116-139.

YANAGITA, T. An experimental framework for the evaluation of dependency liability of various types of drugs in monkeys. *Bull. Narcotics* 1: 25-57, 1973.

The International Journal of the Addictions, 19(2), 153–173, 1984

Paraprofessional Versus Professional Drug Counselors: Diverse Routes to the Same Role

Leona S. Aiken,* PhD

Leonard A. LoSciuto, PhD

Mary Ann Ausetts, MA

Institute for Survey Research, and
Psychology Department
Temple University
Philadelphia, Pennsylvania 19122

Barry S. Brown, PhD

National Institute on Drug Abuse
Rockville, Maryland 20857

Abstract

The backgrounds and roles of ex-addict (EXA) and non-ex-addict (NEA) paraprofessional methadone maintenance and drug-free outpatient counselors were contrasted with those of degreed professional counselors (PRO). There was no evidence of differential assignment of clients to counselors based on drug use, drug treatment, criminal, educational, and employment histories. The three counselor groups were remarkably similar in their participation in 11 areas of job activities ranging from counseling duties per se through administrative

*To whom requests for reprints should be sent at the Institute for Survey Research, Temple University, Philadelphia, Pennsylvania 19122.

 0020-773X/84/1902-0153$3.50/0

support functions. The only reliable difference was the greater involvement of EXAs in counseling and community education activities which took them outside the program.

This study contrasts the roles, functions, and activities of the three different counselor groups who currently provide treatment in drug abuse programs. The first group consists of professional counselors who hold at least a bachelor's degree and who do not have addict backgrounds (PROs). Second are ex-addict paraprofessional counselors who often do not hold a bachelor's degree (EXAs). Third are non-ex-addict paraprofessionals who neither hold a bachelor's degree nor have a history of drug addiction (NEAs). The employment of individuals with such diversity of training and experiential backgrounds in drug programs stems from the 1960s. The proliferation of drug treatment programs led to the hiring of ex-addicts in an advisory and counseling capacity (Deitch, 1974; Flores and Rice, 1974); a more general service expansion in the face of professional manpower shortages, to the exployment of non-ex-addict paraprofessionals (Gartner and Riessman, 1974; Grosser, 1969; Social and Rehabilitation Service, 1974).

It is conceivable that the diversity of backgrounds of the three counselor groups had led to role specialization in terms of counselor-related tasks and clients served. It was the major purpose of this study to examine these roles, both to enrich our knowledge of drug counseling as it is now practiced and to provide input for policy and program staff at federal and local levels. The second purpose was methodological, that is, to determine whether the tasks performed and clients served were so diverse across couselor groups as to undermine the examination of differential effectiveness of these counselor groups. When either the treatment or clients or both differ across comparison groups, the internal validity of any design evaluating outcomes is threatened (Cook and Campbell, 1979; Luborsky, Singer, and Luborsky, 1975). Such a problem exists throughout the literature on the evaluation of treatment provided by paraprofessionals versus professionals (Nietzel and Fisher, 1981).

For this study, counseling in both methadone maintenance and drug-free outpatient programs was examined. The programs chosen were primarily ones in which the three counselor groups were simultaneously employed. This was a critical point of design, since it permitted potentially maximum divergence of roles to occur. In programs employing only one type of counselor, there would, of course, be no opportunity for diversification, since whatever counselors were employed would have to perform all the functions of the counselor role. To maximize the distinction between the PRO and EXA groups, it was also required that EXAs not hold a bachelor's degree.

Finally, the present study was also designed to have strong statistical power in terms of the sample sizes of counselor and clients, since much of the comparative literature of professionals versus paraprofessionals suffers from the comparison of very few counselors in each group. In an area in which null results have been commonly found (Durlak, 1979), the interpretation of these null results is burdened severely by the problem of Type 2 error (Nietzel and Fisher, 1981).

METHOD

Programs

Fifteen programs, nine methadone maintenance and six drug-free outpatient programs, participated. In addition, a 16th program with separate methadone maintenance and drug-free units was also employed. The 16 programs were in five major cities or surrounding areas–New York; Washington, DC; Chicago; Los Angeles; and San Francisco.

Respondents and Procedures

Counselors, clients, and administrators were interviewed in person for 1, 1.5, and 1 hour each, respectively, with clients paid $10 for participation. The counselors–31 PRO, 20 NEA, 31 EXA–were all full-time workers with a caseload of approximately 25 or more clients for whom they had primary responsibility for the treatment regimen. The clients–116 of PROs, 71 of NEAs, and 115 of EXAs–were randomly chosen by the study staff from the caseloads of each counselor, with the aim being to interview four clients of each counselor; the number of clients interviewed fell 8% short of this goal. Administrative interviews were conducted with the director of each program; in 13 programs, a second individual with heavy administrative responsibilities was available and was interviewed, yielding 29 administrator interviews in all.

Content of Interviews

The topics covered in all interviews are more extensive than described here, including attitudinal and treatment outcome data reported by both counselors and clients.

Counselor Interview

Counselors were asked both open- and closed-ended questions in structured interviews concerning their job activities, with the bulk of the questions eliciting counselors' estimates of the frequency of their involvement in 41 activities which spanned 11 areas of potential counselor functioning. The areas and the activities in each area are listed in Table 1. These activities were derived from lists generated by Kozel and Brown (1973) and Teare (1974), and from unstructured interviews by study staff with drug counselors. The list spanned a broad range from the counselor as caregiver to counselor as high-level administrator.

Table 1

Mean Participation Levels of Three Counselor Groups in 41 Job-Related Activities[a]

Activity	Counselor group			Group comparison	
	PRO	NEA	EXA	ANOV[b]	Tukey A[c]
I. Community Education: $F(2,78) = 5.14, p < .01$[d]					
01. Give talks about drug abuse to community groups.	0.74 (.20)	0.95 (.27)	1.81 (.30)	5.19*	PRO < EXA
02. Inform community groups about the services your program provides.	1.67 (.34)	1.70 (.47)	2.26 (.33)	0.87	–
II. Clerical and Service Duties: $F(8,146) = .36, p > .20$					
03. Fill out forms which deal with client admission, progress, and/or discharge.	4.58 (.18)	4.50 (.27)	4.40 (.16)	0.24	–
04. Carry out clerical tasks such as filing, typing letters, covering the telephone switchboard.	4.16 (.28)	3.80 (.41)	3.90 (.31)	0.33	–
05. Do maintenance tasks in the agency such as cleaning, making repairs.	1.42 (.29)	1.65 (.44)	1.32 (.32)	0.21	–
06. Perform messenger services between the treatment center and other centers or offices.	1.87 (.31)	2.11 (.43)	1.90 (.33)	0.11	–
III. Control and Enforcement: $F(6,140) = .65, p > .20$					
07. Discipline clients when necessary by keeping down noise, breaking up fights, or removing verbally abusive clients from the center.	2.61 (.31)	2.35 (.42)	3.13 (.13)	1.31	–
08. Inform police of drug-dealing activities, either by clients or by others.	0.26 (.14)	0.30 (.22)	0.16 (.13)	0.20	–
09. Take responsibility for coordinating and controlling traffic at the center.	3.76 (.35)	3.45 (.50)	3.30 (.40)	0.37	–

IV. Socializing with Clients: $F(6,150) = 1.87, p < .10$					
10. Provide social activities for clients under the auspicies of the program, e.g., a picnic for clients of the program.	1.23 (.27)	1.15 (.39)	1.39 (.30)	0.15	–
11. Meet clients on their own time in public places for socializing, e.g., having lunch with a client, going to a ball game with a client.	0.42 (.19)	1.40 (.34)	1.71 (.31)	6.52*	PRO < EXA
12. Meet clients on their own time to socialize with them in their own homes or the clients' homes.	0.06 (.04)	0.20 (.16)	0.34 (.15)	1.53	–
V. Counseling in the Community: $F(10,130) = 1.89, p = .05$					
13. Visit clients at their place of employment in the community.	0.42 (.17)	1.00 (.31)	0.55 (.20)	1.71	–
14. Accompany clients into the community when they have job interviews.	0.29 (.13)	0.30 (.25)	0.28 (.11)	0.01	–
15. Go into the community and visit a client in the hospital if he has become hospitalized.	1.03 (.19)	1.18 (.25)	1.93 (.24)	4.93*	PRO < EXA
16. Go into the community to appear in court on a client's behalf if the client is called to court.	0.77 (.18)	1.50 (.37)	1.52 (.25)	2.99	–
17. Spend time becoming familiar with community resource agencies in order to know exactly where to send clients for these services in the community.	2.77 (.26)	3.10 (.36)	2.97 (.34)	0.26	–
VI. Personal Aid to Clients: $F(8,146) = .98, p > .20$					
18. Accompany clients to community resource agencies where the clients can get help, e.g., a social work agency, a daycare facility	0.71 (.19)	1.35 (.34)	1.41 (.28)	2.38	–
19. Give personal care to clients, e.g., helping them with housework or cooking, buying food for them.	0.42 (.22)	0.55 (.34)	0.40 (.20)	0.10	–
20. Go into a client's neighborhood to help him deal with people with whom he may be having problems, e.g., someone who is leaning on him to repay a loan.	0.03 (.03)	0.25 (.17)	0.30 (.14)	1.51	–
21. Go into clients' homes to discuss their problems with other members of their families.	0.73 (.21)	0.70 (.25)	1.17 (.28)	1.09	–

(continued)

Table 1 (continued)

Activity	Counselor group			Group comparison	
	PRO	NEA	EXA	ANOV[b]	Tukey A[c]
VII. Administration of Clients: $F(8,142) = 1.28, p > .20$					
22. Decide whether a client will be accepted into your treatment program.	1.19 (.34)	2.11 (.51)	1.61 (.37)	1.21	–
23. Assume responsibility at the center for deciding whether clients should remain in the program.	2.29 (.31)	2.21 (.40)	2.47 (.33)	0.14	–
24. Attend staff meetings that deal with client treatment.	3.71 (.17)	4.05 (.09)	4.00 (.07)	2.33	–
25. Make the decision about support services (e.g., vocational training or psychiatric workups) for clients.	3.68 (.26)	3.74 (.30)	3.48 (.29)	0.21	–
VIII. Administration of Program: $F(2,146) = .26, p > .20$					
26. Supervise other workers, e.g., assigning clients, making out work schedules.	1.61 (.39)	1.11 (.38)	1.35 (.38)	0.38	–
27. Carry out tasks that have to do with money matters of the agency, e.g., keeping track of costs of the agency, making up budgets.	0.29 (.19)	0.26 (.26)	0.06 (.06)	0.58	–
28. Participate in tasks that have to do with the staffing of the agency, e.g., finding people to work, deciding who should be hired or fired.	0.58 (.17)	0.63 (.26)	0.57 (.20)	0.02	–
29. Participate in reviewing and revising policies of the program.	1.65 (.26)	1.68 (.41)	1.55 (.30)	0.05	–
30. Evaluate the effectiveness of services provided by the treatment program.	2.19 (.34)	1.80 (.39)	1.77 (.33)	0.48	–
IX. Counseling in Treatment Center: $F(14,134) = .62, p > .20$					
31. Tell clients about the programs, services, and kinds of help your agency can give them.	4.48 (.15)	4.67 (.16)	4.48 (.12)	0.43	–
32. Discuss with the client problems his family and friends may be having with regard to drugs.	3.84 (.27)	4.11 (.17)	4.03 (.21)	0.34	–

33. Conduct group counseling sessions.	1.90 (.35)	1.50 (.43)	1.68 (.36)	0.27	–
34. Talk to clients about their childhood.	4.00 (.20)	3.47 (.26)	3.57 (.29)	1.19	–
35. Explain the advantages and disadvantages of methadone and abstinence to clients.	3.90 (.23)	3.85 (.33)	3.90 (.27)	0.01	–
36. Review urine results of clients regularly.	4.16 (.21)	3.89 (.30)	4.19 (.19)	0.45	–
37. Thoroughly discuss the specific reasons and circumstances that led the client to drug use.	3.71 (.27)	3.60 (.40)	4.06 (.29)	0.61	–
X. Psychological Assessment: $F(4,154) = .70$, $p > .20$					
38. Administer psychological tests and examinations to clients, e.g., personality tests, job preference tests	0.68 (.29)	0.45 (.25)	0.35 (.20)	0.49	–
39. Interpret psychological tests and examination results, and make recommendations on the basis of their outcome.	0.87 (.30)	0.35 (.24)	0.83 (.27)	0.87	–
XI. Staff Training: $F(4,140) = .77$, $p > .20$					
40. Explain to new counselors the procedures and rules of the program, e.g., how to fill out forms used by the program.	1.59 (.27)	1.85 (.36)	1.50 (.27)	0.33	–
41. Participate as instructors in training programs which deal with drug abuse counseling.	0.87 (.25)	1.05 (.31)	0.63 (.21)	0.64	–

[a] 0 = never, 1 = once or twice a year, 2 = three or four times a year, 3 = once or twice a month, 4 = once or twice a week, 5 = just about every day. Standard errors are given in parentheses.
[b] Value of F test in one-factor analyses of variance applied to individual items.
[c] Results of Tukey A comparisons ($\alpha = .05$) among means of three counselor groups, following significant one-factor analysis of variance.
[d] F approximation to Wilk's lambda for differences among counselor groups on the set of items in the topical area.
*$p \leqslant .01$.

Table 2

Background Measures on Which Clients of the Three Counselor Groups Were Contrasted

A. Drug history
   1. Drugs or drug categories considered
      a. Marijuana/hashish
      b. Drugstore items containing drugs, like cough syrup with codeine
      c. Inhalants such as glue
      d. Hallucinogens such as LSD
      e. Barbiturates such as phenobarbital, secobarbital (Seconal), pentobarbital (Nembutal)
      f. Sedatives or tranquilizers such as chlordiazepoxide (Librium), diazepam (Valium), chloral hydrate
      g. Cocaine
      h. Heroin
      i. Illegal methadone
      j. Opiates or drugs with the same effect such as codeine, morphine, opium, meperidine (Demerol)
      k. Amphetamines and other stimulants
      l. Alcohol to excess
   2. Measures taken on each drug or category of drugs
      a. Number of years of any use
      b. Number of years of continuing use (once a week or more often)
      c. Frequency of use of each drug in year prior to treatment entry
      d. Frequency of use of each drug in 30 days just prior to treatment entry

B. Treatment history
   1. Percent ever in treatment before current treatment episode
   2. Number of prior treatment episodes
   3. Number of attempts to detoxify
   4. Number of times in chemical support modality (methadone maintenance, propoxyphene napsylate [Darvon N])
   5. Number of years in treatment
   6. Number of heroin-related treatment episodes
   7. Number of court-related treatment episodes

C. Educational history
   1. Highest grade completed in school
   2. Percent of clients receiving any schooling in year before treatment
      a. Percent receiving vocational training
      b. Percent receiving other than vocational training
   3. Number of months in school in year before treatment
      a. Number of months in vocational training in year before treatment
      b. Number of months in school in year before treatment
   4. Percent of clients receiving any schooling in the 30 days before treatment
      a. Percent of all clients receiving any vocational training in 30 days before treatment
      b. Percent of all clients receiving any schooling other than vocational training in 30 days before treatment

(continued)

Table 2 (continued)

D. Employment history
   1. Employment of males and females
      a. Percentage of clients who ever held a legal job, one for which they got paid and paid taxes
      b. Percentage of clients who held at least one job in the year prior to treatment entry
      c. Number of months employed in year prior to treatment entry
      d. Percentage of clients who worked at least 1 day in the 30 days prior to treatment entry
      e. Number of days worked, including Saturdays and Sundays, at a legal job in the 30 days prior to treatment entry
      f. Percentage of clients employed at entry into treatment
   2. Time as housewives for female clients
      a. Percentage who had ever been a housewife
      b. Percentage who had been a housewife in the year prior to treatment entry
      c. Number of months mainly a housewife in year before entry into treatment
      d. Percentage mainly housewives in the 30 days prior to treatment entry

E. Criminal involvement
   1. Percent ever arrested
   2. Number of arrests in year prior to treatment entry
   3. Percent of all arrests which were drug-related in year before treatment
   4. Number of days in jail in year before treatment
   5. Percent arrested in 30 days prior to treatment entry
   6. Number of days in jail in 30 days before treatment entry
   7. Percent of clients in treatment due to an arrest

Counselors were also questioned concerning their work experience, education and training, and their own drug use and drug treatment histories.

Administrator Interview

Administrators responded to questions concerning the same 41 activities as had counselors. They indicated the relative involvement of the three counselor groups in each activity, as well as their own views as to which counselor groups should be more or less involved. This questioning gave a second perspective to the on-the-job description generated by the counselors themselves.

Client Interview

Five areas of client backgrounds in addition to demographics were explored in the present study: drug use, treatment, educational, employment, and criminal history. Both long-term and recent history were considered, the latter by examining the year before treatment entry, as well as just the 30 days prior to treatment entry. All background measures on which clients of the three counselor groups were contrasted are given in Table 2.

Clients provided a third perspective on the functions of counselors. Of the 11 areas listed in Table 1, four involve direct counselor-client interactions, that is, counseling in the community, counseling in the treatment center, personal aid to clients, and socializing with clients. Clients indicated whether or not, or the frequency with which, the counselor had engaged in the activities in these areas with them.

RESULTS

The results are organized into four sections. First, the backgrounds of the counselors are described. Then, in order to answer the question of comparability of assignment of clients to counselors in the three groups, client demographics and backgrounds across the groups are contrasted. The third and fourth sections address the functioning of counselors in the program from the perspective of counselors and administrators, respectively. In the third section, descriptions by counselors of their interactions with clients are corroborated by data from clients and administrators. The fourth section, on administrators' views, is mainly narrative in nature, rather than a statistical description of administrator views due to the small number of administrator interviews. A summary and comments are presented at the end of each section, with a general discussion following presentation of outcomes.

Counselor Background

Counselor background was explored from the point of view of demographics, work experience, formal education and training, and drug use and drug treatment history.

Demographics

The three counselor groups differed substantially in ethnic composition, the PROs being 67% White/Anglo, while the other two groups were about 70% Black, χ^2 (2) = 18.02, $p < .01$. Further, while PROs and NEAs were 48% and 60% male, respectively, EXAs were 81% male, χ^2 (2) = 7.08, $p < .05$. Finally, PROs were substantially younger, on the average, than the other groups, with mean ages of 30, 36, and 39 years for PROs, NEAs, and EXAs, respectively, $F(2,78) = 11.12, p < .001$.

Work Experience

Professional counselors averaged about a 1.5-year tenure in their current positions, compared to 3 years for NEAs and slightly over 2 years for EXAs, $F\ (2,78) = 3.74, p < .05$. In terms of previous experience as counselors in any social service programs, 81%, 85%, and 61% of PROs, NEAs, and EXAs, respectively, had such experience, though EXAs' average of 16 months previous work in drug counseling per se was longer than that of PROs (7 months) or NEAs (13 months). (These latter differences did not reach conventional significance levels.)

Education and Training

Educational backgrounds of the three groups, of course, mirrored the definitional criteria for these groups. In addition to the bachelor's degree, 42% of PROs held master's degrees and another 29% had at least some graduate training. Most degrees were in the social sciences at the bachelor's and master's levels, though not one counselor held a master's in counseling per se. Fully 95% of NEAs and 84% of EXAs had high school diplomas, post-high school certificates, or at most some college training, with NEAs averaging 41 college credits and EXAs about 21 credits, $F\ (1,49) = 8.00, p < .01$. Generally, while completed study units were certainly more prevalent among PROs, both paraprofessional groups had some coursework considered relevant to counseling—for example, social deviance and personality theory—with averages of 10, 6, and 2 such courses, for PROs, NEAs, and EXAs, respectively, $F(2,76) = 7.70, p < .001$. All three groups also reported having taken counseling courses, though these courses might have been at any level, even weekend seminars, so long as they were given "in school." Counting all such courses, the groups did not differ significantly in the number of counseling courses taken.

In-service training within drug treatment programs was a substantial source of education for NEAs, with 80% of the group reporting such training, as opposed to 58% and 42% for PROs and EXAs, respectively ($\chi^2\ [2] = 7.71, p < .05$). In all, then, the main source of education and training was markedly associated with counselor group, being the academic setting for PROs, the drug treatment setting for NEAs, and apparently life experience for EXAs.

Counselors indicated whether they had received any training whatever in nine areas relevant to the drug counselor role: drug effects, counseling techniques, specific therapy methods, drug laws, program administration, client control, outreach counseling, clerical functions of counselors, and vocational guidance. For no topic did the three groups differ in incidence of having received training.

Drug Use and Drug Treatment

The drug use history of all counselors was explored by asking how often, if ever, counselors had tried a series of drugs. Forty-five percent of PROs, 15% of NEAs, and, of course, all EXAs reported having used various drugs. EXAs had all been frequent opiate users, and 29 of the 31 EXAs had been in drug treatment, with a median stay in all treatment of 22 months. No PROs or NEAs reported a history of addiction.

Summary and Comment

General expectations regarding the demographic and other background differences between paraprofessional and professional counselors were supported in the current sample. In the context of substantial demographic contrast between PROs and EXAs there is a noteworthy similarity between NEAs and EXAs. PROs are much more likely to be White/Anglo, to be female, and to be younger than EXAs and NEAs. It would seem justifiable to conclude that the two paraprofessional groups do, in fact, reflect the community served, whereas the professionals do not. With reference to training and education, the PROs are characterized, by definition, by formal academic training, while NEAs are educated in drug treatment through in-service training. PROs have the shortest tenure working with drug abuse clients of the three goups. Due to the relatively low rate of in-service training by EXAs, coupled with minimal formal education, we see the apparent implicit assumption of the drug treatment system that EXAs have somehow mastered drug treatment approaches through their own drug use and drug treatment experience.

Client Background

Demographics

Of the 116, 71, and 115 clients of PROs, NEAs, and EXAs, respectively, approximately two-thirds in each client group were male, χ^2 (2) = .14, $p \geqslant .20$. The groups also did not differ in ethnic composition, χ^2 (4) = 2.83, $p \geqslant .20$; half the clients in each group were Black, with another third White and the remainder Spanish-American. Clients of the three counselor groups differed significantly, though only slightly, in age, F (2,299) = 3.70, $p < .05$, with mean ages of 29, 32, and 30 years for clients of PROs, NEAs, and EXAs, respectively.

Client Background

The drug use, treatment, educational, employment, and criminal histories of the three groups were contrasted on the measures listed in Table 1, providing substantial opportunity for the detection of differences, should they have existed. No differences were found between the client groups in terms of educational and employment history. In the area of drug abuse, there was only one group effect. In the drug-free modality only, clients of PROs used alcohol to excess more often in the 30 days prior to treatment than did clients of NEAs ($p < .05$). This difference apparently was not longstanding, since it was not detected in other measures of longer-term alcohol use.

Again in the drug-free modality, a single difference between clients of PROs and NEAs was detected in the area of treatment history, in that clients of PROs had had an average of one more treatment episode than clients of NEAs ($p < .01$). Finally, in the area of criminal history, more clients of EXAs than of PROs or NEAs had been in jail in the year prior to treatment entry ($p < .05$). More critical for evidence concerning the possibility of differential assignment of clients to counselors was that the client groups differed neither in the number in treatment because of an arrest ($p \geqslant .20$) nor the number having spent any time in jail in the month prior to treatment ($p \geqslant .20$).

Summary and Comment

In the main, the demographics, the drug use and treatment histories, the educational and employment histories, and the criminal histories were substantially the same across the clients of the three counselor groups. The four differences detected among 97 measures of demographics and background history were what would have been expected by chance alone and did not themselves present a cohesive picture of differential assignment of clients to one or another counselor group.

Functions and Activities: Counselor Perspective

Hours Worked per Week and Income

The expectation that paraprofessionals might work longer hours and for less pay than professionals was supported. The EXAs reported working significantly more hours per week than did PRO counselors, $p < .05$ (see Table 3). Further, while median annual incomes of the three groups were highly similar–$10,934, $10,500, and $10,068 for the PRO, NEA, and EXA groups, respectively–23% of PROs earned $15,000 or more per year, as contrasted with only 13% of the EXA and 5% of the NEA groups.

Caseload and Hours Devoted to Counseling

Caseloads did not differ significantly in size across groups, ranging from just under 32 clients per NEA counselor to 34 per EXA counselor and 43 per PRO

Table 3

Hours Worked and Caseloads of the Three Counselor Groups[a]

	Counselor group			
Aspect of job	PRO	NEA	EXA	p[b]
1. Total regular hours worked each week	38.45 (.43)	37.75 (1.42)	39.16 (.46)	–
2. Average hours worked overtime per week	1.90 (.61)	3.90 (1.17)	5.26 (1.14)	.05
3. Total hours worked per week	40.35 (.75)	41.65 (1.37)	44.42 (1.31)	.05
4. Number of clients for whom respondent is primary counselor	43.03 (5.36)	31.75 (4.56)	34.00 (3.69)	–
5. Average hours per week in individual counseling	19.55 (1.59)	18.55 (2.07)	14.74 (1.30)	–
6. Average hours per week in group counseling	1.23 (.29)	1.90 (.52)	2.94 (.62)	.05

[a]Means; standard errors given in parentheses.
[b]Significance level of F test in one-factor ANOV.

counselor. As seen from Table 3, Items 3, 5, and 6, EXAs but not NEAs spend proportionally less of their workweek in counseling sessions, with proportions of 0.52, 0.49, and 0.40 of total work time spent in counseling sessions by the PRO, NEA, and EXA groups, respectively. The PRO counselors tended to spend slightly more time in counseling sessions with individual clients than did EXAs, $F(2,79) = 2.60, p < .10$. In contrast, EXAs spent significantly more time than PROs in group counseling sessions, $F(2,79) = 3.31, p < .05$. The NEA group fell between the PRO and EXA groups in both individual and group counseling times.

Job Activities Other Than Direct Counseling

Counselors were asked to describe, in open-ended fashion, the main job activities, other than direct counseling sessions, on which they spent their time. The many activities reported were classified into 12 areas, closely paralleling those listed in Table 1. The groups were remarkably consistent in the activities mentioned. Spearman rank-order correlations of the frequencies of mentioning activities in each category across counselor groups were .97 for PROs versus EXAs, .97 for PROs versus NEAs, and .98 for NEAs versus EXAs.

Activities List

Further contrasts among groups were based on closed-ended questions concerning each of the 41 job activities in the 11 areas listed in Table 1. Counselors indicated for each activity the frequency of their involvement on a six-point scale from "never" to "just about every day." A two-stage approach was taken to analysis. First, a one-factor MANOVA was performed for each of the 11 areas, with responses to the activities within the category as dependent measures and counselor category as the stratification factor. These tests were followed by a series of protected one-factor ANOVAs on the responses to each of the 41 activities.

The outcomes of the MANOVAs are given in Table 1, with F approximations to Wilk's lambda reported for each area. In only 3 of the 11 areas were significant differences or trends toward differences noted among counselor groups. These areas were: I. Community Education ($p < .10$), IV. Socializing with Clients ($p < .10$), and V. Counseling in the Community ($p = .05$). Responses to the 31 activities in the eight nondifferentiating areas were remarkably similar across counselor groups (for 24 of these activities, $F < 1$).

Where differences were found among counselor groups, in either the MANOVA or the ANOVA tests, these differences were invariably in activities which took the counselor out of the program. In the area of Community Education, EXAs were significantly more involved than either PROs or NEAs ($p < .01$ and $p < .05$, respectively, for differences between groups in the MANOVA context). These differences in the multivariate analysis were due to the greater involvement of EXAs in giving talks to community groups (see Table 1), with this difference corroborated by administrators.

In the area of Counseling in the Community, EXAs again were significantly more involved than either PROs or NEAs ($p < .05$ in both cases for differences between groups in the MANOVA context). These differences were due primarily to Activity 15, that of visiting clients in the hospital, with administrators corroborating the counselors' self-reports.

A similar trend was noted in counselors' self-reports of the frequency of their appearances in court on the clients' behalf, with PROs lower than the other group ($p < .10$). Both these trends were corroborated in administrators' and clients' reports of counselor activity.

In the area of socializing with clients, there was a tendency for a difference among the groups to surface in the overall MANOVA test ($p < .10$), with the pairwise difference between EXAs and PROs reaching conventional significance levels ($p < .05$). EXAs reported meeting clients on their own time in public places for socializing–for example, having lunch with a client, going to a ball game with a client–significantly more often than did professionals ($p < .01$), with administrator and client reports corroborating this finding. Clients of

EXAs more often than did clients of PROs reported that their counselors met them on their own time to socialize in their own or their counselors' homes ($p < .05$). Counselors and administrators reported the same pattern as had clients, though the counselor comparison was nonsignificant.

Summary and Comment

Whatever differences were found among counselor groups were most marked between the PROs and EXAs, with NEAs falling in between and typically resembling PROs over EXAs. Overall, the main difference noted among counselor groups in the activities performed was the greater activity of EXAs over the PROs outside the treatment program. This difference was found in three areas of counselor functioning: community education, socializing with clients, and counseling in the community. While these significant differences emerged, it is important to note the differences among counselors within groups. For example, not all EXAs gave talks to community groups. Fully a third of the EXAs had never done so and in this regard were similar to the 58% of PROs who had never done so. The difference between the groups emerged in that there was a substantial percentage of EXAs who spoke at least once or twice a month (36%), while far fewer professionals (10%) spoke to community groups with this frequency.

In the area of socializing with clients, a similar result emerged. Slightly over half (55%) of EXAs reported never socializing with clients in public places, in contrast with three-quarters (77%) of PROs who never did so. It is the 42% of EXAs versus the 6% of PROs who socialized with clients at least once a month which led to the overall difference between the groups.

What is being suggested here is that some but not all EXAs conduct some portion of their treatment activity in the community. A large percentage, however, more heavily concentrate their efforts within the treatment program. This notion of two types of EXA roles was supported by statistical analysis. Discriminant analyses were performed to determine the extent to which individual counselors would be classified as similar to their own versus other counselor groups. In the discriminant analyses for community education and socializing with clients, a substantial subset of EXAs were classified as being statistically more similar to the PROs than to other EXAs. In the classification analysis based on community education activities, 36% of EXAs were statistically clustered with PROs; 48% were so classified based on the socializing with clients activities.

Administrators' Views of Counselor Functions

Interview Results

Another perspective on the functions and activities performed by the different counselor groups was gained from interviews with administrators.

Specifically, each of 41 activities was inquired about with the following question: "Of the three counselor groups in which we are interested—that is, professionals, non-addict paraprofessionals, and ex-addict paraprofessionals—which group, if any, is more involved in [activity]?" In addition, administrators were asked which groups they thought should be involved more than the others in each activity.

While asked to differentiate among counselor groups in their involvement in each activity, administrators often reported that either all counselors or no counselors were involved in a given task. There was substantial agreement between counselors and administrators as to the tasks in which counselors were involved. The correlation across tasks between the number of administrators who said that all counselors were involved in a task and the mean response level of all counselors to the task was $r\,(39) = .78, p < .001$.

In 4 of the 11 areas, administrators were univocal in their reponse that either all or none of the counselors were performing a particular task, and further, that all or none should be involved in the task in question. These areas were clerical and service duties, control and enforcement, providing personal aid to clients, and administration of clients.

At the other end of the spectrum was the area of psychological testing, the one area in which administrators favored a single counselor group. A slight majority (54%) of the 29 administrators felt that PROs should be the one counselor group interpreting psychological tests, and 46% felt that only PROs should administer the tests. Most of the remainder of administrators felt that no counselors should be involved in either administering of interpreting psychological tests. This view mirrors the very low rate of counselor-reported involvement in psychological testing (see Table 1).

In the area of counseling, administrators felt that all activities but two were appropriate for all counselor groups. Eight of the 29 administrators felt that only PROs should run group counseling sessions; and seven, that only PROs should talk to clients about their childhood.

Administrators' reports of differential counselor involvement in community education, counseling in the community, and socializing with clients mirrored the differences reported by the counselors themselves. However, the only support by administrators for existing differential involvement was in community education, with administrators' choice of EXAs occasioned by their special credibility.

Summary and Comment

The predominant picture gleaned from administrators was that where it was appropriate for counselors to be involved, it was all the counselors and not just one or another group who should be involved. Ex-addicts were favored only for community education. PROs were clearly favored only in the area of psychological testing, an area in which advanced training was seen as being required. The only other support for having PROs uniquely involved in an activity was that a minority of administrators felt PROs to be better suited to running group counseling sessions and to exploring with clients their childhoods. It is noteworthy that this support of PROs did not generalize across other activities involved in counseling.

DISCUSSION

Based simply on the number of comparisons made among the three groups of counselors and among the clients of these counselors, more differences would have been expected to emerge by mere chance than were observed in the present study. In all, there was a remarkable lack of difference noted among both the groups of counselors and their clients. Concluding in favor of the null hypothesis, however, requires a careful consideration of the power associated with the statistical comparisons. In other words, one must ask whether a nonnegligible difference which actually exists among the groups could be detected with the design employed. The power of the present design was assessed in accord with the formulation of Cohen (1977). For power analysis of the present study, an effect (or difference among counselor groups) which accounted of 10% of the variance of a particular measure ($\eta^2 = 10\%$) was considered as a meaningful difference from the point of view of differentiating the roles of the groups, whereas smaller differences which would account for only a few percent of the variance in counselor roles were not. With the number of counselors in the present study, and employing the conventional level of significance $\alpha = .05$, the power of this design for detecting such effects is 80%, a level of power deemed acceptable by Cohen (1977). An analogous consideration of statistical power for comparisons among clients indicated power approaching 100% for comparisons among clients on continuous variables and over 80% for discrete variables. On this basis it is concluded that the reliable finding of negligible difference across counselor groups and clients groups is an accurate reflection of the population, rather than a failure of the statistical design to have sufficient power to detect actually existing differences.

The roles of counselors in programs may be differentiated in two ways. Counselors may perform qualitatively different roles from one another. Or they may perform the same functions to different degrees. In terms of qualitative differences among roles, the only noteworthy characteristic of the role of any one counselor group is that the ex-addicts more often report that they are involved in activities in the community: providing community education, visiting hospitalized clients, and socializing with clients. This effect is diminished in its salience by the finding that it is not uniformly characteristic of EXAs to be more active in the community, but rather that it is an active subgroup of EXAs who are involved outside the program.

With regard to in-program activities, the quantitative differences among the groups, where significant, are not large. In all, there is no evidence that counselors of the three groups differed in the content of the counseling provided to clients within the program, based on the activities in the category of counseling in the treatment center. In this regard, a detailed review of the training of the three counselor groups revealed that not even PROs had substantial training in clinical or counseling techniques; of the 13 professionals who held master's degrees, none held degrees in counseling.

Perhaps the clearest indication that the drug treatment system does not distinguish among the counselors of the three groups in terms of their counseling qualifications is that there is no evidence of differential client assignment to one or another counselor group. Should any counselor group be considered more apt than the others, one would expect that clients with more severe addictions, substantially longer treatment histories, and perhaps substantially more criminal involvement would be assigned to one counselor group. No evidence of differential assignment was amassed in this sample of approximately 300 clients.

From the perspective of formulating research designs to evaluate the relative effectiveness of the three counselor groups, homogeneity of clients across groups is critical. As was pointed out before, internally valid comparisons of the therapeutic process and outcomes require that the clients being treated be equivalent across the counselor groups compared. The results of the present study indicate that this necessary condition can be argued to have been met for the treatment modalities considered, even in the absence of random assignment of clients to groups.

Perhaps the differences among the counselor groups which are emplicitly assumed to exist are not in their roles per se. Rather, differences may exist in the attitudes toward drug addiction and the expectations for clients they bring to the treatment process and in the nature of the relationships established with clients. Such questions have been raised concerning paraprofessionals versus professional counselors in other treatment fields in an attempt to understand the process of paraprofessional intervention (Durlak, 1979). The questions will be explored from both the counselor and client perspectives in a subsequent comparison of the three counselor groups distinguished in the present investigation (Lo Sciuto et al., 1984).

Given the noteworthy similarity among counselor groups, particularly EXAs and PROs, in both their roles in the programs and in the clients they treat, one might well wonder why ex-addict counselors have not been employed more widely in related service delivery systems. Lack of acceptance outside the drug treatment community, coupled with positive pressure from within the drug treatment community, may be the prevailing forces, and an investigation of this phenomenon is warranted.

As a final note, it is important to consider the nature of the ex-addict counselor population considered in this investigation. The EXAs represent the opiate-abusing population–male, urban, minority–which formed the basis of our conception of the drug abuse problem of the early '70s. To the extent that the current drug-abusing population is shifting away from this traditional pattern–that is, to polydrug use, to female use, to White as well as minority populations–the nature of future EXAs will necessarily change. This shift may well have implications for the roles served by EXAs in drug treatment programs and for their acceptance in other areas of the service delivery system.

ACKNOWLEDGMENT

This research was supported by NIDA Contract No. 271-76-4410 to the first and second authors, with data collection accomplished in 1977.

REFERENCES

COHEN, J. *Statistical Power Analysis for the Bahavioral Sciences.* New York: Academic Press, 1977.

COOK, T.D., and CAMBELL, D.T. *Quasi-experimentation: Design and Analysis Issues for Field Settings.* Chicago: Rand McNally, 1979.

DEITCH, D.A. The end of the beginning: Dilemmas of the paraprofessional in current drug abuse treatment. In E. Senay, V. Shorty, and H. Alksne (eds.), *Developments in the Field of Drug Abuse: Proceedings of the National Drug Abuse Council, 1974.* Cambridge, MA: Schenkman, 1974.

DURLAK, J.A. Comparative effectiveness of paraprofessional and professional helpers. *Psychol. Bull.* 86(1): 80-92, 1979.

FLORES, V.J., and RICE, K.A. Training viewpoints on paraprofessional counslors. In E. Senay, V. Short, and H. Alksne (eds.), *Developments in the Field of Drug Abuse: Proceedings of the National Drug Abuse Council, 1974.* Cambridge, MA: Schenkman, 1974.

GARTNER, A., and RIESSMAN, F. The paraprofessional movement in perspective. *Pers. Guidance* 53(4): 253-256, 1974.

GROSSER, C. Manpower development program. In C. Grosser, W.E. Henry, and J.G. Kelly (eds.), *Nonprofessionals in the Human Services*, San Francisco, CA: Jossey-Bass, 1969.

KOZEL, N.J., and BROWN, B.S. The counselor role as seen by ex-addict counselors, non-addict counselors, and significant others. *J. Consult. Clin. Psychol.* 41(3): 315, 1973.

LO SCIUTO, L.A., AIKEN, L.S., AUSETTS, M.A., and BROWN, B.S. Paraprofessional versus professional drug abuse counselors: Attitudes and expectations of the counselors and their clients. *Int. J. Addict.* In press, 1984.

LUBORSKY, L., SINGER, G., and LUBORSKY, L. Comparative studies of psychotherapies. *Arch. Gen. Psychiatry* 32(8); 995-1008, 1975.

NATIONAL INSTITUTE ON DRUG ABUSE. *Data from the National Drug Abuse Treatment Utilization Survey (NDATUS).* NIDA Statistical Series F, No. 6, April 1978.

NIETZEL, M.J., and FISHER, S.G. Effectiveness of professional and paraprofessional helpers: A comment on Durlak. *Psychol. Bull.* 89(3): 555-565, 1981.

SOCIAL AND REHABILITATION SERVICE. *Overview Study of Employment of Paraprofessionals–National Study of Social Welfare and Rehabilitation Workers, Work, and Organizational Contexts* (Research Report No. 3). Washington, DC: Department of Health, Education, and Welfare, 1974.

TEARE, R.J. Employment of subprofessionals: Staff and organizational adaptation and implications for service delivery. In *Overview Study of Employment of Paraprofessionals–National Study of Social Welfare and Rehabilitation Workers, Work, and Organizational Contexts* (Research Report No. 3). Washington, DC: Department of Health, Education, and Welfare, 1974.

The International Journal of the Addictions, 19(2), 175–198, 1984

The Effect of Perceived Neighborhood Setting on Self-Reported Tobacco, Alcohol, and Marijuana Use among Inner-City Minority Junior High School Youth

William R. Blount, PhD

Richard Dembo, PhD

Department of Criminal Justice
University of South Florida
Tampa, Florida 33620

Abstract

The relationship between neighborhood setting and drug use appears to be drug specific. For alcohol and tobacco a knowledge of peer (friends') use was highly predictive of personal use, independent of how tough or drug involved the neighborhood was thought to be, but quite dependent on neighborhood perceptions for personal marijuana use, becoming more predictive as the neighborhood was perceived as tougher and more drug involved. Knowledge of spare-time activities was predictive of tobacco and marijuana use (independent of neighborhood) but not predictive for alcohol use. The data suggest that because the relationships are complex, intervention/prevention strategies must not only be drug specific but must proceed on many fronts simultaneously. Some suggestions are offered, along with a discussion of findings which may help identify non-users and users in the same population.

 0020-773X/84/1902-0175$3.50/0

Sociocultural views of nonmedical drug use among inner-city youths argue that this behavior is learned, motivated, peer oriented, and adaptive, reflecting a commitment to a life-style that is socially and culturally valued. The sociocultural view can be seen as one consequence of the research response to the dominant concern of the 1960s and early 1970s over heroin use in the slums and the relationship between addiction and crime. In seeking to probe the drug-taking patterns of different groups in the ghetto, researchers uncovered a wide variation in the place of illicit drugs in the cultural, social, and economic dimensions of slum life (Blumer, Sutter, Ahmed, and Smith, 1967; Sutter, 1966, 1969; Finestone, 1957; Feldman, 1968, 1973, 1974, 1977; Preble and Casey, 1969). The thrust of this work indicated that the use of heroin and other drugs by inner-city youths was an important way of confirming one's toughness, and a key route to prestige and social position in the street life. Drug use is seen as a means of affirming oneself, rather than a mode of escape or retreat (see Merton, 1957; Cloward and Ohlin, 1960).

Kaplan's (1978, 1980) study of the relationship between self-derogation and deviant behavior (including alcohol, marijuana, and narcotics use) uncovered evidence of an interaction effect between social class and self-derogation in regard to participation in deviant activities among the Houston youths he studied. His finding that self-derogation led to deviant behavior among middle-class youths but not among lower-class youths supported his hypothesis of a conditional relationship between the two variables. The hypothesis was based on the notion that the deviant behavior patterns are more compatible with the normative structure of the lower class, whereas this behavior is not compatible with the norms of the middle class.

The work of Kaplan and that of Kaufman (1978) focused on the interactive effect of social class; their line of argument asserts that the environment in which one lives may not directly influence behavior. Rather, behavior results from a complex interplay between personality and social setting. Kaufman (1978), for example, found a much higher rate of severe psychopathology among opiate addicts from high social classes than in opiate addicts from low social classes, indicative, it would seem, of the individual psychological response to one's own perception of one's own deviance. Since opiate addiction was perceived as nondeviant by the lower-class addicts, the severe psychological reaction to a recognition of that addiction was not present, or at least to a significantly lesser extent (48% vs 3%).

This line of reasoning led Dembo, Schmeidler, Burgos, and Taylor (forthcoming) to an examination of the relationship between perceived environmental setting and demographic, neighborhood orientation, and drug use context variables in regard to inner-city junior high school youth's drug use. They were looking specifically for a test of environmental setting effects on the correlates of drug use. Using a procedure similar to that developed by Single, Kandel, and

Faust (1974), a Guttman analysis was performed on data available concerning the frequency of use of the seven categories of drugs (alcohol, marijuana, LSD or similar substances, depressants, narcotics, solvents, and stimulants). The resulting scale placed youths into four categories according to the most "extreme" drug reported to have been used in the last six months: (1) all use denied ($N = 437$; 52.6%), (2) use of alcohol admitted ($N = 194$; 23.3%), (3) use of marijuana–and usually alcohol–admitted ($N = 146$; 17.6%), and (4) claimed use of other drugs–and usually alcohol and marijuana as well ($N = 54$; 6.5%).

Dembo et al. found that demographic variables were not significantly or consistently related to drug involvement over three neighborhood settings, but other variables were. Youths' participation in street culture spare-time activities was significantly related to drug involvement in all three settings and differentially so, being most predictive in the toughest and most drug-oriented neighborhood setting. Youth's friends' use of alcohol and marijuana was much more highly predictive of personal drug involvement than street culture spare-time activities, but was not differentially so across neighborhood settings. Dembo et al. felt that their results suggested that the degree of perceived toughness/drug orientation of the neighborhood operated as a conditioning factor in understanding the correlates of drug involvement.

The present study was concerned with explaining the same relationships but doing so for specific drugs. Of the drugs used in the original study, the vast majority of the sample responded positively to tobacco, alcohol, and marijuana. Of those who responded (each question was asked separately), 43% admitted to tobacco use, 56% admitted to alcohol use, and 29% admitted to marijuana use. The positive response rate to any of the other categories was less than 8% each. Thus, in an attempt to determine if specific drugs related differently to the environment than did an overall measure of drug involvement, the most fruitful avenue was the choice of tobacco, alcohol, and marijuana for these data. That two substances were generally legal and the third illegal also added a dimension to the study, although for this age group, the use of tobacco and alcohol was illegal also. There was reason to believe that the relationships between the use of tobacco, alcohol, and marijuana and neighborhood context variables would differ, if for no other reason than both adult and juvenile perceptions of the substances as "drugs" differ, as do their attitudes toward use of these substances (see, e.g., Tuchfeld, Clayton, and Logan, 1982; Weitzel and Blount, 1982).

Recognizing that one's environment consists of both the physical setting and one's attitudes toward that setting and thoughts concerning how one fits into the scheme of things, both the original study and the present one were concerned with inner-city youths' *perceptions* of (attitudes toward) their neighborhood. Thus, rather than attempt to make any actual measurements relative to differences between one geographical neighborhood setting and another, these two studies allowed the subjects to define neighborhood differences through their own perceptions. This was felt to be justified in that the relationship of the subjects' perceptions and actual differences did not have to be established, and this was considered a fair trade-off for the use of inner-city youths exclusively, where the actual physical differences between neighborhoods might not be as great as those studied by Kaplan (1978, 1980) or Kaufman (1978), if they existed at all. (We know for a fact that the present data had a rather constricted range of socioeconomic status for the families represented by the respondents.)

We also appreciate that there are a wide range of psychological, sociological, economic, and cultural variables that may be related to inner-city youths' drug use. Further, we recognize the restrictions relative to conclusions of causal sequences imposed by a cross-sectional sample such as that used here, as opposed to a longitudinal design. Nevertheless, the data provided an excellent opportunity to study the relationships between an inner-city youth's perception of the neighborhood in which he lived and the correlates of his own drug-taking behavior.

METHOD

The data were gathered in the second wave of a two-part survey of youths attending a South Bronx, New York City, junior high school in the winter of 1976. School officials and local school board members invited the study in hopes that insight gained into the youths' backgrounds, attitudes/values, and experiences with drugs might lead to the development of effective and engaging drug abuse prevention programs. Although a recent New York statewide epidemiological survey had been completed (Lipton, Stephens, Babst, Dembo, Diamond, Spielman, Schmeidler, Bergman, and Uppal, 1977), no relevant data on New York City youths' drug use were available to school officials and community leaders to facilitate their program development work.

The questionnaires were developed from extensive ethnographic work among youths living in neighborhoods similar to those covered by the school. Drafts of the instruments were pretested among panels of youths attending schools other than the one where the survey was conducted, resulting in the development of two protocols which were easy to complete and culturally relevant. Administered in the social studies classrooms of the students, the questionnaires took one period each to complete (see Note 1).

Description of the Sample

Over 97% of the students in class at the time of the survey participated. These youths represented 78% of the 1,344 students enrolled in the school. Efforts taken to ensure confidentiality were helpful in obtaining the high response rate achieved on this voluntary survey. Students were asked not to identify themselves on the forms, and they were provided with seals to secure their answers from persons other than the researchers.

As indicated in Table 1, somewhat more girls than boys were represented in the study, and the youths averaged 13 years of age. Most of the youths were Puerto Rican or Black, and a majority of the youths indicated they lived with both their parents, although 38% claimed to reside with their mothers.

The questionnaires included questions probing father's and mother's educational and occupational levels. Analyses of these data indicated that the youths tended to inflate the skill level of their fathers' occupations. Responses to the level of education questions converged with the fieldwork experience and that of school personnel in reflecting the low to moderate socioeconomic status (SES) range of families represented by students in the school. Accordingly, the educational level of each youth's household head was used to measure SES. These data were somewhat limited in their utility as this information was not available for 41% of the students. These youths either did not respond to this question or claimed they did not know the amount of formal education their parents had received.

Description of the Variables

In order to use as much data as possible, factor scores were developed using a zero (the Z score for each cluster) for a nonresponse. However, mean value substitution was not performed for youngsters who did not answer all the items in a given set. Since the amount of missing data on these variables was small, relatively few cases were affected by this procedure. (Analyses uncovered no demographic or drug use differences to exist between youths not answering any of the questions in each set and those responding to one or more of the items. Similar findings of no difference were found when youths who were included in the regression analyses discussed later were compared to the youths excluded from those analyses.)

Factor scores were derived in such a manner that the higher the score, the greater the adherence to the attitude, perception, or behavior named by the cluster. Table 2 presents a list of the major variables. Since the demographic variables are explained in Table 1, this discussion centers on the others.

Neighborhood Orientation/Involvement Variables

An extensive range of questions were used to probe the youths' orientations to, and involvement in, various aspects of their neighborhood. Twelve questions probed the youths' frequency of participation in a wide range of spare-time activities. These included hanging out, fighting, doing homework for school, and reading magazines. Principal factor analysis of the interrelationships among the

Table 1

Background Characteristics

	Respondents		No response	
	%	N	%	N
Sex				
Male	46.9	478		
Female	53.1	542	2.4	25
	100.0	1,020		
Ethnicity				
Black	42.6	430		
Puerto Rican	44.8	453		
Other Hispanic	3.1	31	3.4	35
White	6.4	65		
Other (mainly Oriental)	3.1	31		
	100.0	1,010		
Live with				
Both parents	58.6	587		
Mother	37.7	378	4.1	43
Father	.7	7		
Neither parent	3.0	30		
	100.0	1,002		
Head of household education level				
8th grade or less	13.2	82		
Some high school	17.9	111		
H.S. graduate	34.6	214		
Some college	11.9	74		
College graduate	14.8	92		
Graduate or professional study	7.6	47		
	100.0	620		

	Respondents				No response	
	Mean	SD	Range	N	%	N
Age at interview	12.97	1.11	10-18	1,032	1.3	13
Age 1st used[a]						
Tobacco	10.25	2.58	1-16	363	61.1	570
Alcohol	9.40	3.29	1-16	435	52.2	475
Marijuana	11.71	2.51	1-17	215	77.3	732

[a]"Age 1st used" data are tainted by some very low reported ages. For example, the percent responding at age 6 and below for 1st use were 8% for tobacco, 19% for alcohol (including 6% at ages 1 or 2), and 4% for marijuana. The marijuana data appeared least affected. Data are in years.

Table 2

Schemata of Variables Used

A. Demographic variables
   1. Ethnicity
   2. Age
   3. Sex
   4. Parent(s) lived with
B. Neighborhood Orientation /Involvement variables
   1. Participation in street culture spare-time activities
   2. Participation in print media/stay-at-home spare-time activities
   3. Survival orientation
   4. Status of drug-using, gang-involved persons by peers
C. Drug Use Context variables
   1. Availability of drugs in the school
   2. Availability of drugs in the neighborhood
   3. Friends' use of alcohol and marijuana
   4. Friends' use of "hard drugs"
D. Neighborhood Setting variable
   1. Toughness/drug use
E. Frequency of Substance Use variables
   1. Alcohol
   2. Tobacco
   3. Marijuana

replies to these items, followed by a varimax rotation of the resulting clusters, isolated two factors which were statistically and substantively meaningful.

Participation in Street Culture Spare-Time Activities. Having an eigenvalue of 1.44, this cluster loaded highly and positively on such activities as hanging out; going to dances, parties, and gigs; going to the movies; and fighting. It was negatively loaded on doing homework for school and staying at home with one's family.

Participation in Print Media/Stay-at-Home Spare-Time Activities. This cluster, with an eigenvalue of 1.10, strongly and positively emphasized such spare-time pursuits as reading magazines, newspapers, and books other than for school. It loaded positively as well on doing homework and being at home with the family.

A third cluster, having an eigenvalue of 1.38, was derived from a varimax factor analysis of 13 questions probing the youths' attitudes toward their neighborhood. *Survival Orientation* indicated a perceived difficulty in coping. This cluster was strongly and positively weighted on items reflecting the felt difficulty of surviving in the neighborhood without joining a gang, the feeling that one did not have much of a chance in making a success in life, and believing it was hard getting oneself together growing up in that neighborhood.

The fourth and final variable in this group was called *Status of Drug-Using, Gang-Involved Persons by Peers.* The youths were asked seven questions regarding the esteem given to different person types by young people their age. Principal factor analysis uncovered a cluster, having an eigenvalue of 1.87, that was strongly and positively loaded on the esteem the youths felt was given to the following types of young people in their neighborhood: the junkie, pot head, occasional pot smoker, and the member of a gang. An item probing the status of "good student" was highly weighted in a negative direction on this factor.

Drug Use Context Variables

A variety of measures were used to probe the degree to which drug use was a part of the social networks in which the youths operated. Two clusters, derived from factor analyses of three item sets that are more extensively discussed elsewhere (Dembo, Burgos, Babst, Scheidler and La Grand, 1978; Dembo, Farrow, Schmeidler and Burgos, 1979), were used to identify different aspects of this experience.

Availability of Drugs in the School. The youths were asked to indicate "how easy" it was to obtain each of the following categories of drugs in this setting: depressants, alcohol, narcotics, solvents, stimulants, LSD or similar drugs, and marijuana/hashish. Principal factor analysis isolated a cluster, having an eigenvalue of 3.75, which loaded highly and positively on each of these seven drug categories.

Availability of Drugs in the Neighborhood. A related set of questions probed the youths' ratings of the ease of obtaining each of the seven drug categories in the neighborhood in which they lived. A principal factor analysis cluster, which had an eigenvalue of 4.34 and was weighted strongly and positively on each of the categories, was chosen as a good summary measure of this dimension.

Reflecting the experience that personal drug taking has been found to be strongly and positively related to the drug use of friends (Johnson, 1973; Kandel, 1973, 1975), the youths were asked a series of questions regarding their friends' drug taking. Varimax factor analysis uncovered two measures of this behavior.

Friends' Use of Alcohol and Marijuana. This varimax cluster, having an eigenvalue of 1.19, was highly and positively loaded on the youths' indication of the frequency with which their friends used these two substances.

Friends' Use of "Hard Drugs." This varimax factor, with an eigenvalue of 2.78, had high and positive weightings on friends' use of depressants, narcotics, LSD or similar drugs, stimulants, and solvents.

The Neighborhood-Setting Variable

Critical to the analyses was the development of a measure of the youths' perception of the neighborhoods in which they were living. Our research interests precluded an examination of the kind and degree of various community life experiences existing in the various neighborhoods where the youths and their families lived. However, our fieldwork uncovered little evidence of a strong sense of community in the areas where we pursued our work. The "neighborhood *perceived*" appeared to be the most salient dimension for us to focus on in addressing the life-styles reflected in the youths' immediate environment. Thus, 13 items were developed to tap views of the degree of "toughness" and drug use existing in their neighborhoods (after Dembo, 1973). Our fieldwork indicated these 13 experiences were salient features of the neighborhoods in which the present population lived. Principal factor analysis of the youths' replies to these items was undertaken first, and the three factors emerging from this study of the data were, then, varimax rotated. One main factor resulting from this analysis, with an eigenvalue of 2.13, appeared to be a good reflection of the concept sought. Labeled *Toughness/Drug Use*, the cluster had high, positive loadings on items probing how "tough" it was to get along in one's neighborhood, whether it contained a lot of gangs, whether people tended to get into fights, whether it was hard avoiding "trouble" growing up in the neighborhood, and whether young people were into getting high on pot and popping pills. A question probing how "peaceful" it was to live in the neighborhood was strongly and negatively weighted on this factor. In order to identify environmental settings of different degrees of perceived toughness/drug use, the factor score range was objectively divided into three equal-sized groups ("low," "medium," and "high" Toughness/Drug Use).

Frequency of Substance Use Variables

As indicated earlier, subjects were asked to respond to several separate question sets concerning their use of eight substances: alcohol, marijuana (including hashish), LSD or similar substances, depressants, narcotics, solvents, stimulants, and tobacco. The frequency-of-use question set provided options of: never used, not used in last 6 months, used once in last 6 months, used 2 to 5 times in last 6 months, used 6 to 10 times in last 6 months (or about once a month), used 11 to 30 times in the last 6 months (or about once a week), and used more than 30 times in last 6 months (Note 2). Only tobacco, alcohol, and marijuana revealed much involvement, the positive response rate for each of the other categories being less than 8%. For tobacco, 43% ($N = 362$) admitted some use (33% in last 6 months); for alcohol, 56% ($N = 475$) admitted some use (41% in the last 6 months); and for marijuana, 29% (N = 246) admitted some use (24% in the last 6 months). Percentages for each response option for tobacco (839 respondents) were, from never used to used more than 30 times in last 6 months, respectively: 56.9%, 9.8%, 4.6%, 7.4%, 3.8%, 2.5%, and 15.0% (206 youths did not respond). For alcohol (852 respondents), the percentages were: 44.3%, 14.8%, 12.8%, 15.2%, 6.3%, 2.6%, and 4.0%, respectively (193 youths did not reply). For marijuana (847 respondents; 198 nonrespondents), the percentages were: 70.7%, 5.2%, 3.8%, 8.3%, 2.4%, 1.8%, and 7.8%, respectively.

RESULTS

In order to increase the validity of the substance use responses, three internal consistency procedures were instituted prior to further data analysis. Since subjects had responded to several sets of questions concerning these substances it was possible to eliminate the inconsistent and obviously erroneous responses. First, any subject who claimed to have used five or more of the seven substances (tobacco was excluded) more than 30 times each in the last 6 months was eliminated. Second, subjects who responded with some frequency of use other than "none" on one question set and selected a "never used" response on another question set for the same substance were also eliminated. Finally, subjects were removed who selected an "age at first use" which was actually older than their chronological age. This process removed 61 subjects from the tobacco respondents, 94 from alcohol, and 55 from marijuana, leaving usable Ns of 778, 758, and 792, respectively.

Race

Since at least one previous analysis of these data indicated that ethnicity interacted with variables similar to those used here in predicting drug involvement (Dembo, Burgos, Des Jarlais, and Schmeidler, 1979), race analyses were completed first. Nonsignificant differences were found for the reported frequency of tobacco use, alcohol use, and marijuana use (for alcohol, F [4, 741] = 0.84, NS; for tobacco, F [4, 751] = 1.06, NS; for marijuana, F [4, 772] = 1.00, NS). Further, reported frequencies of alcohol, tobacco, and marijuana use were compared with race for each of the neighborhood settings, also with nonsignificant results (Note 3). Finally, the perceived neighborhood Toughness/Drug Use score was compared across ethnicity and was nonsignificant as well (F[4,998] = 1.55, NS). For the present data then, race was not productive in the prediction of reported alcohol, tobacco, or marijuana use, and played a secondary role, at best, in understanding this behavior for our population. Therefore, the additional analyses included all ethnic respondents.

Frequency of Use and Neighborhood Setting

Significant chi squares for alcohol (χ^2 [12] = 21.39, $p < .04$), tobacco (χ^2 [12] = 33.54, $p < .001$), and marijuana (χ^2 [12] = 29.84, $p < .003$) were found when frequency of use across the three neighborhood categories was explored. The alcohol and tobacco results were obviously the result of the large sample size. The largest percent differences were in the "never used" category. The results for tobacco were: 67% for the Low Toughness/Drug Use category and 52% for the High Toughness/Drug Use category (r^2 = .0272). For alcohol, 55% occured in the Low Toughness/Drug Use category and 44% in the High Toughness/Drug Use category (r^2 = .0180). While a similar argument could be made for the marijuana data in that only about 3% of the variance was accounted for (r^2 = .0317), one difference was large enough (17%) to force the conclusion that there was a significantly higher percent of reported marijuana use in the High Toughness/Drug Use category than in the low category (respective "never used" percentages were 83.2, 76.8, and 66.3% for low, medium, and high categories).

Predicting Frequency of Alcohol Use

Several analyses were done in an attempt to discover which variables would aid in the prediction of the youths' reported alcohol use. First, regression analyses were completed for each of the three Toughness/Drug Use categories and for the pooled data partialling out the effects of the Toughness/Drug Use variable. Having eliminated race, the three remaining demographic variables (age, sex, and home composition) were then introduced into the analyses, followed by the four Neighborhood Orientation/Involvement variables and finally the four Drug Use Context variables. Next, an analysis of variance examination was made of the homogeneity of the regression coefficients (*b*s) generated in this way. As Table 3 indicates, only the effect of the pooled coefficients was significant, F (11, 616) = 23.10, $p < .001$; the effect of the separate coefficients being nonsignificant, F (22, 594) = 1.14, NS. These results would lead us to expect only modest (if any) indications of differential effect of neighborhood setting on the correlates of alcohol use. This expectation was borne out, as Table 4 illustrates.

In attempting to predict alcohol use across neighborhood settings, demographic variables were not predictive, showing no statistical significance in any of the neighborhood settings. The "life-style" variables (Neighborhood Orientation/Involvement) were slightly more illustrative, at least in the sense that Survival and Participation in Street Culture Spare-Time Activities were significantly related in self-reported alcohol use, even if only in the high Toughness/Drug Use setting. This suggested that a knowledge of the youth's perception of

Table 3

ANOVA Test of Homogeneity of the Regression Coefficients (bs) for Alcohol Use

Source of variation	*SS*	*df*	*MS*	*F*	*p*
Pooled coefficients for the 3 Toughness contexts	529.969	11	48.179	23.10	.001
Residual from pooled coefficients	1293.841	616	2.084		
Separate coefficients	582.167	33			
Differences between separate coefficients	52.198	22	2.373	1.14	NS
Residual from separate coefficients	1231.643	594	2.074		
Total	1813.810	627			

what it took to survive in his neighborhood and his "on-the-street" activities would improve the ability to predict his reported alcohol use, but only in neighborhoods perceived to be very "tough."

One of the Drug Use Context variables was the most informative. Friends' Use of Alcohol and Marijuana was most important in predicting individual self-reported alcohol use. While there was some evidence of differential predictability (such that such knowledge would be quite valuable in the low and medium settings, and less valuable in the high settings), this evidence was weak.

Friends' Use of "Hard Drugs" was significantly negatively related to reported alcohol use but only for the medium toughness category.

Predicting Frequency of Tobacco Use

Identical analyses to those already described were conducted for frequency of tobacco use. Table 5 illustrates results identical to those found for alcohol (see Table 3) for the analysis of variance examination of the homogeneity of the regression coefficients. Only the effect of the pooled coefficients was significant, F (11, 622) = 20.95, $p < .001$, again leading us to expect minimal differential influences of perceived neighborhood setting on the correlates of tobacco use. This expectation was confirmed (see Table 6).

As was true for alcohol, the demographic variables of age, sex, and home composition did not interact with neighborhood setting to predict tobacco use. The only exceptions were that females reported more tobacco use in the medium Toughness/Drug Use settings, and youths from "nonintact" homes reported more tobacco use for the low Toughness/Drug Use setting.

Again, the Participation in Street Culture Spare-Time Activities (from the Neighborhood Involvement/Participation variable set) was predictive, and this time it was predictive across all neighborhood settings, suggesting that a knowledge of "on-the-street" activities would improve the ability to predict self-reported tobacco use in any neighborhood.

Table 4

Stepwise Regression Coefficients of Alcohol Use on Youths' Demographic Characteristics, Neighborhood Orientation/Involvement, and Drug Use Context Variables[a, b]

Variables	All neighborhoods combined[c] ($N = 630$) Coefficient		r	Low Toughness /Drug Use setting ($N = 228$) Coefficient		r	Medium Toughness/Drug Use setting ($N = 201$) Coefficient		r	High Toughness/Drug Use setting ($N = 201$) Coefficient		r
Low Toughness/Drug Use setting[d]	.022	(.006)	−.115									
High Toughness/Drug Use setting[d]	.092	(.025)	.134									
Demographic												
Age	.051	(.032)	.143	−.016	(−.010)	.080	.060	(.038)	.184	.102	(.063)	.156
Sex	−.007	(−.002)	−.004	.222	(.069)	.052	−.054	(−.016)	−.014	−.119	(−.032)	−.060
Home composition	.031	(.010)	.094	.272	(.089)	.170	−.192	(−.063)	.008	.028	(.008)	.074
Neighborhood Orientation/ Involvement												
Survival	−.265**	(−.112)	−.084	−.223	(−.089)	−.066	−.097	(−.042)	−.084	−.522***	(−.209)	−.224
Status of drug-using, gang-involved persons by peers	.128	(.067)	.212	.066	(.033)	.121	.215	(.102)	.199	.122	(.061)	.200
Participation in street culture spare-time activities	.324***	(.157)	.344	.203	(.104)	.290	.250	(.117)	.280	.495***	(.228)	.398
Participation in print media, stay-at-home spare-time activities	−.091	(−.040)	−.098	−.182	(−.081)	−.132	.104	(.045)	−.006	−.157	(−.073)	−.102
Drug Use Context												
Availability of drugs in the school	.188*	(.100)	.205	.144	(.080)	.179	.219	(.108)	.114	.238	(.128)	.258

(continued)

Table 4 (continued)

Variables	All neighborhoods combined (N = 630)			Low Toughness /Drug Use setting (N = 228)			Medium Toughness/Drug Use setting (N = 201)			High Toughness/Drug Use setting (N = 201)		
	Coefficient		r	Coefficient		r	Coefficient		r	Coefficient		r
Availability of drugs in the neighborhood	.140	(.076)	.230	.132	(.073)	.244	.114	(.059)	.082	.165	(.087)	.263
Friends' use of alcohol and marijuana	.788***	(.366)	.483	.820***	(.375)	.474	.823***	(.378)	.410	.694***	(.325)	.519
Friends' use of "hard drugs"	–.204**	(–.097)	–.024	–.025	(–.009)	–.058	–.548***	(–.272)	–.173	–.018	(–.010)	.077
Self-reported alcohol use												
Constant	2.181			1.716			2.519			2.292		
R^2	0.307			0.279			0.283			0.394		
F for R^2	20.989***			7.586***			6.772***			11.152***		
df	13,616			11,216			11,189			11,189		

[a] Standardized coefficients in parentheses.
[b] The variables used in this analysis were coded as follows: age: 11 or under = 1, 12 years = 2, 13 years = 3, 14 years = 4, 15 years = 5, 16 years or over = 6; sex: male = 1, female = 2; home composition: living with both parents = 1, living with father or mother = 2, living with neither parent = 3; the survival, image of different person types, street culture spare-time activities, print media/stay-at-home spare-time activities, availability of drugs in the school, availability of drugs in the neighborhood, and friends' use of alcohol/marijuana and other substances factor scores were constructed such that the lower the score, the less the adherence to the attitude/value dimension, or involvement in the behavior, reflected in the factor; the higher the score, the greater the adherence to the attitude/value dimension or involvement in the behavior.
[c] The b weights represented are those resulting after the effects of neighborhood setting have been partialled out.
[d] Dichotomized variables coded 1 and 0 for each neighborhood setting.
*$p < .05$.
**$p < .01$.
***$p < .001$.

Table 5

ANOVA Test of Homogeneity of the Regression Coefficients (bs) for Tobacco Use

Source of variation	*SS*	*df*	*MS*	*F*	*p*
Pooled coefficients for the 3 Toughness contexts	829.996	11	75.45	20.95	.001
Residual from pooled coefficients	2238.969	622	3.60		
Separate coefficients	898.965	33			
Differences between separate coefficients	68.969	22	3.14	0.87	NS
Residual from separate coefficients	2170.000	60	3.62		
Total	3068.965	633			

In the Drug Use Context variable set, Friends' Use of Alcohol and Marijuana was again most predictive of tobacco use and again was predictive regardless of neighborhood setting.

Friends' Use of "Hard Drugs" was significantly negatively related to self-reported tobacco use, but only in the medium toughness setting.

Predicting Frequency of Marijuana Use

Analyses indentical to those described for alcohol and tobacco were conducted for the frequency of marijuana use variable. Table 7 indicates that the analysis of variance examination of the homogeneity of the regression coefficients provided evidence for interactive effects of neighborhood setting on reported marijuana use. Significant differences were found for both the pooled coefficients, F (11, 637) = 31.77, $p < .001$, and the effect from the separate coefficients, F (22, 615) = 1.80, $p < .025$. Table 8 illustrates those effects.

Similar to the alcohol and tobacco data, the demographic characteristics were of little assistance in predicting self-reported marijuana use across the neighborhood settings. It did appear that the older the adolescent, the heavier his involvement with marijuana, but only in the medium Toughness/Drug Use neighborhood setting. Similarly, adolescents from "nonintact" homes reported heavier involvement with marijuana, but only in the high toughness setting.

The "life-style" variables (Neighborhood Orientation/Involvement) were again more productive. The Status of Drug-Using, Gang-Involved Persons by Peers was important in the high setting, Participation in Street Culture/Spare-Time Activities was important in all three neighborhood settings but not differentially so, and Participation in Stay-at-Home Spare-Time Activities was important in the high Toughness/Drug Use setting.

Finally, the Drug Use Context variables indicated that Friends' Use of Alcohol and Marijuana was not only highly predictive of self-reported marijuana

Table 6

Stepwise Regression Coefficients of Tobacco Use on Youths' Demographic Characteristics, Neighborhood Orientation/Involvement, and Drug Use Context Variables[a]

Variables	All neighborhoods combined (N = 636)			Low Toughness /Drug Use setting (N = 228)			Medium Toughness/Drug Use setting (N = 206)			High Toughness/Drug Use setting (N = 202)		
	Coefficient		r	Coefficient		r	Coefficient		r	Coefficient		r
Low Toughness/Drug Use setting	.184	(.040)	–.115									
High Toughness/ Drug Use setting	.495*	(.103)	.180									
Demographic												
Age	–.030	(–.014)	.077	.015	(.008)	.085	–.033	(–.016)	.102	–.078	(–.034)	.047
Sex	.385*	(.085)	.118	.273	(.069)	.075	.963***	(.225)	.267	–.101	(–.019)	–.001
Home composition	.254	(.062)	.157	.495*	(.132)	.235	.198	(.053)	.151	.126	(.028)	.064
Neighborhood Involvement/Participation												
Survival	–.204	(–.066)	–.048	–.134	(–.043)	–.027	–.277	(–.097)	–.157	–.206	(–.060)	–.101
Status of drug-using gang-involved persons by peers	.106	(.043)	.192	–.075	(.031)	.121	.188	(.074)	.173	.160	(.057)	.147
Participation in street culture spare-time activities	.600	(.220)	.392	.481**	(.194)	.372	.502**	(.184)	.342	.650**	(.215)	.395

Participation in print media, stay-at-home spare-time activities	–.110	(.037)	–.081	–.100	(–.036)	–.093	–.122	(–.042)	–.034	–.095	(–.031)	–.066
Drug Use Context												
Availability of drugs in the school	–.056	(–.023)	.050	.055	(.024)	.083	.127	(.052)	–.001	–.329	(–.127)	–.014
Availability of drugs in the neighborhood	.122	(.047)	.131	.048	(.021)	.157	.119	(.050)	.008	.119	(.046)	.090
Friends' use of alcohol and marijuana	.947***	(.336)	.440	.930***	(.341)	.454	.816***	(.303)	.345	1.161***	(.388)	.469
Friends' use of "hard drugs"	–.307**	(–.114)	–.074	–.070	(–.020)	–.086	–.549***	(–.232)	–.186	–.187	(–.073)	–.031
Self-reported alcohol use												
Constant	1.3528			1.2610			0.5357			2.9448		
R^2	0.295			0.279			0.307			0.292		
F for R^2	19.99**			7.60***			7.82			7.13		
df	13,622			11,216			11,194			11,190		

[a] See notes to Table 4.
$*p < .05$.
$**p < .01$.
$***p < .001$.

Table 7

ANOVA Test of Homogeneity of the Regression Coefficients (bs) for Marijuana Use

Source of variation	*SS*	*df*	*MS*	*F*	*p*
Pooled coefficients for the 3 Toughness contexts	721.299	11	65.573	31.77	.001
Residual from pooled coefficients	1314.565	637	2.064		
Separate coefficients	800.983	33			
Differences between separate coefficients	79.687	22	3.622	1.80	.025
Residual from separate coefficients	1234.881	615	2.008		
Total	2035.864	648			

use, it was differentially so across neighborhood settings, such that the relationship became stronger as the perception of the neighborhood became "tougher" and more drug involved.

Friends' Use of "Hard Drugs" was again significantly negatively related to reported marijuana use, and again only in the medium category.

DISCUSSION

Since the present study was initiated in an attempt to determine if specific drugs related differently to the environment in predicting drug use than did an overall drug involvement measure, it is appropriate to address that issue first. The answer, and quite dramatically so, was yes. The previous study (Dembo, Schmeidler, Burgos, and Taylor, forthcoming; which excluded tobacco) found an interaction between Participation in Street Culture Spare-Time Activities and Neighborhood Setting in the prediction of drug involvement, such that this prediction was best for the high Toughness/Drug Use setting. The present study indicated that this result was due almost entirely to the marijuana variable, the relationship being virtually nonexistent in the alcohol data. Second, the previous study found a very strong but not differential relationship between Friends' Use of Alcohol and Marijuana and reported overall Drug Involvement. This result was replicated in the present study, but only for alcohol. The marijuana data showed a dramatic interaction occasioned by the youth's perception of his environment, such that the tougher and more drug involved he perceived his surroundings, the stronger the relationship between friends' use and his personal involvement with marijuana. Both of these findings (which have strong implications for prevention strategies) were unavailable when an overall measure was employed.

The similarities and differences for the three substances also invite comment. Alcohol and marijuana were clearly different. Knowledge of Street Culture Spare-Time Activities was important in predicting marijuana use across

Table 8

Stepwise Regression Coefficients of Marijuana Use on Youths' Demographic Characteristics, Neighborhood Orientation/Involvement, and Drug Use Context Variables[a]

Variables	All neighborhoods combined ($N = 651$)			Low Toughness/Drug Use setting ($N = 235$)			Medium Toughness/Drug Use setting ($N = 207$)			High Toughness/Drug Use setting ($N = 209$)		
	Coefficient		r	Coefficient		r	Coefficient		r	Coefficient		r
Low Toughness/Drug Use setting	−.004	(−.001)	−.154									
High Toughness/ Drug Use setting	.142	(.037)	.171									
Demographic												
Age	.170**	(.101)	.206	.042	(.032)	.118	.374***	(.229)	.372	.054	(.028)	.141
Sex	−.114	(−.031)	.007	.030	(.011)	.007	−.002	(.000)	.033	−.439	(−.101)	−.083
Home composition	.281**	(.085)	.169	.265	(.099)	.206	.167	(.053)	.147	.438*	(.114)	.132
Neighborhood Orientation/ Involvement												
Survival	−.055	(−.022)	.017	−.069	(−.031)	−.024	.131	(.056)	.025	−.267	(−.092)	−.099
Status of drug-using gang-involved persons by peers	.209**	(.105)	.272	.012	(.007)	.117	.228	(.108)	.300	.337*	(.145)	.250
Participation in street culture spare-time activities	.525***	(.240)	.423	.458***	(.262)	.420	.468***	(.209)	.370	.532***	(.208)	.421
Participation in print media, stay-at-home spare-time activities	−.327***	(−.137)	−.206	−.148	(−.074)	−.129	−.257	(−.106)	−.150	−.565***	(−.221)	−.254
Drug Use Context												
Availability of drugs in the school	−.014	(−.007)	.089	.042	(.026)	.139	.083	(.040)	.035	−.193	(−.089)	.030

(continued)

Table 8 (continued)

Variables	All neighborhoods combined ($N = 651$) Coefficient		r	Low Toughness /Drug Use setting ($N = 235$) Coefficient		r	Medium Toughness/Drug Use setting ($N = 207$) Coefficient		r	High Toughness/Drug Use setting ($N = 209$) Coefficient		r
Availability of drugs in the neighborhood	−.042	(.022)	.155	.120	(.076)	.224	.035	(.017)	.031	−.041	(−.019)	.092
Friends' use of alcohol and marijuana	.783***	(.342)	.501	.653***	(.338)	.476	.784***	(.346)	.455	.990***	(.385)	.523
Friends' use of "hard drugs"	−.207*	(−.094)	−.035	−.097	(−.039)	−.083	−.424***	(−.206)	−.152	−.110	(−.051)	.023
Self-reported alcohol use												
Constant	1.140			1.239			0.518			1.907		
R^2	0.377			0.330			0.411			0.412		
F for R^2	29.645***			10.010***			12.356***			12.557***		
df	13,637			11,223			11,195			11,197		

[a] See notes to Table 4.
*$p < .05$.
**$p < .01$.
***$p < .001$.

all neighborhood settings, but it was useful for alcohol only in the neighborhoods perceived to be the toughest and most drug oriented. Further, although significant for both alcohol and marijuana, Friends' Use of Alcohol and Marijuana was quite different in predicting alcohol as opposed to marijuana use, being equally important in all neighborhood settings for alcohol but increasing substantially for marijuana use in predictive power as neighborhoods were perceived to be more and more tough and drug involved.

There are obvious differences, therefore, in the influence of peers on alcohol and marijuana use; these influences are fairly independent of neighborhood setting for alcohol but are very dependent on the perception of neighborhood for marijuana. That is, if a youth perceives his neighborhood to be tough and drug oriented, he is much more likely to report marijuana use for both himself and his peers than if he perceives his neighborhood to be not so tough. He is likely to report alcohol use for himself and his peers regardless of his perceptions of his neighborhood.

Interestingly, tobacco showed a middle ground between alcohol and marijuana. Like alcohol, a knowledge of Friends' Use of Alcohol and Marijuana was important for predicting tobacco use but not differentially so across neighborhood settings (i.e., knowing how the youth perceived his neighborhood did not influence predictability). Like marijuana, a knowledge of the youth's Spare-Time Street Culture Activities was quite important in predicting tobacco use, and, also like marijuana, such predictability was not altered by a knowledge of the youth's perception of his neighborhood.

The latter finding is at least logical. One of the prime activities in the street culture is "hanging out," and one of the main activities while hanging out is smoking. Smoking (tobacco as well as dope) is thus engrained in these activities. Not so alcohol, it would seem. It is apparently unacceptable to certain peer groups to stand around and drink on street corners (to say nothing of pool hall owners, restaurateurs and movie house managers), at least at age 13. You can smoke, but not drink. (The high category is an exception, as in that case either behavior seems acceptable.)

Finally, it is appropriate to speculate on the lack of relationship with the other variables used in the present study. That the demographic variables were unpredictive is consistent with the findings of Kandel (1975), Kandel, Kessler, and Margulies (1978), and Jessor and Jessor (1977), whose results highlight the fact that drug use tends to be influenced by attitude/value and interpersonal factors. However, at least on the surface, the individual's perception of drug-using, gang-involved peers, and the availability of drugs would seem to exert some influence on his own behavior. It is possible that they do and that the effect is simply too weak or our measure too crude to reveal it.

IMPLICATIONS FOR INTERVENTION

The implications for intervention then, seem clear. First one must recognize that it is not physical environment per se that is so important, but how the target youth interacts with the people in it and how he perceives those people in relation to himself. Hence users and nonusers coexist in the same physical space. How they can be differentiated (identified, predicted) is a crucial area for additional research. The present data offer demonstrated differences in attitudes and the influence of their peers as beginning points.

The relationships are complex rather than simple and so also must be the intervention strategies. These must exist on several levels at one time: at a minimum with both the target youth as an individual and with his associates. Further, community-based behavioral alternatives which are at least non-drug centered if not totally drug-free are mandatory. Recreational centers, professionally staffed with persons acceptable to the target youth, are an obvious beginning, along with honest discussions of drug use in schools, especially for users.

Viewing the youth and his environment as a system would seem required to coordinate efforts in all aspects of his life in order to help avoid dysfunctional drug use. The system approach employed by the U.S. Department of Transportation in their efforts to combat the drinking driver in the '70s is an excellent example.

Second, one must tailor the intervention strategies to the particular drug of interest. The drugs are different. The reactions to them are different and the intervention strategies must also be different.

SUMMARY AND CONCLUSIONS

A knowledge of an adolescent's friends' use of alcohol and marijuana is extremely important in predicting his personal alcohol, tobacco, and marijuana use. For tobacco and alcohol this relationship was fairly constant across neighborhood settings. For marijuana, the relationship was also strong but indicated a rather dramatic interaction (indirect) influence with the environment, such that the relationship was weakest for the low Toughness/Drug Use setting and strongest for the high Toughness/Drug Use condition.

Further, the use of "life-style" and "context" variables (as opposed to demographic) appears to be the most productive in this line of research.

ACKNOWLEDGEMENTS

This research was supported in part by a grant from the University of South Florida Research and Creative Scholarship Fund. We are grateful for the assistance given us by the principal, teachers, and parents of the junior high school, who must remain anonymous. The reactions of many youngsters to earlier versions of the survey instruments were valuable to our research effort. The support and encouragement of the New York State Office of Drug Abuse Services, and especially Douglas S. Lipton, Director of the Division of Cost Effectiveness and Research, are appreciated. Bill Burgos was invaluable in all phases of the study. Ken Marion, Dean Babst, Sharon Diamond, Carol Spielman, and Phyllis Bergman were helpful in processing the data. Jim Schmeidler provided valuable data processing and statistical assistance throughout the project and on the present paper. However, these persons are not responsible for the views that are expressed in the paper or the ways in which the data were examined. We would also like to thank Dr. Louise G. Richards, Division of Research, National Institute on Drug Abuse, for initially suggesting that we pursue the line of analysis of which this paper is one product.

NOTES

1. As implied, the data were gathered in two parts. The school system would not permit merger of the separate administrations. Thus we were unable to relate items from one data set to the data presented here (such as substance use by other family members, relationships with parents, attitudes toward school, self-image, etc.).
2. Six months was used as a time frame because recall problems were minimized and 6 months is a substantial length of time for this age group. The latter was most important due to the known infrequency of use of such substances by the age group in question. The addition of the qualifiers of "once a month," "once a week," etc. (which appeared on the questionnaire) made this sequence of use categories not only quite meaningful to the subjects but also easy for them to respond to. See Lipton et al. (1977) for additional details of this development process.
3. For alcohol: low Toughness/Drug Use, $F\ (4, 254) = .87$, NS; medium Toughness/Drug Use; $F\ (4, 232) = .67$, NS; high Toughness/Drug Use; $F\ (4, 238) = .61$, NS. For tobacco: low Toughness/Drug Use; $F\ (4, 259) = .081$, NS; medium Toughness/Drug Use; $F\ (4, 239) = 1.20$, NS; high Toughness/Drug Use; $F\ (4, 237) = 1.46$, NS. For marijuana: low Toughness/Drug Use; $F\ (4, 268) = .66$, NS; medium Toughness/Drug Use, $F\ (4, 241) = .12$, NS; high Toughness/Drug Use; $F\ (4, 247) = .85$, NS.

REFERENCES

BLUMER, H., SUTTER, A., AHMED, S., and SMITH, R. *The World of Youthful Drug Use*. Berkeley, CA: University of California at Berkeley, School of Criminology, 1967.

CLOWARD, R.A., and OHLIN, L.E. *Delinquency and Opportunity*. New York: Free Press, 1960.

DEMBO, R. Critical factors in understanding adolescent aggression. *Soc. Psychiatry* 8: 212-219, 1973.

DEMBO, R., BURGOS, W., BABST, D.V., SCHMEIDLER, J., and LA GRAND, L.E. Neighborhood relationships and drug involvement among inner city junior high school youths: Implications for drug education and prevention programming. *J. Drug Educ.* 8: 231-252, 1978.

DEMBO, R., BURGOS, W., DES JARLAIS, D., and SCHMEIDLER, J. Ethnicity and drug use among urban junior high school youths. *Int. J. Addict.* 14: 557-568, 1979.

DEMBO, R., FARROW, D., SCHMEIDLER, J., and BURGOS, W. Testing a causal model of environmental influences on the early drug involvement of inner city junior high school youth. *Am. J. Drug Alcohol Abuse* 6: 313-336, 1979.

DEMBO, R., SCHMEIDLER, J., BURGOS, W., and TAYLOR, R. Environmental setting and early drug involvement among inner city junior high school youths. *Int. J. Addict.* Forthcoming.

FELDMAN, H.W. Ideological supports to becoming and remaining a heroin addict. *J. Health Soc. Behav.* 9: 131-139, 1968.

FELDMAN, H.W. American way of drugging. *Society*, May-June, 1973, pp. 32-38.

FELDMAN, H.W. *Street Status and the Drug Researcher: Issues in Participant-Observation.* Washington, DC: Drug Abuse Council, 1974.

FELDMAN, H.W. A neighborhood history of drug switching. In R.S. Weppner (ed.), *Street Ethnography.* Beverly Hills, CA: Sage, 1977.

FINESTONE, H. Cats, kicks and color. *Soc. Probl.* 5: 3-13, 1957.

JESSOR, R., and JESSOR, S.L. *Problem Behavior and Psychosocial Development: A Longitudinal Study of Youth.* New York: Academic Press, 1977.

JOHNSON, B.D. *Marijuana Users and Drug Subcultures.* New York: Wiley, 1973.

KANDEL, D.B. Adolescent marijuana use: Role of parents and peers. *Science* 181: 1067-1070, 1973.

KANDEL, D.B. Some comments on the relationship of selected criteria variables to adolescent illicit drug use. In D.J. Lettieri (ed.), *Predicting Adolescent Drug Abuse: A Review of Issues, Methods and Correlates.* Rockville, MD: National Institute on Drug Abuse, 1975.

KANDEL, D.B., KESSLER, R.C., and MARGULIES, R.Z. Antecedents of adolescent initiation into stages of drug use: A developmental analysis. In D.B. Kandel (ed.), *Longitudinal Research on Drug Use.* Washington, DC: Hemisphere, 1978.

KAPLAN, H.B. Social class, self-derogation and deviant behavior. *Soc. Psychiatry* 13: 19-28, 1978.

KAPLAN, H.B. *Deviant Behavior in Defense of Self.* New York: Academic Press, 1980.

KAUFMAN, E. The relationship of social class and ethnicity to drug abuse. In D.E. Smith, S.M. Anderson, M. Buxton, N. Gottlieb, W. Harvey, and T. Chung (eds.), *A Multicultural View of Drug Abuse.* Cambridge, MA: Shenkman Press, 1978.

LIPTON, D.S., STEPHENS, R.C., BABST, D.V., DEMBO, R., DIAMOND,S.C., SPIELMAN, C.R., SCHMEIDLER, J., BERGMAN, P.J., and UPPAL, G.S. A survey of substance use among junior and senior high school students in New York State, winter 1974-75. *Am. J. Drug Alcohol Abuse* 4: 153-164, 1977.

MERTON, R. Social structure and anomie. In R.K. Merton (ed.), *Social Theory and Social Structure.* Glencoe, IL: Free Press, 1957.

PREBLE, E., and CASEY, J.J., Jr. Taking care of business–The heroin user's life on the street. *Int. J. Addict.* 4: 1-24, 1969.

SINGLE, E., KANDEL, D.B., and FAUST, R. Patterns of multiple drug use in high school. *J. Health Soc. Behav.* 15: 344-357, 1974.

SUTTER, A.G. The world of the righteous dope fiend. *Issues Criminol.* 2: 177-222, 1966.

SUTTER, A.G. Worlds of drug use in the street scene. In C.R. Cressy and D.A. Ward (eds.), *Delinquency, Crime, and Social Process.* New York: Harper and Row, 1969.

TUCHFELD, B.S., CLAYTON, R.R., and LOGAN, J.A. Alcohol, drug use and delinquent and criminal behaviors. *J. Drug Issues* 12: 185-198, 1982.

WEITZEL, S.L., and BLOUNT, W.R. Incarcerated female felons and substance abuse. *J. Drug Issues* 12: 259-273, 1982.

The International Journal of the Addictions, 19(2), 199–219, 1984

A Comprehensive Care Program for Pregnant Addicts: Obstetrical, Neonatal, and Child Development Outcomes

Frederic Suffet, MA

Richard Brotman, PhD

Center for Comprehensive Health Practice
New York Medical College
New York, New York 10029

Abstract

This study reports the results of a comprehensive care program for pregnant addicts, one that provides medical, counseling, and child development services. Findings include the following. Women who enroll while pregnant generally stay through childbirth, and most deliveries are free of complication. Most newborns are of normal gestational age and birthweight, and these outcomes are directly related to length and amount of prenatal care. Neonatal withdrawal is directly related to prenatal maternal methadone dose. Child development, as measured by the Bayley Scales, is usually in the normal range, although mean scores for cognitive development decrease through age 2. Female babies generally have higher cognitive and motor scores than males, and their cognitive scores decline less sharply than those of the males. Developmental scores are directly related to neonatal maturity, especially birthweight. Prenatal maternal methadone dose tends to be negatively related to developmental scores for boys but not for girls.

 0020-773X/84/1902-0199$3.50/0

INTRODUCTION

The well-being of the drug-addicted mother and her newborn had been a problem of long-standing concern. Reports on the problem began to filter into the medical literature even before the turn of the century (Cobrinik et al., 1959). However, it was not until the past few decades, with the spread of the present heroin "epidemic," that such reports began to appear with ever-greater frequency. This is not surprising, since the general increase in the heroin-using population implied an increase in the number of female addicts. For example, the addict population of New York City increased from the 1960s to the early 1970s (Des Jarlais and Uppal, 1980), by which time a fourth of it was reported to be female (New York City Narcotics Register, 1973), a figure that was soon reflected in national treatment statistics (National Institute on Drug Abuse, 1977).

The increase in the number of addicted women was accompanied by a rise in the number of addict births. The New york City Department of Health reported 227 addict births in 1966 (a rate of 1.5 per 1,000 live births) and 1,043 addict births in 1976 (a rate of 9.5 per 1,000 live births [Whiting et al., 1978]). Also in New York City, a study conducted at Metropolitan Hospital, in the disadvantaged East Harlem section of the borough of Manhattan, found that the ratio of addict to nonaddict births at the hospital had increased from 1:164 in 1960 to 1:47 by 1969 (Stone et al., 1971).

The latter study also documented the adverse effects of addict births. For instance, an unusually high incidence of such obstetrical complications as anemia, toxemia, and shortened labor was found. Furthermore, 30% of the infants were premature by gestational age, 49% were below normal birthweight, and 67% showed signs of addiction. This in part was to be expected, since few of the women had had even a minimal amount of prenatal care, the lack of which has been shown to be associated with an increased risk of low birthweight (Eisner et al., 1979). Of course, minimal prenatal care was hardly unique to female addicts; it was (and still is) typical among many women who are poor (Watson and Hollander, 1978). What was unique was their addiction and its effects on the newborn, and this was something that most hospitals and drug programs were not well prepared to handle (Friel and Saltonstall, 1973; Ryan, 1977; Taleporos et al., 1978).

By the mid-1970s it had become clear that special programs were needed to address the special needs of this population. Thus, programs to provide care to pregnant addicts were established with National Institute on Drug Abuse support in Detroit, Houston, New York City, Philadelphia, San Rafael, California, and Washington, DC (Beschner and Brotman, 1977).

The New York City program, called the Pregnant Addicts and Addicted Mothers Program (PAAM), was inaugurated in February 1975 under the auspices of the Center for Comprehensive Health Practice of New York Medical College. Originally supported by two successive 3-year demonstration grants from the National Institute on Drug Abuse, PAAM now operates under contract to the New York State Division of Substance Abuse Services.

Programs goals relevant to the present study are for the pregnant addict to have a normal pregnancy and deliver a healthy newborn, and for the baby to develop normal cognitive and motor abilities during early childhood. We shall thus report obstetrical, neonatal, and child development outcomes, using for this purpose pregnancy data on the women who joined PAAM during its first 5 years (through January 1980) and neonatal and child development data obtained on their children through the end of PAAM's sixth year (January 1981). (Outcomes concerning other goals, such as reduction of substance abuse and improvement of various areas of social functioning, were reported in an earlier paper [Suffet et al., 1981].) Before we examine these data, let us describe the program and the treatment population.

PROGRAM DESCRIPTION

PAAM is an outpatient facility located in the New York Medical College and Flower Hospital complex in East Harlem. Its treatment philosophy stresses comprehensive care, meaning that a full range of services is provided on-site. These—more fully described later—include addiction treatment and obstetrical, pediatric, psychiatric, and general medical care; individual and group counseling; and child development services (parent education classes, developmental assessment, and a preschool nursery). PAAM is open weekdays from 8:30 A.M. to 4:30 P.M. and weekends from 8:00 A.M. to 11:00 A.M. A 24-hour program hotline is available for patients to call in case of an emergency.

Any pregnant women, regardless of stage of pregnancy, is eligible to join PAAM if she is at least 18 years old (or 16 or 17 with the consent of a parent or legal guardian), and if she is currently addicted to illicit opiates or is receiving prescribed methadone. A nonpregnant woman is eligible if she meets the age criterion, has a child under a year old, and is currently addicted to illicit opiates or is receiving prescribed methadone and can document an addiction history of at least a year. A woman with a multiple addiction who meets the eligibility criteria is referred to an inpatient detoxification facility and may enroll in PAAM after starting on methadone, if necessary, and detoxifying from nonopiates.

Women who join PAAM must meet certain minimum requirements for program participation. These include: following a schedule of examinations set by the medical staff (prenatal and postnatal examinations for herself and pediatric examinations for her newborn); visiting the program at least 5 days a week for methadone, if it is prescribed, and refraining from the use of illicit drugs; having at least one individual counseling session a week; and attending parent education classes weekly. Persistent failure to meet these requirements may result in termination from the program; and such illegal acts as assault, theft, or selling drugs will automatically result in termination if committed on program premises.

PAAM's original treatment capacity was 110 cases, and this has gradually been increased to the present level of 130. A case may include not only the woman who is the "index" patient and her infant, but also any older children she has, as well as her legal or consensual spouse. Pediatric and child development services are available for the children, and the spouse may receive any services geared to adults. The present average annual cost per case, paid for by contract funds, Medicaid, and patient fees, is $4,600. This covers the following services for the woman, her newborn, and other persons included in the case.

Medical Services

Pregnant patients are cared for by the PAAM obstetrician. They deliver at one of New York Medical College's affiliates, Metropolitan Hospital (and formerly at another affiliate, Flower Hospital). Inpatient neonatal care is managed by the PAAM pediatrician, who also provides follow-up care for the children born on the program and treats any older children the women may have. The program psychiatrist provides specialized care as needed in individual cases. General medical care is given by the PAAM internist, who also sets methadone schedules. Most pregnant patients are maintained on methadone through childbirth, usually at 40 mg or less daily. After giving birth, a woman is encouraged to detoxify if possible.

Counseling Services

Individual counseling begins as soon as a woman joins PAAM. Initial sessions focus on emergency needs and also serve to clarify expectations regarding program participation. Later sessions deal with specific problems defined by the treatment staff according to information obtained in the intake interview. If a woman has a legal or consensual spouse, she is encouraged to have him join her in family counseling sessions. Counselors act as patients' advocates, assisting them in dealings with the welfare office, landlords, day care centers, and so on.

Group counseling is provided in the course of weekly "life skills" classes. Some topics are basic to daily living (e.g., nutrition, leisure activity), others are based on questions that come up routinely in individual counseling (e.g., birth control, sleep problems), while still others address concerns often expressed by patients (e.g., crib death).

Child Development Services

Weekly parent education classes are held during the prenatal and postpartum periods. Prenatal classes are usually attended by 20 or more pregnant patients and cover such topics as physical and emotional changes during pregnancy, fetal growth and development, nutrition and hygiene during pregnancy, preparation for childbirth, labor and delivery, and infant care. Within a month of giving birth, a woman joins a group for postpartum classes, which she is expected to attend until her child reaches 2 years of age. There are six to eight groups at any time, each comprised of 8 to 10 women with children of approximately the same age. The classes focus on childrearing techniques and on developmental stages during the first 2 years of a baby's life (Lief, 1981).

The preschool nursery is for children age 2 to 5. Usually, about 30 children participate in the nursery, which includes guided group play designed to teach the youngsters how to relate to age mates and individual instruction designed to remedy such problems as poor attention span. Group sessions, dealing with such topics as discipline and sibling rivalry, are held weekly for mothers of children in the nursery.

In addition to the parenting classes and preschool nursery, the child development component of PAAM includes periodic assessment, via the Bayley Scales of Infant Development (Bayley, 1969), of the children's cognitive and motor development through 2 years of age.

TREATMENT POPULATION

A total of 278 women were admitted to PAAM during the program's first 5 years. Their demographic characteristics are shown in Table 1. Most were in their 20s, of minority group background, not high school graduates, living with a male partner and in some cases with children or parents, and residing in Manhattan.

As indicated in Table 2, 85.3% of the women were pregnant at admission. The remaining 14.7% had given birth within the year prior to enrollment. Of those who were pregnant, 84.4% delivered while on the program. The others either aborted, miscarried, or left PAAM before giving birth. Fifteen women who delivered on PAAM later gave birth to another child on the program. Ten of them had left PAAM after the initial delivery but returned when they became pregnant again. Of those who were not pregnant at admission, three later had a child on PAAM, and one who miscarried also later had a child. In sum, there were 219 PAAM births, including one set of twins, for a total of 220 babies.

PRENATAL CARE

Four variables on the nature and extent of prenatal care provided in the 219 pregnancies that resulted in PAAM deliveries are shown in Table 3.

Table 1

Demographic Characteristics (N = 278 Unless Otherwise Noted)

Variable	Categories	Percent	*N*
Age	19 or under	5.4	15
	20 to 24	48.6	135
	25 to 29	35.3	98
	30 or over	10.8	30
Race/ethnicity	Black	48.6	135
	Hispanic	33.8	94
	White	16.9	47
	Other	0.7	2
Education (*N* = 276)[a]	Not high school graduate	66.7	184
	High school graduate	22.1	61
	Some college	10.5	29
	College graduate	0.7	2
Marital status	Single	68.7	191
	Married	15.5	43
	Separated	11.2	31
	Divorced	2.5	7
	Widowed	2.2	6
Male cohabitant	None	45.3	126
	Legal spouse	12.2	34
	Consensual spouse/boyfriend	42.4	118
Others in household (*N* = 276)[a]	None	32.6	90
	Parent(s)	21.0	58
	Child(ren)	41.7	115
	Other(s)	28.3	78
Place of residence	Manhattan	64.0	178
	Bronx	24.1	67
	Queens	7.6	21
	Brooklyn	2.9	8
	Outside New York City	1.4	4

[a]Two cases are omitted due to incomplete data.

Table 2

Pregnancy Course

Variable	Categories	Percent	N
Pregnancy status at admission (*N* = 278)	Pregnant	85.3	237
	Not pregnant	14.7	41
Outcome for those pregnant at admission (*N* = 237)	Delivered on PAAM	84.4	200
	Aborted	3.4	8
	Miscarried	3.0	7
	Left while pregnant	9.3	22

Table 3

Prenatal Care (N = 219 Unless Otherwise Noted)

Variable	Categories	Percent	*N*
Gestational duration at first visit	13 weeks or less	11.4	25
	14 to 26 weeks	52.1	114
	27 weeks or more	36.5	80
Days of care	49 or less	24.2	53
	50 to 99	22.8	50
	100 to 149	28.3	62
	150 or more	24.7	54
Number of prenatal visits ($N = 218$)[a]	4 or less	21.6	47
	5 to 9	29.8	65
	10 to 14	33.5	73
	15 or more	15.1	33
Methadone dose at delivery ($N = 216$)[b]	None	8.8	19
	5 to 20 mg	38.4	83
	25 to 40 mg	44.0	95
	45 mg or more	8.8	19

[a] One case is omitted due to incomplete data.
[b] Three early cases are omitted in which the patient was receiving methadone from a program other than PAAM, and in which precise dosage information was unavailable.

Gestational duration at first visit is a measure of promptness in seeking care. In the majority of cases, care began for the mothers in the second or third trimester ($\bar{X} = 23.6$ weeks, SD = 8.1).

Days of care refers to the interval between the start of prenatal care and delivery. In three-fourths of the cases the period of care was at least 50 days ($\bar{X} = 107.6$, SD = 65.9).

Number of prenatal visits refers to the number of times the patient was examined by the PAAM obstetrician before giving birth. In nearly four-fifths of the cases there were at least five visits ($\bar{X} = 9.1$, SD = 5.3).

Methadone dose at delivery indicates the amount of methadone the woman was receiving at PAAM at the time she gave birth. The dose usually remained stable during the last trimester, and the majority of those on methadone were receiving 40 mg or less ($\bar{X} = 29.1$, SD = 14.1).

OBSTETRICAL OUTCOMES

Distributions on six obstetrical outcome variables are shown in Table 4. The *N*s vary for two reasons. First, 13 babies were born at hospitals other than our two affiliates, Flower and Metropolitan, and in these cases complete records were not always available. Second, hospital charts at the two affiliates, from which obstetrical data were coded, sometimes did not contain notations on these items.

Table 4

Obstetrical Outcomes

Variable	Categories	Percent	N
Premature rupture of membranes (N = 191)	No	63.9	122
	Yes, 24 h or less	30.9	59
	Yes, over 24 h	5.2	10
Blood pressure (N = 192)	Normotensive	87.5	168
	Hypertensive	12.5	24
Fetal heart rate (N = 187)	Normal	91.4	171
	Abnormal	8.6	16
Meconium passage (N = 200)	No	91.5	183
	Yes	8.5	17
Delivery mode and presentation (N = 219)	Vaginal and vertex	86.3	189
	Vaginal and breech	3.2	7
	Cesarean	10.5	23
Number of complications (N = 201)	None	65.6	132
	1	27.4	55
	2	6.5	13
	3	0.5	1

Premature rupture of the membranes refers to the interval, if any, between the time the membranes rupture and the onset of labor. An interval of over 24 hours is likely to be associated with amniotic infection, and such an interval was observed in 5.2% of the cases.

Blood pressure was counted as high if at least one intrapartum reading of 140 or more over 90 or more was obtained. A reading in this range is a possible sign of toxemia and was obtained in 12.5% of the cases.

A fetal heart rate of less than 111 or greater than 159 beats a minute is considered abnormal and an indicator of fetal distress. A reading at one or the other of these extremes was obtained in 8.6% of the cases.

Meconium passage during labor, observed in 8.5% of the cases, also is considered a sign of fetal distress. There were an additional 12 cases in which the baby was meconium stained. Thus, there were a total of 29 cases, or 14.5%, involving meconium passage or staining.

Delivery mode was by cesarean section 10.5% of the cases. A breech presentation in a vaginal birth, typically associated with a difficult delivery, occurred in 3.2% of the cases.

Complications of labor and delivery were absent in nearly two-thirds of the cases, and in the remainder there was usually no more than one complication. The most common complication, occurring in 45 cases (20.5%), was premature delivery. Apart from that, one to six instances of each of the following were observed: abruptio placenta, cephalopelvic disproportion, hepatitis, hypertension, laceration of the perineum, placenta previa, pneumonia, postpartum hemorrhage, postpartum fever, precipitous delivery, prolapsed cord, septicemia, urinary tract infection, and uterine atony. These complications are generally consistent with those reported on other groups of pregnant addicts (Finnegan, 1982; Stone et al., 1971; Stryker, 1977; Wilson et al., 1973).

NEONATAL OUTCOMES

Eight variables describing the condition of the 220 babies born to mothers in the PAAM treatment population are shown in Table 5. The *N*s do not always equal 220 because complete records were not always obtainable on those who were delivered at hospitals other than our affiliates.

A gestational age at birth of less than 37 weeks is considered premature, and this condition occurred in 20.5% of the cases. (For all cases, $\bar{X} = 38.2$ weeks, SD = 2.9.)

A birthweight of 2,500 g or less considered low, and slightly more than a fourth of the infants were of low birthweight. (For all cases, $\bar{X} = 2{,}822.9$ g, SD = 523.7.)

In general, our findings on gestational age and birthweight are similar to those reported on other populations of pregnant addicts receiving adequate prenatal care (Davis, 1977; Finnegan, 1978) and are considerably improved over outcomes for pregnant addicts receiving little or no prenatal care (Davis, 1977; Finnegan, 1978; Stone et al., 1971).

Table 5

Neonatal Outcomes (N = 220 Unless Otherwise Noted)

Variable	Categories	Percent	*N*
Gestational age at birth	37 weeks or more	79.5	175
	36 weeks or less	20.5	45
Birthweight	2,501 g or more	72.7	160
	2,500 g or less	27.3	60
Withdrawal status	Absent	29.9	44
(*N* = 192)	Present and not treated	58.9	113
	Present and treated	18.2	35
Sex	Male	54.5	120
	Female	45.5	100
Congenital anomaly	No	96.8	213
	Yes	3.2	7
Apgar score at 1 min	7 or more	91.0	191
(*N* = 210)	6 or less	9.0	19
Apgar score at 5 min	7 or more	95.7	201
(*N* = 210)	6 or less	4.3	9
Infant death	No	97.7	215
	Yes	2.3	5

Withdrawal status was assessed by the Neonatal Narcotic Withdrawal Index (Green and Suffet, 1981). The index was first used some months after PAAM began, and thus the full series is not represented in the table. Also excluded are most of the infants born at hospitals other than our affiliates, since they could not be assessed on the index. However, five of these cases are included under the category "present and treated," as we learned that the babies were treated pharmacologically for withdrawal.

About fourth-fifths of the infants showed signs of withdrawal, and of these less than a fourth were treated pharmacologically (with paregoric). This reflects the PAAM philosophy of being conservative in medicating newborns in order not to compound the effects of intrauterine drug exposure. Infants in withdrawal were typically managed by swaddling and by increasing the frequency of feedings.

The sex distribution shows a preponderance of male babies, a fact noted in a previous PAAM report (Green et al., 1979).

Congenital anomalies, found in seven cases, include one each of the following: anencephalia, branchial cyst, extra manual digit, hernia, preauricular skin tag, posterior cleft palate, and retracted testicle.

Apgar scores of 6 or less are indicative of neonatal asphyxia, a condition found in 9.0% of the cases at 1 minute ($\bar{X}$ = 7.9, SD = 1.4) and in 4.3% at 5 minutes ($\bar{X}$ = 9.0, SD = 1.2). These results parallel those reported by Davis (1977) for newborns of pregnant addicts in her Clinic A (high care) group, and are better than those for her Clinic B (low care) group.

There were five infant deaths. Three babies died in the hospital soon after birth—one of hyaline membrane disease and one of septicemia, and one was anencephalic—and two were crib deaths at several months of age. The 2.3% mortality rate is about equal to the rate reported for all births in East Harlem and Central Harlem (Watson and Hollander, 1978), two neighborhoods in which many PAAM patients reside, and is lower than the rate one would expect for infants of untreated pregnant addicts (Stone et al., 1971).

EFFECTS OF PRENATAL CARE ON NEONATAL OUTCOMES

While some of our neonatal outcome findings suggest the benefits of PAAM care, it is instructive to examine more closely the effects of prenatal care on neonatal outcomes. In order to do this, Pearson product-moment correlations were computed for the four measures of prenatal care versus three key outcome measures: gestational age at birth, birthweight, and withdrawal status. The results are shown in Table 6.

Two care variables—days of care and number of prenatal visits—are significantly correlated with gestational age and birthweight. In other words, more extensive care, however measured, is related to favorable outcomes on the

Table 6

Product-Moment Correlations of Prenatal Care Variables Versus Neonatal Outcomes

	Neonatal outcomes		
Prenatal care variable	Gestational age at birth	Birthweight	Withdrawal status
Gestational duration at first visit	.059 (220)	−.120 (220)	−.039 (192)
Days of care	.248* (220)	.332* (220)	.014 (192)
Number of prenatal visits	.266* (219)	.361* (219)	.005 (191)
Methadone dose at delivery	−.132 (217)	.002 (217)	.236* (191)

*$p < .001$, two-tailed test.

measures of neonatal maturity. This finding is in accord with results obtained in another program for pregnant addicts (Finnegan, 1978). A question, to be addressed later, is why gestational duration at first visit, which is highly correlated with days of care ($r = .867, p < .001$) and number of visits ($r = .715, p < .001$), is unrelated to gestational age and birthweight. Methadone dose at delivery shows a significant correlation with withdrawal status, which is in accord with findings reported by others (Ostrea et al., 1976; Strauss et al., 1976a).

To further examine the relationship between prenatal care and neonatal outcomes, a stepwise regression analysis was performed on the 216 full-data cases, deploying the four measures of prenatal care as independent variables and the two measures of neonatal maturity as dependent variables. The findings, as shown in Table 7, reveal that all four prenatal care variables contribute significant increments to the proportion of variance explained in gestational age at birth, and three (all except methadone dose) do so with respect to birthweight. An important point is that gestational duration at first visit, which appears unrelated to the neonatal outcomes in the zero-order correlations, is shown to act as a "suppressor" variable (Nunnally, 1967), whose significant effect, especially on gestational age, now emerges. The substantive meaning of this finding is that it is vital not only to be seen often for care, but also to start care as early in pregnancy as possible.

A stepwise regression analysis also was performed using withdrawal status as the dependent variable and relating it to the four prenatal measures. Only methadone dose explained a significant proportion of the variance ($R = .229$, $R^2 \times 100 = 5.2$, $F = 10.42, p < .01$). None of the others explained more than 0.3% of the variance.

Table 7

Summary of Stepwise Regression Analysis: Gestational Age at Birth and Birthweight Related to Four Prenatal Care Variables (N = 216)

Dependent variable	Independent variables in order of entry	Cumulative multiple correlation (R)	Cumulative % of variance explained ($R^2 \times 100$)	Increment in % of variance explained	F for increment
Gestational age at birth	Number of prenatal visits	.277	7.7	7.7	17.76***
	Gestational duration at first visit	.446	19.9	12.2	32.62***
	Days of care	.649	42.1	22.2	81.27***
	Methadone dose at delivery	.659	43.2	1.1	3.94*
Birthweight	Number of prenatal visits	.360	13.0	13.0	31.95***
	Gestational duration at first visit	.408	16.7	3.7	9.36**
	Days of care	.532	28.3	11.6	34.43***
	Methadone dose at delivery	.532	28.3	< 0.1	0.14

*$p < .05$.
**$p < .01$.
***$p < .001$.

CHILD DEVELOPMENT ASSESSMENTS

The development of children born on PAAM was assessed via the Bayley Scales of Infant Development at 3, 6, 12, 18, and 24 months of age. Assessments were done by a child development specialist, usually in the presence of the mother.

The Bayley Scales are composed of two sets of behavioral tasks. The first, called the Mental Development Index (MDI), is designed to assess such cognitive aspects of development as perceptual abilities, orienting, and manual or fine motor coordination. The second, called the Psychomotor Development Index (PDI), is designed to assess such gross motor coordination abilities as sitting upright, balancing, and walking. The tasks in each set are age-graded for difficulty.

The number of tasks passed, or "correctly" performed by a child, is compared to a norm, set at 100, for children of that age, yielding an index score for the child.

We have examined the Bayley scores of PAAM children in terms of age point, sex, neonatal outcomes, and maternal methadone dose.

Age Point

The mean MDI and PDI scores at each of the five age points are presented in Table 8. The *N*s decline for two reasons. First, because of attrition in the treatment population, an increasing proportion of children had left the program by each point. Second, many of the children born more recently, although still on PAAM at the end of its sixth year, were not old enough to be tested at the later points. In addition, the five babies who died were never tested.

The patterns of the two sets of scores are different. The MDI, after a slight increase between 3 and 6 months, shows a continuous decline thereafter. The PDI, in contrast, decreases from 3 to 12 months, and then increases through 18

Table 8

Mean Bayley MDI and PDI Scores at Five Age Points

	Score	
Age point	MDI	PDI
3 months		
$\bar{X}$	106.3	112.1
SD	13.5	15.5
N	131	131
6 months		
$\bar{X}$	108.1	105.0
SD	19.4	14.5
N	106	106
12 months		
$\bar{X}$	105.7	99.0
SD	12.4	14.7
N	99	99
18 months		
$\bar{X}$	97.7	101.3
SD	17.3	16.1
N[a]	48	47
24 months		
$\bar{X}$	89.3	106.5
SD	17.0	19.1
N	35	35

[a] *N*s vary because the PDI could not be completed on one child.

and 24 months. The overall drop in MDI scores among addicted women's children by 24 months of age has been found by other investigators (Kaltenbach et al., 1979; Lodge, 1977). A study by Strauss et al. (1976b) found that MDI scores remained fairly stable from 3 to 6 to 12 months, but that PDI scores showed a decline similar to ours. Strauss and his colleagues found that the decline was in part attributable to the difficulty some children had in passing the locomotion items, such as walking. A review of the 12-month protocols for PAAM children revealed the same thing, although the increase in PDI scores at 18 and 24 months indicates that they overcome this difficulty.

Some studies have compared addict and nonaddict children of similar socioeconomic background at single age points, and the findings indicate that the former usually have lower scores (Lodge et al., 1975; Strauss et al., 1979; Wilson et al., 1981). At least three studies have compared addict to nonaddict children on the Bayley Scales at more than one age point (Kaltenbach et al., 1979; Rosen and Johnson, 1982; Strauss et al., 1976b). While addict children were generally found to have lower scores, in two of the studies such declines over time as were observed tended to characterize both groups. Since in each study both addict and nonaddict children came from disadvantaged backgrounds, the preponderance of the evidence suggests that the decrease is due in part to social environmental factors common to both groups. However, because all comparison studies, whether done at single or multiple age points, have found that addict children usually perform more poorly than their nonaddict peers, the findings indicate that the former grow up under an additional disadvantage. But whether this is primarily a social factor—that is, early childhood exposure to the addiction life-style—or a specific effect of intrauterine exposure to opiates and other drugs, remains an open question. Given the knowledge that has accumulated in recent years on the physical and behavioral consequences to offspring of prenatal maternal drug ingestion (Brazelton, 1970; Finnegan, 1981; Hutchings, 1978, 1980; Wilson, 1975), the latter possibility cannot be discounted.

Sex

Although the earlier developmental maturity of girls than boys, even at a young age, has long been known (Hutt, 1972), the studies of addicted women's children that have been cited here usually did not include sex comparisons on the Bayley scores. Such comparisons were made with the PAAM data, on the expectation that female babies would produce higher scores than males. The mean MDI and PDI scores for boys and girls at each age point are presented in Table 9, and the findings indicate that the expectation was warranted: On all 10 comparisons the females' scores are higher. Although the difference is statistically significant on only three comparisons, the overall pattern tends to confirm that boys and girls exhibit different rates of developmental maturation.

Table 9

Mean Bayley MDI and PDI Scores at Five Age Points, by Sex

	Score and sex			
	MDI		PDI	
Age point	Male	Female	Male	Female
3 months				
$\bar{X}$	104.9	107.9	112.1	112.2
SD	14.5	12.4	16.7	14.2
N	68	63	68	63
6 months				
$\bar{X}$	106.5	109.7	104.5	105.6
SD	18.4	20.4	16.2	12.6
N	53	53	53	53
12 months				
$\bar{X}$	102.7	108.8*	95.7	102.3*
SD	12.8	11.2	14.5	14.2
N	50	49	50	49
18 months				
$\bar{X}$	95.8	100.0	101.1	101.4
SD	19.2	15.4	19.0	12.7
N	24	24	24	23
24 months				
$\bar{X}$	82.0	99.2**	103.0	111.2
SD	14.9	14.8	20.2	17.0
N	20	15	20	15

*$p < .05$ for male-female difference.
**$p < .01$ for male-female difference.

It is also worth noting that while the MDI scores for both sexes decline from 6 to 24 months, the drop is much sharper for boys. This suggests that there may be some consistent difference in socialization patterns, and, in fact, PAAM child development specialists report that PAAM mothers tend to favor female babies and treat them less restrictively than they do the boys.

Neonatal Outcomes

Since the PAAM data set includes information on the children's condition at birth, it is logical to ask how neonatal variables relate to the Bayley scores. Table 10 presents a product-moment correlation matrix of three key neonatal outcomes versus MDI and PDI scores at all five age points. All 10 correlations between gestational age at birth and Bayley score are positive, although only the two at 6 months are statistically significant. Birthweight is even more marked in its effect: All 10 correlations are positive, and nine are statistically significant.

Table 10

Product-Moment Correlations of Bayley MDI and PDI Scores Versus Neonatal Outcomes

Age point and score	Neonatal outcomes: Gestational age at birth	Birthweight	Withdrawal status
3 months			
MDI	.136	.308***	.009
	(131)	(131)	(119)
PDI	.172	.229**	.009
	(131)	(131)	(119)
6 months			
MDI	.292**	.492***	–.162
	(106)	(106)	(98)
PDI	.275**	.435***	.040
	(106)	(106)	(98)
12 months			
MDI	.100	.117	–.113
	(99)	(99)	(90)
PDI	.156	.298**	–.078
	(99)	(99)	(90)
18 months			
MDI	.131	.304*	–.171
	(48)	(48)	(46)
PDI	.159	.356*	.020
	(47)	(47)	(45)
24 months			
MDI	.313	.465**	–.073
	(35)	(35)	(33)
PDI	.160	.375*	–.042
	(35)	(35)	(33)

*$p < .05$, two-tailed test.
**$p < .01$, two-tailed test.
***$p < .001$, two-tailed test.

Withdrawal status, in contrast, shows no consistent pattern of correlations, except that most are low and none is significant. Clearly, then, whatever other factors may be at work, degree of maturity at birth has a persistent effect on early development.

Maternal Methadone Dose

The well-known fact that males show greater intrauterine vulnerability than females (Hutt, 1972), considered against the apparent behavioral effects on young children of maternal prenatal methadone use (Hutchings, 1982), suggests the possibility that fetal sensitivity to methadone exposure may vary by sex of the fetus. A study reported in the animal research literature (Hutchings et al., 1979) supports this possibility. It found that among offspring of female rats prenatally administered methadone, there are differential performance effects according to sex on certain conditioning tasks. Therefore, one might expect maternal methadone dose to produce differential effects on the development of male and female babies as measured by the Bayley Scales, with males presumably affected in a more negative direction.

In order to test this hypothesis, product-moment correlations of maternal methadone dose at delivery versus MDI and PDI scores at all age points were computed separately for boys and girls. The results are shown in Table 11.

Table 11

Product-Moment Correlations of Bayley MDI and PDI Scores Versus Maternal Methadone Dose, by Sex

Age point and score	Maternal methadone dose when sex is: Male	Female
3 months		
MDI	−.172	−.036
	(66)	(63)
PDI	−.320*	.025
	(66)	(63)
6 months		
MDI	−.120	.024
	(52)	(53)
PDI	−.182	.016
	(52)	(53)
12 months		
MDI	−.162	.089
	(49)	(49)
PDI	−.408*	−.030
	(49)	(49)
18 months		
MDI	−.293	−.002
	(23)	(24)
PDI	.137	.223
	(23)	(23)
24 months		
MDI	−.183	.199
	(20)	(15)
PDI	−.314	−.308
	(20)	(15)

*$p < .01$, two-tailed test.

Among the boys 9 of the 10 coefficients are negative, with two being statistically significant. Among the girls, on the other hand, only four coefficients are negative and none is significant. Moreover, on every comparison, the correlation for males is closer to the −1.0 extreme. The findings thus lend support to the hypothesis that maternal methadone dose produces differential neurobehavioral effects on boys and girls, although the possibility that unknown social factors play an explanatory role cannot be ruled out.

CONCLUSION

The findings of this study have certain implications for program policy. First, it is clear that assembling in a single program the multiple services relevant to the needs of pregnant addicts is a feasible undertaking, and that such a program will attract and retain patients. The latter point is demonstrated by the fact that women who join PAAM while pregnant generally stay on the program through childbirth, and most stay until the child is at least a year old.

Second, it is apparent that comprehensive care generates a series of positive consequences. Deliveries are usually free of complication, and most newborns are healthy. Furthermore, the earlier in pregnancy women join the program and the more often they are seen for prenatal care, the more favorable are neonatal outcomes. In turn, favorable neonatal outcomes are associated with sound early childhood development. All this not only emphasizes the value of the PAAM approach but also indicates the need for any program that treats pregnant addicts to develop outreach and early case finding mechanisms.

Third, the importance of keeping prenatal methadone doses as low as practicable is indicated by the finding that dosage is directly related to neonatal withdrawal. Moreover, since more severe withdrawal is likely to require pharmacotherapy, the longer hospitalization of the newborn this often necessitates (Green and Suffet, 1981) interferes with the mother-infant bonding process at a crucial point. And the finding suggesting that higher doses may adversely affect the early development of male babies provides yet another reason for taking a conservative approach to methadone dosage.

Finally, with respect to staff training, we have found that reviewing the findings of this and other PAAM studies with the treatment staff enables them to see how their individual efforts relate to the overall pattern of outcomes; and because the outcomes are generally positive, the value of their efforts is reinforced. Such a review, moreover, permits staff to focus attention on areas in which further program development may be desirable, albeit within the limits imposed by funding constraints, the characteristics of the treatment population, and other such factors. For example, although in a recent study (Suffet and Brotman, 1981) we found that at 1 year of age PAAM children performed significantly better on several developmental measures than did children of a comparable group of non-PAAM addict mothers, the decline in Bayley scores found in the present study, particularly on the MDI, underscores the need to continue to seek ways of combating the effects on children of a milieu characterized by poverty and parental addiction.

ACKNOWLEDGMENTS

Preparation of this paper was supported by National Institute on Drug Abuse grant H81 DA 01987, and by New York State Division of Substance Abuse Services contract C148127. We are indebted to the many members of the PAAM staff who assisted in the research by collecting and coding data, and helping to interpret the results.

REFERENCES

BAYLEY, N. *Bayley Scales of Infant Development.* New York: Psychological Corporation, 1969.

BESCHNER, G., and BROTMAN, R. (eds.). *Symposium on Comprehensive Health Care for Addicted Families and Their Children.* Rockville, MD: National Institute on Drug Abuse, 1977.

BRAZELTON, B. Effect of prenatal drugs on the behavior of the neonate. *Am. J. Psychiatry* 126: 1261-1266, 1970.

COBRINIK, R.W., HOOD, R.T., and CHUSID, H. The effect of maternal narcotic addiction on the newborn infant: Review of the literature and report of 22 cases. *Pediatrics* 24: 288-304, 1959.

DAVIS, M. The quality of prenatal treatment of narcotic addicted women as a factor in neonatal outcome. In G. Beschner and R. Brotman (eds.), *Symposium on Comprehensive Health Care for Addicted Families and Their Children.* Rockville, MD: National Institute on Drug Abuse, 1977.

DES JARLAIS, D.C., and UPPAL, G.S. Heroin activity in New York City, 1970-1978. *Am. J. Drug Alcohol Abuse* 7: 335-346, 1980.

EISNER, V., BRAZIE, J.V., PRATT, M.W., and HEXTER, A.C. The risk of low birthweight. *Am. J. Public Health* 69: 887-893, 1979.

FINNEGAN, L.P. Management of drug dependent women. *Ann. N.Y. Acad. Sci.* 311: 135-145, 1978.

FINNEGAN, L.P. The effects of narcotics and alcohol on pregnancy and the newborn. *Ann. N.Y. Acad. Sci.* 362: 136-157, 1981.

FINNEGAN, L.P. Outcome of children born to women dependent upon narcotics. *Adv. Alcohol Subs. Abuse* 1: 55-101, 1982.

FRIEL, L., and SALTONSTALL, M. *Drug-Addicted Infants in Massachusetts.* Boston: Massachusetts Committee on Children and Youth, 1973.

GREEN, M., SILVERMAN, I., SUFFET, F., TALEPOROS, E., and TURKEL, W.V. Outcomes of pregnancy for addicts receiving comprehensive care. *Am. J. Drug Alcohol Abuse* 6: 413-429, 1979.

GREEN, M., and SUFFET, F. The Neonatal Narcotic Withdrawal Index: A device for the improvement of care in the abstinence syndrome. *Am. J. Drug Alcohol Abuse* 8: 203-213, 1981.

HUTCHINGS, D.E. Behavioral teratology: Embryopathic and behavioral effects of drugs during pregnancy. In G. Gottlieb (ed.), *Studies on the Development of Behavior and the Nervous System*, Vol. 4. New York: Academic Press, 1978.

HUTCHINGS, D.E. Neurobehavioral effects of prenatal origin: Drugs of use and abuse. In R.H. Schwarz and S.J. Yaffe (eds.), *Drug and Chemical Risks to the Fetus and Newborn.* New York: Alan R. Liss, 1980.

HUTCHINGS, D.E. Methadone and heroin during pregnancy: A review of behavioral effects in human and animal offspring. *Neurobehav. Toxicol. Teratol.* 4: 429-434, 1982.

HUTCHINGS, D.E., TOWEY, J.P., GORINSON, H.S., and HUNT, H.F. Methadone during pregnancy: Assessment of behavioral effects in the rat offspring. *J. Pharm. Exp. Ther.* 208: 106-112, 1979.

HUTT, C. Sex differences in human development. *Hum. Dev.* 15: 153-170, 1972.

KALTENBACH, K., GRAZIANI, L.J., and FINNEGAN, L.P. Methadone exposure in utero: Developmental status at one and two years of age. In T. Sonderegger and E. Zimmerman (eds.), *Protracted Effects of Perinatal Drug Dependence*. Fayetteville, NY: ANKHO International, 1979.

LIEF, N.R. Parenting and child services for drug dependent women. In G.M. Beschner, B.G. Reed and J. Mondanaro (eds.), *Treatment Services for Drug Dependent Women*, Vol. 1. Rockville, MD: National Institute on Drug Abuse, 1981.

LODGE, A. Developmental findings with infants born to mothers on methadone maintenance: A preliminary report. In G. Beschner and R. Brotman (eds.), *Symposium on Comprehensive Health Care for Addicted Families and Their Children.* Rockville, MD: National Institute on Drug Abuse, 1977.

LODGE, A., MARCUS, M.M., and RAMER, C.M. Behavioral and electrophysiological characteristics of the addicted neonate. *Addict. Dis.* 2: 235-255, 1975.

NATIONAL INSTITUTE ON DRUG ABUSE. *Annual Summary Report, 1975: Data from the Client Oriented Data Acquisition Process (CODAP), Series E, No. 1.* Rockville, MD: NIDA, 1977.

NEW YORK CITY NARCOTICS REGISTER. *Analysis of Narcotic Addiction Trends Through June 1973.* New York: New York City Health Department, 1973.

NUNNALLY, J. *Psychometric Theory*. New York: McGraw-Hill, 1967.

OSTREA, E.M., CHAVEZ, C.J., and STRAUSS, M.E. A study of factors that influence severity of neonatal narcotic withdrawal. *J. Pediatr.* 88: 642-645, 1976.

ROSEN, T.S., and JOHNSON, H.C. Children of methadone-maintained mothers: Follow-up to 18 months of age. *J. Pediatr.* 101: 192-196, 1982.

RYAN, V.S. *Hospital Treatment of the Pregnant Addict.* Detroit: National Women's Drug Research Coordinating Project, 1977.

STONE, M.L., SALERNO, L.J., GREEN, M., and ZELSON, C. Narcotic addiction in pregnancy. *Am. J. Obstet. Gynecol.* 109: 716-723, 1971.

STRAUSS, M.E., ANDRESKO, M., STRYKER, J.C., and WARDELL, J.N. Relationship of neonatal withdrawal to maternal methadone dose. *Am. J. Drug Alcohol Abuse* 3: 339-345, 1976a.

STRAUSS, M.E., LESSEN-FIRESTONE, J.K., CHAVEZ, C.J., and STRYKER, J.C. Children of methadone-treated women at five years of age. In T. Sonderegger and E. Zimmerman (eds.), *Protracted Effects of Perinatal Drug Dependence*. Fayetteville, NY: ANKHO International, 1979.

STRAUSS, M.E., STARR, R.H., OSTREA, E.M., CHAVEZ, C.J., and STRYKER, J.C. Behavioral concomitants of prenatal addiction to narcotics. *J. Pediatr.* 89: 842-846, 1976b.

STRYKER, J.C. A unique situation–Two people must be considered: An overview of the Hutzel Hospital program. In G. Beschner and R. Brotman (eds.), *Symposium on Comprehensive Health Care for Addicted Familes and Their Children.* Rockville, MD: National Institute on Drug Abuse, 1977.

SUFFET, F., and BROTMAN, R. *Final Report: Maternal Addiction and Child Development Program.* New York: Center for Comprehensive Health Practice, New York Medical College, 1981.

SUFFET, F., BRYCE-BUCHANAN, C., and BROTMAN, R. Pregnant addicts in a comprehensive care program: Results of a follow-up survey. *Am. J. Orthopsychiatry* 51: 297-306, 1981.

TALEPOROS, E., SUFFET, F., and BROTMAN, R. *The Prevalence of Addict Births in New York City and the Response of Treatment Agencies.* New York: Center for Comprehensive Health Practice, New York Medical College, 1978.

WATSON, A.L., and HOLLANDER, G. *The Communities of Harlem: A Plan for Health Care.* New York: New York City Health Systems Agency, 1978.

WHITING, M., WHITMAN, S., BERGNER, L., and PATRICK, S. Addiction and low birth weight: A quasi-experimental study. *Am. J. Public Health* 68: 676-678, 1978.

WILSON, G.S. Somatic growth effects of perinatal addiction. *Addict. Dis.* 2: 333-345, 1975.

WILSON, G.S., DESMOND, M.M., and VERNIAUD, W.M. Early development of infants of heroin-addicted mothers. *Am. J. Dis. Child.* 126: 457-462, 1973.

WILSON, G.S., DESMOND, M.M., and WAIT, R.B. Follow-up of methadone treated and untreated narcotic-dependent women and their infants: Health, developmental, and social implications. *J. Pediatr.* 98: 716-722, 1981.

The International Journal of the Addictions, 19(2), 221–232, 1984

Note

Infectious Complications of Illicit Drug Use*

Ronald R. Blanck,† DO

Norman W. Ream, MD

Joseph S. Deleese, MD

Department of Medicine
Brooke Army Medical Center
Fort Sam Houston, Texas 78234

INTRODUCTION

Despite all the attention given illicit drug use by government and private agencies, major social and medical consequences continue. Medical complications, in particular, occur disproportionately and atypically in the unique drug-using population. This paper identifies retrospectively cases of illicit-drug-associated medical complications seen in the United States Army teaching hospitals from 1970 through 1976. Those complications due to infectious causes are discussed.

*The opinions or assertions contained herein are the private views of the authors and are not to be construed as reflecting those of the Department of the Army or the Department of Defense.

†To whom reprint requests should be addressed: Chief, Medical Corps Career Activities Office, U.S. Army Medical Department Personnel Support Agency, 1900 Half Street, SW, Washington, DC 20324.

 0020-773X/84/1902-0221$3.50/0

POPULATION

Records were reviewed on 266 patients identified by final hospital diagnoses as having both a significant medical problem and a history of illicit drug use (generally confirmed by positive urine testing). Their mean age was 19.8 years (range 17-38). All but six patients were male, indicative of the military population seen; 206 (77.4%) were White, 55 (20.7%) Black, and 5 (1.9%) other. About half (55.2%) had been evacuated from overseas posts, chiefly Vietnam and Germany. Home of record and social background were not available.

DRUGS

Heroin was the most commonly used drug. Only 24 (9.0%) patients did not admit to its use. Amphetamines and/or barbiturates were used by 71 (26.7%); and opiates other than heroin, lysergic acid diethylamide, propoxyphene, and other drugs were also reported as used. Marijuana use was common, while tobacco and alcohol use was noted in almost all patients. The method of drug administration was intravenous or subcutaneous in 241 (90.6%) and exclusively sniffing (snorting) or smoking in 25 (9.4%)–this despite the large extent of non-needle drug use in Vietnam (Lloyd, 1973). The prominent role of the needle in medical complications is thus emphasized by this study.

MEDICAL COMPLICATIONS

Medical complications of illicit drug use can be separated into infectious and noninfectious groups. Contamination with biologic agents induces the former, while immunologic reactions, mechanical processes, and pharmacologic effects comprise the latter. Table 1 shows those diseases identified in our patients, while the following sections present our data and descriptions of those infections considered to be complications of illicit drug use.

Infective Endocarditis

Infective endocarditis was identified in 31 heroin users. All used heroin intravenously. Their presenting symptoms and physical findings are shown in Tables 2 and 3. The duration of complaints before presentation was difficult to ascertain but appears to be between 3 and 10 days. Such an interval is shorter than the usual prodrome of endocarditis but consistent with the predominance of staphylococcal endocarditis seen in our population (Pelletier and Petersdorf, 1977). Although symptoms were nonspecific, physical findings were frequently helpful. Fever on presentation was greater than 102°F in 20 and over 100°F in 6 of the 26 patients with temperatures recorded. Murmurs were useful in early

Table 1

Medical Complications Identified (N = 266)

Complication	N	%
Infectious		
Endocarditis	31	11.7
Hepatitis, viral	184	69.2
Pneumonia (including tuberculosis)	8	3.0
Sepsis	3	1.1
Local	12	4.5
Malaria	3	1.1
Noninfectious		
Pulmonary edema	14	5.3
Renal disease	2	0.8
Neurologic disorders	3	1.1
Acute pyrogenic reactions	6	2.3

Table 2

Infective Endocarditis Presenting Symptoms (N = 31)

Complaint	N	%
Chills	14	45.2
Malaise	10	32.3
Cough, nonproductive	9	29.0
Headache	6	19.4
Chest pain, pleuritic	5	16.1
Fever	5	16.1
Dyspnea	4	12.9
Nausea	4	12.9
Vomiting	4	12.9
Rhinorrhea	4	12.9
Meningismus	3	9.7
Myalgias	3	9.7
Hemoptysis	2	6.5
Anorexia	2	6.5
Ear ache	2	6.5

Table 3

Infective Endocarditis Presenting Physical Findings (N = 31)

Sign	N	%	Sign	N	%
Fever	26	100[a]	Rales	6	19.4
Murmur	20	64.6	Splenomegaly	5	16.1
Systolic	19	61.3	Arthritis	3	9.7
Diastolic	1	3.2	Otitis media	2	6.5

[a] Initial temperature recorded on 26.

Table 4

Infective Endocarditis Murmurs (N = 31)

	Murmur present		
	Diagnostic	Nondiagnostic	Murmur absent
Right lesions			
Admission	11	5	5
Postadmission	8	0	3
Left lesions			
Admission	4	0	6
Postadmission	6	0	0

diagnosis and are categorized in Table 4. The presence on first examination of diagnostic murmurs in right-sided disease and the occasional absence of murmurs initially in left-sided disease is unusual but has been reported (Banks et al., 1973; Graham et al., 1973; Joseph et al., 1973; Sapira, 1968). While the presence of fever was initially helpful, it frequently persisted during antibiotic therapy (greater than 7 days in 5 patients) and did not correlate with clinical improvement. Decrease in constitutional symptoms and a feeling of "well-being," though difficult to quantify, seemed to be more sensitive indicators of therapeutic response.

The causative organisms and involved valves documented by cathetherization are listed in Table 5. Complications and therapy are also listed in Table 5. Septic pulmonary emboli were the most common embolic complication, as might be expected, with the high incidence of right-sided disease. While systemic emboli were seen with left-sided disease, they also occurred with only right-sided valve involvement, presumably through large pulmonary shunts. The presence of systemic emboli, therefore, does not necessarily mean left-sided disease (Louria, 1974; Louria et al., 1967; Sapira, 1968). Seven of the 21 patients on methicillin developed urine abnormalities, and 2 of the 7 patients on nafcillin developed leucopenia which led to the use of alternate antibiotics.

Finally, outcome is shown in Table 5. Appropriate antimicrobial therapy seems to have been effective since only 4 of our patients required valve replacement. The low mortality in our study (6.5%) and in other studies, compared to other reported mortalities of up to 85%, may have been due to a high index of suspicion and early diagnosis combined with vigorous medical and surgical therapy (Banks et al., 1973; Garvey and Neu, 1978; Menda and Gorback, 1973).

Viral Hepatitis

In this study, 184 cases of acute symptomatc hepatitis were identified, making it the most commonly recognized major medical complication. Twenty-

Table 5

Thirty-One Cases of Infective Endocarditis in the Illicit Drug User

Case no.	Valve	Organisms	Therapy	Complications	Outcome
1	Tricuspid	Staphylococcus aureus	Methicillin	Septic pulmonary emboli	Recovered, no surgery
2	Aortic	Alpha Hemolytic Streptococcus	Penicillin, Streptomycin	Congenital aortic stenosis pulmonary edema	Aortic valve replacement, recovered
3	Tricuspid	Staphylococcus aureus	Methicillin	Septic pulmonary emboli	Recovered, no surgery
4	Tricuspid	Staphylococcus aureus	Methicillin, Cleocin	Septic pulmonary emboli, empyema	Recovered, no surgery
5	Tricuspid	Staphylococcus aureus	Methicillin	Septic pulmonary emboli	Recovered, no surgery
6	Tricuspid	Staphylococcus aureus	Keflin	Septic pulmonary emboli	Recovered, no surgery
7	Mitral	Streptococcus faecalis	Penicillin, Streptomycin	Renal emboli, pancytopenia	Recovered, no surgery
8	Mitral	Staphylococcus aureus	Methicillin, Keflin	Pneumonia	Recovered, no surgery
9	Tricuspid	Pseudomonas aeruginosa	Gentamycin, Carbenicillin, Nafcillin	Septic pulmonary emboli	Tricuspid valve replacement, recovered
10	Tricuspid	Staphylococcus aureus	Methicillin	Septic pulmonary emboli	Recovered, no surgery
11	Mitral	Staphylococcus aureus	Methicillin	Right hemiparesis	Recovered, no surgery
12	Tricuspid	Staphylococcus aureus	Dicloxacillin	Septic pulmonary emboli, septic arthritis	Recovered, no surgery
13	Aortic	Alpha Hemolytic Streptococcus	Penicillin, Streptomycin	Aortic cusp rupture	Aortic valve replacement, death 18 days postop
14	Tricuspid	Staphylococcus aureus	Methicillin, Nafcillin	Septic pulmonary emboli, hepatitis	Recovered, no surgery, postnecrotic cirrhosis
15	Aortic	Candida parapsilopsis	Amphotericin B, 5-fluorocytosine	None	Recovered, no surgery
16	Tricuspid	Staphylococcus aureus	Methicillin	Septic pulmonary emboli	Recovered, no surgery

(continued)

Table 5 (continued)

Case no.	Valve	Organisms	Therapy	Complications	Outcome
17	Tricuspid	Staphylococcus aureus	Methicillin, Nafcillin, Vancomycin	Septic pulmonary emboli	Recovered, no surgery
18	Mitral	Staphylococcus aureus	Methicillin, Nafcillin	Cerebral emboli	Recovered, no surgery
19	Tricuspid	Staphylococcus aureus	Methicillin	Septic pulmonary emboli	Recovered, no surgery
20	Tricuspid, aortic	Staphylococcus aureus	Methicillin	Septic pulmonary emboli, retinal microabscesses	Recovered, no surgery
21	Pulmonic	Staphylococcus aureus	Keflin	Septic pulmonary emboli, splenic infarction	Recovered, no surgery
22	Tricuspid	Staphylococcus aureus	Methicillin	Osteomyelitis of symphysis pubis	Recovered, no surgery
23	Tricuspid	Staphylococcus aureus	Lincomycin, Methicillin, Nafcillin	Septic pulmonary emboli, septic arthritis	Recovered, no surgery
24	Tricuspid	Staphylococcus aureus	Nafcillin, Vancomycin	Septic pulmonary emboli	Recovered, no surgery
25	Mitral, aortic	Staphylococcus aureus	Methicillin, Nafcillin	Systemic emboli to brain, liver, spleen, kidneys, skin; congestive heart failure	Aortic valve replacement, mitral valve replacement

26	Pulmonic, tricuspid	Alpha Hemolytic Streptococcus, Nisseria sica, Bacteroides melaninogenicus, Bacteroides species	Penicillin, Streptomycin	Septic pulmonary emboli	Recovered, no surgery
27	Aortic	Staphylococcus aureus	Methicillin	Infarction of one distal phalanx, right hand; conjunctival emboli; congestive heart failure	Aortic valve replacement, recovered
28	Tricuspid	Staphylococcus aureus	Keflin, Methicillin	Septic pulmonary emboli	Recovered, no surgery
29	Tricuspid	Staphylococcus aureus	Methicillin, Chlor-amphenicol	Septic pulmonary emboli	Recovered, no surgery
30	Tricuspid	Staphylococcus aureus	Methicillin	Septic pulmonary emboli, pleural and pericardial friction rubs	Recovered, no surgery
31	Tricuspid	Staphylococcus aureus	Methicillin, Gentamycin	Septic pulmonary emboli	Recovered, no surgery

three of the 184 patients had a history of one previous hepatitis episode and 1 patient had a history of two previous episodes of symptomatic hepatitis. Of the 117 patients with acute hepatitis tested for hepatitis B surface antigen (HBsAg), 51 (43.6%) were positive. Our slightly lower incidence of positivity compared to other studies may be due to a different environmental exposure, particularly in those acquiring the disease outside of the United States, or to the use of early tests for antigen with high false-negative results (Alter and Michael, 1958; Altshul et al., 1952; Grady et al., 1972; Sutnick et al., 1971).

Despite nonparenteral transmission of both hepatitis A and B, as well as the frequent nonparenteral use of drugs in the population studies, only 7 (3.8%) of our group of hepatitis patients did not use needles (Garibaldi et al., 1972; Hersh et al., 1971; Wright, 1975). A possible explanation for the small group of nonneedle drug users with hepatitis is that the needle users might have used drugs longer, increasing the likelihood of viral exposure (Sapira et al., 1968).

The presenting symptoms and physical findings are shown in Tables 6 and 7. Most patients were asymptomatic within 1 week, and, as reported in similar studies, laboratory values began to fall within 2 weeks (Boyer, 1976; Deinhardt, 1976; Silverberg, 1977). The presenting symptoms of HBsAg-positive hepatitis were present for a mean of 13.8 days, compared to a mean of 8 days for HBsAg-negative hepatitis.

Bilirubin and SGOT were generally higher in the HBsAg-positive group, as seen in Table 8. Only 1 patient with type B hepatitis died, suggesting the generally good immediate prognosis of acute hepatitis and, in this group, its rare contribution to the mortality of illicit drug users. There was no specific follow-up done.

Table 6

Viral Hepatitis Presenting Symptoms

	$HBsAg^-$ ($N = 66$)		$HBsAg^+$ ($N = 51$)	
Symptom	*N*	%	*N*	%
Dark urine	48	72.7	41	80.4
Fatigue and malaise	38	57.6	30	58.8
Anorexia	34	51.5	25	49.0
Nausea and vomiting	32	48.5	16	31.4
Abdominal pain	21	31.8	16	31.4
Decreased taste for cigarettes	16	24.2	15	29.4
Light stools	12	18.2	11	21.6
Pruritis	7	10.6	3	5.9
Myalgias	1	1.5	5	9.8
Arthralgias	–	–	3	5.9

Table 7

Viral Hepatitis Presenting Physical Findings

	HBsAg$^-$ (N = 66)		HBsAg$^+$ (N = 51)	
Finding	N	%	N	%
Scleral icterus	46	69.7	37	72.5
Jaundice and icterus	24	36.4	28	54.9
Enlarged and tender liver	14	21.2	16	31.4
Enlarged spleen	4	6.1	3	5.9
Upper right quadrant tenderness	5	7.6	6	11.8

Table 8

Viral Hepatitis Laboratory Values on Admission

Lab test	HBsAg$^-$ (N = 66)	HBsAg$^+$ (N = 51)
White blood cell count (mm^3)		
Mean	7,522	6,779
SD	2,606	1,998
Hematocrit (vol %)		
Mean	45.2	46.9
SD	6.2	3.4
Bilirubin (mg/dL)		
Mean	4.7	6.5
SD	4.1	4.2
Serum glutamic oxaloacetic transaminase (international units)		
Mean	789	1,450
SD	690	1,189

Pulmonary Infections

Eight of our patients had pneumonia. One patient had primary tuberculosis, 3 had *Staphylococcus aureus* pneumonia, 1 had mixed *Staphylococcus aureus* and Klebsiella-Enterobacter infection, and 3 had small infiltrates with no organisms identified. This is almost certainly less than the true incidence of pneumonia in the group of drug users from whom we drew our complications, possibly because the common pneumonias were treated locally rather than being sent to a medical center. Also, the drug users in our group may have been less debilitated and better able to mobilize pharyngeal aspirations than most drug users. Even in those not debilitated, however, opiates have a depressant effect on the cough reflex and may predispose to pulmonary infections. Although pneumonia due to aspiration of gastric contents has been reported and might be expected in drug users, we found no diagnosed cases unassociated with other diseases (Joseph et al., 1973; Siegel, 1972).

The staphylococcal pneumonias in our patients may have been hematogeneously spread, as 2 patients had coexisting staphylococcal sepsis without evidence of endocarditis. The patient with the mixed pneumonia was the only one of this group to die.

Sepsis

Although septic pulmonary emboli and systemic emboli occasionally occur in the absence of endocarditis, we considered sepsis as a distinct entity only in those without embolic phenomena but with positive blood cultures and signs of generalized infection.

There were 3 cases of sepsis in our series, which comprise 8% of the infectious complications found, excluding hepatitis. Since sepsis might be considered to be midway on a spectrum between localized cellulitis, abscesses, and septic thrombophlebitis, on the one hand, and endocarditis, on the other, it is not surprising that the variety of offending organisms is similar in the three instances. All of our cases were due to *Staphylococcus aureus*. As with staphyloccal endocarditis, penicillinase-resistant antibiotics are indicated, and with such therapy, all of our patients survived.

Local Infections

We found 6 cases of cellulitis, 4 of local abscess, and 2 of septic thrombophlebitis, all localized to injection sites and unassociated with other infections. Two patients had local cultures positive for *Staphylococcus aureus*, 1 for *Neisseria* species and *Staphylococcus epidermidis*, and the rest had negative or no cultures. Treatment was with penicillin, ampicillin, or erythromycin, plus heat and incision and drainage when appropriate. This is probably far less than the true incidence of local infections of drug users, but such infections are frequently treated locally on an ambulatory basis, so did not appear in our population. Infected injection sites may be a source of more distant infections such as sepsis and endocarditis (Hussey and Katz, 1950). In fact, 1 of our 3 cases of sepsis had a preexisting staphylococcal cellulitis.

Miscellaneous Infections

We identified 2 patients with plasmodium vivax malaria and 1 with plasmodium falciprim malaria. All shared needles, injecting themselves with heroin presumably not "cut" with quinine, but the patients themselves had been in malaria areas so they may have been primarily infected.

Although tetanus has been noted as a particular complication of the needle-using group, it was not found in our population, perhaps because of stringent immunization requirements in the military (Cherubin, 1967, 1971; Louria, 1974; Louria et al., 1967).

Osteomyelitis, commonly reported to occur in drug users, and a variety of less common infections, were also not found in our group (Briggs et al., 1967; Forlenza et al., 1979; Goldin et al., 1973; Kido et al., 1973; Louria, 1974).

REFERENCES

ALTER, A.A., and MICHAEL, M. Serum hepatitis in a group of drug addicts. *N. Engl. J. Med.* 259: 387, 1958.

ALTSHUL, A., FOSTER, P.D., and PALEY, S.S. Incidence of hepatitis among narcotic addicts in Harlem Hospital. *Arch. Intern. Med.* 89: 24, 1952.

BANKS, T., FLETCHER, R., and ALI, N. Infective endocarditis in heroin addicts. *Am. J. Med.* 55: 444, 1973.

BOYER, J.L. The diagnosis and pathogenesis of clinical variants in viral hepatitis. *Am. J. Clin. Pathol.* 65: 898, 1976.

BRIGGS, J.H., MC KERRON, C.G., and SOUHAMI, R.L. Severe systemic infections complicating "mainline" heroin addictions. *Lancet* 2: 1227, 1967.

CHERUBIN, C.E. The medical sequelae of narcotic addiction. *Ann. Intern. Med.* 67: 23, 1967.

CHERUBIN, C.E. Infectious disease problems of narcotic addicts. *Arch. Intern. Med.* 128: 309, 1971.

DEINHARDT, F. Epidemiology and mode of transmission of viral hepatitis A and B. *Am. J. Clin. Pathol.* 65: 890, 1976.

FORLENZA, S.W., AXELROD, J.L., and GRIECO, M.H. Pott's disease in heroin addicts. *J. Am. Med. Assoc.* 241: 379, 1979.

GARIBALDI, R.A., HATCH, F.E., and BISNO, A.L. Nonparenteral serum hepatitis. *J. Am. Med. Assoc.* 220: 963, 1972.

GARVEY, G.J., and NEU, H.C. Infective endocarditis: An evolving disease. *Medicine* 57: 105, 1978.

GOLDIN, R.H., CHOW, A.W., EDWARDS, J.E., and LOUIS, J.S. Sternoarticular septic arthritis in heroin users. *N. Engl. J. Med.* 289: 616, 1973.

GRADY, G.F., BENNETT, A.J.E., and CULHANE, P.O. Eight years of surveillance of patients hospitalized with hepatitis. *J. Infect. Dis.* 126: 87, 1972.

GRAHAM, D.Y., REUL, G.J., and MARTIN, R. Infective endocarditis in drug addicts: Experiences with medical and surgical treatment. *Circulation*, 48 (Suppl. 3): 37, 1973.

HERSH, T., MELNICK, J.L., and GOYAL, R.K. Nonparenteral transmission of viral hepatitis Type B (Australia antigen associated serum hepatitis). *N. Engl. J. Med.* 285: 1363, 1971.

HUSSEY, H.H., and KATZ, S. Infections resulting from narcotic addiction: Report of 102 cases. *Am. J. Med.* 9: 186, 1950.

JOSEPH, W.L., FLETCHER, H.S., and GIORDANO, J.M. Pulmonary and cardiovascular implications of drug addiction. *Ann. Thorac. Surg.* 15: 263, 1973.

KIDO, D., BRYAN, D., and HALPERN, M. Hematogenous osteomylitis in drug addicts. *Am. J. Roentgenol.* 118: 356, 1973.

LLOYD, S.J. A clinical evaluation of 81 heroin addicts in Vietnam. *Milit. Med.* 138: 298, 1973.

LOURIA, D.B. Infectious complications of nonalcoholic drug abuse. *Ann. Rev. Med.* 25: 219, 1974.

LOURIA, D.B., HENSLE, T., and ROSE, J. The major medical complications of heroin addiction. *Ann. Intern. Med.* 67: 1, 1967.

MENDA, K.G., and GORBACK, S.L. Favorable experience with bacterial endocarditis in heroin addicts. *Ann. Intern. Med.* 78: 25, 1973.

PELLETIER, L.L., and PETERSDORF, R.G. Infective endocarditis: A review of 125 cases from the University of Washington hospitals, 1963-1972. *Medicine* 56: 287, 1977.

SAPIRA, J.D. The narcotic addict as a medical patient. *Am. J. Med.* 45: 555, 1968.

SAPIRA, J.D., JANINSKI, D.R., and GORODETZKY, C.W. Liver disease in narcotic addicts: The role of the needle. *Clin. Pharmacol. Ther.* 9: 725, 1968.

SIEGEL, H. Human pulmonary pathology associated with narcotic and other addictive drugs. *Hum. Pathol.* 3: 55, 1972.

SILVERBERG, M. Acute viral hepatitis: Modern knowledge. *Pediatr. Ann.* 6: 299, 1977.

SUTNICK, A.I., CERDA, J.J., and TOSKES, P.P. Australia antigen and viral hepatitis in drug abusers. *Arch. Intern. Med.* 127: 939, 1971.

WRIGHT, R.A. Hepatitis B and the HBsAg carrier. *J. Am. Med. Assoc.* 232: 717, 1975.

INFORMATION FOR AUTHORS SUBMITTING MANUSCRIPTS

Send a clear double-spaced typewritten original and one duplicate to Ms. Nancy Reid-Rappolt, Editorial Assistant, *International Journal of the Addictions,* c/o Winch, Smith, Ostermann and Mates, MD's, 4141 Geary, Suite 326, San Francisco, California 94118. Also send one duplicate to the Chief Editor, Dr. Stanley Einstein, Building 113/41, East Talpiot, Jerusalem, Israel. DOUBLE-SPACE the entire manuscript; do not use single spacing anywhere, including references.

Include authors' academic degrees and present affiliation. If applicable, cite auspices under which work being reported was done. Specify address to which requests for reprints should be sent.

Begin your TITLE with a word useful in indexing. A 75- to 100-word ABSTRACT should be provided, which precedes each article. A summary is then not necessary. Major and minor headings may be used in the text; indicate major headings by typing in capitals.

Use METRIC UNITS of measure. If measurements were made in English units, give metric equivalents.

Cite all TABLES and FIGURES in the text. Tables should have titles, and figures should have brief legends. In tables, give each column a heading. Indicate units of measure in parentheses in the heading for each column. Do not use vertical rules. Do not use horizontal rules other than those in the heading and at the bottom. Submit PHOTOGRAPHS as glossy prints, untrimmed and unmounted; identify each with pencil lightly on the back and indicate top.

ARTWORK will not be returned unless specifically requested, and will be disposed of three months after publication.

REFERENCES in the text should be enclosed in parentheses and include the author's surname and the date of the item cited. Keep footnotes to a minimum. Footnotes should be collected at the end of the manuscript in their numerical order of appearance.

The BIBLIOGRAPHY (double-spaced) should be given at the end of the article in alphabetical order. Journal references should include authors, title, name of journal abbreviated according to *Chemical Abstracts List of Periodicals*, inclusive page numbers, and date. Book references should include authors, title, place of publication, publisher, and date.

AUTHOR RESPONSIBILITY: It is the sole responsibility of the author(s) to obtain written permission from the author(s), publisher(s), etc. for figures, tables, or any other information excerpted from previously published works which are used in the manuscript(s) considered for publication. It is understood that the manuscript(s) considered for publication in the *International Journal of the Addictions* have not been previously published nor are they under simultaneous publication consideration elsewhere.

Statements and opinions expressed in the articles and communications herein are those of the author(s) and do not necessarily express those of the Editor or publisher.

THE INTERNATIONAL JOURNAL OF THE ADDICTIONS

Volume 19 Number 2 1984

CONTENTS

Editorial: Considering the Risks of "Populations at Risk": S. Einstein . . iii

Drug-Induced Ego States. I. Cocaine: Phenomenology and Implications: J. V. Spotts and F. C. Shontz 119

Paraprofessional Versus Professional Drug Counselors: Diverse Routes to the Same Role: L. S. Aiken, L. A. LoSciuto, M. A. Ausetts, and B. S. Brown 153

The Effect of Perceived Neighborhood Setting on Self-Reported Tobacco, Alcohol, and Marijuana Use among Inner-City Minority Junior High School Youth: W. R. Blount and R. Dembo 175

A Comprehensive Care Program for Pregnant Addicts: Obstetrical, Neonatal, and Child Development Outcomes: F. Suffet and R. Brotman 199

Note

Infectious Complications of Illicit Drug Use: R. R. Blanck, N. W. Ream, and J. S. Deleese 221

MARCEL DEKKER, INC., New York and Basel

CODEN: INJABN 19(3) i-vi, 233-366 (1984)
ISSN: 0020-773X

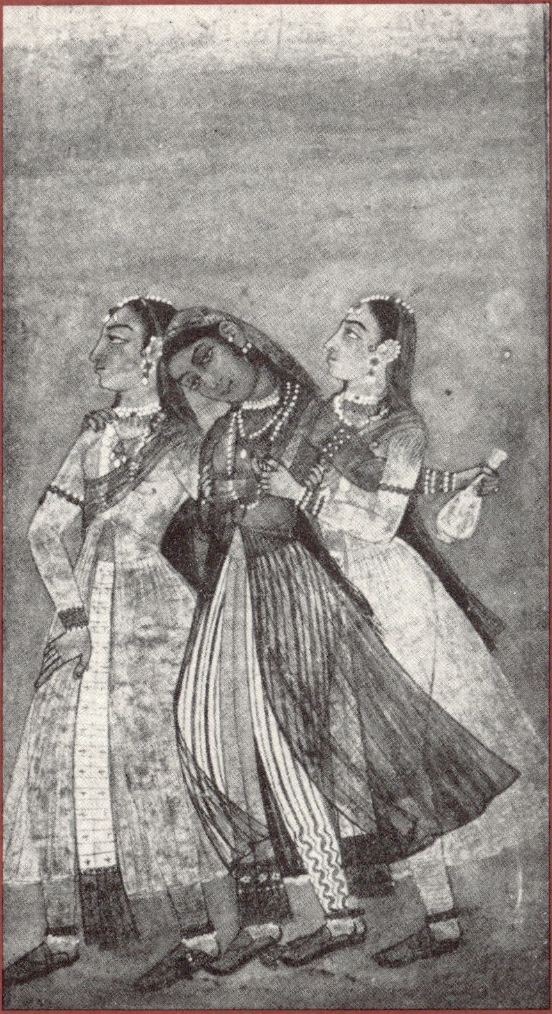

THE INTERNATIONAL JOURNAL OF THE Addictions

Volume 19 Number 3 1984

THE INTERNATIONAL JOURNAL OF THE ADDICTIONS

May 1984

Aims and Scope. This journal is a comprehensive medium for worldwide communication among both concerned laymen and professionals in research, training, and treatment in the field of addiction and substance misuse.

Indexing and Abstracting Services. Articles published in *The International Journal of the Addictions* are selectively indexed or abstracted in:

• Adolescent Mental Health Abstracts • ASCA • Bibliographic Index of Health Education Periodicals (BIHEP) • BioSciences Information Service of Biological Abstracts (BIOSIS) • Classified Abstract Archive of the Alcohol Literature • Current Contents/Clinical Practice • Excerpta Medica • Index Medicus • International Pharmaceutical Abstracts • ISI/BIOMED • Journal of Abstracts of the All-Union Institute of Scientific and Technical Information of the USSR • Psychological Abstracts • Science Citation Index • Selected List of Tables of Contents of Psychiatric Periodicals • Social Sciences Citation Index • State Central Scientific Medical Library/International Book Exchange–USSR

Articles published in *The International Journal of the Addictions* are listed in Selected List of Tables of Contents of Psychiatric Periodicals.

Manuscript Preparation and Submission. See inside back cover of this issue.

Subscription Information. *The International Journal of the Addictions* is published eight times annually in February, April, May, July, August, September, November, and December by Marcel Dekker, Inc., 270 Madison Avenue, New York, New York 10016. The subscription rate for Volume 19 (1984), containing eight numbers, is $225.00 per volume (prepaid). The special discounted rate for individual professionals and students is $112.50 per volume. To secure this special rate, your order must be prepaid by personal check. Add $20.00 for surface postage outside the United States. For airmail to Europe, add $32.48; to Asia, add $40.48.

Mailing Address. *Please mail payment with order to:* Marcel Dekker Journals, P. O. Box 11305, Church Street Station, New York, New York 10249.

Contributions to this journal are published free of charge. Second-class postage paid at New York, New York and at additional mailing offices.

Library of Congress Catalog Card Number 66-9896

Cover illustration courtesy of the Picture Collection, The Branch Libraries, New York Public Library.

THE INTERNATIONAL JOURNAL OF THE Addictions

The International Journal of the Addictions, 19(3), iii–v, 1984

Editorial

Drug Use Intervention and Control Mechanisms

In many parts of the world the elements of the traditional "holy trinity" of treatment, information dissemination (prevention/drug education), and law enforcement remain the basic tools and the agreed upon options for drug use intervention. Relevant research, when carried out, is aimed at improving these three unrelated and unrelating efforts (happenings?). This brief note is designed to explore drug use intervention and control mechanisms. After many decades of international, national, and regional efforts to control selected chemical substances and specific types of substance users and subpopulations, as well as areas of the world, we are faced with the reality that, at least on the surface, unacceptable drugs—their use and users—continue to exist and even to increase notwithstanding our efforts.

The major purpose of this note is not to help you the reader to evaluate the differential effectiveness of the tools of law enforcement (fines, taxes, licensing; court-ordered treatment, incarceration; control over chemical purity; control over the development and distribution of medicines, social substances, experimental drugs; and even death penalties), its representatives, its institutions, or its world view concerning drug use. Rather this note is designed to suggest that if a commitment is to be made to effectively control drug use (which may indeed be an unrealistic objective), then we owe it to ourselves to expand our notions of *control* beyond that of law enforcement.

Schema 1 is designed to help the reader to recognize that:

1. There are an almost unlimited number of control mechanisms available, each one being significantly different from the others.
2. A gradient of foci for intervention exists, and each of these foci is not necessarily suitable for each type of control mechanism.
3. Both the existing *variations of control* and the foci of control are dynamic and not static; their meaning(s), importance, and availability for intervention change over time.

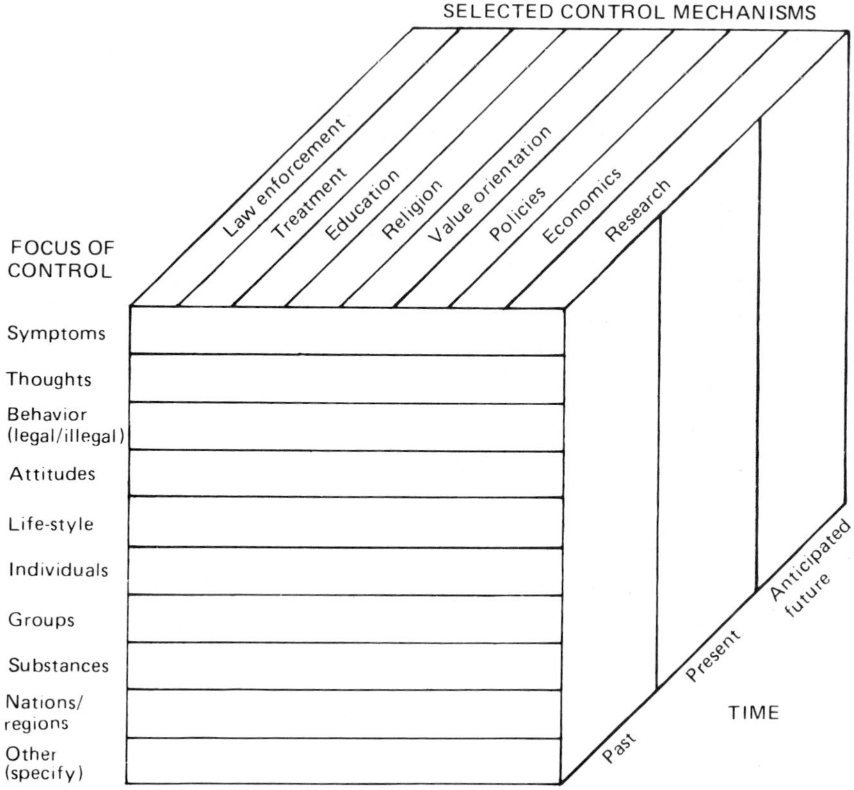

Schema 1. The interface between foci of control, selected mechanisms of control, and time.

4. Effective intervention planning demands that the planner fully understand the interface between the technology of control, the focus of control, and the temporal factors within which the control efforts are made possible or impossible.

For example, the use of treatment to control an individual's unacceptable drug-related behavior—on the part of the therapist who does not share and/or understand the patient's world view, within a complaining society which has vested interests in "numbing" segments of its members—is inappropriate, irrelevant, and morally questionable; and yet this approach is utilized increasingly all over the world.

An educational ideology cannot be effective if it sets as a high priority the exploration of oneself and the known world as well as yet unknown worlds; and it seemingly arbitrarily puts a "blockade" around certain "drugs" and attributes magical qualities and effects to them, which it then denigrates; and it removes the "known-visible" drug user from participating in this process. This ideology is obviously defeating its own self-selected mandate.

A religious belief system which transmits the notion of "God said it; I believe it, and that's it," in a world of secular and religious anomie, may not be sufficient to embrace and fulfill the increasing numbers of young and old who continue to seek instant solutions in this world. One could continue to be arbitrarily critical of the potential effectiveness of each of the control mechanisms which are potentially available for drug use intervention. That is not the purpose of this note! Rather it is to remind you the reader, in your various roles, that if *control* seems to be a reasonable approach to drugs, their use, and the users, as well as the abstainers, then it is incumbent upon you to help to develop or select the most appropriate conditions for the most effective interface of the suitable factors. To do otherwise is to support, as well as to possibly suffer from, empty rituals.

There is nothing innately advantageous or disadvantageous about control efforts of the law enforcement variety or any of the other mechanisms of control. There are known as well as "unknown" costs/consequences associated with each type of effort.

We owe it to ourselves to better understand what we are supporting, rejecting, or even not really caring about.

S. Einstein, PhD
Jerusalem, Israel

The International Journal of the Addictions, 19(3), 233–252, 1984

Paraprofessional Versus Professional Drug Abuse Counselors: Attitudes and Expectations of the Counselors and Their Clients

Leonard LoSciuto, PhD

Leona S. Aiken,* PhD

Mary Ann Ausetts, MA

Institute for Survey Research and Department of Psychology
Temple University
Philadelphia, Pennsylvania 19122

Barry S. Brown, PhD

National Institute on Drug Abuse
Rockville, Maryland 20857

Abstract

Three groups of methadone maintenance and drug-free outpatient counselors, ex-addict paraprofessionals (EXAs), non-ex-addict paraprofessionals (NEAs), and degreed professional counselors (PROs), were contrasted in terms of their views of drug abuse and drug treatment, their attitudes toward and expectations for their clients, and in terms of their clients' attitudes toward them. Across groups, counselors agreed on the major cause of drug abuse, the critical factor in treatment, the

*To whom requests for reprints should be sent at the Institute for Survey Research, Temple University, Philadelphia, Pennsylvania 19122.

 0020-773X/84/1903-0233$3.50/0

> definition of treatment success, and their expectations for client success. While clients of the three groups viewed their counselors as equally able to understand them and were equally confident of the counselors, the clients of EXAs saw their counselors as more knowledgeable about critical issues of drugs and the street scene, were more willing to bring personal problems to their counselors, and expected and desired more participation from their counselors in both counseling-related and personal problems.

In terms of training and drug use background there are currently three categories of counselors providing services to drug abuse clients. First are professional counselors who hold at least a bachelor's degree and who are not former addicts (PROs). Second are ex-addict paraprofessional counselors who do not hold a bachelor's degree but who do have a history of drug addiction (EXAs). Third are non-ex-addict paraprofessional counselors who neither hold a bachelor's degree nor have a history of drug addiction (NEAs). The distinct drug use histories and training backgrounds of these counselor groups might lead to a divergence of views concerning drug addicts, drug use, and drug addiction. Reciprocally, one might expect the clients of these three groups of counselors to diverge in their feelings about the credibility and compatibility of their counselors, and in their beliefs about the capacity and even the willingness of their counselors to help them. These views, in turn, may influence effectiveness of treatment.

There are few empirical studies in the drug abuse field in which the views of counselors in these three groups or those of their clients are contrasted. This is surprising in light of current interest in the differential effectiveness of professional versus paraprofessional service providers (Durlak, 1979; Neitzel and Fisher, 1981), as well as an older substantial literature within the psychotherapy context on the impact of therapist and client variables on psychotherapy outcomes (see reviews by Gurman, 1977; Luborsky, Chandler, Auerbach, Cohen, and Bachrach, 1971; Meltzoff and Kornreich, 1970; Parloff, Waskow, and Wolfe, 1978).

The basis for the paraprofesssional movement in the field of drug abuse has been the belief that the ex-addict counselor could have a greater understanding of the drug abuse client and of the problems to be faced in making changes in that life functioning. The ex-addict counselors' own experiences may well create greater empathy, on the one hand; lessened opportunity for his or her being conned by clients, on the other; and furthermore, a clearer articulation of what can be expected for and achieved by clients through treatment. Further, the experiences of ex-addict counselors may lead their clients to have greater faith in the ability of their counselors to help them. Within a more general psychotherapy context, positive relationships have been reported in some (but not all) studies of therapists' expectancies for their clients' outcomes and the maintenance of therapeutic relationships (Heller and Goldstein, 1961), and between therapists' liking of clients and therapeutic outcomes (Gottschalk, Mayerson, and Gottlieb, 1967; Strupp, Wallach, Wogan, and Jenkins, 1963). Also within the psychotherapy context is some literature, albeit inconsistent, to suggest that clients' expectancies (Goldstein and Shipman, 1961; Gurman, 1977) and positive orientation to their counselors (Lipkin, 1954) are positively related to outcomes.

What literature exists which contrasts the views of professional versus paraprofessional drug counselors in predominantly subjective, rather than empirically based, in nature. Subjective evaluations have characterized professional counselors as substantially different from paraprofessionals. Professional counselors have been described as formal, impersonal, and calculating (Chappel, Charnett, and Norris, 1974; Scher, Keavitt, Rothman, Kaplan, Weinstein, and Weisfeld, 1973; Suchotliff and Seligman, 1974), while paraprofessionals, especially ex-addict paraprofessionals, have been characterized as empathic, understanding, and spontaneous (Brown and Thompson, 1976; Dash, 1973; Reinstein, 1973; Social and Rehabilitation Service, 1974; Suchotliff and Seligman, 1974; Zimmerman and Coghlan, 1972). Paraprofessionals have also been characterized as more comfortable with their clients and more optimistic about their clients' prognosis (Reinstein, 1973), as well as more dedicated to their clients (Gay, Smith, Wesson, and Sheppard, 1972). In marked contrast with these subjective evaluations are the results of two empirical studies. These latter studies reveal convergence of views held by ex-addict and non-addict counselors toward heroin addicts (Brown, Jansen, and Bass, 1974) and toward the ideal counselor (Kozel and Brown, 1973).

Empirical studies of client views of their professional versus paraprofessional counselors are also rare. Two such studies paint paraprofessionals in a better light than professionals. For example, Ball, Graff, and Sheehan (1974) report that a higher percentage of clients in a methadone maintenance program saw paraprofessional (62%) as opposed to professional staff (40%) as helpful. Further, ex-addicts were viewed by a group of heroin addicts as a more credible source of information about street drugs than were professional caregivers, for example, psychologists and social workers (Sinnett, Hagen, and Harvey, 1975). These empirical studies reflect the same view as do more subjective descriptions of clients' apparent feelings toward ex-addict versus professional counselors (e.g., Baider, 1973; Baldwin, Liptzin, and Goldstein, 1973; Chapell et al., 1974; Dash, 1973; Scher et al., 1973; Suchotliff and Seligman, 1974; Wolf, Panyard, and Snowden, 1973).

The purpose of the present study was to characterize counselor and client attitudes and expectations within the three distinct counselor groups delineated in the opening paragraph—that is, PRO, NEA, and EXA. Both methadone maintenance and drug-free outpatient programs were examined, with programs chosen being primarily those in which the three groups were simultaneously employed. This was important in order to avoid possible confounding of types of clients or style of program approach with counselor group.

It should be noted here that the present study was also designed to have adequate statistical power in terms of sample sizes of both counselors and clients. This was required so that any null results legitimately could be interpreted as suggesting convergence of attitudes or expectations, rather than as a failure to detect differences due to lack of statistical power.

METHOD

The methods employed are described in detail in Aiken, LoSciuto, Ausetts, and Brown (1982), and are briefly summarized here.

Programs

Nine methadone maintenance and six drug-free outpatient programs participated, as well as a 16th program with separate drug-free outpatient and methadone maintenance units. These programs were situated in five major cities: Washington, DC, New York, Chicago, Los Angeles, and San Francisco.

Respondents and Procedure

Interviews were conducted with 31 PROs, 20 NEAs, and 31 EXAs, all of whom were full-time counselors and all of whom had caseloads of at least 25 clients. With the aim of enlisting four clients randomly chosen from each counselor's caseload, 116 clients of PROs, 71 clients of NEAs, and 115 clients of EXAs were also interviewed for a 92% response rate of clients sampled. Twenty-nine administrators including all program directors and 13 other individuals with heavy administrative responsibility were also interviewed.

Content of Interviews

The topics covered in all interviews are more extensive than described here; they included background information for all respondents, job descriptions of counselors, and client outcome data.

Counselor Interviews

Counselors, through the use of structured interviews made up of both closed-ended and several open-ended questions, indicated their beliefs about how drug abuse starts and gave their own definitions of treatment success and their expectations that clients would successfully complete treatment. They also expressed views on the characteristics of drug abuse clients and the nature of appropriate interactions between counselors and clients.

Client Interviews

Client interviews were structured around question frames complementary to those administered to counselors. Clients estimated the frequency with which their counselors provided certain services for them and gave their perceptions of their counselors' willingness to become involved in a number of activities with them. Clients indicated how desirous they were that their counselors perform such services for them. Clients were also asked how likely they would be to discuss certain personal problems with their counselors and/or ask for their counselors' help. Clients' perceptions of their counselors' views about the nature of and expectations for drug abuse clients were also sought, as well as some overall opinions on clients' relationships with their counselors. Data on clients' own expectations and quality of life were also collected. Finally, background information was solicited for each client regarding education, work, criminal, drug use, and drug treatment histories.

Administrator Interviews

Administrators were asked for their views of counselor-client relationships. They were asked whether one counselor group or another received and/or issued more complaints with regard to clients, and whether these complaints were justified in their own view.

RESULTS

First, the backgrounds of the counselors and the clients are briefly reviewed. (Backgrounds are examined in substantially greater detail in Aiken et al., 1982.) These overviews provide a backdrop against which any differences in attitudes and expectations of the various counselor and client groups might be considered. Second, the attitudes and expectations of the three groups of counselors are contrasted. Third, the client perspective on counselors and drug counseling is compared across counselor groups. In a fourth section, comments are presented concerning the interaction of counselors and clients, from the point of view of program administrators. The emphasis in all sections is on differences in attitudes and expectations among the three counselor groups, rather than on the attitudes and expectations per se.

Counselor and Client Backgrounds

Counselor Background

Professional counselors (PROs) were 67% White/Anglo, half male, and on average 30 years old; non-ex-addict paraprofessional counselors (NEAs), 70% Black, 60% male, and on average 36 years old; and paraprofessional counselors (EXAs), 70% Black, 81% male, and on average 39 years old, χ^2 (4) = 18.02, $p <$ .01 for race; χ^2 (2) = 7.08, $p < .05$ for sex; $F(2,78) = 11.12, p < .001$ for age. Counselor groups differed in their tenure in their current positions: 1.5 years for PROs, 3 years for NEAs, and slightly over 2 years for EXAs, $F(2,78) = 3.74, p < .05$. Of the PRO counselors, in accord with the definition for this study, all held bachelor's degrees, with 42% additionally holding master's degrees and another 29% having some graduate training. Of the EXAs and NEAs, respectively, 95% and 84% had high school diplomas, post-high school certificates, or at most some college training. Drug experience differed widely across groups, with 45% of PROs, 15% of NEAs, and all EXAs reporting the use of various drugs, with heavy opiate abuse by all EXAs. In all, 29 of the 31 EXAs had been in drug treatment, with a median stay of 22 months.

Client Background

Client backgrounds were compared across demographics, drug use and treatment histories, educational and employment histories, and criminal histories, with comparisons made on 97 measures in all (listed in Aiken et al. [1982]).

Clients assigned to the three counselor groups did not differ in either sex or ethnic composition ($p > .20$), being two-thirds male, half Black, a third White, and the remainder Spanish-American. The groups differed slightly in age, $F(2,299) = 3.70, p < .05$. with mean ages of 29, 32, and 30 years, for clients of PROs, NEAs, and EXAs, respectively.

The complete educational and employment histories of the three client groups were equivalent, as were their educational and employment experiences over the year, and more specifically, in the 30 days just prior to treatment entry. While more clients of PROs than of NEAs had spent at least 1 day in jail during the pretreatment year (52%, 39%, 36%), χ^2 (2) = 6.28, $p < .05$, the groups did not differ in the percentages of clients who were in treatment because of an arrest ($p > .20$).

In the areas of drug use and drug treament histories, only two differences were noted. First, in the drug-free modality, clients of PROs, more often than those of NEAs, reported excessive alcohol use in the 30 days prior to treatment ($p < .05$), but not for any longer time period. Second, in the drug-free modality, clients of PROs reported, on average, one more treatment episode than clients of NEAs ($p < .01$), though the groups did not differ on a variety of treatment history variables, including the number of years in treatment, the number of attempts to detoxify, and the number of heroin-related and court-related treatment episodes.

In all, the four differences detected among 97 measures of demographics and background history were the number that would have been expected by chance alone. There appeared to be no systematic differential assignment of clients to counselor groups.

Counselors' Attitudes and Expectations

Each aspect of counselors' attitudes was examined with a series of items. Each series of items was treated in two ways. First, separate analyses of variance were performed on the responses to each item in a set and counselor group as the stratification variable. Second, the set of items was treated in a single analysis of variance for reliability (Winer, 1972), with counselor groups as "judges," the individual items as elements being judged, and the mean response of a counselor group to an item as the dependent measure. The resulting reliability coefficients indicate the extent of similarity among counselor groups in their profile of responding over the items in the set. Differences among counselor groups across all the items of a series were also assessed from the reliability analyses, in those cases in which items were rated individually, rather than ranked.

Beliefs About How Drug Abuse Starts

Counselors first rank ordered six potential reasons why drug abuse starts: curiosity, bad home life, poverty, being discriminated against, peer group pressures, and some personality problems. There was remarkable agreement among the three counselor groups, in that all rated peer group pressures as most important and poverty and discrimination at least important. There was no difference in the mean ranking assigned to each item across groups ($p > .10$ in all cases). Finally, the analysis of variance of interjudge agreement yielded a reliability coefficient of .97 (Winer, 1972), supporting the notion that the three groups of counselors viewed the causes of drug abuse in a common fashion.

Factors Important to Treatment Success

Counselor groups were also in substantial agreement when asked to rank the relative importance of four factors in accounting for treatment success or failure: the client, the client's family and friends, the counselor, and supporting drugs. The client was ranked by all three counselor groups as most important, and supporting drugs were ranked as the least important, with an interjudge reliability coefficient on mean rankings of .99. The only difference, albeit weak, noted among the counselor groups was a tendency for PROs, on average, to rank counselors as less important than the other groups, $F\ (2,79) = 2.90, p < .10$.

Counselors' Definitions of Treatment Success

Counselors supplied their own definitions of treatment success, in response to the open-ended question "Please explain in your own words what treatment success means to you." All criteria mentioned were tabulated. The most commonly given definition involved becoming and remaining drug free, reflected in 29%, 31%, and 23% of the comments of PROs, NEAs, and EXAs, respectively. Similar percentages of reasons mentioned in the three groups (respectively, 25%, 26%, 20%) included a change in life-style to a "normal, mainstream" existence. Surprising, in face of the federal criteria of treatment success which include employment and freedom from crime, was the consistently low rate of mentioning these criteria across the counselor groups: 15%, 15%, and 12% for becoming employable and/or employed, and 7%, 3%, and 4% for staying away from crime, among PROs, NEAs, and EXAs, respectively. The only group difference of note was that EXAs mentioned internal states of adjustment (e.g., coping, feelings of self-sufficiency, self-awareness) as important more often than the other groups, that is, 32% of EXA, versus 16% and 15% for PROs and NEAs, respectively, $\chi^2\ (2) = 6.51, p < .05$.

Counselor Expectations of Treatment Outcomes

Counselors rated on a four-point scale the likelihood of each of 10 potential treatment outcomes, a year after clients had left treatment: remaining drug free, getting legal jobs, holding legal jobs, staying away from crime, having good physical health, having good mental health, having good family lives, having good lives in general, being productive members of society, and having no need for treatment. Differences among counselor groups emerged on only one item, that of having good mental health, $F\ (2,77) = 3.10, p < .05$, with NEA counselors less optimistic than either PROs or EXAs, who did not differ in their views. The pessimism of the NEAs appeared somewhat general, in that NEAs had lower mean expectation levels on all but three of the items (getting a legal job, holding a legal job, and staying away from crime), a result not expected by chance alone ($p < .05$). The pessimism was hardly dramatic, however, since in no case except mental health did a item difference approach significance ($p > .10$ in all cases).

Ex-addict counselors tended to be more optimistic than the other groups that their clients would remain drug free $F\ (2,77) = 2.90, p < .10$, though all three counselor groups believed it unlikely that clients would have no need for treatment, with NEAs and EXAs giving this possible outcome their lowest likelihood rating; PROs, their second lowest rating. In all, differences among the counselor groups were not at all marked, with an interjudge reliability coefficient of .64 over the mean expectation levels assigned to the 10 items by the three counselor groups.

Counselors' Perceived Characteristics of Drug Abuse Clients

Counselors were asked whether they agreed or disagreed with each of 19 statements about the current status of the average drug abuse client in their program: that the average drug abuse client in the program was mentally ill, physically ill, an unfortunate victim of society, unaware of mental problems, criminal by nature, morally weak, basically no better or worse than other people, capable of real and permanent change, hostile, reachable, culturally disadvantaged, smarter than most people, discriminated against unfairly, likely to steal, likely to be dangerous, resistant to treatment, just needing a break, likely to become alcoholic if drugs aren't available, and childish. There was substantial agreement among the three counselor groups across the 19 items, with an interjudge reliability coefficient of .93. For many of the items, there was no marked tendency to either agreement or disagreement. However, on three items clear convergence to a single pole was noted; all counselor groups believed that clients were not criminal by nature, that they were reachable, and that they were capable of permanent change.

Counselor-Client Interactions

Counselors, in a final question frame, expressed their agreement with 10 statements concerning three aspects of interaction with clients: client control, relationships with clients, and counselor background required for treating clients. (Due to the length of the items, they are listed in Table 1.) Once again, strong differences did not surface. On none of the relationship items, including those that involved socializing with clients (Items 5, 6, 7), was there a difference among groups. Not surprisingly, one difference which did emerge was that EXAs agreed more than PROs or NEAs that personal experience with the same problems as a client is needed for an understanding of the client, $F\ (2{,}79) = 8.37$, $p < .001$. However, even EXAs, on the average, tended to disagree with this item. On the other hand, all three counselor groups disagreed with the background items which suggested specifically the necessity for coursework in counseling and social work, in order to deal with clients (Item 9), and more generally the need for a lot of education in order that clients will think counselors can help them (Item 10). In sum, on these counselor background related items, on

Table 1

Attitude Items Concerning Counselor Interaction with and Treatment of Clients

A. Control Items
1. Clients will take advantage of you if you get too friendly with them.
2. You've got to keep tight control over your clients or they will walk all over you.

B. Relationship Items
3. You've got to get to know a client personally before you can really help him.
4. It is important to build up trust with families and friends of clients so that they won't be afraid to give information about the clients.
5. It's good to get out and socialize with the clients in their own neighborhoods if you want to help them.
6. Going places informally with clients, such as to ball games or picnics, is important.
7. It is the counselor's job to help his client at the program site, not to go out in the community.

C. Counselor Background Items
8. Unless you have a lot of education, most clients think you can't help them.
9. There is no substitute for coursework in counseling or social work for learning how to deal with clients.
10. You can't really understand a client's problems unless you've had the same problems yourself.

which perhaps the most dramatic differences might be expected, convergence, rather than divergence, among counselor groups was noted.

Summary of Counselors' Views of Clients

Though differences in backgrounds of the three groups of counselor groups were evident, these differences did not lead to divergence among the counselor groups across a spectrum of issues related to drugs and drug treatment. Counselors of all three groups agreed that peer group pressure was the major cause for the onset of drug abuse, that the client was the critical factor in treatment success or failure, and that treatment success involved becoming and remaining drug free and, additionally, assuming a "normal, mainstream" life-style. Counselors also had similar expectations for the success of their clients after the clients left treatment. Though NEAs seemed slightly more pessimistic than the other groups, all groups believed it unlikely that clients would have no need for later treatment. Counselors also agreed in their views on the current status of clients in treatment, believing that clients were not criminal by nature, that they were reachable and capable of permanent change. Perhaps the most remarkable agreement among counselor groups was that all groups felt that extensive coursework was not necessary for working with clients. Finally, although EXAs were in less disagreement than the other groups with the idea that personal experience with the same problems as a client is required for an understanding of the client, even EXAs tended to disagree with this notion. Overall, then, counselor groups could not be differentiated on the basis of their views of drug abuse, drug abusers, or drug treatment.

Clients' Attitudes and Expectations

Clients were stratified into three groups, clients of PROs, NEAs, and EXAs by virtue of the group membership of their primary counselor. To ensure that clients' expressed views of the three counselor groups were not contaminated by input from other counselors, clients were explicitly asked questions only about their primary counselors. Data were treated in a fashion analogous to those for counselors.

Clients' Views of Their Counselors

Clients expressed their level of agreement with 30 statements concerning their counselors. These statements, listed in Table 2, covered three areas: (1) the counselor's knowledge of drugs and the street; (2) the counselor's competence, including the ability to understand and help the client; and (3) the quality of the relationship between client and counselor. Marked differences in attitudes emerged in clients' responses to items concerning their counselors' knowledge of drugs and the street. On all five items in this area (see Items 1 through 5, Table 2), clients of EXAs were more likely to believe their counselors to be knowledgeable than were clients of other counselors ($p < .001$ in all cases). This difference did not, however, carry over with great strength into clients' more general views of the competence of their counselors. Only one difference in this direction emerged across the 12 items concerned with counselor competence to understand and help the client (Items 6 through 17, Table 2). Clients of EXAs agreed more strongly than clients of PROs or NEAs that they "get something out of the counseling sessions" (Item 14, $F(2,286) = 3.12$, $p < .05$), though clients of all groups on the average agreed with this item. The only other difference which emerged was that clients of professional counselors were more likely to view their counselors as intelligent than were clients of NEAs (Item 6, $F(2,294) = 3.48$, $p < .05$), though clients of all groups, on average, agreed that their counselors were intelligent. There were no differences among the client groups or their views of their relationships with their counselors (Items 18 through 30, Table 2), considered either on the basis of mean responses across the 13 items, $F(2,24) = 1.35$, $p < .20$, or in analyses of variance applied separately to each item. Further intergroup agreement was high, with an intergroup reliability coefficient of .91.

Table 2

Items Used to Examine Clients' Views of Their Counselors

A. Counselor Knowledge of Drugs and the Street
1. My counselor knows a lot about drugs.
2. My counselor knows a lot about the street.
3. My counselor understands people with drug problems.
4. My counselor knows how tough it is to get off drugs.
5. My counselor knows how to handle problems on the street for his clients.

B. Counselor Competence to Understand and Help the Client
6. My counselor is intelligent.
7. My counselor doesn't seem to understand me.
8. My counselor seems "uptight" when he talks to me.
9. I can talk with my counselor about deep personal feelings.
10. My counselor makes things clearer for me.
11. I have confidence in my counselor.
12. My counselor doesn't seem sure of himself.
13. Talking with my counselor helps me to understand myself better.
14. I feel as though I really get something out of the counseling sessions.
15. My counselor completely understands my feelings.
16. My counselor's way of speaking confuses me.
17. My counselor tries to help me make decisions about a job.

C. Quality of Counselor-Client Relationship
18. In counseling sessions, my counselor listens to my ideas and plans without putting me down.
19. I don't trust my counselor.
20. My counselor seems like a "real human being."
21. My counselor has a good sense of humor.
22. My counselor always insists on being "right."
23. My counselor makes me feel as though my problems are really important.
24. My counselor is very patient.
25. I feel the counselor really wants to help me.
26. My counselor treats me as an individual.
27. My counselor makes me feel more like a "case" than an individual.
28. I feel comfortable in talking to my counselor.
29. My counselor seems to look down on me.
30. My counselor makes me feel as though he will jump on me if I say the wrong things.

Clients' Perceptions of Counselors' Views of Clients

A mark of the clarity of the therapist-client relationship is the accuracy with which clients understand their therapists' views of them. To this end, clients were asked to estimate how their primary counselors would respond to the 19 items measuring perceived characteristics of drug addict clients. As with counselor responses, the average reponses of clients on many items indicated neither strong agreement nor strong disagreement. The most clearly polarized responses for clients matched those of their counselors, in that they occurred on the same three items and in the same direction as had been produced by counselors. Clients felt their counselors believed that they (the clients) were not criminal by nature, that they were reachable, and that they were capable of real and permanent change. Correlations between the mean responses of clients and counselors in a group across the 19 items were substantial, $r\ (17) = .81$, .66, and .78 for PRO, NEA, and EXA counselors and clients, respectively, $p < .01$ in all cases, indicating that clients had relatively accurate views of their counselors' feelings about drug abuse clients.

There was some small amount of variation among the three client groups on individual items. Clients of EXAs believed that their counselors saw them as somewhat more antisocial than did clients of PROs. The clients of EXAs rated their counselors as agreeing more highly that their clients were likely to steal than did clients of PROs, $F\ (2{,}287) = 3.56$, $p < .05$. Clients of EXAs also indicated that their counselors, on average, disagreed less strongly than did clients of PROs with the idea that clients are likely to be dangerous, $F\ (2{,}283) = 3.13$, $p < .05$. Even with these two differences, there was very high agreement across the three client groups as to their counselors' views, with an interjudge reliability coefficient of .98 over the 19 items.

Problems Clients Would Bring to Their Counselors

Clients were presented with a series of 10 problems on situations and asked how likely it was that they would discuss the problem with their counselors. The 10 problems were chosen to be broadbased, covering a wide range of likely situations encountered by drug addicts, from those involving personal relationships to those resulting from criminal activity. The problems were as follows: (1) your (wife/husband/girlfriend/boyfriend) left you; (2) your mother or any other close relative was sick and needed medical attention; (3) someone was threatening you because you couldn't pay off a loan; (4) your landlord said he would evict you; (5) you needed to borrow $100 quickly; (6) you were about to lose a job that you like; (7) you were having problems getting along with your family; (8) you had a problem with the law; (9) one of your children was in trouble in school; and (10) you were using drugs heavily again. Further, if the client was likely to discuss a problem with the counselor, he was then asked how likely he would be to ask the counselor for help with the problem. At times in the counseling context, of course, discussing the problem and asking for help might be one and the same. In other situations (e.g., needing money, family problems, problems with a landlord), direct counselor intervention, in addition to discussion, might be sought by the client.

There was broad variation across problems in the percentages of clients who thought it either likely or very likely that they would discuss the problem with their counselors. The problem with the highest likelihood of being brought to counselors, across all counselor groups, was having a problem with the law, mentioned as likely or very likely to be brought to counselors by 89% of all clients. This was followed closely by the problem of heavy drug use, mentioned by 83% of all clients; and the loss of a job, mentioned by 78% of clients. These problems are, interestingly, those with which drug abuse programs were originally designed to cope. In contrast, the least likely problems to be brought to counselors involved the more private, less clearly treatment-related problems of need to borrow money, mentioned by 30% of clients as a problem they would likely bring to counselors; being threatened due to nonpayment of a loan, mentioned by 40% of clients; and a client's child having a problem in school, mentioned by 42% of clients. In all, there was substantial agreement among the clients of the three counselor groups on the types of problems which they were most (and least) likely to bring to their counselors, with an intergroup reliability coefficient of .98.

However, it should be noted that there were also significant differences among the three client groups in the general willingness of clients to bring any problems whatever to their counselors. When aggregated over all 10 problems, the average percentage of clients who said it was likely that they bring a problem to the counselor was somewhat higher for EXAs (65%) versus clients of PROs (61%) and NEAs (60%), $F\ (2,18) = 4.58, p < .05$. This overall difference was reflected most on items of a personal nature, most notably in regard to borrowing money, with 29%, 23%, and 35% of clients of PROs, NEAs, and EXAs, respectively, indicating that they would bring this problem to their counselors $F\ (2,293) = 5.69, p < .01$, for difference among groups in mean likelihood rating on a four-point likelihood scale.

Clients' Perceptions of Counselor Willingness to Help, and Clients' Desire for Help

Clients were also asked whether they thought their counselors would be willing to participate in certain activities with and for them, and then, whether the clients desired such participation. Six were clearly counseling related: (1) visit you at work, (2) go with you on a job interview, (3) visit you in the hospital, (4) go to court to testify for you, (5) go with you to an agency where you could get help, and (6) have members of your family come to this program for counseling about your problems. The other five were of a more personal nature: (7) give you personal help, such as helping with housework or cooking or buying food for you, (8) come to your neighborhood to help you deal with people with whom you are having problems, (9) come to your home to discuss your problems with you or the people you live with, (10) meet you in a public place for socializing (e.g., to have lunch or to go to a ball game), and (11) socialize with you in your home or the counselor's home.

Considering the six counseling-related items alone, on average 86%, 88%, and 92% of clients of PROs, NEAs, and EXAs, respectively, believed their counselors would help them with the problem, $F\ (2,10) = 7.94$, $p < .01$, with the average percentage of EXAs significantly higher than for the other groups ($p < .05$ for both differences by Newman Keuls analysis). While these differences for counseling-related items were not dramatic, the differences were notable for the personal problems, with an average of 59%, 70%, and 76% of clients of PROs, NEAs, and EXAs, respectively, believing their counselors would help them, $F\ (2,8) = 25.52$, $p < .001$, and all groups differentiated from one another ($p < .05$ at least by Newman Keuls analysis for all pairwise comparisons). This pattern of results was repeated in clients' indications of whether they would want their counselors to help them. For counseling items, on average, 71%, 70%, and 78% of clients of PROs, NEAs, and EXAs, respectively, would have wanted their counselors to help with the problems, $F\ (2,10) = 6.27$, $p < .05$, with the percentage of EXAs significantly greater than for the other two groups ($p < .05$ for both differences by Newman Keuls analysis). For non-counseling-related items, on average, 40%, 48%, and 53% of the clients of PROs, NEAs, and EXAs, respectively, would have wanted their counselors to help with the problems, $F\ (2,8) = 15.88$, $p < .005$, with all groups differentiated from one another ($p < .05$ at least by Newman Keuls analysis for all pairwise comparisons).

Clients' Expectations for the Future

Clients indicated their expectations for their own lives after leaving treatment, responding to the same 10 items as had counselors. Clients' expectations were remarkably similar across groups, with an interjudge reliability coefficient of .99 and no difference among groups in average expectation level considered over all 10 items, $F\ (2,18) = 1.23$, $p > .20$, or on each individual item taken separately ($F < 1$ in all cases).

Clients' expectations were substantially higher than those of their counselors. In a two-factor analysis of variance of counselor group (PRO, NEA, EXA) by respondents (clients, counselors), with items as the unit of analysis and the mean rating to each item as the dependent measure, client ratings were significantly higher than those of counselors, $F(1,18) = 110$, $p < .001$. The absence of the two-factor interaction, $F\ (2,36) = 1.86$, $p > .10$, indicated equivalent elevations of clients' over counselors' expectations in all three groups. Client expectations across the 10 items were not significantly correlated with those of counselors, $r\ (8) = .60, .46, .30$, for clients for PROs, NEAs, and EXAs, respectively, $p > .05$ in all cases. The very high expectations of clients across the 10 items resulted in truncation of range. What was consistent between counselors and clients in all groups were the lowest levels of optimism about the need for further treatment.

Summary of Clients' Views of Counselors

Clients of EXAs felt their counselors were more knowledgeable about drugs and the street than clients of the other groups, and felt that they got more out of counseling sessions than clients of the other groups. This was so even though the three groups of clients reported their relationships with their counselors to be equally positive and had equivalently high expectations for the outcomes of treatment. Clients of the three groups also held congruent beliefs about how their counselors felt about them. Clients of EXAs reported that they would be slightly more likely than clients of the other groups to bring a variety of problems to their counselors, though the clients of all groups appeared to agree highly on the types of problems they would be more or less likely to bring to counselors. Clients of EXAs also perceived their counselors as more willing than counselors of the other groups to participate in a number of counseling-related activities. All three groups of counselors were differentiated in their perceived willingness to help with more personal problems of clients, which problems would draw the counselor into the social milieu of the client; here EXAs were seen as most willing; PROs, as least willing. The same pattern of differentiation among counselor groups was evidenced in the desires of clients to have their counselors help with the problems. In sum, while clients of the three groups viewed their counselors as equally able to understand them and were equally able to understand them and were equally confident of the counselors, the clients of EXAs saw their counselors as more knowledgeable about critical issues of drugs and the street scene, were more willing to bring personal problems to their counselors, and expected and desired more participation from their counselors in both counseling-related and personal problems.

Administrators' Observations of Counselor-Client Relationships

Program administrators gave observations of client-counselor interactions from both the perspective of the counselor and that of the client. With regard to counselors, administrators were asked which of the three counselor groups voiced most complaints about clients, what the nature of these complaints was, and whether or not the complaints were legitimate. Remarks from the administrators lent some corroborating evidence that counselors were for the most part favorably disposed to their clients. The comments indicate few negative feelings, and these feelings were not well differentiated by counselor group. Over half of the administrators saw no differences between the counselor groups regarding their complaints about clients. While a few more administrators saw PROs as complaining more than NEAs or EXAs, the differences were not impressive. The most frequent complaint to administrators of all counselor groups was that clients were "gaming" or conning and manipulative, that they were unreliable (e.g., in showing up for appointments), and that they would not live up to the rules of the program. The administrators saw those complaints as largely legitimate, although they pointed out that it was sometimes the inability of the counselor to get through to the client which encouraged such behavior.

Administrators also were asked which of the three counselor groups was the object of most complaints from clients, what the nature of these complaints was, and whether or not they (the administrators) saw these complaints as legitimate. Administrators were also asked to describe in their own words how the different counselor groups worked with clients and the differences, if any, between the groups in their attitudes toward clients.

The results of this questioning generally corroborated what has already been seen—that clients and counselors seem to get on very well. It should be emphasized here that the complaint questions were designed to elicit relative rather than absolute frequencies of complaints for purposes of comparing counselor groups. However, when administrators were asked to identify the most frequently complained about group, no one group stood out as receiving more complaints than another. When administrators were asked to identify the most frequent client complaint about EXAs, it was that they were seen as too often using themselves as a central reference and not allowing for the individual characteristics and needs of the clients. The most frequent complaint by clients about PROs, on the other hand, was that the PROs were sometimes rather distant and removed from the clients because they themselves have not been addicted. Administrators reported that the number of such complaints about either group is small, however. Also, administrators tended to think that these few complaints were not particularly well justified, and that the groups work equally well with clients. In general, the group differences are quite small, and the overall level of satisfaction with counselors in each group by clients seems quite high if one uses complaint to administrators in conjunction with administrators observations as an index.

DISCUSSION

The similarities in responses of the three groups of counselors are much more impressive than are the differences, considering the disparities in demographic, educational, and experiential backgrounds of these three groups of individuals. The groups conceive of the etiology of drug abuse, the nature of drug abusers, the factors critical for drug treatment, and the lasting outcomes of treatment as essentially the same. These results extend the findings of Brown et al. (1974) and Kozel and Brown (1973) of agreement among divergent counselor groups on the nature of heroin addicts and on the role of the ideal counselor.

Concluding in favor of the null hypothesis is problematic, if the statistical power of the design is inadequate. The power of the counselor comparisons on any single item was assessed by the formulation of Cohen (1977). At the conventional level of significance of $\alpha = .05$, the power of the design for detecting effects accounting for at least 10% of the variance is .8, a level of power deemed acceptable by Cohen. In sum, the lack of difference among groups is not attributable to a failure of the design, but rather appears to reflect true convergence among the counselors in their expressed attitudes.

Had noteworthy differences emerged among the three counselor groups, it would have been of interest to link these differences to divergence among the groups in demographic background or, more importantly, differences in training and experience. In the absence of expressed differences on critical matters of drug use etiology, client characteristics, and treatment outcomes, references to the experiential backgrounds of the three groups seem unwarranted.

It was in the responses of clients that certain differences emerged—differences which generally favored ex-addict counselors. Clients of EXAs saw their counselors as more knowledgeable about drugs and the street than did clients of the other groups and were most positive about what they got out of counseling sessions. These clients also expressed a slightly higher likelihood of bringing a variety of personal problems to their counselors than did the others. Clients of the three counselor groups differed reliably in their beliefs about whether their counselors would support them in both counseling- and non-counseling-related activities, with clients of EXAs expecting the most support; and clients of PROs, the least. Parallel differences were found among clients in their desire to have their counselors participate in these activities.

The differences in perceived willingness and desire for support seem important indicators of the social distance between clients and counselors and of clients' beliefs in their counselors' commitment to them. These differences also have implications for client and counselor behavior. Fishbein and Ajzen (1975), in their consideration of the relationships between attitudes and behavioral intentions, theorized that the attitudes held by an individual toward another individual should influence the general level of favorability of that person's behavioral intentions to the individual. If clients differ in their perceptions of their counselors' intentions to help them, then inferring from Fishbein and Ajzen's model, the clients must at some level differ in what they believe to be the feelings the counselors hold toward them. Such feelings might well also underlie the differential desire of clients to have their counselors help them. Behavioral intentions are now generally regarded as better predictors of actual behavior than are mere declarations of attitudes. This is perhaps to be expected since they are one step closer to behavior, although emanting from affective states.

These differences seem to corroborate more subjective evaluations of professional versus paraprofessional counselors, which paint the professional counselors as more distant from and the paraprofessionals as more comfortable with and dedicated to their clients. While these differences appear neither in counselors' expressed attitudes toward clients nor in general attitude statements of clients about their counselors, they are consistently evident in clients' comments about potential interactions with counselors with reference to a variety of client needs. How these feelings impact upon client outcomes cannot be anticipated from the somewhat ambiguous literature on the relationship between client and therapist variables and ultimate patient outcomes in the psychotherapy context.

ACKNOWLEDGMENT

This research was supported by NIDA contract number 271-76-4410 to the first and second authors.

REFERENCES

AIKEN, L.S., LO SCIUTO, L., AUSETTS, M.A., and BROWN, B.S. Paraprofessional versus professional drug counselors: Diverse routes to the same role. *Int. J. Addict.* 19(2): 153-173, 1984.

BAIDER, L. Group work with addicts and therapists: Observations in a drug addiction clinic. *Drug Forum* 3(1): 91-102, 1973.

BALDWIN, B.A., LIPTZIN, M.B., and GOLDSTEIN, B.B., Jr. Youth services: A multifaceted community approach to drug abuse. *Hosp. Comm. Psychiatry* 24(10): 695-697, 1973.

BALL, J.C., GRAFF, H., and SHEEHAN, J.J., Jr. The heroin addicts' view of methadone maintenance. *Br. J. Addict.* 69(1): 89-95, 1974.

BROWN, B.S., JANSEN, D.R., and BASS, U.F. Staff attitudes and conflict regarding the use of methadone in the treatment of heroin addiction. *Am. J. Psychiatry* 131(2): 215-219, 1974.

BROWN, B.S., and THOMPSON, R.F. The effectiveness of formerly addicted and non-addicted counselors on client functioning. *Drug Forum* 5(2): 123-129, 1976.

CHAPPEL, J.N., CHARNETT, C.V., and NORRIS, T.L. Paraprofessional and professional teamwork in the treatment of drug dependence. In E. Senay, V. Shorty, and H. Alksne, (eds.), *Developments in the Field of Drug Abuse: Proceedings of the National Drug Abuse, Council, 1974.* Cambridge, MA: Schenkman, 1974, pp. 297-306.

COHEN, J. *Statistical Power Analysis for the Behavioral Sciences.* New York: Academic Press, 1977.

DASH, R. MMTP: A patient-oriented view. In *Proceedings of the Fifth National Conference on Methadone Treatment*, Vol. 1. Rockville, MD: National Association for Prevention of Addiction to Narcotics, U.S. National Institute of Mental Health, 1973, pp. 8-10.

DURLAK, J.A. Comparative effectiveness of paraprofessional helpers. *Psychol. Bull.* 86(1): 80-92, 1979.

FISHBEIN, M., and AJZEN, I. *Belief, Attitude, Intention and Behavior: An Introduction to Theory and Research.* Boston, MA: Addison-Wesley, 1975.

GAY, G.R., SMITH, D.E., WESSON, D.R., and SHEPPARD, C.W. Outpatient barbiturate withdrawal using phenobarbital. *Int. J. Addict.* 7(1): 17-26, 1972.

GOLDSTEIN, A.P., and SHIPMAN, W.G. Patient expectancies, symptom reduction and aspects of the initial psychotherapeutic interview. *J. Clin. Psychol.* 17(2): 129-133, 1961.

GOTTSCHALK, L.A., MAYERSON, P., and GOTTLIEB, A. Prediction and evaluation of outcome in an emergency brief psychotherapy clinic. *J. Nerv. Ment. Dis.* 144(2): 77-96, 1967.

GURMAN, A.S. The patient's perception of the therapeutic relationship. In A.S. Gurman and A.M. Razin (eds.), *Effective Psychotherapy: A Handbook of Research.* New York: Pergamon Press, 1977.

HELLER, K., and GOLDSTEIN, A.P. Client dependency and therapist expectancy as relationship maintaining variables in psychotherapy. *J. Consult. Clin. Pshchol.* 25(5): 371-375, 1961.

KOZEL, N.J., and BROWN, B.S. The counselor role as seen by ex-addict counselors, nonaddict counselors, and significant others. *J. Consult. Clin. Psychol.* 41(2): 315, 1973.

LIPKIN, S. Clients' feelings and attitudes in relation to the outcome of client-centered therapy. *Psychol. Monogr.* 68 (1, Whole No. 372), 1954.

LUBORSKY, L., CHANDLER, M., AUERBACH, A., COHEN, J., and BACHRACH, H. Factors influencing the outcome of psychotherapy: A review of quantitative research. *Psychol. Bull.* 75(3): 145-185, 1971.

MELTZOFF, J., and KORNREICH, M. *Research in Psychotherapy.* New York: Atherton Press, 1970.

NEITZEL, M.T., and FISHER, S.G. The effectiveness of professional and paraprofessional helpers: A comment on Durlak. *Psychol. Bull.* 89(3): 555-565, 1981.

PARLOFF, M.B., WASKOW, I.E., and WOLFE, B.E. Research on therapist variables in relation to process and outcome. In A.F. Bergin and S.L. Garfield (eds.), *Handbook on Psychotherapy and Behavior Change.* New York: Wiley, 1978.

REINSTEIN, M.J. The role of drug counselors in a hospital drug-cure program. *Hosp. Comm. Psychiatry* 24(12): 839-841, 1973.

SCHER, J., LEAVITT, A., ROTHMAN, R., KAPLAN, J., WEINSTEIN, J., and WEISFELD, G. Professionally directed existential group therapy in methadone maintenance rehabilitation. In *Proceedings of the Fifth National Conference on Methadone Treatment*, Vol. 2. Rockville, MD: National Association for Prevention of Addiction to Narcotics, U.S. National Institute of Mental Health, 1973, pp. 1191-1202.

SINNETT, E.R., HAGEN, K., and HARVEY, W.M. Credibility of sources of information about drugs to heroin addicts. *Psychol. Rep.* 37(3): 1239-1242, 1975.

SOCIAL AND REHABILITATION SERVICE. *Research Report No. 3: Overview Study of Employment of Paraprofessionals–National Study of Social Welfare and Rehabilitation Workers, Work, and Organizational Contexts.* Washington, DC: Department of Health, Education, and Welfare, 1974.

STRUPP, H.H., WALLACH, M.S., WOGAN, M., and JENKINS, J.W. Psychotherapists' assessment of former patients. *J. Nerv. Ment. Dis.* 137(3): 222-230, 1963.

SUCHOTLIFF, L., and SELIGMAN, E. The myth of the ex-addict staff. *Drug Forum* 4(1): 47-51, 1974.

WINER, B.J. Statistical principles in experimental design. New York: McGraw-Hill, 1972.

WOLF, K., PANYARD, C., and SNOWDEN, L. "Behavioral contracting" as a technique for facilitating effective professional/paraprofessional interaction. In *Proceedings of the Fifth National Conference on Methadone Treatment*, Vol. 1. Rockville, MD: National Association for Prevention of Addiction to Narcotics, U.S. National Institute of Mental Health, 1973, pp. 243-251.

ZIMMERMAN, R.S., and COGHLAN, A.J. The (mis)use of ex-addicts in drug abuse treatment programs. *Drug Forum* 1(4): 367-372, 1972.

The International Journal of the Addictions, 19(3), 253-263, 1984

Drug Taking by Nigerian Students in American Universities: Prevalences for Four Commonly Used Drugs

Onuegbu Emmanuel Achalu, PhD

David F. Duncan,* DPH

Department of Health Education
Southern Illinois University at Carbondale
Carbondale, Illinois 62901

Abstract

A standardized-item survey of drug taking was administered to 239 Nigerian students attending three American universities. Alcohol was the most widely used drug in the sample (current use by 64%), followed by tobacco (31.8% current use), cannabis (13.9%), and amphetamine and other stimulants (5.3%). Differences are reported between males and females, and among age groups and college levels. Levels of drug taking were high but no higher than those commonly reported for U.S. college students.

The United States plays host to an increasingly large number of Nigerian students who come to this country to further their education; there are now 17,350 (Boyan et al., 1981). These students have academic, social, financial, and some health problems common to all students in the United States. One health problem in particular concerns the nonmedical use of drugs. This is a widespread area of concern among American publics, and it is regarded as a

*To whom reprint requests should be addressed.

 0020-773X/84/1903-0253$3.50/0

major social problem (Duncan and Gold, 1982). Josephson and Carroll (1974) note that similar concern appears to exist in many other parts of the world.

Despite the concern over the problem of illicit/nonmedical drug use among Nigerians, reliable statistics on its magnitude are virtually nonexistent. Estimates and educated guesses vary greatly depending on their origin and purpose (Anumonye, n.d.).

An exhaustive literature search reveals that there have been no direct studies on licit and/or illicit drug use among foreign or Nigerian students in the United States. However, Oghojafor (1979), in studying preferred treatment for "Brain Fag Syndrome," reports that about 98% of those surveyed believe that Nigerian students in the United States use Indian hemp, and 95.7% and 93.6%, respectively, believe that Nigerian students use amphetamine and dextroamphetamine (stimulants). It is therefore of practical importance to conduct such research, and Nigerian students in American colleges and universities are felt to constitute a good sample of a specific cohort that can be studied economically by the present researchers.

The purposes of the study were to determine (1) the extent of drug use among Nigerian students attending three selected American universities, (2) the types of drugs most frequently used by these students, and (3) whether living in the United States influenced Nigerian students' drug-taking behavior. Analysis was limited to four major drug categories: tobacco, alcohol, cannabis, and amphetamines and other stimulants.

Table 1

Sample Characteristics

Characteristic	Descriptor	%
Sex	Male	83.7
	Female	15.9
Age	26 or older	38.5
	25 or younger	61.5
	(range 19-37)	
Class level	Graduate	21.8
	Senior	28.5
	Junior	20.5
	Sophomore	15.8
	Freshman	13.4
Time in U.S.	61 months or more	10.4
	31-60 months	37.7
	13-30 months	28.0
	1-12 months	23.9
	(range 2-144 months)	

METHODS

The sample consisted of 239 Nigerian students of both sexes, who were attending three American universities. Of the students who participated in this study, 50.2% were from Alabama A&M University, Normal, Alabama; 20.5% from North Texas State University, Denton, Texas; and 29.3% from Southern Illinois University at Carbondale, Illinois. Table 1 provides a summary of sample characteristics.

Data were collected using a standardized-item, self-administered survey questionnaire developed and tested for reliability and validity by the World Health Organization in cooperation with the United Nations Fund for Drug Abuse Control and titled *A Methodology for Student Drug-Use Surveys* (Smart et al., 1980). Questionnaires were personally distributed and gathered by the primary investigator. Reporting was descriptive in nature; no tests of significance were applied.

RESULTS

Prevalence of Tobacco Use

A substantial majority (62.3%) stated that they had either smoked, chewed, or sniffed a tobacco product in their lifetime. Less than one-half (41.8%) said they had smoked, chewed, or sniffed a tobacco product in the past 12 months. Seventy-six respondents (31.8%) said they had smoked, chewed, or sniffed a tobacco product during the past 30 days. More than one-third, or 38.5%, said they had first used a tobacco product when they were between 11 and 18 years old; 19.2% said they were 19 years or older at the time of first use. About 5% had smoked, chewed, or sniffed a tobacco product when they were only 10 years old or less.

While a majority (71%) of the males indicated they had smoked, chewed or sniffed a tobacco product in their lifetime, only 18.4% of the females had done so. Nearly one-half (49.7%) indicated they strongly disapproved and 31% said they disapproved of people 18 years or older who smoke 20 or more cigarettes a day. Only 18% said they did not disapprove.

Prevalence of Alcohol Use

A substantial majority (91.2%) of the respondents said they used alcoholic beverages in their lifetime, while a small number (7.5%) said they had never used any alcoholic beverages. Over two-thirds (79.1%) stated they had used alcoholic beverages in the past 12 months; 19.2% indicated they had not, while 1.7% did not respond.

Table 2

Current Prevalence of Alcohol Use

Response	N	%
No, did not use	81	33.9
Yes, on 1-5 days	82	34.3
Yes, on 6-19 days	28	11.7
Yes, on 20 or more days	43	18.0
Missing data	5	2.1
	239	100.0

As shown in Table 2, a large majority (64%) had drunk alcoholic beverages during the past 30 days: 46% on 1 to 19 days, and 18% on 10 or more days.

A majority (52.2%) said that they first had a drink when they were bêtween 11 and 18 years old; 21% indicated they were 19 years or older; 18% had their first drink when they were 10 years old or younger. Roughly equal proportions of males (92.4%) and females (92.1%) indicated they had drunk alcoholic beverages in their lifetime.

Prevalence of Cannabis Use

Over two-thirds of the sample (68.6%) said they had never taken cannabis, while 30.6% indicated they had taken the drug; 79.5% said they had not used cannabis in the past 12 months, and 19.2% admitted using the drug in the past 12 months. A small number of respondents (13.9%) had used cannabis in the past 30 days (see Table 3).

A majority of the respondents (16.8%) said they first used cannabis when they were 19 years or older; 12.1% were between 11 and 18 years, and 1 person (.4%) was 10 years old or younger when first using the drug.

Table 3

Current Prevalence of Cannabis Use

Response	N	%
No, did not use	200	83.6
Yes, on 1-5 days	19	8.0
Yes, on 6-19 days	3	1.3
Yes, on 20 days or more	11	4.6
Missing data	6	2.5
	239	100.0

A higher percentage of males (35.7%) than females (5.3%) had taken cannabis in their lifetimes. Strong disapproval of people 18 years or older trying cannabis once or twice was expressed by 46.9% of the sample; 27.6% disapproved, and 23.8% did not disapprove. Nearly half the sample (45.6%) strongly disapproved of people smoking cannabis occasionally, 27.2% disapproved and 24.7% did not disapprove. Over two-thirds (68.2%) strongly disapproved of people 18 years or older smoking cannabis regularly; 21.8% disapproved, and only 8.8% did not disapprove. Regarding availability of cannabis, 46.4% said it was easy to get cannabis, 26.8% said it was difficult, and 22.2% said it was probably impossible (see Table 4).

In response to the question whether cannabis was used in Nigeria, a substantial majority (77.8%) indicated they had never used the drug in Nigeria, while a small number (18%) said they had. Concerning their willingness to admit cannabis use, a substantial majority (68.6%) said they would have admitted it if they had actually used cannabis, 23.8% indicated they would not have, and 4.6% said they were not sure.

Prevalence of Amphetamine and Other Stimulant Use

About 80% of the respondents indicated they had never taken any amphetamines, and 19.7% said they had taken these drugs. A substantial majority, 88.3% said they had not used amphetamines or other stimulants in the past 12 months, while 10.4% said they had. As shown in Table 5, amphetamines and other stimulants had been used in the past 30 days by 5.3% of the respondents. Of these, the majority had used the drug on 5 days or less.

About 9% of the respondents indicated they first used amphetamines when they were 19 years or older; 9.1% were between 11 and 18 years old, and only 1 person was 10 years old or younger when first using the drug. Lifetime use of amphetamines and other stimulants was reported by 19.1% of the males and 23.7% of the females.

Table 4

Responses Concerning the Perceived Availability of Cannabis in the United States

Response	*N*	%
Probably impossible	53	22.2
Very difficult	31	13.0
Fairly difficult	33	13.8
Fairly easy	59	24.6
Very easy	52	21.8
Missing data	11	4.6
	239	100.0

Table 5

Current Prevalence of Amphetamine and Other Stimulant Use

Response	*N*	%
No, did not use	223	93.4
Yes, on 1-5 days	8	3.3
Yes, on 6-19 days	1	0.4
Yes, on 20 or more days	4	1.6
Missing data	3	1.3
	239	100.0

Table 6

Respondents' Levels of Difficulty in Obtaining Amphetamines and Other Stimulants in the United States

Response	*N*	%
Probably impossible	76	31.8
Very difficult	42	17.5
Fairly difficult	42	17.5
Fairly easy	43	18.0
Very easy	18	7.6
Missing data	18	7.6
	239	100.0

Table 7

Respondents' Sources of Introduction to Drug Use

Response	*N*	%
Don't know	123	51.6
Friends	65	27.2
Others	14	5.9
Family	13	5.4
Casual acquaintance	13	5.4
Physician (doctor)	6	2.5
Drug pusher	2	0.8
Pharmacist or druggist	2	0.8
Other health practitioner	1	0.4
	239	100.0

Questioned on stimulant use in Nigeria, 82.9% of the respondents indicated they had not used amphetamines and other stimulants in Nigeria, 14.6% reported they had, and 2.5% did not respond. As shown in Table 6, 35% of the total respondents said that in the United States it was difficult to get amphetamines and other stimulants; 31.8% said it would probably be impossible, while 25.6% said the drug was easy to obtain.

Asked to name the amphetamines or other stimulants that they had taken most recently, 13 (5.5%) reported "speed"; 9 (3.8%), coffee; 4 (1.7%), diet pills; 3 (1.3%), dextroamphetamine sulfate; 3 (1.3%), kola nut; 2 (.8%), "uppers"; and 1 (.4%), "phospherine." In addition, a number of nonstimulant drugs were listed in answer to this question: Mandrax, Phenergan, "yellow jackets," and "angel dust" were each listed by two respondents (.8%); and "China" was listed by 1 (.4%).

Other Nonmedical Drugs

When asked to name any other drug taken without a physician's advice in the past year, 2 people (.8%) indicated hashish, and 1 each (.4%) stated codeine, Dagga, and Proplus. When asked to name any other drugs that people are now taking to make them feel good or intoxicated, 3.4% named Indian hemp, and less than 1% each indicated LSD, quaalude, alcohol, Mandrax, "black beauties," "angel dust," and codeine. More than a fourth of the respondents (27.2%) said they were introduced to nonmedical drug use by friends, 5.4% by a casual acquaintance, 5.4% by a family member, and 2.5% by a physician. A small number (.8% each) were introduced by either a drug pusher or a pharmacist, as shown in Table 7.

A large number (15.9%) indicated that their first nonmedical use of drugs was motivated by curiosity; 10.9% took the drug for the relief of cold, hunger, or fatigue; 6.3% to be sociable; and 5% for enjoyment. Small percentages stated that their motivation was acceptance by others, religious custom, enhancement of sex, treatment of health disorder, relief of psychological stress, or improvement of work performance (see Table 8).

When asked whether living in the United States influenced their drug-taking behavior, a large majority (72.4%) said no, 10.5% said yes, and 15.5% indicated they had no opinion.

Comparisons of Drug Use Prevalences

As summarized in Table 9, prevalences of use for the four drugs under study varied considerably, with the highest prevalence for alcohol and the lowest for amphetamines and other stimulants.

Table 8

Responses Concerning Respondents' Reasons for Drug Use

Response	*N*	%
Did not respond	109	45.6
Curiosity	38	15.9
Relief of cold, hunger, or fatigue	26	10.9
To be sociable	15	6.3
Enjoyment	12	5.0
Treatment of health disorder	11	4.6
Religious custom	7	2.9
To be accepted by others	6	2.5
Relief of psychological stress	6	2.5
Improvement of work performance	6	2.5
Enhancement of sex	3	1.3
	239	100.0

Sex Differences

In general, more males than females were involved in the use of two drugs—tobacco and cannabis; more females than males had used amphetamines and other stimulants; and roughly equal proportions of both sexes had used alcohol. The prevalence rates are reported in Table 10.

Age Differences

A higher proportion of people 25 years or younger reported using tobacco, amphetamines, and other stimulants at some time, compared to a smaller proportion of those 26 years or older. Also, roughly the same proportion of people 25 years or younger and 26 years or older reported using alcohol and cannabis.

Table 9

Prevalences of Use for the Four Selected Drugs

Drug	Lifetime prevalences (%)	Annual prevalences (%)	Current prevalences (%)
Alcohol	91.2	79.1	64.0
Tobacco	62.3	41.8	31.8
Cannabis	30.6	19.2	13.9
Stimulants	19.7	10.4	5.3

Table 10

Lifetime Prevalences of Use for Four Selected Drugs, by Sex

Drug	Male (%)	Female (%)
Alcohol	92.4	92.1
Tobacco	71.0	18.4
Cannabis	35.7	5.3
Stimulants	19.1	23.7

Differences Related to College Level

Overall, freshmen had higher rates of use for tobacco, compared with other college levels, followed by graduate students, seniors, juniors, and sophomores, in that order. Sophomores and freshmen had almost the same rates for alcohol use, followed by graduate students, juniors, and seniors. The highest rate of use for cannabis was among seniors, there were no differences between juniors and graduate students, and the lowest rates of use for cannabis were among freshmen. For the use of stimulants, sophomores had a higher rate, followed by juniors and graduate students. Seniors and freshmen had roughly the same rates of stimulant use. The rates of use of the illicit drugs (cannabis and stimulants) were lowest among freshmen (see Table 11).

Age at First Use for Four Drugs

A substantial majority of the respondents reported using tobacco, alcohol, and stimulants when they were between 11 and 18 years old. As for cannabis, however, more respondents (16.8%) reported first trying it when they were 19 years or older. A particularly important finding is that 18% of the respondents first used alcoholic beverages when they were 10 years old or younger, and 5.1% tried tobacco products at the same age (see Table 12).

Table 11

Lifetime Prevalence of Use for Four Drugs, by College Level

Drug	Freshmen (%)	Sophomores (%)	Juniors (%)	Seniors (%)	Graduates (%)
Alcohol	96.8	97.4	91.7	86.6	94.2
Tobacco	68.8	50.0	61.2	64.7	65.4
Cannabis	15.6	23.7	32.7	38.8	32.7
Stimulants	15.6	23.7	22.9	16.2	21.2

Table 12

Ages of Respondents at First Use for Four Drugs

Drug	Never used drug (%)	10 years or younger (%)	11-18 years (%)	19 years or older (%)
Tobacco	36.8	5.1	38.5	19.2
Alcohol	7.5	18.0	52.2	21.0
Cannabis	69.9	0.4	12.1	16.8
Stimulants	81.3	0.4	9.1	8.8

CONCLUSION

The findings from this study showed that the overall prevalence of drug use, especially alcohol, among this sample was high but not higher than that reported in the literature concerning American college students. While the study is by no means exhaustive, it does provide information to add to an otherwise inadequate body of literature on drug use among Nigerian college students at home or abroad. Whether the results obtained are truly representative of all the Nigerian students studying in U.S. institutions is uncertain; the findings do supply a baseline for future research on drug use. A further study of another U.S. sample would be desirable, as would be studies of Nigerian students at universities in England and in Nigeria to allow comparisons.

When respondents were asked whether they used cannabis and amphetamines in Nigeria, 43 people (18%) admitted using cannabis, while 35 people (14.6%) admitted using amphetamines. When asked about lifetime use, 73 respondents (30.6%) said they used cannabis, while 47 people (19.7%) admitted using amphetamines. Furthermore, when asked whether living in the United States encouraged them to take drugs, a large majority (72.4%) said no, 10.5% said yes, and 15.5% indicated they had no opinion. In fact, there was obviously a substantial increase in the number of users of cannabis, which suggests there might have been some influence since coming to the United States. The use of amphetamines increased also but not as impressively as cannabis use. Finally, when asked to name the amphetamines or other stimulants they had taken most recently, two respondents listed a few nonstimulant drugs, indicating that they did not recognize the true effects of these drugs.

REFERENCES

ANUMONYE, A. *Nigerian Drug Scene.* Lausanne, Switzerland: International Council on Alcohol and Addictions, no date.

BOYAN, D.R., JULIAN, A.C., and REW, J. (eds.). *Open Doors 1980/81: Report on International Educational Exchange*. New York: Institute of International Education, 1981.

DUNCAN, D.F., and GOLD, R.S. *Drugs and the Whole Person*. New York: Wiley, 1982.

JOSEPHSON, E., and CARROLL, E.E. *Drug Use: Epidemiological and Sociological Approaches*. New York: Wiley, 1974.

OGHOJAFOR, A.L. *Psychiatric and traditional healing modalities for "brain fag syndrome."* Unpublished dissertation, Southern Illinois University, 1979.

OKIGBO, C.C. *Nigerian students in the United States: Factors related to their expatriation*. Unpublished dissertation, Southern Illinois University, 1981.

SMART, R.G., HUGHES, P.H., JOHNSTON, L.D., ANUMONYE, A., KHANT, U., MORA, M.E.M., NAVARATNAM, V., POSHYACHINDA, V., VARMA, V.K., AND WADUA, K.A. *A Methodology for Student Drug-Use Surveys*. Geneva: World Health Organization, 1980.

The International Journal of the Addictions, 19(3), 265–286, 1984

An Empirical Examination of the Social Bond Theory of Drug Use

R. Thomas Dull,* PhD

Department of Criminal Justice
Memphis State University
Memphis, Tennessee 38152

Abstract

The purpose of the present study was to investigate the relationship between control theory, measured through a created social bond scale, and the respondents' self-admitted drug use (alcohol, marijuana, tobacco, amphetamines, and barbiturates). An analysis was conducted of self-reported drug use data from a general Texas adult population. This analysis included a series of bivariate cross-comparison correlations between the independent variable (social bond) and the dependent drug variables. The relationship between the independent and dependent variables was further examined by calculating the correlation and level of significance within selected categories of several demographic (age, race, sex, education, income, and marital status) variables. The results showed a significant positive correlation between reduced social bonding and greater drug use. However, while these relationships were significant, they were relatively weak and of little explanatory value. It was concluded that Hirschi's social bond theory fails to provide an adequate explanation for the use of drugs within the framework of this analysis.

*Address all correspondence to the author at 405 Mitchell Hall, Memphis State University, Memphis, Tennessee 38152.

 0020-773X/84/1903-0265$3.50/0

INTRODUCTION

Control theory is found in its most current and clearly defined form in Hirschi's *Causes of Delinquency* (1969). Hirschi's social bond concepts have been somewhat reconceptualized, but basically substantiated, by the works of Hindelang (1973) and Conger (1976). Hirschi's social control theory has several dimensions along which the bond of the individual to society varies, including attachment, commitment, involvement, and belief (Gibbons, 1979).

> Attachment has to do with the strength of ties to others such as parents or peers, while commitment designates the person's devotion to conformist lines of conduct. Individuals also vary in involvement, that is, in the degree to which they are engaged in activities that restrict the time they have available for deviant activities. They also differ in belief, that is, the strength of their attitudes toward conformity. (Gibbons, 1979, p. 120)

In examining belief, Hirschi (1969) contends that

> . . . there is variation in the extent to which people believe they should obey the rules of society, and furthermore, that the less a person believes he should obey the rules the more likely he is to violate them. (1969, p. 26)

Control theory should not be viewed as deterrence theory, for it is more of a general explanation of deviance that is basically restricted to informal social control which comes from individuals being bonded to groups and institutions (Akers et al., 1979).

Hirschi's self-report study (1969), conducted in Richmond, California, obtained data on delinquent activities and social control variables. The findings of this research basically confirmed his social bond hypothesis. Youths who showed less attachment to parents, school, peers, social institutions, and conventional activities tended to be more delinquent. While Hirschi was not specifically interested in utilizing control theory as an explanation of drug use, he did note that students who expected little formal education are more likely to engage in these practices. Thus, activities such as smoking and drinking are, at least in part, indicative of lack of commitment to the educational system.

It has fallen to others to attempt to substantiate the use of control theory and its explanatory value in the area of drug use (Burkett and Jensen, 1975; Levine and Kozak, 1979; Mercer, Hundleby, and Carpenter, 1978; Suchman, 1968–for more detailed analysis of these studies and those that follow, the reader is referred to the Resource Chart, Table 1). Aultman and Wellford (1978), using a path analysis model, concluded that the control variables of an adolescent's relations with parents and peers were most important in explaining delinquency. They suggested that future research should focus on various dimensions of these bonds.

Suchman's (1968) research suggested that lack of commitment to conventional social values and institutions is the primary determinant of drug use and of involvement in the drug subculture. Bruce Johnson (1973) argues that lack of commitment has an indirect effect on drug use by predisposing those who have broken social commitment bonds to identify and become involved with drug-using groups.

The findings of research by Burkett and Jensen (1975) consistently showed that those with low stakes in conformity (scored low on school and family involvement and on attachment to parents and school) are more likely to use marijuana. Those who maintain strong attachment to conventional others and are involved in conventional activities are far less likely to use marijuana. The Burkett and Jensen findings were consistent with their hypothesis that the belief in certainty of apprehension for marijuana use is inversely related to self-reported use. However, it also appears that conventional ties, such as family and school, may serve as sources of control independent of one's belief in certainty of apprehension.

> Of particular importance is involvement with other users. Use is unlikely given the absence of group supports. This holds both for youth who maintain conventional ties and for those with weak ties. Further, involvement with nonusing peers is related to patterns of use as well as the belief that one will get caught should he try. The effectiveness of the law as a deterrent, then, is questionable given peer involvement and reinforcement for beliefs which effectively discount or support the certainty of apprehension as a viable reason for nonuse. (Burkett and Jensen, 1975, p. 522)

Levine and Kozak (1979) suggest that inadequate and deficient parental attachment, and attachment to delinquent companions are important factors in determining the use of alcohol and drugs among both prepubertal and teenage students (see Note 1). Mercer et al. (1978) evaluated adolescents' perceptions of the family as a unity and related these dimensions to the use of tobacco, alcohol, and marijuana. It was found that the parental attachment factors of warmth, support, and interest related negatively and significantly to the use of alcohol and tobacco by males. For the females, these factors related negatively and significantly to the use of all three drugs.

Several studies have suggested that drug use is not related to lack of commitment to conventional institutions or involvement in conventional activities

Table 1

Resource Chart:

Reference	Year study was done	Number of subjects	Type of subjects	Data-collecting technique
Suchman (1968)	1967	497	College students	Interviews, observations, and questionnaires
Johnson (1973)	1970	3,500	College students	Questionnaires
Ginsberg and Greenley (1978)	1971-1974	1,502	College students	Longitudinal questionnaires
Finnell and Jones (1975)	1972	335	College students	Questionnaires and ACT scores
Mercer, Hundley and Carpenter (1978)	1974	286	9th grade students	Questionnaires
Aultman and Wellford (1979)	1975	1,500	Junior/senior high school students	Questionnaires
Burkett and Jensen (1975)	1975	1,056	Senior high school students	Questionnaires
Levine and Kozak (1979)	1977	796	5th grade through high school students	Questionnaires

Control Theory and Drug Use

Statistical technique	Theory variable (source of control)	Drug variable	Results
Test of significance coefficient of association	Commitment to conventional institutions and social values	Alcohol, marijuana, and LSD	Significant relationship with moderate to strong association
Percentage breakdowns	Involvement in conventional activities and commitment to subculture	Marijuana, cocaine, heroin, barbiturates, amphetamines	Tenative support for theory
Multiple regression and path analysis	Commitment to conventional institutions and involvement in conventional activities	Marijuana	Not significantly related
F test of significance; Scheffe's method	Commitment to education and attachment to school	Alcohol and marijuana	Not significantly related
Correlational and regression techniques	Various social bond elements tested with a OFAM scale (Overall Family Attitude Measure)	Alcohol, marijuana, and tobacco	Significant relationship with moderate association
Multiple regression and path analysis	Attachment: ties to parents and peers	Use and selling of various drugs	Significant and causal relationship
Ordinal level measure of association (gamma)	Involvement in school and attachment to school and family	Marijuana	Significant relationship with relatively strong associations
Percentage	Attachment: ties to parents and peers	Alcohol and marijuana	Tenative support for theory

(Finnell and Jones, 1975; Ginsberg and Greenley, 1978). Finnell and Jones (1975) found no significant relationships between regular use of alcohol beverages and marijuana and the academic performance of college students. The Ginsberg and Greenley (1978) longitudinal study of marijuana use is probably the most critical indictment against the use of control theory as an explanation for marijuana use. They found that, contrary to earlier conclusions based solely on cross-sectional data, marijuana use at follow-up is neither directly nor indirectly related to initial lack of commitment to conventional institutions. In addition, the degree of involvement in conventional activities was found to be unrelated to marijuana use.

Almost without exception, empirical tests which have been developed to assess the predictive powers of theories designed to account for drug use have utilized either adolescent, high school, or college samples. Thus, we must exercise caution in generalizing these results to other situations, especially nonstudent populations. Our present study utilizes a general population rather than a sample from a restricted juvenile population. This is especially crucial today when the drug users of 20 years ago, the zenith of marijuana's popularity, are now well beyond adolescence.

The present study explores the relationship between social bond theory, as enunciated by Hirschi's (1969) various social bond elements, and the use of drugs. An analysis of zero-order correlations regressing social bond against the various types of drug use (alcohol, marijuana, tobacco, amphetamines, and barbiturates; see Note 2) is conducted, as is a similar analysis of social bond and the two composite drug categories (UserE and UserP). A major section of the paper analyzes the various demographic categories (sex, age, race, school, income, and marital status) to see if either specific or composite drug use is associated with the elements of the bond. Finally, we conduct a sixth-order partial correlation of social bond with the drug types, in which we control for the demographic variables of sex, race, age, school, income, and marital status. A clarifying note, for our unaware readers: An increase in bond scale value indicates a decrease in the degree and level of social bonding. This permits positive correlations to signify a positive linear relationship between the lack of social bonding and the increased use of drugs.

The criterion used in determining whether a "powerful explanation" exists is the traditional statistical criterion of explained variation. Such a technique focuses on the "explanatory power" of the presumed independent variable as a function of the percent of variance shared between variables. Costner (1965) refers to this use of measures of association as "proportionate reduction in error"; that is, the amount of variation within one variable which can be "predicted" from a knowledge of another variable. This mode of determining explanatory power is dependent on two factors. First, the relationship between the two variables must not be due to chance error (traditionally defined at a probability level of .05). Second, any amount of explained variation must be causally meaningful (i.e., at least 10% of the total variation in the dependent variable). A "powerful explanatory theory" is, then, that theory which is capable of predicting a relatively large amount of variation in either specific forms of drug use or in drug use per se.

METHODOLOGY

Self-report questionnaires were mailed to a systematic random sample of 2,000 individals drawn from the population of persons holding valid driver's licenses in the state of Texas. Every *n*th name was taken in order to provide the size sample desired. Over 90% of Texas residents, age 17 and over, are part of this population (Teske and Jeffords, 1979).

The survey data examined in the present study are derived from one portion of the 1981 *Texas Crime Poll* (Kercher and Dull, 1981) conducted by the Survey Research Program at Sam Houston State University. The Survey Research Program conducts this statewide survey annually. The format of the *Texas Crime Poll* remains basically the same each year, with a number of trend questions replicated so as to permit the measurement of changes in public opinion. Other items or sections of the *Poll* are topical and are included only once. The general, or topical, section of the 1981 *Texas Crime Poll* included the questions for the present study.

Upon completing the original draft of the questionnaire, the instrument was pretested. A purposive sample of individuals was selected for the pretesting. The sample was designed to represent various educational, ethnic, racial, and rural/urban backgrounds.

Prior to the first mailing, all Spanish-surname individuals in the sample were identified. A Spanish-language version of the questionnaire, along with an explanatory letter in Spanish, was included with both the first and second mailings. This was done so that the large number of Spanish-speaking and -reading Mexican-Americans residing in Texas would not be excluded from the opportunity to respond to the survey.

Procedure

In implementing the mail-out self-report survey, a multistage procedure was utilized in order to obtain the highest possible return rate. One week prior to the mailing of the first set of questionnaires, each person in the sample was sent a presurvey sensitizing postcard. The purpose of this postcard was to alert the prospective respondents to the fact they had been randomly chosen to participate in this statewide study and that they should expect the survey package within approximately 1 week. It was hoped that the presurvey postcard would prepare the respondents for the survey instrument and reduce the initial rejection rate due to confusing the survey with "junk mail."

One week after the sensitizing postcard was sent, the first set of questionnaires were mailed. Each person in the sample received a survey package consisting of a self-administered questionnaire, a personalized letter explaining the purpose of the poll, a presharpened pencil, and a stamped, addressed, typeset return envelope. The address label and the survey instrument were numbered so that those returning surveys could be removed from the follow-up process.

Two weeks after mailing the questionnaire, all nonrespondents were sent a follow-up postcard asking them to complete and return the questionnaire. The postcard reminded the respondents of the survey's importance and asked that they take the time necessay to fill it out. Two weeks after the follow-up postcard, a second survey package was forwarded to those respondents who had still not returned their survey. As with the first mailing, this package contained a personally addressed cover letter, survey instrument, a pencil, and a self-addressed envelope. As before, the address label and the survey instrument were numbered so that those returning surveys could be removed from the follow-up process.

Finally, 1 week after the second survey package, a final reminder postcard was sent to those respondents who had failed to return the survey instrument. This postcard, again, reminded the respondent of the survey's importance and asked if they would return the instrument at their earliest convenience.

The cut-off date for returns used for analysis in the present study was approximately 10 weeks after the mailing of the first questionnaire, which is consistent with the cut-off dates used with earlier *Crime Polls*. Of the 2,000 Texas residents who were surveyed for this study, 1,449 completed usable questionnaires, 28 of which were in Spanish. This represents a return rate of 72.5% of the original total sample. When the 100 nonforwardables and the individual ascertained to be deceased were subtracted from the total sample of 2,000 the actual sample of potential respondents dropped to 1,899. The adjusted return rate, then, was 76.3%.

Independent and Dependent Variables

The creation of the control theory scale was a multistep procedure. This scale is titled the Social Bond Scale since it represents Hirschi's (1969) delineation of control theory. Respondents were asked to rate (very important = 1, occasionally important = 2, of little importance = 3, and of no importance = 4) a series of items that represented various social bond elements (Hirschi, 1969; Note 3). Items were derived from a previously tested instrument (Marshall et al., 1981) that had attempted to develop items that represented each of the four elements of Hirschi's social bond concept. Hirschi suggested that the elements of the social bond include attachment, belief, commitment, and involvement. Later evaluation in this present study suggested that separate elements of the bond were present within the survey instrument items.

The second step was to examine the items through a principal component factor analysis process. There were two reasons for adopting a factor analysis approach. First, we desired to know if the elements of the social bond represented unique and separate dimensions. If the items all clustered in a single block or dimension, then we do not have separate elements of the bond but a single composite measure of social bond. The second purpose for the factor analysis was to obtain a more parsimonious scale. By utilizing only items that received high factor loading scores (.60 and higher), we were able to reduce the number of items (thus more parsimonious) without seriously reducing the explanatory power of the scale (Note 4). After the factors were rotated using a varimax criterion with Kaiser normalization, the items clustered into three separate dimensions, with two items in each dimension having factor loading values of .60 or greater (see Table 2 and Note 5).

The Social Bond Scale was the cumulative score for the six remaining items. A respondent's rating of very important for an item received a score of 1. On the other extreme, a respondent's rating of no importance for an item received a score of 4. A respondent could obtain a total scale score ranging from 6 (individual's bond to society is very strong) to 24 (individual's bond to society is weak or broken).

There were seven dependent variables utilized in this study. The distinct drug use dependent variables were alcohol, tobacco (Note 6), marijuana, amphetamines, and barbiturates. In addition, two composite drug use categories were created. The composite drug use categories were total number of drugs tried in a lifetime (UserE) and total number of drugs used during the last year (UserP).

Table 2

Factor Analysis—Rotated Loadings

Element	Item	Factor 1	Factor 2	Factor 3
Belief	A	.767		
Belief	B	.715		
Involvement	C		.786	
Involvement	D		.659	
Commitment	E			.861
Commitment	F			.848

Data Analysis

In the present study all of the independent and dependent variables under analysis are either interval, dummy, or high ordinal levels of measurement. It was determined that for all statistical comparisons, interval-level statistics would be utilized.

The practice of using ordinally measured variables with statistical methods, such as regression analysis, is supported by Labovitz (1967, 1970), who demonstrated that true magnitudinal positions are not severely misrepresented and that regression is, by its nature, a very robust statistic. Borgatta (1968) and Boyle (1970) also support the use of interval techniques with ordinal data. This study found greater explained variation for the created trichotomous dependent variables than was found in an alternate approach using dichotomous dependent variables (drug use, drug nonuse). This higher predictive ability would suggest the use of three-level ordinal dependent variables and follows from evidence that increased categories better represent the nature of the data. A recent study (Bollen and Barb, 1981) analyzed simulated data and examined differences in the correlation between two normally distributed continuous variables and the same two variables collapsed. They concluded that analysis of categorical data by techniques with continuous assumptions is a reasonable approach to the level-of-measurement problem. In addition, others have recently used interval-level statistics in this regard, Akers et al. (1979) being a case in point.

Several studies (Blalock, 1972; Gillespie, 1977; Suits, 1957) have examined the use of dummy variables within regression analysis. Suits (1957) and Blalock (1972) suggest that it is acceptable to use dummy independent variables within the regression equation. A more recent article by Gillespie (1977) supports the use of dummy criterion variables with interval-level techniques, such as regression analysis.

For the present study the method of analysis involved a bivariate cross-comparison correlation of the independent variable (control or social bond theory) with our seven dependent variables (specific drug use types and composite drug categories). Pearson's product-moment correlation coefficient was the statistic used for these bivariate correlations. In addition, partial correlations were analyzed, controlling for each of the following demographic variables: age, race, sex, education, income, and marital status. The relationship between the independent and dependent variables is further examined later by calculating the correlation and level of significance within selected categories of the control variables. A corresponding test of significance, utilizing the t test, was conducted for each of the bivariate comparisons.

RESULTS

Unelaborated Relationships

Table 3 offers some support for Hirschi's proposition, in that there was a significant positive correlation between reduced social bonding (commitment, involvement, and belief) and greater drug use. As suggested by Hirschi's study, alcohol (r = .16) was more strongly correlated than the use of tobacco (r = .10). Lack of social bonding was most highly correlated with the use of marijuana (r = .24), in which it was capable of explaining almost 6% (r^2 = .058) of the total variance of marijuana use. Since this study used an adult sample, versus Hirschi's juvenile sample, we might expect the use of marijuana to be more indicative of a social act of nonconformity, than either alcohol or tobacco use. These results suggested that social bond theory may be better in explaining illegal delinquent behavior than drug behavior, which may or may not be illegal.

In all cases except for marijuana, the bond variable was capable of explaining no more than 3% for any of the other specific drug types. Thus, while there was some association between the social bond elements and the use of specific drugs, at this level of analysis, the association was not strong enough to fulfill the requirement necessary for a "powerful explanatory" theory.

The results of the zero-order correlations between social bond and the two composite drug use categories are shown in Table 4. The relationship between increases in bond scores (decreased level of social bonding) and increases in number of drugs used (UserE and UserP) suggests that bond theory may be more valuable in explaining composite drug use than specific types of drug use. Unfortunately, even this restrictive use of the independent bond variable is questionable, since the amount of explained variance (UserE, r^2 = .053; UserP, r^2 = .040) was only moderately better than for the individual drug types. The results derived from direct zero-order correlations of social bond theory failed to provide an adequate explanatory level to be deemed a "powerful explanatory" theory.

Table 3

Zero-Order Correlations of Bond with Five Types of Drugs

Drug types (dependent variables)	Frequency (N)	r	r^2	p
Alcohol	1,246	.16	.026	.000
Marijuana	1,248	.24	.058	.000
Tobacco	1,246	.10	.010	.000
Amphetamines	1,248	.17	.029	.000
Barbiturates	1,247	.07	.005	.008

Table 4

Zero-Order Correlations of Bond with Two Composite Drug Scales

Composite scale (dependent variables)	Frequency (N)	r	r^2	p
UserE	1,248	.23	.053	.000
UserP	1,247	.20	.040	.000

Elaborated Relationships

This failure to provide a powerful explanation for either specific types of drug use or composite drug use does not rule out the possibility of a stronger association within the demographic categories.

Sex

Table 5 suggests that the use of drugs by females was more strongly influenced by the reduction of social control through the breakdown of the bonding elements.

As the female's bond to society weakens there is an increase in marijuana use ($r = .25$; $r^2 = .063$); in the past use of drugs, as defined by UserE ($r = .24$; $r^2 = .058$); and in the present use of drugs, as defined by UserP ($r = .24$; $r^2 = .058$). While this may suggest that female drug use is more clearly interpreted through social control theory, one should not become overly enthusiastic about explained variance values of approximately 6%. From these results it can be determined that while social bond is not a strong predictor of drug use, it does a better job of explaining female, rather than male, drug use.

Table 5

Zero-Order Correlations of Bond with Drug Types within Sex Categories (Significant Correlation Values of .20 and Greater)

Drug type	Sex	Frequency (N)	r	r^2	p
Marijuana	Male	656	.23	.053	.001
Marijuana	Female	592	.25	.063	.001
UserE	Female	592	.24	.058	.001
UserP	Female	592	.24	.058	.001

Age

Since Hirschi (1969) found strong relationships between juveniles' lack of social bonding and delinquency patterns, it could be expected that the younger age categories within this study would display similar bonding correlations with drug use. In addition, the younger an individual is, the less likely he is to have developed attachment and commitment to the social order and the various social institutions. It can be suggested that these bonds of commitment, involvement, and belief tend to form over time and that younger individuals will have experienced less social bonding. In this study, however, no bond-drug correlations were discovered with any age category under the age of 25 (see Table 6). There were moderately low correlations for the 26-30 age category with the use of amphetamines (r = .21; r^2 = .044), barbiturates (r = .20; r^2 = .040) and UserE (r = .26; r^2 = .068). An interpretation of this higher correlation for certain types of drug use, by the 26-30 age category, is not readily apparent. One can only assume that for individuals of this age, the weakening of societal bonds results in an increased use of amphetamines and barbiturates. It may be that amphetamines and barbiturates have become an acceptable reaction of young adults to the loss of commitment, attachment, involvement, and belief.

Race

Hirschi (1969) found that a significantly greater percentage of Blacks had police records as compared with Whites. However, he also discovered that approximately the same percentage of Black and White males admitted commiting one or more delinquent acts during the preceding year. These findings support the labeling argument that true racial or social class differences with respect to self-reported delinquency are very small.

Table 6

Zero-Order Correlations of Bond with Drug Types within Age Categories (Significant Correlation Values of .20 and Greater)

Drug type	Age	Frequency (N)	r	r^2	p
Amphetamines	26-30	190	.21	.044	.005
Barbiturates	26-30	190	.20	.040	.01
UserE	26-30	190	.26	.068	.001
UserE	31-40	286	.21	.044	.001
UserE	41-50	203	.21	.044	.005
UserP	41-50	203	.20	.040	.005

Table 7

Zero-Order Correlations of Bond with Drug Types within Race Categories (Significant Correlation Values of .20 and Greater)

Drug type	Race	Frequency (N)	r	r^2	p
Alcohol	Black	85	.28	.078	.005
Amphetamines	Mexican-American	160	.23	.048	.025
Marijuana	White	990	.23	.048	.001
Marijuana	Black	85	.28	.078	.005
Marijuana	Mexican-American	160	.26	.068	.001
UserE	White	990	.21	.044	.001
UserE	Mexican-American	160	.30	.090	.001
UserP	White	988	.21	.044	.001
UserP	Black	86	.20	.040	.025

Hirschi concludes that "the official reaction hypothesis aside, there is no reason to believe that the causes of crime among blacks are different from those among whites" (1969, p. 79). If control theory forms the basis of explanation of most forms of aberrant or unusual behavior, we should expect to find the cause of drug use among the various races to be similar. The results given in Table 7 can be seen to add support to this hypothesis. Each of the three racial categories (Black, Mexican-American, and White) showed positive correlations between bond score and certain types of drug use. Blacks showed the strongest correlations between bond values and marijuana (r = .28; r^2 = .078), and alcohol (r = .28; r^2 = .048) and UserE (r = .30; r^2 = .90). Whites showed a stronger relationship than any other racial group between bond theory and present use of drugs (UserP, r = .21; r^2 = .044). Three significant correlations of greater than .20 were discovered for each of our racial categories. These results supported the argument that no specific racial group's drug use was substantially better explained through bond theory.

Education

Hirschi (1969) found a positive association between loss of commitment to education and the activities of smoking and drinking. This suggests that a relationship exists between bond values and specific types of drug use for those with lower levels of education. A juvenile's weakening of educational commitment would directly result in the weakening of his bond to society and would also be linked to an increased use of drugs. It should be expected that the loss of educational commitment would militate against additional schooling. If this scenario does take place, one would expect to be able to measure this effect within our adult sample. An additional argument is grounded in the fact that our educational variable is basically a measure of time spent in school. Realizing this fact provides the link between educational aspirations and involvement in conventional activities. It can be shown that involvement limits one's opportunity to commit deviant acts (use of drugs) and thus permits us to get away from the assumption implicit in many theories that these deviant opportunities are simply randomly distributed through the population. Since time and energy are inherently limited, time spent in academic involvement is time spent away from nonconventional activities. Supporting results would show higher correlations between social bond values and drug use for those who obtained lower levels of education.

The lowest education category (grades 1-11) presented a stronger correlation between bond value and alcohol use than any other educational level (see Table 8). This within-category correlation did support the Hirschi hypothesis. However, the overall results, presented in Table 8, did not seem to support Hirschi's findings. As an example, those with advanced college degrees (suggesting a high commitment to and involvement in education) showed a strong correlation between bond and marijuana use (r = .34; r^2 = .116). The fact that almost 12% of the marijuana variance was directly explainable through the independent bond variable cast doubt on the lower-educational hypothesis.

It must be kept in mind that involvement in or commitment to education or the educational system is only one of several components of the social bond theory. It is quite possible that other forms of attachment, commitment, involvement, and belief have interacted to overshadow any lower-educational-level variation. Possibly the only conclusion that can be made from the present

Table 8

Zero-Order Correlations of Bond with Drug Types within School Categories (Significant Correlation Values of .20 and Greater)

Drug type	Schooling	Frequency (N)	r	r^2	p
Alcohol	Grades 1-11	233	.23	.048	.001
Amphetamines	High school	340	.26	.068	.001
Marijuana	High school	340	.28	.078	.001
Marijuana	Some college	384	.21	.044	.001
Marijuana	Adv. college	83	.34	.116	.005
UserE	Grades 1-11	233	.22	.044	.005
UserE	High school	340	.27	.073	.001
UserE	Some college	384	.22	.044	.001
UserE	Adv. college	83	.23	.048	.025
UserP	High school	340	.26	.068	.001
UserP	Adv. college	81	.20	.040	.025

results is that there is little support for Hirschi's proposition of a direct link between components of control theory and the use of drugs.

Income

It seems rational to suggest that the larger an individual's income, the greater is his commitment to the social order, since income is usually derived from conventional sources. In addition, we would suggest that larger incomes are a product of time invested in the conventional social order (i.e., involvement). Income is also commonly used as a measure of social class, which again reflects commitment and belief in the moral order. Hirschi's (1969) study, however, was more concerned with the aspirations for wealth than the actual income level of the respondent since his sample was a juvenile sample. The closest direct comparison to income for Hirschi was the commitment to high-status occupations, which in itself may be more closely related to educational level than income. One is making a major assumption to claim that Hirschi's finding that "the higher the aspiration, the lower the rate of delinquency" is comparable to "the higher the income, the stronger an individual's bond to society and thus the lower the rate of drug use." If social bond theory is harmonious with this second hypothesis, we would suggest that Table 9 lends support to both the hypothesis and the theory.

For those respondents making less than $6,000, there were significant correlations between the weakening of the social bond and the dependent

Table 9

Zero-Order Correlations of Bond with Drug Types within Income Categories (Significant Correlation Values of .20 and Greater)

Drug type	Income	Frequency (N)	r	r^2	p
Alcohol	<$6 K	114	.31	.096	.001
Amphetamines	<$6 K	114	.21	.044	.025
Amphetamines	$6-$15 K	317	.24	.053	.001
Marijuana	<$6 K	114	.29	.084	.005
Marijuana	$6-$15 K	317	.23	.048	.001
Marijuana	$15-$25 K	338	.24	.053	.001
Marijuana	>$50 K	86	.36	.130	.005
UserE	<$6 K	114	.34	.116	.001
UserE	$6-$15 K	317	.29	.084	.001
UserE	>$50 K	86	.21	.044	.05
UserP	<$6 K	115	.27	.073	.005
UserP	$6-$15 K	317	.22	.048	.001
UserP	$15-$25 K	336	.21	.004	.001

variables; alcohol (r = .31; r^2 = .096), amphetamines (r = .21; r^2 = .044), marijuana (r = .29; r^2 = .084), UserE (r = .34; r^2 = .116), and UserP (r = .27; r^2 = .073). The testing of the social bond concepts as indicators of drug use held up fairly well for the subcategory of individuals making $6,000 or less. These r^2 values are substantial enough to suggest that control theory may be a possible "powerful explanatory" theory for those individuals making less than $6,000.

Marital Status

Since Hirschi (1969) was involved with the study of juveniles, he was not concerned with the marital status of his respondents. However, since the act of separation or divorce means the breaking of a conventional commitment, these two categories, along with those who have become widowed, have had to break strong attachments. Individuals within these categories should have had their bond to society and its institutions weakened. It can also be added that marriage in itself is considered a social institution. The results of the present study showed that divorced and widowed respondents' bond scores were significantly correlated with a variety of drug types (see Table 10).

The highest levels of explained variation between social bond and drug use were found within the marital statuses of divorced and widowed. For widowed respondents, social bond correlated high with alcohol (r = .33; r^2 = .109), UserE (r = .29; r^2 = .084) and UserP (r = .30; r^2 = .090). The divorced category showed even stronger correlations for UserE (r = .38; r^2 = .144), UserP (r = .39; r^2 = .152), and marijuana (r = .44; r^2 = .194). The latter ability to predict

Table 10

Zero-Order Correlations of Bond with Drug Types within Marital Status Categories (Significant Correlation Values of .20 and Greater)

Drug type	Marital status	Frequency (N)	r	r^2	p
Alcohol	Widowed	36	.33	.109	.025
Amphetamines	Divorced	84	.23	.048	.05
Marijuana	Married	893	.21	.044	.001
Marijuana	Single	189	.23	.048	.005
Marijuana	Divorced	84	.44	.194	.001
UserE	Single	189	.27	.073	.001
UserE	Divorced	84	.38	.144	.001
UserE	Widowed	37	.29	.084	.05
UserP	Divorced	84	.39	.152	.001
UserP	Widowed	36	.30	.090	.05

between 14% and 19% of the variation within certain dependent drug variables from a knowledge of the social bond variable suggested a causally meaningful relationship. However, while this theoretical relationship may be meaningful, it was still limited to a specific marital status group and applied only to certain dependent drug-type variables.

It was earlier concluded that the social bond variable failed to provide an adequate level of explanatory power, for either specific types of drug use or composite drug use, and therefore could not be deemed a "powerful theory." Further examination of the theory within categories of demographic variables failed to alter that assessment. Yet, we must note that it is still possible that social bond is more highly correlated with drug use but that intervening (control) variables have suppressed the true effect of the social bond variable.

Table 11 presents a sixth-order partial correlation of social bond with the seven dependent variables, controlling for sex, race, school, income, age, and marital status. After partialling out the effect of the control variables, all drug-type correlations remained strongly significant. However, one must remember that a relationship that is significant, but weak, has a useless explanatory function. The theory has failed to meet our "powerful explanatory" standard since no explained variation (r^2) value was greater than 4%.

These results do not necessarily discredit Hirschi's (1969) findings or his social bond theory. We must remember that Hirschi proposed a control theory of delinquency. His further conclusion that the theory forms the basis of explanation for most forms of aberrant or deviant behavior, however, must be questioned in light of these findings. Finally, it can be concluded from the evidence of this study that Hirschi's social bond theory fails to provide an adequate explanation for the use of those drugs within the framework of this analysis.

Table 11

Sixth-Order Partial Correlations of Bond with Drug Types, Controlling for Sex, Race, School, Income, Age, and Marital Status

Drug type (dependent variables)	Frequency (N)	Partial r	r^2	p
Alcohol	1,246	.12	.014	.000
Marijuana	1,248	.20	.040	.000
Tobacco	1,246	.08	.006	.002
Amphetamines	1,248	.13	.017	.000
Barbiturates	1,247	.06	.004	.022
UserE	1,248	.18	.032	.000
UserP	1,247	.16	.026	.000

THE STUDY AND ITS LIMITATIONS

In analyzing these results, one must be cautious in the interpretation of these findings. Therefore, some discussion of the possible limitations present in this study should be advanced.

While our sampling frame represents over 90% of Texas residents, there is a problem regarding those who do not hold Texas driver's licenses. We might expect that our sample will underrepresent older persons, women, certain races, illegal aliens, and a number of other groups less likely to hold driver's licenses. In addition, we might expect that a proportion of heavy drug users may lose their driver's licenses because of their drug use. These individuals would, thus, not have been a part of the sampling frame. Our sample, also, includes only residents aged 17 and over. This will render comparability with any drug study that used teenage or adolescent populations somewhat problematic.

While a general adult sample was used in this study, it was a sample taken exclusively from the State of Texas. There is evidence to suggest that drug behavior in other areas of the country may be dissimilar to the drug behavior in the State of Texas (Fishburn et al., 1979). It is possible that the causal factors behind drug use are regionally effected.

In conducting a study of drug use, the utilization of a self-report questionnaire will raise a number of methodological problems. Two fundamental issues in any self-report study concern the questions of reliability and validity. To better understand the extent to which a self-report method is reliable, one must explore several issues. Are large numbers of offenses concealed? Do individuals take the opportunity to exaggerate their deviant or drug behavior for fun or fantasy? How do problems of recall and memory fade affect reliability?

It should also be noted that our conceptualization of the theoretical concepts and the method of measuring use and nonuse of drugs is only one of a number of possible approaches to the conceptualization of these terms. Our constructed social bond scale is only one of a number of possible measures that could be used to represent social bond theory, and drug use may be refined by including amount and frequency of use.

There is a great need for follow-up and additional research in the empirical examination of social bond theory and drug use. It is recommended that future studies use a national sample and that replications of this study attempt further refinement of the theoretical concepts, as well as more sensitive construction of the drug use variables. Any follow-up study should especially focus on a drug use variable that takes into consideration the amount and frequency of drug use. In addition, other drugs should be examined to explore whether social bond theory may be more applicable to other types of drugs and their use.

NOTES

1. The importance placed on group support and peer involvement by some control theorists tends to suggest a relationship between social bonding theory and the social network perspective (Wister and Avison, 1982). The social network model assumes that congruence of beliefs is associated with attraction to one another. This mutual attractiveness and similarity of beliefs are the primary variables responsible for peer group formation. Finally, the social network perspective suggests that peer group pressures are the important agents in determining whether one will use drugs and the extent of that use (see Akers et al., 1979; Johnson, 1973; Kandel, 1973, 1978a, 1978b). The basic difference between the two approaches is that social bond theory does not view peer group formations or pressures as primarily responsible for drug use. Instead, it is one's low stake in conformity (lack of social bonding) that is responsible for deviant or drug behavior and, in addition, leads to the acquisition of delinquent friends (peer group formation). Under the control model the relation between drug use and peer group formation is spurious. While there are similarities between these two approaches, the causal ordering between stakes in conformity and drug use of companions is reversed from one model to the other.
2. The most frequently examined drugs in the study of control theory have been alcohol and marijuana. In addition, a few control theorists have included in their studies drugs such as amphetamines, barbiturates, cocaine, heroin, LSD, and tobacco. The researchers of this study selected what was believed to be the five most commonly used drugs within the general population. This was done in order to obtain a user sample large enough to be of statistical value. In retrospect, we would have had a more appropriate testing of social bond theory if we had included in the investigation several of the illegal but less popular drugs, such as heroin, cocaine, and LSD. The majority of the drugs examined in this study are legal substances. This raises serious questions concerning the "meaning" which the subjects attribute to these substances and the "meaning(s)" attributed to these substances by those to whom they are bonded. This raises some concern as to the validity and relevancy of our interpretation of the data.
3. The control theory scale involves items directly related to Hirschi's (1969) elements of the social bond. After an examination of the questionnaire which Hirschi utilized (see *Causes of Delinquency*, pp. 245-299, Appendices), a number of questions were selected that tested the following elements of the social bond: involvement in school and church, attachment to family, belief or values related to law and American traditions, and commitment to social and financial success.
4. This procedure supports Hirschi's theoretical position by presenting statistical evidence that individual unique elements of the social bond actually exist. The creation of a more parsimonious scale lends support to the power of the theory by maintaining its explanatory ability in spite of a reduced number of measurable items. In control theory the question, according to Hirschi (1969), is "Why don't people commit crimes?" If we can reduce the number of factors, or elements, or items which measure these elements, we have improved both the measuring device and the theory.
5. Items A through E were drawn from the following questions: Item A–"How important do you consider being an American?" (belief); Item B–"How important do you consider keeping American traditions?" (belief); Item C–"How important do you consider church membership?" (involvement); Item D–"How often do you attend church?" (involvement); Item E–"How important do you consider financial success?" (commitment); and Item F–"How important do you consider social success?" (commitment).

6. The tobacco variable was created by including the response to three items: cigarettes, cigars, and pipes. If a respondent stated that he had smoked any of these three tobacco products, he was coded as a tobacco user. Failure to use any of these three items resulted in the coding of the respondent as a non-tobacco user.

REFERENCES

AKERS, R.L., KROHN, M.D., LANZA-KADUCE, L., and RADOSEVICH, M. Social learning deviant behavior: A specific test of a general theory. *Am. Sociol. Rev.* 44(August): 635-655, 1979.

AULTMAN, M.G., and WELLFORD, C.F. Towards an integrated model of delinquent causation: An empirical analysis. *Sociol. Soc. Res.* 63(2): 316-325, 1978.

BLALOCK, H.M. *Social Statistics.* New York: McGraw-Hill, 1972.

BOLLEN, K.A., and BARB, K.H. Pearson's *r* and coarsely categorized measures. *Am. Sociol. Rev.* 46: 232-239, 1981.

BORGATTA, E.F. My student the purist: A lament. *Sociol. Q.* 9: 29-34. 1968.

BOYLE, R. Path analyses and ordinal data. *Am. J. Sociol.* 75(January): 461-480, 1970.

BURKETT, S.R., and JENSEN, E.L. Conventional ties, peer influences, and the fear of apprehension: A study of adolescent marijuana use. *Sociol. Q.* 16(Autumn): 522-533, 1975.

CONGER, R.D. Social control and social learning models of delinquent behavior: A synthesis. *Criminology* 14: 17-40, 1976.

COSTNER, H.L. Criteria for measures of association. *Am. Sociol. Rev.* 30: 341-353, 1965.

FINNELL, W.S., and JONES, J.D. Marijuana, alcohol, and academic performance. *J. Drug Educ.* 5(1): 13-21, 1975.

FISHBURN, P., ABLESON, H., and CISIN, I. *National Survey on Drug Abuse: Main Findings: 1979.* Rockville, MD: National Institute on Drug Abuse, 1979.

GIBBONS, D.C. *The Criminological Enterprise: Theories and Perspectives.* Englewood Cliffs, NJ: Prentice-Hall, 1979.

GILLESPIE, M.W. Log-linear techniques and the regression analysis of dummy dependent variables: Further bases for comparison. *Sociol. Meth. Res.* 6(1): 103-122, 1977.

GINSBERG, I.J., and GREENLEY, J.R. Competing theories of marijuana use: A longitudinal study. *J. Health Soc. Behav.* 19(March): 22-34, 1978.

HINDELANG, M.J. Causes of delinquency: A partial replication and extension. *Soc. Probl.* 20: 471-487, 1973.

HIRSCHI, T. *Causes of Delinquency.* Berkeley, CA: University of California Press, 1969.

JOHNSON, B.D. *Marijuana Users and Drug Subculture.* New York: Wiley, 1973.

KANDEL, D. Adolescent marijuana use: Role of parents and peer. *Science* 181: 1067-1070, 1973.

KANDEL, D. Homophily, selection, and socialization in adolescent friendships. *Am. J. Sociol.* 84: 427-436, 1978a.

KANDEL, D. Similarity in real-life adolescent friendship pairs. *J. Pers. Soc. Psychol.* 36: 306-312, 1978b.

KERCHER, G.A., and DULL, R.T. *Texas Crime Poll, 1981.* Huntsville, TX: Survey Research Program, Criminal Justice Center, 1981.

LABOVITZ, S. Some observations on measurement and statistics. *Soc. Forces* 46(2): 151-160, 1967.

LABOVITZ, S. The assignment of numbers to rank order categories. *Am. Sociol. Rev.* 35: 515-524, 1970.

LEVINE, E.M., and KOZAK, C. Drug and alcohol use, delinquency, and vandalism among upper class pre- and post-adolescents. *J. Youth Adolescence* 8(1): 91-101, 1979.
MARSHALL, R.O., WILLIAMS, F.P., and DULL, R.T. *Alcohol and Marijuana Use in Texas*. Huntsville, TX: Survey Research Program, Criminal Justice Center, 1981.
MERCER, W.G., HUNDLEY, J.D., and CARPENTER, R.A. Adolescent drug use and attitudes toward the family. *Can. J. Behav. Sci. Rev.* 10(1): 79-90, 1978.
SUCHMAN, E.A. The hang-loose ethic and the spirit of drug use. *J. Health Soc. Behav.* 9: 146-155, 1968.
SUITS, D. The use of dummy variables in regression equation. *J. Am. Statist. Assoc.* 52: 548-551, 1957.
TESKE, R.H.C., and JEFFORDS, C.R. *Texas Crime Poll, Spring 1979.* Huntsville, TX: Survey Research Program, Criminal Justice Center, 1979.
WISTER, A.V., and AVISON, W.R. "Friendly Persuasion": A social network analysis of sex differences in marijuana use. *Int. J. Addict.* 17(3): 523-541, 1982.

The International Journal of the Addictions, 19(3), 287–294, 1984

Conditioned Abstinence in Alcoholics: A Controlled Experiment

Lasse Eriksen,* PhD

K. Gunnar Götestam, MD, PhD

Department of Psychiatry
University of Trondheim
Östmarka Hospital
N-7001 Trondheim, Norway

Abstract

The existence of conditioned abstinence symptoms in 16 abstinent alcoholics was investigated by comparing their subjective, physiological, and behavioral responses while viewing slides of alcohol-related and non-alcohol-related stimuli. The alcoholics were randomly assigned to one of two groups. The first group viewed a set of six alcohol-related slides the first day and a set of six non-alcohol-related slides the following day. The second group looked at the same slides, but the order of presentation was reversed. Alcohol-related slides produced significantly greater increases in subjectively reported alcohol craving and anxiety scores. There were no differences between the two sets with regard to physiological measures or subjective reports of heart rate. The global observations showed significant differences between the alcohol-related and non-alcohol-related slides.

*To whom requests for reprints should be sent at Östmarka Hospital, P.O. Box 3008, N-7001 Trondheim, Norway.

 0020-773X/84/1903-0287$3.50/0

The existence of conditioned abstinence reactions to drug-related stimuli in drug-free drug addicts has been reported by Teasdale (1973), Sideroff and Jarvik (1980), and Hugdahl and Ternes (1981) (see Table 1).

The present study (conducted in 1980) investigated the possibility that alcohol-related slides produce significant changes in physiological measures (heart rate), subjective ratings (craving, anxiety, and heart rate), and global observations (tension and relaxation) compared to non-alcohol-related stimuli.

METHOD

Subjects

The patient volunteers were 18 alcoholics, being treated of their own free will at an alcoholism treatment center as inpatients. The inclusion criteria were: male, inpatient at least 1 week before the study started and being sober during the same time period, and being sober during the study (breath tests were administered and all subjects were found to be sober). The exclusion criteria were: ever having been treated for heart diseases and not following the experimenters' instructions. One alcoholic who volunteered for the study was not included because of a drinking episode. Thus, 17 subjects participated in the study. One of these did not follow the instructions and was therefore excluded. The mean age of the 16 male alcoholics remaining in the study was 39.6 (range 24-52 years). The mean duration of their alcohol problems was 12.9 years (range 2-25). All subjects were Norwegians and Protestants. Only one subject was under pharmacological treatment during the study.

Apparatus and Assessments

Heart Rate

An EKG apparatus (Phillips Cardiopan 531) was used. Speed selection was 25 mm/sec and amplitude was 10 mV/sec. The peripheral electrodes were put on the left arm and leg. The baseline for heart rate was recorded 1 min before the first slide. Then heart rate was recorded 10 sec before, during, and after each slide (the slide was shown on the screen for 10 sec with 1 min to fill in the subjective rating scale afterward). The heart rate for each slide was scored as a mean of the recording 10 sec before, during, and after each slide.

Subjective Rating Scales (visual analogue scales)

The subject rated himself by putting a mark on a sheet which contained a 10-cm line (one end indicating "not at all" and the other indicating "very

Table 1

Studies on Conditioned Abstinence in Human Addicts[a]

Author	Date	Type *S*s	No. of *S*s	Stimuli medium	Assessment modalities	Results[b]
Teasdale	1973	Male heroin addicts (drug free)	6	Slides	Subjective (tests)	Tension +, confusion +, craving +
					Physiological	(Apparatus broken down)
Sideroff and Jarvik	1980	Heroin addicts (drug free)	8	Videotape	Subjective (check-list)	Craving +, anxiety +, depression +, hostility 0
		Controls (drug free)	8			
Hugdahl and Ternes	1981	Opiate addicts (drug free)	5	Slides, videotape, and objects	Physiological	SSRR +
		Methadone maintenance addicts	5			
		Controls (drug free)	5			
Eriksen and Götestam	(present study)	Alcoholics (drug and alcohol free)	16	Slides	Subjective (self-rating scale)	Craving +, anxiety +, heart rate 0
					Behavioral	Tension +, relaxation –
					Physiological	Heart rate 0

[a] Excludes studies in which conditioning of conditioned abstinence was the goal.
[b] + = statistically significant increase; – = statistically significant decrease; 0 = no difference between groups.

much"). In the rating for perceived heart rate change, "no change" was in the middle of the scale. In between the three ratings, two distractor ratings were placed, asking how interesting the subjects found the slides and how much they liked them. Since the subjects talked about the distractor ratings at the end of the session, it seems that these ratings actually did serve as distractors.

Global Observations

One of the experimenters observed and recorded the subject with regard to whether he looked relaxed, tensed, or neither when the slides were shown. Furthermore, every verbal expression and gross body movement of the subject was recorded while the slides were shown.

Stimuli

As a check of the relevance of the slides (see Table 2), all the subjects were asked what their favorite drink was. Each subject's favorite drink appeared at least once in the alcohol-related stimuli. (No pretests were made with the slides, as that was considered to affect the results.)

Table 2

The Two Sets of Slide Stimuli[a]

Slide no.	Alcohol-related stimuli	Non-alcohol-related stimuli
1	A state liquor shop	A building with shops
2	A glass of beer and a bottle of beer	A glass of milk and a carton of milk
3	A bottle of vodka being poured into a glass with ice	A teapot and a tea box
4	A bottle of 60% pure alcohol, a bottle of beer, and a glass on a kitchen table	A coffee pot, a carton of milk, and a box of cocoa on a kitchen table
5	A man starting to drink from a large bottle of wine	A man reading a newspaper sitting at a table with a glass of milk, a carton of milk, and a coffee pot
6	Two men sitting at a table with large cocktails	Two men sitting at a table reading newspapers with a glass of milk, an empty glass, a carton of milk, and a coffee pot

[a]The slides were selected on the basis of clinical experience and were roughly matched.

Design and Statistics

The subjects were randomly assigned to the two groups (nine in one group and eight in the other). Two series of slides were shown, with one group viewing the alcohol-related slides first and the other group viewing the non-alcohol-related slides first, to control for order effects.

t Tests for correlated groups were used. Because of the hypothesis and experimental design, the expectation was only in one direction; therefore, one-tailed tests were applied. A 5% level of significance was used.

Procedure

Instructions

The subjects were informed that the study consisted of showing slides and measuring the reactions to these slides. They were also informed about criteria for participation and duration and time of the study. They were told that participation in the study could give more understanding about their alcohol problems. They were promised a meeting after the study for an explanation of the study and its results (this was conducted directly after all data were collected). The subjects were told not to discuss the study with other clients in the center while the study was being conducted (it was not possible to control this, but no one was able to describe the goal of the study, when asked before each session).

The Experiment

The subjects were scheduled for participation according to their own choice. Each subject participated in two sessions, held 24 hours apart. Initially, the first part of the instructions was read out loud by one of the experimenters. An alcohol breath test was then taken and the EKG electrodes were placed on the subject's leg and arm. Then the second part of the instructions was read. Here the subject was told that he soon would be shown a series of slides. The subject filled in one rating scale sheet as an exercise. One minute before the first slide was shown, baseline heart rate was recorded. Then the EKG measures were taken 10 sec before, during, and after each slide. The subject was instructed to mark the first sheet with the five ratings. After 1 min a new slide was shown. The subject's behavior was observed and recorded by one of the experimenters while the slide was shown. The same procedure was repeated for all six slides in each session for both groups and days.

RESULTS

Heart Rate

Mean heart rate was calculated for each slide, and a daily mean was determined. No significant difference in heart rate was found when alcohol-related slides and non-alcohol-related slides were shown (see Table 3). There was no difference in heart rate in the groups with regard to the order in which the slides were shown.

Subjective Ratings

Mean scores were calculated for each day and each person.

Craving for Alcohol

A significant difference between alcohol-related and non-alcohol-related slides was found for craving for alcohol ($p < .005$; see Table 3). There was no difference in craving for alcohol in the groups with regard to the order in which the slides were shown.

Table 3

Means of Heart Rates, Subjective Ratings, and Global Observations of Each Subject and Slide Series

		Slides					
		Alcohol related		Non-alcohol related			
Assessment		*M*	(SD)	*M*	(SD)	*t*	*p*
Physiological measure (EKG)	Heart rate per min	80.81	(13.27)	77.75	(14.80)	1.27	NS
Subjective measures (ratings)	Craving of alcohol	3.59	(2.60)	2.06	(1.73)	3.64	<.005
	Anxiety	2.51	(2.16)	1.88	(1.43)	2.03	<.05
	Heart rate	5.26	(2.00)	5.26	(1.70)	0.17	NS
Behavioral measures (global observations)	Tensed	1.94	(0.38)	0.81	(0.28)	2.02	<.05
	Relaxed	2.94	(0.38)	4.69	(0.29)	2.73	<.01

Anxiety

A significant difference between alcohol-related and non-alcohol-related slides was found for anxiety ($p < .05$; see Table 3). There was no difference in anxiety in the groups with regard to the order in which the slides were shown.

Heart Rate

No difference between alcohol-related and non-alcohol-related slides was found for heart rate (see Table 3). There was no difference in heart rate in the groups with regard to the order of viewing the slides.

Global Observations

Verbal Expressions

No verbal expression or gross body movement whatsoever was observed when the slides were shown.

Relaxation and Tension

A significant difference between the alcohol-related and the non-alcohol-related slides was found, with regard to both tension ($p < .05$) and relaxation ($p < .01$) (see Table 3). The first group (alcohol-related slides the first day) was responsible for most of the difference between the alcohol-related and the non-alcohol-related slides.

DISCUSSION

In the present study significant differences between alcohol-related and non-alcohol-related slides were found with regard to subjective alcohol craving and anxiety, and the global observations "tensed" and "relaxed." This is in line with Ludwig and Wikler's (1974) theory, especially the considerable difference in subjective alcohol craving, which Ludwig and Wikler predicted as the most potent measure.

A methodological weakness with regard to the global observations is the lack of interrater reliability scores.

It is very difficult to assess the importance of the conditioned abstinence phenomenon in relapse in alcoholics, since many other factors may also play important roles. Thinking of conditioned abstinence as a major factor in relapse seems plausible (Mathew et al., 1979), and hence it will be important to try to decrease or extinguish it as a part of a treatment program for alcoholics. Several behavioral procedures could be applied to reduce or eliminate conditioned abstinence reactions; for example, extinction, aversive methods, relaxation, systematic desensitization, self-instructions, and assertiveness or self-control techniques (Eriksen et al., 1982; Miller, 1976).

Training of staff and therapists in these techniques seems warranted. Future research should apply other types of physiological apparatus to test for physiological differences and should apply one or more of the previously mentioned techniques to change or reduce conditioned abstinence in alcoholics.

ACKNOWLEDGMENT

We wish to thank Eli Haugstvedt and Kjell Ludvigsen for assistance in conducting the experiment.

REFERENCES

ERIKSEN, L., BATES, S., and GÖTESTAM, K.G. Behavioral treatment of alcoholism–A review. *J. Psychiatr. Treatm. Eval.* 4: 25-31, 1982.

HUGDAHL, K., and TERNES, J.W. An electrodermal measure of arousal in opiate addicts to drug-related stimuli. *Biol. Psychol.* 12: 291-298, 1981.

LUDWIG, A.M., and WIKLER, S. "Craving" and relapse to drink. *Q. J. Stud. Alcohol* 35: 108-130, 1974.

MATHEW, R.J., CLAGHORN, J.L., and LARGEN, J. Craving for alcohol in sober alcoholics. *Am. J. Psychiatry* 136: 603-606, 1979.

MILLER, P.M. *Behavioral Treatment of Alcoholism*. New York: Pergamon Press, 1976.

SIDEROFF, S., and JARVIK, M.E. Conditioned responses to a videotape showing heroin-related stimuli. *Int. J. Addict.* 15: 529-536, 1980.

TEASDALE, J. Conditioned abstinence in narcotic addicts. *Int. J. Addict.* 8: 273-292, 1973.

The International Journal of the Addictions, 19(3), 295–326, 1984

The Phenomenological Structure of Drug-Induced Ego States. II. Barbiturates and Sedative-Hypnotics: Phenomenology and Implications

James V. Spotts,* PhD

Greater Kansas City Mental Health Foundation
Kansas City, Missouri 64108

Franklin C. Shontz, PhD

Department of Psychology
University of Kansas
Lawrence, Kansas 66045

Abstract

Empirically derived descriptions of experiential states, induced by heavy, chronic consumption of drugs, provide valuable information for treatment personnel as well as for scientists studying drug abuse or pharmacology. A 7-year program of research has studied persons committed to heavy, long-term use of several prominent substances of abuse. This report results from that research and provides a phenomenological description of the psychological state induced by heavy, chronic use of barbiturates and sedative-hypnotics. Interview, Q-sort and semantic differential data indicate the barbiturate state is intensely unpleasant: a state in which users lose desired characteristics, take on

*To whom correspondence should be addressed: Assistant Director, Greater Kansas City Mental Health Foundation, 600 East 22nd Street, Kansas City, Missouri 64108.

0020-773X/84/1903-0295$3.50/0

undesired characteristics, engage in self-destructive acts, and emerge in worse condition than before entering it. Explaining why people choose to enter such a state is difficult. Several theoretical alternatives for doing so are considered. Psychotherapy with these individuals must deal with the theme of abandonment/rejection that permeates their lives and with the diffuse hostility, expectations of failure and defeat, self-destructive tendencies, and feelings of hopelessness that they display. Suggestions are presented for treatment of individual cases.

INTRODUCTION

Biomedical research enhances our understanding of the pharmacology of a variety of drugs. Such research can define drug parameters, identify adverse side effects or medical hazards, and specify long-term physical consequences of drug use. However, it cannot tell why one person develops a commitment to a particular drug, heroin, for example, while another develops a commitment to amphetamine. It cannot describe the experience an individual seeks by taking a particular substance; nor can it tell why some persons express a preference for one class of drugs (e.g., opiates) but chronically abuse another (e.g., barbiturates). These are psychological issues.

A number of theories link the pharmacological properties of drugs to user characteristics. Some lack generality because they focus upon a single substance or class of substances, usually opiates (Ausubel, 1961, 1964; Dole and Nyswander, 1967; Lindesmith, 1947, 1980, Rado, 1933; Savitt, 1963). Others disregard differences in the effects produced by various substances. For example, they may attribute all drug abuse to loss of self-esteem (Kaplan, 1980a, 1980b), conditioning (Wikler, 1965, 1973, 1980), social deviance (Hill, 1980), learning (Frederick, 1972, 1980), or addiction to pleasure (Bejerot, 1972, 1980).

Most such theories derive from research in which "objective" measures are correlated with drug use in large groups of subjects, who vary widely in level and chronicity of drug use. This research yields quantifiable data, but it yields no understanding of the experiential states that heavy, chronic drug users seek. All major drugs of abuse have powerful psychological effects, and the experiences induced by barbiturates and sedative-hypnotics differ from those induced by cocaine, amphetamine, and the opiates. Failure to understand these experiences may lead to oversights in the development of theories to explain drug abuse or the design of treatment techniques to alleviate its adverse consequences. Yet, to our knowledge, empirically derived descriptions of the psychological states induced by the major drugs of abuse have not yet been published.

Such descriptions are important to pharmacology because drug abusers take substances for their psychic effects, and these may be different from what is intended medically. A case in point is phencyclidine (PCP), a drug originally intended for use as a surgical anesthetic but now used illicitly for its psychological effects. The study of heavy, chronic use is especially important because heavy chronic users take drugs in doses, at frequencies, and for periods of time that exceed medically prescribed levels and often produce unanticipated effects. Finally, it is important to recognize that with heavy use, even drugs of similar classes, such as amphetamine and cocaine (both sympathomimetics), can produce different psychological effects (Spotts and Shontz, 1980a).

Understanding the ego states induced by *heavy, chronic use* of specific drugs is also important in the treatment of chronic drug abusers. It gives practitioners some appreciation of the psychological state the individual is trying to attain and provides some clues about the life state from which the individual is attempting to escape.

The following description of the ego state induced by barbiturates and sedative-hypnotics is the second of two reports, the first of which describes the ego state induced by heavy, chronic use of cocaine. In these reports, the ego is defined as the point or focus of consciousness (Jung, 1958). The term *ego state* refers to the distinguishing properties of the field of consciousness within which the ego is located at a given time.

Barbiturates and Sedative-Hypnotics

Barbiturates and sedative-hypnotics are the most widely prescribed drugs in the United States (Smith, Wesson, and Seymour, 1979) and have been used extensively to treat anxiety, nervousness, and insomnia. They have also been used as surgical premedicants and to treat neuromuscular disorders, epilepsy, status epilepticus, hyperbilirubinaemia, cerebral edema, intracranial hypertension, emotional disorders, and other conditions (Harvey, 1980; Hoff and Smith, 1977; Marshall and Shapiro, 1977; Smith, 1977; Stern, Khanna, Levy, and Yaffe, 1970; Yatsu, 1976). Though widely used in medicine, these drugs are also common substances of abuse (Wesson and Smith, 1977). Most produce physical dependence, psychological dependence, and tolerance. CNS depressants and the barbiturates in particular are high on the list of suicide poisons in the United States, Canada, Great Britain, France, Germany, and other industrial nations (Cimbura, McGarry, and Daigle, 1972; Ettlinger, 1964; Glatt, 1962; Gold, 1965; Le Breton and Garat, 1965; Lindelius, 1979; McGuire, Bird, Gottschalk, Heiser, and Dinovo, 1973; Rupprecht, 1950; Whitlock, 1975). Withdrawal from these drugs can be dangerous and should be undertaken under close medical supervision, for it can produce delirium, psychosis, convulsions, and death (Brownstein and Pacella, 1943; Essig, 1967; Fraser, Shaver, Maxwell, and Isbell, 1953; Heston and Hastings, 1980; Lloyd and Clark, 1959; Osgood, 1947; Schnoll and Fishkin, 1972; Swanson and Okada, 1963; Wikler and Essig, 1970; Wulff, 1959).

The psychological state induced by heavy use of the barbiturates and sedative-hypnotics has a definite structure which distinguishes it from other drug-induced states. In this report it is designated the *barbiturate state* because barbiturates are the prototype CNS depressant, and sedative-hypnotics produce similar effects (Essig, 1964, 1965, 1966; Harvey, 1980).

Research Context

The men studied are part of an ongoing program of research, which intensively examines individuals who comprise carefully matched groups of heavy, chronic users of cocaine, amphetamine, opiates, barbiturates, and sedative-hypnotics, as well as a comparable group of men committed to the nonuse of drugs. The research employs the Representative Case Method (Shontz, 1965, 1977) and assumes that more can be learned about the structure, dynamics, and motivations for drug abuse from the intensive study of carefully selected, pure user types than from less intensive, large-scale surveys of heterogeneous user groups. For ethical and moral reasons, no serious investigator would administer dangerous doses of drugs to human subjects for long periods of time. Therefore, heavy users provide information about drug effects that can be obtained in no other way.

METHODS

The Experts

The nine consultants (participants) in this subproject were selected from more than 260 male drug users who reported themselves to be knowledgeable about the barbiturates and sedative-hypnotics. All the men selected had experimented with a wide variety of drugs. All had developed a personal commitment to the barbiturates or sedative-hypnotics and had used them long enough to be expert as to their effects. Each man was studied individually for 12-15 days over a period of 4-5 months; data collection for all nine took approximately 1.5 years.

The men were approximately 29 years of age (range: 22-48 years), of above average intelligence, and with almost 12 years of education. The majority were White and came from small, intact middle-class families (Table 1). Three were married and two were divorced; only two marital relationships produced children. These men were reared in traditional Catholic and Protestant families, but none showed any interest in religious beliefs or activities.

As in the other studies in this research program, participants were drawn from all sectors of society and included persons in heterogeneous legal and illegal occupations: a middle-class blue-collar worker; a professional thief; a scion of a wealthy family; a musician; an entrepreneur; a social misfit; a gambler and pimp; an ambitious, achievement-oriented individual; and a two-worlder (Brotman and Freedman, 1969) who maintained full-time legal employment to mask another illegal occupation. Variation of life-style ensured that findings about drug effects were not due to selection of a single psychological type.

All but two of these men had practiced intravenous injection of barbiturates, but by the time of our studies most had shifted to oral ingestion to avoid the painful and persistent abscesses that can accompany intravenous use (Table 2).

Table 1

Personal/Family Characteristics of Participants (N = 9)

1. Personal Characteristics	
Age	
Median	29
Range	22-48
Intelligence	
Revised Beta	
Mean IQ	105.8
SD	8.87
WAIS	
Mean Verbal IQ	109.1
SD	12.56
Mean Performance IQ	104.4
SD	12.44
Mean Full Scale IQ	107.6
SD	12.88
Educational achievement (yr)	
Mean	11.5
Range	9-14
Marital status	
Single	3
Married	4
Divorced	2
Socioeconomic background	
Median	Middle class
Range	Lower-upper class[a]
Race	
Black	1
White	8

(continued)

Table 1 (continued)

2. Family Characteristics	
Parents' marital status	
Intact[b]	6
Divorced	2
Parent deceased	1
Parents' educational achievement (yr)	
Father	
Median	13
Range	7-20
Mother	
Median	12
Range	8-18
Siblings	
Brothers	
Median	0
Range	0-3
Sisters	
Median	2
Range	0-7
Birth order	
Median	2
Range	1-7

[a]A five-class typology (upper, upper-middle, middle, lower-middle, lower) based on the father's occupation and income using a modification of status assessment procedures developed by Hollingshead (1965).
[b]An intact marital relationship does not necessarily mean a healthy one, but only one in which the parents remained together until the participant was age 15 or older.

Two indices of *chronicity of drug use* were calculated. The first was Age of Last Use Minus Age of First Use of drug(s) of commitment. This index provides a crude measure of duration but fails to account for variations in frequency of use over time or for contingency factors; that is, times when the substance is unavailable, or when the individual cannot afford it, or when use is voluntarily terminated. Therefore, a second index, Estimated Years of Daily Use (total days of lifetime use, converted to years), was also employed. Both indices confirm that the men studied had consumed these substances for extended periods (Table 2).

In other research series, the heavy, chronic users of cocaine, opiates, and amphetamine had used their drugs of choice regularly for 3 to 7 years or more. However, barbiturate and sedative-hypnotic users practiced heavy, regular use of these drugs for periods ranging from 4 to 36 months (median: 12.0 months), then shifted to another drug (typically opiates) for 1-3 months, then returned to the drugs of commitment. Most reported that periods of abstinence were

Table 2

Participant Drug Use Characteristics

1. Presenting Characteristics	
Primary method of administration	8 oral 1 intravenous
Chronicity of use (yr)[a]	
Median	11
Range	8-22
Estimated years daily use of drug of commitment[b]	
Median	6.0
Range	5.0-12.0
Estimated typical daily dosages	
Median	225 mg[c]
Range	120-630 mg[d]
Number of drug overdoses reported	27
Median	3
Range	0-7
Number in treatment at time of investigation	3
Longest voluntary termination of use of drug of commitment (mo)	
Median	0
Range	0.0-2.7
2. Historical Background of Use	
Age first ever use of illegal substance[e]	
Median	16
Range	11-17
Age first ever use of drug of personal commitment	
Median	17
Range	14-26
Number of different drugs ever used	
Median	35
Range	22-53
Abuse of drugs by parents	3 alcoholic fathers
Abuse of drugs by siblings	1 addict brother
Introduced to drug of personal commitment by	2 parents 5 friends 2 acquaintances

[a]Age of last use of drug of personal commitment minus age of first use.
[b]Total days lifetime use converted to years.
[c]Since the men studied practiced heavy, chronic use of several different barbiturate/sedative-hypnotics, their typical daily doses were converted to therapeutic phenobarbital equivalents (Koda-Kimble et al., 1978) to assure dosage comparability.
[d]120 mg is a relatively low dosage and appears at the bottom of the drug use range because participants were selected to depict the entire drug use continuum from low to high.
[e]Defined as the use of illicit substance(s) or illicit use of licit substances other than alcohol.

necessary because (at their dosage levels) these drugs were too debilitating, both physically and mentally, to be used for extended periods.

Daily use ranged from 120 to 630 mg therapeutic phenobarbital dose equivalents (median: 225 mg) per day. In therapeutic dosages, 30 mg of phenobarbital is equivalent to 100 mg secobarbital, amobarbital, and pentobarbital. This amount of phenobarbital is also equivalent to 75 mg methaqualone and 5-10 mg diazepam (Koda-Kimble, Katcher, and Young, 1978). It should be noted that therapeutic dose equivalents are not the same as withdrawal dose equivalents (Smith, Wesson, and Seymour, 1979). Median estimates reveal that these men had used barbiturates or sedative-hypnotics for almost 50% of their lives since they began use of drugs. Data in Table 2 demonstrate that they qualify as heavy, chronic users.

Seven men reported a total of 24 overdoses on these drugs in which they would have died had others not intervened; they also reported three overdoses on other drugs. The nonchalance with which they discussed these near-fatal episodes left the impression that they cared little whether they lived or died. Half the men reported hepatitis and serious abscesses associated with intravenous use of barbiturates. Three reported going into comas (one of 4 days duration) that required hospitalization, when using these drugs; and four reported a total of six seizures or convulsions when the drugs were temporarily unavailable.

These men began their first use of illicit substances at about age 16 (range: 11-17) and their first use of barbiturates and/or sedative-hypnotics at about 17 (range: 14-26). Nearly all used alcohol before trying other substances. They had experimented with a variety of drugs, particularly sedative-hypnotics. Most settled upon regular use of a preferred drug—secobarbital, amobarbital and secobarbital, methaqualone, diazepam, etc.—but continued to experiment with other sedative-hypnotics hoping to find one that might better meet their needs.

Abuse of illicit drugs by parents was limited. Three of these men's fathers were alcoholics, and three mothers were regular users of barbiturates or sedative-hypnotics, obtained by prescriptions. Some had introduced their sons to these drugs as children.

The nine men reported a total of 25 siblings (7 brothers and 18 sisters). The relatively large number of siblings is due to the fact that two men were reared in families of seven children each. One of the men described a brother as an opiate addict, a second described a sister as an alcoholic, and a third described his sister as a rehabilitated barbiturate user. Five members (three brothers and two sisters) of one of the larger families were described as occasional recreational drug users. Thus, 32% of the siblings were described as having some experience with illicit drugs; the remainder were described as nonusers. The majority of the men indicated that they were introduced to their drugs of commitment by close friends.

Instruments and Procedures

These descriptions of the barbiturate state constitute a reconstruction of phenomenological experience, based on many kinds of data. The procedures used to collect these data included intensive and extensive interviews covering drug use history, use patterns, the social context of use, reasons for selecting the drug(s) of choice, and drug preferences, as well as three exhaustive checklists of possible effects of barbiturates. Items on one list described physical effects, the second list contained items describing psychological effects, and the third contained items describing withdrawal (Table 3). Each person was read each item and asked whether he experienced that effect at his use level and, if so, what percentage of the time he experienced it. He was then requested to add comments to explain, clarify, or elaborate his answer. Complete drug use interviews required 3-4 days per person.

Another important source of data was the Q-sort. This instrument contains 60 descriptive statements about the self, representing positive and negative

Table 3

List of Drug Effect Items

	Physical	
Dilation of pupils	Hemiparesis	Tremors
Feel drunk	Increased salivation	Dysrhythmia
Angioneurotic edema	Sore gums	Hepatitis
Lowered body temperature	Diarrhea	Dry mouth
Sluggish reflexes	Delerium	Loss of taste
Decreased movement	Arrhythmia	Anorexia
Enuresis, nocturia	Facial numbness	Constriction of pupils
Nystagmus	"Burns"	Ataxia (poor motor control)
Weight loss or gain	Feel heavier	Respiratory problems
Insensitivity to pain	Relaxation of body	Choreiform movements
Perspire more or less than usual	Drowsiness	Double vision
"Needles and pins" in extremities	Nausea, vomiting	Chest congestion
Slow but shallow respiration	Convulsions	Elevated temperature
Hangover	Allergic reactions	Palpitations
Overdose	Coma	Constipation
Rush	Loss of voice	Increased or decreased appetite
Indigestion	Slurred speech	Loss of balance
Chilling	Vertigo	Increased or decreased urination
Glassy-eyed	Nasal drip	Decreased audio acuity
Edema	Headaches	Urticaria
	Dizziness	
	Bad taste	

(continued)

Table 3 (continued)

	Psychological	
Loss of inhibitons	Become hostile, mean	Pleasurable, drowsy feeling
Sense of wellbeing	Inability to work	Unable to think clearly
Relief from unbearable tension and anxiety	Feel relaxed and at ease	Have greater self-control
Loss of anger, hostility, or resentment	Increased sexual drive	Become inconsiderate of others' needs
Feeling of indestructibility	Less self-control	Loss of psychological tensions
Loss of worries, fears, anxieties	Memory difficulties	Inability to concentrate
Dreams: wild, pleasant, or none	Errors in judgment	Decreased sexual performance
Impotence, difficulty with erection	Hallucinations	Time slowed down/ speeded up
Impaired fine motor coordination	Shrinking genitalia	Do not think about consequences of actions
Confusion, forgetfulness	More impulsive	Less sensitive to others
Increased sexual fantasies	More talkative	Temporal acceleration, deceleration
Peace, relaxation	Sexual stimulation	Little things irritate you that normally do not
Euphoria	Have memory lapses	
	Insensitive to pain	
	Irritability	
	Live for the moment	
	Sense of exhilaration	
	Depressed, despondent	
	Aggressive, quarrelsome	
	Withdrawal	
Restlessness, anxiety	Dysphagia, difficulty in swallowing	Easier urination
Nervousness, apprehension	Agitation	Increased appetite
Tachycardia	Nausea, vomiting	Excessive sweating
Tremulousness, tremors	Insomnia	Abdominal cramps
Muscle twitching	Convulsions	Coma
Hyperpyrexia	Seizures	Delirium
Palpitations	Exhaustion	Cardiovascular collapse
Feel worn out for days	Chills	Numbness of extremities
Dizziness	Tearing	Runny nose
	Yawning	Depression
		Hyperactive reflexes

expressions of traits in 15 content areas, such as achievement, independence, sexuality, etc. Each person used this instrument to describe himself as he usually is, his ideal self, his bad or worst self, and himself when wanting barbiturates or sedative-hypnotics, when under the influence of drugs, after their use, and several other aspects of his personal identity. Q-sorts were administered 14 times at each of three testing sessions, approximately 2 months apart. A complete description of the instrument and procedure appears in Spotts and Shontz (1980a).

A semantic differential measure was also employed. Each person rated nine substances—amphetamine, beer, barbiturates, cocaine, hard liquor, heroin,

LSD, marijuana, and speedball (a combination of cocaine and heroin)—on 26 scales. This instrument is also described in detail in Spotts and Shontz (1980a).

RESULTS

Descriptive Framework

This description covers seven aspects of ego states (Table 4). The first three are *sensorimotor functioning, cognitive functioning,* and *emotionality.* The fourth is *spatiality,* considered in terms of two vectors. On the vertical vector, movement upward indexes elevation toward ethereal or spiritual states, and movement downward indexes depression and dejection (Ellenberger, 1958). On the horizontal vector, movement outward indexes involvement with the environment, and movement inward indexes withdrawal. The fifth dimension is *temporality*, considered in terms of the directional movement (future, past) of life processes and personal tempo, the experience of time. The sixth dimension is *causality*, considered in terms of the extent to which the person regards his world as ordered and lawful, and the extent to which he feels capable of influencing or controlling his life. The seventh dimension is *materiality*, the way

Table 4

Phenomenological Dimensions

Dimension	Components	Behavior
Sensorimotor	Vision, hearing, touch, taste, smell, muscle sense, balance, pain	Responsiveness to environment, coordination of actions, energy level
Cognitive	Intelligence, memory	Judgment, recall, reality testing, rational control
Emotionality	Sexuality, aggression, guilt, pleasure	Sexual activity, argumentation, fights, impulsive acts
Spatiality	Horizontal, vertical, expansiveness-constriction	Increase or decrease in social or environmental contacts, attempts to produce spiritual experiences
Temporality	Past, present, future, personal tempo	Planning, reminiscing, pace of thought and action
Causality	Orderliness of world; control over self or one's existence	Executing plans; dominating, mastering, or manipulating environment
Materiality	Variety of objects in personal world; quality of objects and of medium of movement	Richness vs poverty of life activities; uses or is used by objects; fullness and variety of experience

the person experiences the primary and secondary qualities of the objects in his phenomenal world, the number and variety of such objects, and the textural quality of the life space—rough, sharp, smooth, jagged, etc.—as well as the properties of the medium through which psychological movement takes place (Ellenberger, 1958). These seven dimensions affect the individual's experience of all existential worlds. In the *Eigenwelt*, they influence the sense of self-hood and identity. In the *Mitwelt,* they influence interpersonal relations. In the *Umwelt*, they influence the person's sense of belonging to the world at large (May, 1958).

Phenomenological Structure of the Barbiturate State

Sensorimotor Functioning

The barbiturate state is a cloudy, foggy, and stuporous condition (a dark and turbulent experience) in which all sensorimotor functions are severely impaired. Reflexes are sluggish; vision is distorted; people and objects appear blurry and indistinct. Sounds are muffled; the person has trouble understanding what others are saying. Communication is difficult, both because the user's speech is slurred and because he grasps only segments of others' conversation. Visual-motor coordination is impaired; balance, equilibrium, and gait are unstable. The user feels acutely the downward pull of gravity; his head and extremities feel heavy and leaden, and movement is awkward and cumbersome. He falls into tables, over chairs, and up or down stairs; he walks into walls, doors, street signs, and telephone poles. Behind the wheel of an automobile he is a hazard to himself and others. Barbiturate/sedative-hypnotic users reported the highest incidence of serious auto wrecks and accidents of any group studied. Seven men reported 14 accidents in which the vehicles they were driving were demolished, and numerous less severe auto accidents. One user reported that in the barbiturate state he often deliberately sideswiped parked cars, an act he found particularly pleasurable at the time. These men report that barbiturates produce numbness. Since these drugs are not analgesics (Harvey, 1980), it seems more likely that pain is experienced but is either not troublesome, is misperceived, or is quickly forgotten. Dreaming is all but obliterated when using these drugs.

Cognitive Functioning

In the barbiturate state, thinking is slow, ponderous, and difficult. The person is confused and forgetful, and has difficulty maintaining attention or remembering what he is trying to accomplish. Memory lapses are common. The heavy user may get up to go to the bathroom but forget his intention and be drawn into some other activity. He may awaken in bed with a strange woman, not knowing where he is, how he got there, or what he did the night before. Memory for events may disappear as rapidly as new situations present themselves. The rational, intellectual controls that enable people to analyze, evaluate, and accurately interpret experiences are all but obliterated. Thinking, reality testing, memory concentration, judgment, etc., are seriously impaired, if not abolished, and the heavy user no longer takes into account the hazards, dangers, or consequences of his actions.

Emotionality

Heavy abuse of barbiturates precipitates dissolution of the ego, which first produces a sense of calm but later unleashes an upsurge of emotionality. Initially, users experience relief and relaxation, followed by growing bodily numbness and eradication of fears, worries, and anxieties. With the muting of worries and reduction of experienced pain, many report increased feelings of strength, power, and invulnerability that border on grandiosity. The person begins to feel he can move mountains, overcome any obstacle, achieve any goals. Irritability and impatience increase, and the behavior of other people begins to seem irritating, annoying, even stupid. The user experiences a welling up of anger, rage, and hostility and intense impulses to violence; a need to strike out, hit, or attack things or people, to wreck and destroy.

In this state, the user feels no responsibility for his acts. Some enter a comatose condition which in its extreme could bring about death. Others enter a disoriented, stuporous state in which they blindly strike out, releasing emotions in paroxysmal outbursts of rage. They become belligerent, quarrelsome, and abusive, and provoke senseless fights, arguments, and violent confrontations with friends, acquaintances, or strangers. In such altercations heavy users are often badly beaten by their less disabled adversaries.

The men we studied were extroverted and sexually active. Some reported that their drugs stimulated sexual desire, but most indicated the drugs decreased their interest in sexuality. Almost all agreed that in the drug state both performance and pleasure were impaired. Some reported difficulty obtaining or maintaining an erection, while others reported (rather sheepishly) that on occasions they had fallen asleep during the act.

Spatiality

Even during abstinence, heavy, chronic barbiturate abusers experience spatiality as restricted. They live in narrow and constricted lifespaces with limited free movement (Spotts and Shontz, 1982). In such a world, rise to spiritual heights is out of the question. Horizontal movement is blocked, for every effort to influence the environment seems to meet with failure and frustration. Movement inward is intolerable, for it requires confrontation with malevolent inner forces which seem to threaten destruction. The only open route is down, and in the barbiturate-induced state this is the direction in which movement ultimately occurs. Several men presented vivid accounts of how, with the aid of these drugs, they plummeted downward through depression to a state of near nonawareness and often beyond it to oblivion.

Temporality

For most people, life flows toward the future, without serious impediment, but the time perspective of chronic barbiturate abusers is blocked, for these men are tied to the past, stuck with hapless identities garnered from the experiences of childhood (Spotts and Shontz, 1980b, 1982). Most live in an unhappy present and see themselves as having no future. It is not that they have chosen to live in the moment, but that they see their situation as remediless and live without hope. For such persons, oblivion may seem the only alternative, a state with no past or future, in which time itself is obliterated.

Only one man (a musician) has a definite vocational goal, and only two others have described future plans; the rest are adrift in life, going nowhere. One, a millionaire's son, appears future oriented, but his fate is tied to his father; he cannot break away to create his own existence. Another, a thief, lives in a stuporous fog from day to day. Death or imprisonment is probable in his future, and he is seemingly waiting to see which it will be. A third talks about a future (regular employment, owning a home, raising his family) but has systematically destroyed several opportunities to make it real. Another, though exceptionally bright, is sitting "dead in the water," with no plans, eking out a living as a part-time salesman and taxi driver. Finally, another, an older drug dealer, talks about trying legitimate business but doubts he can escape the attractions and hazards of the drug world.

In the barbiturate state, these men temporarily cut their ties with an oppressive past, but by the same stroke they unweave time and space and destroy temporality. The temporal chaining and continuity of events breaks, and experiences scatter like beads from a broken necklace; connections with past and future disintegrate, and existence shrinks to fragmentary experiences of the moment. The individual feels an impulse and acts. He encounters something in the environment and reacts, frequently with violence or verbal abuse. Without an ego to maintain the normal rhythm, meter, and cadence of existence, time seems to slacken, crawl, plod, and drag along.

Causality

Although barbiturate abusers believe that the world is ordered, regular, and predictable, they do not believe control is possible for themselves. They see other people (particularly nonusers of drugs, whom they idealize) taking control of life: finding mates, pursuing careers, and attaining a modicum of happiness. They admire these people but feel painfully different because they cannot influence their own destinies.

For most of these men, heavy barbiturate use produces substantial though temporary increases in experienced power. The apparent numbness and cessation of fears, anxieties, and self-doubts enable the user, for a brief period, to have the illusion of being powerful and self-confident ("I felt like Superman," "I felt like I could pull telephone poles out of the ground," "I felt invulnerable and knew no one could hurt me"). This illusion is accompanied by aggressive action. To the users' regret, however, the illusion does not outlast the drug state.

When in despair, some men seem to take barbiturates in an effort to perform the last possible act of control: managing fate by demolishing it, destroying consciousness in the hope that it will never return again.

Materiality

When not taking drugs, the barbiturate user's world is cold, gray, and bleak; at worst hostile and rejecting, at best cold and uncaring; a rocky wasteland swept by sudden, violent, emotional storms. Dark clouds hang over everything. Most objects, and there are not many, are hard, heavy, and resistive. Locomotion is slow, difficult, and energy draining, for the individual experiences the constant downward pull of inner forces.

As previously noted, one major effect of heavy barbiturate use is to briefly increase the user's sense of power. Temporarily enabled to overcome the drag of the psyche, the barbiturate abuser—though his body feels heavy and leaden—does feel able to act. For a brief period, he has an illusion of freedom. In the drug state, the world is as bleak and even more hostile than before, but he feels able to move, and since experienced pain has been erradicated he can strike out with impunity. The problem is that, to maintain this illusion, the user must keep moving, because as soon he pauses or stops to rest, he lapses into unconsciousness.

Findings from Q-Sorts

Q-sort data present a revealing picture of the barbiturate state and provide independent confirmation of the phenomenology of the drug state obtained from interviews.

Earlier studies indicate that most heavy, chronic users of cocaine, amphetamine, and opiates see their drugs as increasing the congruence between their usual and ideal selves. Because the drug seems to enhance movement toward the ideal self, it is described in pleasant and positive terms. Q-sort data from barbiturate abusers are strikingly different.

Unlike users of other drugs, barbiturate abusers did not describe a consistent usual self. However, they did describe a clear, though idealized, conception of nonusers; an exaggerated, but unattainable, ideal self; and an articulate picture of their worst self (those parts of themselves they despise and fear most which have never been integrated into the personality).

These men describe themselves when not using drugs as being somewhat like their ideals and somewhat unlike their worst selves, with their ideal selves being polar opposites to their worst selves (usual self vs ideal, $r = .672$; usual self vs worst self, $r = -.574$; and ideal self vs worst self, $r = -.988$—these and all subsequent values are medians for the group, corrected for attenuation). Although they feel alienated from the nonuser society they idealize nonusers and wish they could be more like them (usual self vs nonsuers, $r = .164$; ideal self vs nonusers, $r = .942$). These men described themselves during abstinence as being strong and deep, kind, friendly, and wise; as logical and striving people who desire to achieve and accomplish. However, life history data show that they cannot confirm this self-concept in action. No matter how hard the user tries to make this image real, he fumbles, falters, and ultimately fails. He soon expends his reserves, gives up, marks up another failure in a litany of failures, and turns to drugs. His frustration is intensified by seeing others finding the success and contentment that for him seems unattainable.

Q-sort data indicate that these men experience powerful rage and pressures to attack and injure others. In response to this pressure, however, they are more likely to place themselves into situations where they are injured themselves than to seek out opportunities to injure others.

Unlike users of other drugs, the heavy user of barbiturates is not helped by his drug to become more like his usual self or his ideal. In the *predrug state* these individuals' egos begin to flounder and fail; controls begin to crumple. These men describe themselves when in this state as being unhappy, lonely, and depressed; as weak, nervous, anxious, and apprehensive. They lose their ambition, poise, and consideration for other people. They feel a welling up of hostility, rage, and embitterment, and the desire to strike out against the world in acts of cruelty and violence. With emergence of these feelings they become less like their usual and ideal selves and more like their worst selves (usual self vs wanting drug self, $r = .351$; ideal self vs wanting drug self, $r = -.526$; worst self vs wanting drug self, $r = .798$).

In the *barbiturate state* the men we studied describe themselves as being strikingly different from their usual selves (usual self vs drug self, $r = -.449$), as being identified with their worst selves (worst self vs drug self, $r = .854$), and in outright opposition to their own ideals and society at large (drug self vs ideal, $r = -.693$; drug self vs nonusers, $r = -.632$). In the drug state, these men all but become their worst selves, or shadows (Jung, 1958). They undergo a personality transformation which is similar is some respects to that described by Robert Louis Stevenson in his book *The Strange Case of Dr. Jekyll and Mr. Hyde.* They describe the drug state as a negative, extremely unpleasant condition accompanied by massive losses in self-regard and self-esteem. While in this state these men lose all the psychological characteristics they aspire to (peace, wisdom, kindness, happiness, ambition, satisfaction, and self-control) and take on the characteristics they despise and fear most (they become hostile, arrogant, and impulsive; cruel, explosive, vicious, and violent men who callously use and exploit other people).

With some users of other drugs we studied, the experience immediately following heavy use is one of release, quiescence, or relaxation. However, heavy, chronic barbiturate users uniformly describe the *postdrug state* as a miserable and unhappy one in which they feel worse than they did before using the drug (usual self vs after-drug self, $r = .152$; ideal self vs after-drug self, $r = -.892$). These men describe themselves in the postdrug state as sad and depressed; nervous, anxious, and self-destructive; inept, cruel and hostile; unkind and unfriendly; unhappy, ashamed, and foolish. They become more like their worst self than they were when using the drugs (worst self vs after-drug self, $r = 1.000$).

Even though these individuals show striking similarities in family backgrounds, patterns of adult adjustment, and performance on a variety of psychological tests (Spotts and Shontz, 1982, 1983), it would be incorrect to conclude that these drugs have the same meaning or serve identical purposes in the lives of all heavy users or even the nine men described in this report. These findings depict the major theme or the underlying melody of relationships that emerged from the Q-sort data. Three discernible patterns of relationships emerged on this instrument: the dominant (summarized previously) and two variations (described in the following paragraphs).

The first variation was depicted by two men who could be described as living in *alienation*, in estrangement from other people and the values of the larger society. Both identified with their worst selves, disidentified with their ideal selves, and saw themselves as being different from people who do not use drugs (usual self vs ideal self, $r = -.625$; usual self vs worst self, $r = .618$; ideal self vs worst self, $r = -.866$; usual self vs nonusers, $r = -.522$). Upon abstinence, these men described themselves as lonely, depressed, and unhappy; as nervous, tense, and insecure; as volatile and explosive loners who were feared by others but not respected; as men who lack self-confidence and self-respect. They wished to be at peace with themselves and as happy as other people seemed to be, but they felt little hope of ever achieving these ideals. These men used barbiturates to help them live with their negative identities. In the predrug state they became increasingly depressed, frustrated, and embittered; they felt cheated and rejected, and experienced a welling up of explosive anger, rage, and impulses to violence. Heavy use of barbiturates did not eliminate these feelings but did help make the men's negative self-identities seem more tolerable, providing temporary relief and some sense of peace and contentment ("You just don't suffer as much when you're high on barbs"). After the drug state these men returned to their usual state of depression and malaise but also felt weak, drained, sluggish, foolish, stupid, and more negative toward themselves than before (usual self vs after-drug self, r = .889; ideal self vs after-drug self, r = -.922; worst self vs after-drug self, r = 1.000).

The second variation appeared in the lives of two men who lived in *impotence*. These men described themselves when not using drugs as weak, inadequate, and ineffectual persons; as men who lacked self-confidence, were fearful of women, and were unable to approach their ideals. They see only a modest similarity between themselves and nonusers, for they are failures in their own eyes (usual self vs ideal self, r = .385; usual self vs worst self, r = -.515; ideal self vs worst self, r = -.875; usual self vs nonusers, r = .405). They turn to heavy use of barbiturates and sedative-hypnotics because these drugs muffle their anxieties, wipe out their fears and doubts, and enable them to temporarily escape from their identities as failures. Equally important, these drugs help them experience a brief sense of potency and assertiveness that they seem unable to experience during abstinence. Barbiturates do not transform these men into their evil or worst selves but into a different self that is more aggressive, self-confident, and perhaps more competent than they normally are. Unfortunately, although these men, by pharmacological means, are able to break free from their usual selves, their drug-induced identity does not last. In the postdrug state, they fall back into impotence. Again, they feel weak and nervous, timid and unsure of themselves, depressed and withdrawn; but they now are less like their usual or ideal selves than before taking drugs (usual self vs after-drug self, r = .243; ideal self vs after-drug self, r = -.756; worst self vs after-drug self, r = .499).

Semantic Differential

Semantic differential data reveal other peculiar aspects of the barbiturate experience. On this test heavy, chronic users of cocaine, opiates, and amphetamine tended to describe their drugs in positive terms, such as mighty, bright, beautiful, pleasant, successful, etc. However, barbiturate/sedative-hypnotic users indicated that their drugs of choice are: hazardous, strong, mighty, dangerous, sick, trite, weary, loud, slow, feeble, and wrong. Clearly these terms do not recommend these drugs to others, and the drugs are obviously held in low esteem even by the persons who practice their regular heavy use.

DISCUSSION

Summary of Findings

In low, medically prescribed doses, barbiturates and sedative-hypnotics induce relaxation and sleep, and provide symptomatic relief from anxiety or irritability. However, heavy, chronic use of these drugs produces severe disability. In the barbiturate state, sensorimotor functions are seriously impaired; cognitive functions are crippled; reality testing declines; anger and impulses to violence flood the user; temporality collapses; the user becomes involved in a variety of self-destructive activities and no longer takes into account the consequences of his actions. These men choose to enter a negative and intensely unpleasant state, where they lose all the characteristics they hold dear, take on characteristics they fear and despise most, and emerge in worse condition than before entering it. Aside from a brief (but illusory) sense of power, the barbiturate experience is wholly negative.

Some investigators (Smith, Wesson, and Seymour, 1979; Wesson and Smith, 1977, 1981) report that disinhibition euphoria (disinhibition with exaggerated mood elevation) can make barbiturates and certain sedative-hypnotics appealing as intoxicants. However, none of the men we studied reported euphoria. The most common effect was simply relief. These men readily admitted that they used barbiturates and sedative-hypnotics to gain temporary release from worries, anxieties, frustrations, failures, and problems in living. Paradoxically, however, they also turn to these drugs when deeply depressed. They seek to escape from an intolerable situation, and these drugs allow them to do it.

The trajectory of heavy, chronic barbiturate use is downward and has the characteristics of a Fall, Descent, or Plunge. Massive doses trigger a precipitous Fall toward Oblivion, a state whose characteristic is the "blinking out" of the Light of Consciousness. This state lies below the lowest level of experience and even beyond sleep, for in sleep the person dreams and is sometimes aware of changes in bodily position or noises in adjacent rooms. Oblivion is analogous to the mythological Void, the Abyss, annihilation or death, for in this state all awareness is extinguished (Spotts and Shontz, 1980c).

Some writers contend that the attainment of the self-reflective ego is humanity's greatest achievement, an accomplishment of such magnitude that it is identified in mythology with Creation and the Coming of Light into the Universe (Campbell, 1949, 1974; Jaynes, 1976; Jung, 1956; von Franz, 1978; Whyte, 1950; Wilber, 1981). Self-reflecting consciousness separates human beings from the beasts of the field. With it people modify their behavior, find meaning for existence, transcend the immediate situation, and dream new worlds and create them. Most drug users we studied chose their drug because it seemed to provide support for the ego and its ideals. However, heavy, chronic barbiturate/sedative-hypnotic users apparently view the ego as an enemy and feel compelled to destroy it.

The ego state induced by heavy, chronic use of barbiturates and sedative-hypnotics presents a serious challenge to psychological theories, for the major effects are not explainable by traditional theoretical models based upon homeostasis, tension reduction, reinforcement, pleasure seeking, social status, or desires to enhance self-esteem. The evidence of a strong component of self-destructiveness in the lives of these men is undeniable (Spotts and Shontz, 1980b, 1982, 1983). Yet, self-destructiveness cannot be the whole story, for if it were, these men would have been dead long ago.

Theoretical Explanations

The present authors (Spotts and Shontz, 1980b) have provided a structural/formal model that describes the barbiturate state as one that produces ego-self estrangement, perhaps an ultimate in estrangement, for heavy use of these drugs all but severs ego-self relationships. To explain why users seek this state requires a theory anchored in a historical, developmental, or motivational schema. Spotts and Shontz (1980c) have examined six such models and found that while each captures one or more facets of the psychological situation, none is sufficient to encompass all (Table 5).

Table 5

Summary of the Theoretical Models

Model	Critical concept	Process	Limitation
Existential	Life entrapment	Stagnation	Does not describe origin
Death seeking	Self-destruction	Desire to return to uroboric state	Does not explain why men are still alive
Adaptation	Physical or psychic death avoidance	Inoculation by exposure to less harmful form of death	Does not explain why adaptation is never complete
Growth seeking	Self-actualization	Overcoming obstacles; renewed efforts to succeed	Does not explain why ego fails to respond
Enantiodromia	Self-direction; improved status	Sudden reversal; shock	Does not explain why ego fails to respond
Mythical/ metaphorical	Worship of destructive forces	Masochistic behavior	Seems not to offer positive, life-oriented solution

The first model is *existential* (Ellenberger, 1958). It postulates that heavy, chronic barbiturate/sedative-hypnotic users are trapped in an impossible life situation of stasis or stalemate. Because they cannot go forward or upward or withdraw, they use drugs to move them in the only direction open to them, downward. Although this model aptly describes the psychological situation of stagnation, it tells little about how these men reached that state.

The second formulation is a *death-seeking model* which asserts that these men actively seek death (Berger, 1967; Cusky, 1978; Kennedy, 1974; Kessel, 1967; Menninger, 1938) and are attempting to return to the Magna Mater (Klopfer, 1965); to the Uroboros (Neumann, 1949/1954), the "good, ever nourishing maternal breast" (Lewin, 1950). The death-seeking model captures some of the self-destructiveness of these men but fails to account for why they are still alive. The only way this theory might apply is by postulating corollary concepts such as "chronic suicide" or "gratification in self-destruction" (Howard and Borges, 1971; Menninger, 1938).

The third model, an *adaptation model*, postulates that these men recognize the potentially lethal consequences of chronic barbiturate abuse but take these drugs—in a gamble with death—to avoid overwhelming anxiety or impulses to self-destruction that otherwise might be uncontrollable, or to preclude the psychological equivalent, psychosis (Cusky, 1978; Inciardi, McBride and Pottieger, 1978; Lester and Lester, 1971; Mayo, 1974). The adaptation model asserts that these men (at great personal risk) submit to a temporary psychological death in the hope of warding off, averting, or precluding biological death.

A fourth possibility is a *growth-seeking model*, which hypothesizes that these men are engaged in a fumbling but obstinate effort at personal growth. The faltering ego amasses its feeble resources, reaches out in an attempt to wrest control from part of the environment, fails, withdraws, turns to barbiturates to find respite or release, and, if death does not intervene, begins this fumbling process again upon recovery. The growth-seeking model provides one explanation of why these men doggedly continue their struggle. However, it does not explain their self-hatred and apparently deliberate attempts to bring about failure and self-destruction.

A fifth formulation is based upon the concept of *enantiodromia* (Jung, 1959). This formulation suggests that an unconscious, unifying Self is attempting to: (1) shock, jolt, and mobilize the user into recognizing his certain fate (death) if stagnation and stalemate continue; and (2) point out in unmistakable terms the direction that changes must take if self-destruction is to be avoided. Theoretically, the Self could achieve both by inducing an enantiodromia, a sudden reversal that occurs when a state has gone to such an extreme in one direction (toward self-destruction) that it precipitates its opposite (subsequent integration). This model explains how the psyche might turn the tables on destructive thanatonic forces, if the egos of these men were willing or able to follow its lead.

The last model is *mythical-metaphorical*. According to this model heavy, chronic barbiturate/sedative-hypnotic users are unknowingly like worshippers of Kali or other Dark Goddesses, for they are masochistic and guilt-ridden, and seem to be seeking atonement and extirpation of their status as unlovable persons (and possible subsequent rebirth) through self-sacrifice and death.

Implications for Treatment

Any attempt to provide treatment for the heavy, chronic barbiturate/sedative-hypnotic user must take into account the underlying theme of *abandonment/rejection* that permeates these men's lives. This theme appears in the form of four manifest problems: thinly veiled but *diffuse rage and hostility*, *pervasive expectations of failure and defeat*, *nonreflective self-destructive tendencies*, and *feelings of hopelessness and worthlessness*.

In many ways, the personality structures and early family histories of the men in this research series call to mind descriptions of *borderline* states (Kernberg, 1967, 1977; Masterson, 1976). In some instances, borderline conditions appear superficially to originate in neurosis, but they are actually based on such early and severe disturbances of person-environment relations that they are closer to psychotic states. In some better-organized cases, the borderline person may achieve a seemingly successful social adaptation; in less well organized cases, the person constantly teeters on the brink of disaster. Generally, borderline persons are incapable of genuine love or intimacy (Masterson, 1976). Their existences seem empty to them, and they may feel or act as if they are half alive (Seligman, 1982).

Psychotherapy with such persons is extremely difficult (Masterson, 1972, 1976). They exhibit only a tenuous ability to form a working alliance (transference) with their therapists. If their distancing does break down, the result is likely to be, not transference but infantile dependence. Interpretation by the therapist is not productive because the disturbances being treated have their source in a core conflict that began before language was available to the person. Even borderline persons who seem able to function effectively in society are skating on thin ice; any crisis may precipitate a decompensation that can carry them to the darkest and coldest depths of unconscious life. Like users of barbiturates and sedative-hypnotics, borderline individuals seem not to be in need of relief from anxiety but of reconstruction of almost the whole of their personalities.

The following describes what appears to be the typical course of early psychological development of the men in this series of investigations. Early in life, all evidently experienced enough basic nurturance, through the affect image of the Elementary Mother (Spotts and Shontz, 1982, p. 950), to assure that the ego spark, present at birth, did not go out completely. If they had not, they would have developed blatantly schizophrenic patterns of adjustment; none did.

Only a few found this early period of life satisfying enough to wish return to it as adults. Those who did were the ones who tended to get along somewhat better in later life and to show personality traits similar to those evidenced by opiate users. The rest seem to have adopted either of two attitudinal courses. Some chose to live in *anger*. In some instances this resulted in identification with their own worst self, what would be the Shadow in most people. Others chose the course of living in *despair* and *alienation* or *anomie*, with a constant sense of being an outsider.

The failures in ego development in these men seem to have stemmed from a combination of deficiencies in early relations with parents. Their mothers were timorous, passive-dependent, and ineffectual women who were unable to protect their sons or provide the complementary functions of nurturance and liberation of the ego. These mothers not only deprived their sons of a solid base in love and trust, but also failed to encourage the growth of the skills requisite to the development of a secure sense of personal identity.

Nature is often redundant, and in some instances, where a biological mother fails, a father may perform the Transforming (liberating) function and lure the infantile ego into autonomy (Spotts and Shontz, 1982). In the cases of these men, however, redundancy did not operate. Their fathers were either brutal and abusive or inaccessible and neglecting men who ignored their sons entirely. Consequently, these men grew up feeling loved by neither parent. Their early lives are characterized by a pervasive sense of abandonment, of being aliens in a world that did not want them (Shontz, 1982).

This pattern of early family dynamics left the child with no hope of salvation. Most seem to feel that at some unremembered time they were the perpetrators of an unspecifiable Original Sin or were the innocent victims of a Fall from Grace that was imposed upon them without reason. Some seem to have learned to accept this as their doom; they bear psychic wounds of unknown origin that are endurable but never heal. They feel like born losers, but they want to live in the world and continue struggling.

Others become angry and feel justified in striking back at Fate. The angriest seem to be people who attempted to identify, to whatever extent possible, with their inaccessible or sadistic fathers. Their attempts were doomed to failure, for the earliest affect image of the Great Father is hostile and intimidating, even under favorable circumstances. To a child who lacks support and protection from the Nurturing Mother and has not been helped by the Transforming Mother to develop a clear sense of personal identity, the Father imago is overwhelming (Spotts and Shontz, 1982). Given the early lives of these men, one would hardly be surprised to find that this affect image had the qualities of the voice of God, accusing the first human beings of the unforgivable sin of self-awareness and announcing that they are banished from his sight, to live eternally in a cold, cruel, or at best unwelcoming world. To yield to such a God means to submit, as some of these men do, to an unending sense of alienation. To oppose Him, as some of our men did, means to take upon oneself the character of evil incarnate, for only another divinity, as powerful as Satan, would have the temerity to defy such a force.

These men live with impaired egos that leave them poorly equipped to cope with adult life. They experience constant tension, suffer much, and are plagued and, at times, overwhelmed by doubt, self-hatred, and feelings of worthlessness and inadequacy. The typical heavy user feels he will fail at whatever he attempts and, unconsciously at least, seems to feel he has no right to exist (Spotts and Shontz, 1982). Most, though not all, seem to be at least minimally capable of self-reflection (adopting an abstract approach to the self and the problems of everyday life), but few, if any, are able to sustain it.

Although their life histories show some similarities to those described in borderline conditions, heavy, chronic barbiturate/sedative-hypnotic users differ from borderline persons in at least one significant regard; when stressed, they do not become psychotic. Rather, they use barbiturates and sedative-hypnotics to muffle their anxieties, extinguish the ego, and escape to a consciousnessless state of Oblivion. They also use these drugs to help them vent their anger and frustration in paroxysmal outbursts of rage without feeling personally responsible for their actions.

The high incidence of defeats, fights, accidents, injuries, and drug overdoses they report might suggest to an observer that these men wish to die. This could be true, in a sense. However, the heavy, chronic barbiturate/sedative-hypnotic user does not seek to destroy himself as much as to force someone else (or "chance") to commit the act.

As indicated in the discussion of borderline phenomena, the psychological situations of these men were made worse because ego-damaging events undermined their development before they were capable of using language effectively as an adaptive mechanism. Consequently, the events that shaped their lives are often not verbalizable and not subject to modification later in life by purely verbal means. The development of a capacity for accurate or sustained self-reflection, appraisal, and control requires not only the evolution of self-awareness (which has occurred in these men) but also successful completion of the Second Dragon Fight, in which the ego frees itself from the affect image of the Great Mother (Spotts and Shontz, 1982) and undertakes an apprenticeship to the positive affect image of the Father. Few of these men have undertaken that fight, much less completed it. None demonstrated a stable capacity for self-judgment, and few evidenced an ability to consistently manage their environments. Most seemed to feel that, however negative their fate might be, it was beyond their powers to understand or alter it.

Given the harsh circumstances of their early lives, these men have been unable to develop a concept of personal salvation. Forgiveness means nothing to them, for they do not believe they have done anything wrong enough to deserve their despair. Most never reached the stage at which one learns to hope. Their situation is virtually escape proof. For example, though harsh, punitive, or rejecting, their fathers tended to be economically successful. One was a college president, another was a self-made millionaire, a third was a NASA engineer, and so on. Because the men we studied also want to succeed, they must, to a degree, identify with their fathers' values. To do this, however, they must emulate and identify with the Terrible Father of Childhood for whom they feel anger, resentment, hatred, and even contempt. They therefore feel driven to oppose and reject society (the World of the Fathers) even though it means they forfeit all real chances for personal success.

Psychotherapy. If this analysis is accurate it has important implications for treatment. The most obvious implication is a negative one: that success seems unlikely for therapies that rely primarily on verbal communication. A second implication is that any form of therapy is likely to arouse in these men powerful, infantile, feelings of abandonment and subsequent reactions of either self-destructiveness or rage against the therapist or others. Such individuals expect disappointment and may set out to force the therapist to reject or punish them, may react with rage and fury when their expectations are realized, and may respond with anger or violence toward their therapist or commit masochistic acts of destructiveness against themselves.

Self-destructiveness in these cases is not likely to follow the pattern expected in depression, for these people are not depressed in the usual clinical sense. Deliberate suicide demands a degree of conscious self-judgment of which few of these men are capable. Rather, in such individuals, self-destruction will most probably come about "accidentally," as the result of an impulsive drug overdose, a fight provoked with a stranger in a bar, or an automobile wreck that happens while driving under the influence of drugs.

Anger directed against the world will probably not come in the context of a well-developed set of delusional ideas, as it would in a paranoid state; nor is it likely to appear as a purely impulsive act of unprovoked aggression. It is most likely to seem to the patient to be the desperate act of a person who feels trapped and unable to respond in any other way; it is likely to have a strong component of a wish to be defeated and destroyed as a result of its enactment.

It is our opinion that, while the use of traditional outpatient approaches may be successful with some better-organized individuals, it will be expensive, time consuming, and relatively ineffective in terms of overall costs and benefits.

New therapeutic approaches may be required. They must contend with the sense of abandonment, anger, self-destructiveness, and feelings of hopelessness that pervade these men's lives.

There are at least two approaches to the task of therapy with a heavy, chronic barbiturate/sedative-hypnotic user. With the first, the therapist enters into a relationship in which he becomes a surrogate ego, as it were, for his client, and allies himself with the intact elements of the client's personal structure and begins the slow and uncertain process of attempting repair of a severely damaged ego. This is the more traditional approach described by Masterson (1976), Kernberg (1967, 1977), and others. The second approach attempts the total rebuilding of the personal structure.

If full-scale reconstruction is the goal of therapy the ego must first be taken back to its earliest stages of development. The only approach we can suggest that might accomplish this is a variation of Morita Therapy as described by S. C. Chang (1974, 1978), which requires that the person be removed from the outside world and that his contacts with others be minimized for several weeks. In the variation suggested here, treatment during this period would be designed to promote carefully monitored regression to primitive stages of nonlinguistic experience. Drugs or systematic guided imagery might be used to induce such regression. The images aroused should at first put the patient in touch with restful and peaceful elements of inner life. Later, it may be necessary to deliberately arouse scenes of violence, destruction, and death (if they do not arise spontaneously). Attempts to interpret these images should be minimized, but the patient should be encouraged to learn to use verbal language to describe his experiences and feelings.

Successful treatment of this type may bring about some kind of personal crisis, perhaps a threatened psychotic break, a suicide attempt, or an attack upon the therapist. If this crisis can be managed constructively, personality redevelopment may follow. Obviously, such an approach must be closely monitored and cannot be undertaken without full recognition of the risks involved for all concerned.

A parallel to the psychological situation of the men we studied comes from an unusual source, the modern stage. In Edward Albee's one-act play *Zoo Story* (1960), a younger man (Jerry) comes upon an older one (Peter), sitting on a bench in Central Park. Jerry sits down and aggressively initiates a conversation with Peter, who would prefer to continue reading his book. Jerry learns some facts about the older man's life, then tells Peter about his own isolated existence living in a large, dilapidated roominghouse. Jerry describes his inability to establish meaningful contact with anyone, even the landlady's dog. The play builds in intensity until the younger man provokes the older one into stabbing him with a knife that the younger man has provided (actually, Jerry impales himself). As he is dying, Jerry smiles and says:

Thank you Peter, I mean that, now; thank you very much. Oh, Peter, I was so afraid I'd drive you away. [He laughs as best he can.] You don't know how afraid I was you'd go away and leave me. And now I'll tell you what happened at the zoo. I think . . . I think this is what happened at the zoo . . . I think. I think that while I was at the zoo I decided that I would walk north . . . northerly, rather . . . until I found you . . . or somebody . . . and I decided that I would talk to you . . . I would tell you things . . . and things that I would tell you would . . . Well, here we are. You see? Here we are. Could I have planned all this? No . . . no, I couldn't have. But I think I did. And now I've told you what you wanted to know, haven't I? And now you know all about what happened at the zoo. And now you know what you'll see on your TV, and the face I told you about . . . you remember . . . the face I told you about . . . my face, the face you see right now. Peter . . . Peter? . . . Peter . . . thank you. I came unto you [He laughs, so faintly] and you have comforted me. Dear Peter.

You'd better go now. Somebody might come by, and you don't want to be here when anyone comes. [Jerry takes a handkerchief and with great effort and pain wipes the knifehandle clean of fingerprints.]

Hurry away, Peter. Wait . . . wait, Peter. Take your book . . . book. Right here . . . beside me . . . on your bench . . . my bench, rather. Come . . . take your book. Hurry . . . Peter.

Very good, Peter . . . very good. Now, hurry away. (pp. 61-62; quoted with permission)

Up to a point, the parallel between the men we studied and the situation in Albee's *Zoo Story* is striking. Perhaps chronic barbiturate abusers are searching for someone to put an end to their intolerable suffering. Unlike Peter, however, a trained therapist would know what to expect and would not be a party to the client's suicidal impulses.

The therapist has two tasks. The first is to bring the patient's self-destructive tendencies into the open, in a setting which does not allow them to be acted upon. The second is to help the patient build a stable identity, as someone who has the same right to life as everyone else, and an ego effective enough to support this identity and to enable the client to find some peace, contentment, and success in life.

ACKNOWLEDGMENTS

This research program has been supported continuously by contracts and grants from the National Institute on Drug Abuse. The authors wish to thank Dr. Daniel J. Lettieri for his constant encouragement and helpful suggestions.

REFERENCES

ALBEE, E. *The Zoo Story, the Death of Bessie Smith, the Sandbox: Three Plays Introduced by the Author.* New York: Coward-McCann, 1960.

AUSUBEL, D.P. Causes and types of narcotic addiction: A psychosocial view. *Psychiatr. Q.* 35: 525-531, 1961.

AUSUBEL, D.P. *Drug Addiction: Physiological, Psychological, and Sociological Aspects.* New York: Random House, 1964.

BEJEROT, N. *Addiction: An Artificially Induced Drive.* Springfield, IL: C.C. Thomas, 1972.

BEJEROT, N. Addiction to pleasure: A biological and social-psychological theory of addiction. In D.J. Lettieri, M. Sayers, and H.W. Pearson (eds.), *Theories of Drug Abuse: Selected Contemporary Perspectives.* NIDA Research Monograph No. 30, DHHS Publ. No. (ADM) 80-967. Washington, DC: U.S. Government Printing Office, 1980.

BERGER, F.M. Drugs and suicide in the United States. *Clin. Pharm. Ther.* 8: 219-223, 1967.

BROTMAN, R., and FREEDMAN, A.M. *A Community Mental Health Approach to Drug Addiction.* Juvenile Delinquency Publ. 9005. Washington, DC: U.S. Government Printing Office, 1969.

BROWNSTEIN, S.R., and PACELLA, B.L. Convulsions following abrupt withdrawal of barbiturate: Clinical and electroencephalographic studies. *Psychiatr. Q.* 2: 112, 1943.

CAMPBELL, J. *The Hero with a Thousand Faces.* Bollingen Series No. 17. Princeton, NJ: Princeton University Press, 1949.

CAMPBELL, J. *The Mythic Image.* Princeton, NJ: Princeton University Press, 1974.

CHANG, S.C. Morita therapy. *Am. J. Psychother.* 28: 208-221, 1974.

CHANG, S.C. The psychology of consciousness. *Am. J. Psychother.* 32: 105-116, 1978.

CIMBURA, G., MC GARRY, E., and DAIGLE, J. Toxicological data for fatalities due to carbon monoxide and barbiturates in Ontario—A 4-year survey, 1965-68. *J. Foren. Sci.* 17: 640-644, 1972.

CUSKY, N.R. Self-destruction: Suicide and drugs. In D.J. Lettieri (ed.), *Drug and Suicide: When Other Coping Strategies Fail.* Beverly Hills, CA: Sage Publications, 1978.

DOLE, V.P., and NYSWANDER, M.E. Rehabilitation of the street addict. *Arch. Environ. Health* 14: 477-480, 1967.

ELLENBERGER, H.F. A clinical introduction to psychiatric phenomenology and existential analysis. In R. May, E. Angel, and H.F. Ellenberger (eds.), *Existence: A New Dimension in Psychiatry and Psychology.* New York: Basic Books, 1958.

ESSIG, C. Addiction to nonbarbiturate, sedative, and tranquilizing drugs. *Clin. Pharm. Ther.* 5: 334-343, 1964.

ESSIG, C. Clinical aspects of barbiturate and sedative drug abuse. *Am. J. Hosp. Pharm.* 22: 140-143, 1965.

ESSIG, C. Newer sedative drugs that can cause stages of intoxication and dependence of the barbiturate type. *J. Am. Med. Assoc.* 196: 126-129, 1966.

ESSIG, C.F. Clinical and experimental aspects of barbiturate withdrawal convulsions. *Epilepsia* 8: 21-30, 1967.

ETTLINGER, R.W. Suicides in a group of patients who had previously attempted suicide. *Acta Psychiatr. Scand.* 40: 363, 1964.

FRASER, H.F., SHAVER, M.R., MAXWELL, E.S., and ISBELL, H. Death due to withdrawal of barbiturates. *Ann. Intern. Med.* 38: 1319-1325, 1953.

FREDERICK, C.J. Drug abuse as self-destructive behavior. *Drug Ther.* 2: 49-68, 1972.

FREDERICK, C.J. Drug abuse as learned behavior. In D.J. Lettieri, M. Sayers, and H.W. Pearson (eds.), *Theories of Drug Abuse: Selected Contemporary Perspectives.* NIDA Research Monograph No. 30, DHHS Publ. No. (ADM) 80-967. Washington, DC: U.S. Government Printing Office, 1980.

GLATT, M.M. The abuse of barbiturates in the United Kingdom. *Bull. Nar.* April-June: 19-38, 1962.

GOLD, N. Suicide and attempted suicide in Northeast Tasmania. *Med. J. Australia* 2: 361, 1965.

HARVEY, S.C. Hypnotics and sedatives. In A.G. Gilman, L.S. Goodman, and A. Gilman (eds.), *The Pharmacological Basis of Therapeutics* (6th ed.). New York: Macmillan, 1980.

HESTON, L.L., and HASTINGS, D. Psychosis with withdrawal from ethchlorvynol. *Am. J. Psychiatry* 137: 249-250, 1980.

HILL, H.E. The social deviant and initial addiction to narcotics and alcohol. In D.J. Lettieri, M. Sayers, and H.W. Pearson (eds.), *Theories of Drug Abuse: Selected Contemporary Perspectives.* NIDA Research Monograph No. 30, DHHS Publ. No. (ADM) 80-967. Washington, DC: U.S. Government Printing Office, 1980.

HOFF, J., and SMITH, A. Experimental and clinical use of barbiturates in focal cerebral ischemia. In P. Schmiedck (ed.), *Microsurgery for Stroke.* New York: Springer-Verlag, 1977.

HOLLINGSHEAD, A.B. *The Two-Factor Index of Social Position.* New Haven, CN: Yale University Press, 1965.

HOWARD, J., and BORGES, P. Needle sharing in the Haight: Some social and psychological functions. *J. Psychedelic Drugs* 4: 71, 1971.

INCIARDI, J.A., MC BRIDE, D.C., and POTTIEGER, A.E. Gambling with death: Some theoretical and empirical considerations on drugs and suicide. In D.J. Lettieri (ed.), *Drugs and Suicide: When Other Coping Strategies Fail.* Beverly Hills, CA: Sage Publications, 1978.

JAYNES, J. *The Origin of Consciousness in the Breakdown of the Bicameral Mind.* Boston: Houghton-Mifflin, 1976.

JUNG, C.G. *Symbols of Transformation* (2nd ed.). Princeton, NJ: Princeton University Press, 1956.

JUNG, C.G. Aion. In V.S. deLaszlo (ed.), *Psyche and Symbol: A Selection from the Writings of C.G. Jung.* New York: Doubleday Anchor Books, 1958.

JUNG, C.G. General considerations and prospects. In V.S. deLaszlow (ed.), *The Basic Writings of C.G. Jung.* New York: Modern Library, 1959.

KAPLAN, H.B. Self-esteem and self-derogation theory of drug abuse. In D.J. Lettieri, M. Sayers, and H.W. Pearson (eds.), *Theories of Drug Abuse: Selected Theoretical Perspectives.* NIDA Research Monograph No. 30, DHHS Publ. No. (ADM) 80-967. Washington, DC: U.S. Government Printing Office, 1980a.

KAPLAN, H.B. *Deviant Behavior in Defense of Self.* New York: Academic Press, 1980b.

KENNEDY, P. Not another overdose. *Nursing Times* 70: 1566-1567, 1974.

KERNBERG, O. Borderline personality organization. *J. Am. Psychoanal. Assoc.* 15: 641-685, 1967.

KERNBERG, O. The structural diagnoses of borderline personality organization. In P. Hartocollis (ed.), *Borderline Personality.* New York: International Universities Press, 1977.

KESSELL, N. Self-poisoning. In E.S. Schneidman (ed.), *Essays in Self-Destruction.* New York: Science House, 1967.

KLOPFER, B. Suicide: The Jungian point of view. In N.L. Farberow and E.S. Schneidman (eds.), *The Cry for Help.* New York: McGraw-Hill, 1965.

KODA-KIMBLE, M.A., KATCHER, B.S., and YOUNG, L.Y. *Applied Therapeutics for Clinical Pharmacologists.* San Francisco, CA: Applied Therapeutics, 1978.

LE BRETON, R., and GARAT, J. Suicides par les dérivés barbituriques associés á l álcool éthylique [Suicides by barbiturate derivatives combined with ethyl alcohol]. *Ann. Med.* 45: 78-80, 1965.

LESTER, G., and LESTER, D. *Suicide: The Gamble with Death.* Englewood Cliffs, NJ: Prentice-Hall, 1971.

LEWIN, B.D. *The Psychoanalysis of Elation.* New York: Norton, 1950.

LINDELIUS, R. Trends in suicide in Sweden 1749-1975. *Acta Psychiatr. Scand.* 60: 295-310, 1979.

LINDESMITH, A.R. *Opiate Addiction.* Indianapolis: Indiana University Press, 1947.

LINDESMITH, A.R. A general theory of addiction to opiate type drugs. In D.J. Lettieri, M. Sayers, and H.W. Pearson (eds.), *Theories of Drug Abuse: Selected Contemporary Perspectives.* NIDA Research Monograph No. 30, DHHS Publ. No. (ADM) 80-967. Washington, DC: Government Printing Office, 1980.

LLOYD, E.A., and CLARK, L.D. Convulsions and delirium incident to glutethimide (doriden) withdrawal (case report). *Dis. Nerv. Syst.* 20: 524-526, 1959.

MARSHALL, L.F., and SHAPIRO, H.M. Barbiturate control of intracranial hypertension in head injuries and other conditions: (atrogenic coma). *Acta Neurologia* 56: Suppl., 156-157, 1977.

MASTERSON, J. *Treatment of the Borderline Adolescent: A Developmental Model.* New York: Wiley Interscience, 1972.

MASTERSON, J. *Treatment of the Borderline Adult: A Developmental Model.* New York: Bruner/Mazel, 1976.

MAY, R. Contributions of existential psychotherapy in psychology. In R. May, E. Angel, and H.F. Ellenberger (eds.), *Existence: A New Dimension in Psychiatry and Psychology.* New York: Basic Books, 1958.

MAYO, J.A. Psychopharmacological roulette: A follow-up study of patients hospitalized for drug overdose. *Am. J. Public Health* 64: 616-617, 1974.

MC GUIRE, F.L., BIRD, H., GOTTSCHALK, L.A., HEISER, J.F., and DINOVO, E.D. A comparison of suicide and non-suicide deaths involving psychotropic drugs in four major U.S. cities. *Am. J. Public Health* 66: 1058-1061, 1976.

MENNINGER, K.S. *Man Against Himself.* New York: Harcourt, Brace, 1938.

NEUMANN, E. *The Origins and History of Consciousness.* Bollingen Series No. 42. Princeton, NJ: Princeton University Press, 1949/1954.

OSGOOD, C.W. Convulsive seizures following barbiturate withdrawal. *J. Am. Med. Assoc.* 133: 104-105, 1947.

RADO, S. The psychoanalysis of pharmacothymia (drug-addiction). *Psychoanal. Q.* 2: 1-23, 1933.

RUPPRECHT, H. Vergiftung mit phanodorm-calcium (selbst mordversuch) [Poisoning with phandorm-calcium (suicide attempt)]. *Med. Monatsschr.* 4: 533-534, 1950.

SAVITT, R.A. Psychoanalytic studies on addiction. *Psychoanal. Q.* 32: 43-57, 1963.

SCHNOLL, S.H., and FISHKIN, R. Withdrawal syndrome with methaqualone. *J. Psychedelic Drugs* 5: 79-80, 1972.

SELIGMAN, E. The half-alive ones. *J. Anal. Psychol.* 27: 1-20, 1982.

SHONTZ, F.C. *Research Methods in Personality.* New York: Appleton-Century-Crofts, 1965.

SHONTZ, F.C. Single-organism designs. In P.M. Bentler, D.J. Lettieri, and G.A. Austin (eds.), *Data Analysis Strategies and Designs of Substance Abuse Research.* NIDA Research Issues No. 113, DHEW Publ. No. (ADM) 77-389. Washington, DC: U.S. Government Printing Office, 1977.

SHONTZ, F.C. Retrospective family histories of chronic drug users. In N. Stinnett, J. DeFrain, K. King, H. Lingren, C. Rowe, S. VanZandt, and S. Williams (eds.), *Family Strengths 4: Positive Support Systems.* Lincoln, NE: University of Nebraska Press, 1982.

SMITH, A.R. Barbiturate protection in cerebral hypoxia. *Anesthesiology* 47: 285-293, 1977.

SMITH, D.E., WESSON, D.R., and SEYMOUR, M.A. The abuse of barbiturates and other sedative-hypnotics. In R.I. DuPont, A. Goldstein, J. O'Donnell, and B. Brown (eds.), *Handbook on Drug Abuse*. Washington, DC: U.S. Government Printing Office, 1979.

SPOTTS, J.V., and SHONTZ, F.C. *Cocaine Users: A Representative Case Approach*. New York: Free Press, 1980a.

SPOTTS, J.V., and SHONTZ, F.C. A life theme theory of chronic drug abuse. In D.J. Lettieri, M. Sayers, and H.W. Pearson (eds.), *Theories of Drug Abuse: Selected Contemporary Perspectives.* NIDA Research Monograph No. 30, DHHS Publ. No. (ADM) 80-967. Washington, DC: U.S. Government Printing Office, 1980b.

SPOTTS, J.V., and SHONTZ, F.C. *Studies on the personality and life styles of drug users: Part I: Barbiturate and sedative-hypnotic users.* Executive summary, NIDA Grant No. 1-RO-DAO-01786-02, 1980c.

SPOTTS, J.V., and SHONTZ, F.C. Ego development, dragon fights, and chronic drug abusers. *Int. J. Addict.* 17: 945-976, 1982.

SPOTTS, J.V., and SHONTZ, F.C. Psychopathology and chronic drug use: A methodological paradigm. *Int. J. Addict.* 18: 633-680, 1983.

STERN, L., KHANNA, N.N., LEVY, G., and YAFFE, S.J. Effect of phenobarbital on hyperbilirubinemia and glucuronide formation in newborns. *Am. J. Dis. Child.* 120: 26-31, 1970.

SWANSON, L.A., and OKADA, T. Death after withdrawal of meprobamate. *J. Am. Med. Assoc.* 184: 780-781, 1963.

VON FRANZ, M. *Patterns of Creativity Mirrored in Creation Myths.* Irving, TX: Anchor Press/Doubleday, 1978.

WESSON, D.R., and SMITH, D.E. *Barbiturates: Their Use, Misuse, and Abuse.* New York: Human Sciences Press, 1977.

WESSON, D.R., and SMITH, D.E. Abuse of sedative-hypnotics. In J.H. Lowinson and P. Ruiz (eds.), *Substance Abuse, Clinical Problems and Perspectives.* Baltimore, MD: Williams and Wilkins, 1981.

WHITLOCK, F.A. Suicide in Brisbane, 1956 to 1973: The drug-death epidemic. *Med. J. Australia* 1: 737-743, 1975.

WHYTE, L.L. *The Next Development in Man.* New York: Mentor, 1950.

WIKLER, A. Conditioning factors in opiate addiction and relapse. In D.M. Wilner and G.G. Kassenbaum (eds.), *Narcotics.* New York: McGraw-Hill, 1965.

WIKLER, A. Dynamics of drug dependence: Implications of a conditioning theory for research and treatment. *Arch. Gen. Psychiatry* 28: 611-616, 1973.

WIKLER, A. A theory of opiod dependence. In D.J. Lettieri, M. Sayers, and H.W. Pearson (eds.), *Theories of Drug Abuse: Selected Contemporary Perspectives.* NIDA Research Monograph No. 30, DHHS Publ. No. (ADM) 80-967. Washington, DC: U.S. Government Printing Office, 1980.

WIKLER, A., and ESSIG, C.F. Withdrawal seizures following chronic intoxication with barbiturates and other sedative drugs. *Epilepsy: Mod. Probl. Pharmacol. Psychiatry* 4: 170-184, 1970.

WILBER, K. *Up from Eden: A Transpersonal View of Human Evolution.* Garden City, NY: Anchor Press/Doubleday, 1981.

WULFF, M.H. The barbiturate withdrawal syndrome: A clinical and electroencephalographic study. *Electroenceph. Clin. Neurophysiol.* 14: 1-173, 1959.

WULFF, L.L., and HASTINGS, D. Psychosis with withdrawal from ethchlorvynol. *Am. J. Psychiatry* 14: 1-175, 1959.

YATSU, F.M. Protective effects of barbiturates on cerebral ischemia. In R.L. McLauren (ed.), *Head Injuries.* New York: Grune and Stratton, 1976.

The International Journal of the Addictions, 19(3), 327–334, 1984

Smoking Cessation with Hospital Employees: An Example of Worksite Smoking Cessation

Harold H. Dawley, Jr.,* PhD

Psychology Service
Veterans Administration Medical Center

Department of Medicine and
Department of Psychiatry and Neurology
Tulane University School of Medicine

Wellness Institute, Inc.

Barbara J. Fleischer, PhD

Linda T. Dawley, PhD

Wellness Institute, Inc.
New Orleans, Louisiana

Abstract

Fifteen hospital employees and two patients completed a smoking cessation treatment program of 10 1-hour sessions. At 6-month follow-up, 13 of the employees were still working at the hospital and were able to be contacted. Of those employees who completed treatment and were still employed, seven were not smoking, a success rate of 53%. Worksite smoking cessation programs are viewed not only as cost-effective ways for hospitals to help their employees stop but as a way of encouraging their employees to model more healthy behavior to patients.

*To whom reprint requests should be addressed: Smoking Control and Education Officer, Veterans Administration Medical Center, 1601 Perdido Street, New Orleans, Louisiana 70146.

 0020-773X/84/1903-0327$3.50/0

The importance of controlling and discouraging tobacco smoking in a hospital setting can hardly be overstated. Smoking is widely recognized as the greatest single cause of premature preventable death (Surgeon General, 1974). Ample evidence is also available showing that passive smoking poses risks to nonsmokers with heart disease and similar problems (Aronow, 1978; Aronow, Ferlinz, and Glauser, 1977; Russell, Cole, and Brown, 1973). Yet, despite the hazards of secondhand smoke to hospital patients, little effort has been directed to controlling and discouraging smoking in a hospital setting. The reduction of smoking among hospital employees is one such effort that potentially may significantly reduce and control smoking and contribute to helping patients stop smoking.

Although it is clearly preferable to have people stop smoking prior to the onset of illness, hospitalization is nonetheless seen as an optimal time to stop smoking. During this time patients are away from their usual environments and are more aware of the health implications of smoking. The more that the hospital environment can be modified to discourage smoking, the greater the likelihood that the advantages inherent in this period and setting can be used to help patients stop smoking.

Despite the clear advantages of smoking control and discouragement, relatively few hospitals have taken meaningful steps in this direction. Cigarettes are still sold in most hospitals, with an estimated one-third of the income from canteen sales in the 165 or so Veterans Administration hospitals coming from the sales of tax-exempt tobacco products (American Psychological Assoc., 1980). The Veterans Administration hospital system is also thought to be the largest nonmilitary tax-free outlet for cigarettes in America.

In addition to humanitarian reasons, there are clear economic advantages to be gained by hospitals, and employers in general, through provision of smoking cessation treatment to interested employees. The National Interagency Council on Smoking (1980) estimates that the average one-pack-a-day smoker cost his or her employer $600 in otherwise avoidable expenses. Some estimates have been made that one-fifth of all lost work days in the United States can be attributed to the effects of cigarette smoking (Russell, 1977).

The unique features about smoking cessation efforts for hospital employees are the advantages inherent in worksite smoking cessation programs. The administrative structure of the worksite allows for environmental manipulations to discourage smoking and to encourage participation in smoking cessation programs. Worksite programs for smoking cessation have the potential to reach 50% of the American blue-collar workforce who smoke (Gallup, 1974; Houpt, Orleans, George, and Brodie, 1979). The members of this blue-collor workforce are also the persons who underutilize existing smoking cessation services (Sterling and Weinkham, 1976).

Writers on the topic of smoking generally use the terms *smoking control* and *smoking discouragement* as being synonymous with smoking cessation. Even though these terms are used interchangeably in the literature on smoking, each term has recently been defined with explicitly different meanings. "Smoke-Free" (Dawley, 1982), a comprehensive worksite smoking program, describes *smoking control* as dealing with limiting or restricting smoking to designated areas, *smoking discouragement* as consisting of educational efforts to encourage people to stop smoking, and *smoking cessation* as more formal treatment programs designed to help people stop smoking. This program is based on the assumption that worksite smoking cessation programs operate most effectively when offered in conjunction with worksite smoking control and discouragement efforts.

Dawley, Morrison and Carrol (1981) investigated the smoking control manipulation of placing positively versus negatively worded no-smoking signs for a brief period of time in a hospital waiting area where smoking was previously allowed. Unobtrusive measurements of smoking before and after the sign placement revealed that both types of signs resulted in less smoking. The positively worded no-smoking signs were found to produce better compliance than negatively worded signs. The degree of compliance of patients and employees to no-smoking signs without enforcement was then studied by placing several signs in the hospital canteen eating area, an area where smoking was previously allowed (Dawley, Morrison, and Carrol, 1980). No attempt at enforcement of no-smoking rules was made. Good compliance to these signs was observed initially, followed within 2 weeks by employees, and then patients, increasing their smoking rate to the preintervention level. The results of this study suggest that signs alone without enforcement will not produce compliance. The degree of compliance of patients and employees to no-smoking signs with enforcement was then studied by observing the effect of previously posted smoking and no-smoking signs in the outpatient clinic area of the hospital, along with the placement of additional similar signs in the remainder of the first floor area. These signs were moderately enforced. Observations suggested that this approach was helpful in controlling smoking as well as serving to increase the protection of patients from exposure to passive smoking (Dawley, 1982). A subsequent study (Dawley and Baldwin, 1983) investigated hospital smoking control efforts with good enforcement and discovered a 94-98% compliance rate. An interesting finding of these studies is the apparent myth about smokers' rights. Not one recorded incident of a patient complaining about not being able to smoke in the designated no-smoking areas was recorded over a 2-year period of time.

Bandura's (1977) social learning theory (modeling) is particularly relevant to the problem of discouraging smoking in a hospital setting. Glad and Odessor (1976) showed that people are influenced to smoke mainly because those around them smoke. Dawley, Carrol, and Morrison (1981) investigated the influence of modeled behavior of hospital employees on patients and visitors. A high-status model meant to resemble a "doctor" and a "peer" model meant to model a veteran both smoked in the presence of patients and visitors waiting in a designated no-smoking working area. Their results revealed a highly significant ($p < .02$) effect for modeling reliably increasing smoking rate. This study indicated the importance of employees not smoking in the presence of patients. Generalizing the findings of this study to business settings in general, the importance of supervisory personnel complying with smoking policy is indicated, since they model behavior for employees.

A recent article reviewing what hospitals have done to control smoking states that hospitals across the country are in the same dilemma in that "they recognize their responsibility as health care institutions to discourage smoking, yet problems with enforcing smoking policies, concern for patients' rights and attitudes, and smoking behavior of the hospital staff are major obstacles to doing more to control smoking" (Riffer, 1982).

Offering smoking cessation treatment to hospital employees is seen as a logical extension of smoking control and discouragement efforts, with direct benefits to employees and to the hospital as an employer, and indirect benefits to patients in that more healthy behavior is modeled for them by employees.

METHOD

Subjects and Setting

Employees were solicited for participation in a worksite smoking cessation program via announcements in the hospital's daily bulletin and posters placed throughout the hospital. Two separate groups were offered, the second group 3 months after the first. While primary attention was directed toward soliciting hospital employees, several patients responded to the posters and were included in the group. The first group consisted of eight employees and two patients, while the second group consisted of seven employees who completed treatment. Table 1 presents background of participants. In addition to the 17 *S*s who completed treatment, two employees and one patient withdrew from the first group by the third session, and two employees and one patient withdrew from the second group by the fifth session.

Treatment

Treatment consisted of the packaged smoking cessation part of a comprehensive worksite smoking control, discouragement, and cessation program, identified as SmokeFree (Dawley, 1982). This cessation program uses 10 1-hour group sessions presenting educational material; self-assessment instruments to

Table 1

Demographic Characteristics of Subjects

Characteristic	*N*	Percentage of sample	Characteristic	Mean	SD	Range
Sex			Age	40.5	3.36	30-62
Male	6	35				
Female	11	65	Education (yr)	12.9	0.41	8-17
Marital status			Smoking rate (cigarettes per day)	33.9	1.58	28-45
Single	10	59				
Married	7	41				
Race			Age started smoking	16.0	0.04	15-17
White	11	65				
Black	6	35	No. years smoking	25.1	3.59	15-45
Occupation			Percentage of life smoking	62.2	4.61	50-73
Technical	8	47				
Clerical	6	35				
Professional	3	18				
Significant others smoke?						
Yes	11	65				
No	6	35				

identify why respondents smoke and why they want to stop; lectures on the importance of substitute behavior, weight control, stress reduction; incentives for not smoking; and similar techniques. A heavy emphasis was placed on developing and maintaining group cohesion and support. Significant features of SmokeFree include the designation of the fifth session as the SmokeFree ceremony in which each participant stands before the group and reads aloud his or her personally prepared statement about plans on stopping smoking. Pictures are also taken at this time, as they discard their cigarettes and smoking paraphernalia. The last five sessions emphasized mutual catharsis and support, with a buildup of peer pressure to stay SmokeFree. During this time subjects were taught how to make their environments more conducive to not smoking. Contact was maintained with group participants. Group participants continued to support each other's efforts at not smoking. At 6 months, all participants received a Certificate of Recognition from the hospital director acknowledging their not having smoked for 6 months.

RESULTS

Seventeen participants completed treatment. At end of treatment, 15 of the 17 participants were not smoking (88%). At a 4-month follow-up, 10 of the 16 participants able to be contacted were not smoking (68%). A 6-month follow-up revealed that 7 of 14 participants able to be contacted were not smoking (50%). Looking at employees alone, we see a higher success rate, with 12 of 15 participants contacted (80%) at 4 months and 7 out of 13 (53%) at 6 months still not smoking.

DISCUSSION

Despite the clear moral, legal, and ethical responsibility of hospitals to control and discourage smoking within their settings, relatively little has been done to discourage smoking in hospitals. Even though clear evidence exists that passive smoking is harmful to certain patients (Aronow, 1978), smoking is not controlled in most hospitals. Evidence is also available demonstrating that the average employee who smokes one pack of cigarettes a day cost his or her employer $600 a year in otherwise avoidable expenses (National Interagency Council on Smoking, 1980). One-fifth of all lost work days in the United States can be attributed to the effects of smoking (Russell, 1977). This study directed toward assisting hospital employees in stopping smoking. Of 13 employees who completed treatment and who were still employed at the 6-month follow-up, and thus able to be contacted, seven were still abstinent, a success rate of 58%.

Of significance in this study is the demonstrated potential for worksite smoking cessation programs. The seven employees who were still not smoking at the end of treatment reported that they derived support from other employees who participated in the group with them. They also reported that their public declaration during the SmokeFree ceremony made them feel that they had made a commitment to themselves and the group that they felt obligated to keep. Many added that they felt under pressure not to smoke since most of their co-workers were aware of their pledge not to smoke. Several also reported receiving encouragement to remain off cigarettes from co-workers.

A surprising finding was the effect the seven nonsmoking employees had on fellow workers who were considering stopping smoking. About 25 or so employees contacted the group leader and requested permission to participate in the next smoking group. The successful employees were literally "walking billboards," clearly demonstrating that kicking the tobacco habit was possible.

In summary, worksite smoking cessation programs offer potential for hospitals and employers in general to help their employees stop smoking. Cessation efforts appear to work well when offered in conjunction with smoking control and discouragement efforts. Although there is limited research available on worksite smoking cessation programs, preliminary findings suggest that they are likely to be more effective than community-offered programs. The advantages of peer support during and after treatment, administrative backing and recognition, and other environmental manipulations such as placement of humorous antismoking posters and control of smoking by designating smoking and no-smoking areas make worksite smoking cessation programs particularly effective ways for helping people stop smoking.

REFERENCES

AMERICAN PSYCHOLOGICAL ASSOCIATION. VA Hospital system large tobacco outlet. *Public Service Psychology* (Newsletter of the Division of Psychologists in Public Service), 1980, p. 5.

ARONOW, W.S. The effects of passive smoking on angina pectoris. *N. Engl. J. Med.* 222(1): 21-24, 1978.

ARONOW, W.S., FERLINZ, J., and GLAUSER, F. Effects of carbon monoxide on exercise performance in chronic pulmonary disease. *Am. J. Med.* 63: 904-908, 1977.

BANDURA, A.A. *Psychological Modeling*. Chicago: Aldine, 1977.

DAWLEY, H.H. *SmokeFree: A Program for Worksite Smoking Control, Discouragement and Cessation*. New Orleans: Wellness Institute, 1982.

DAWLEY, H.H., and BALDWIN, J. The control of smoking: Smoking rate in designated smoking and no-smoking areas. *Int. J. Addict.* 18: 1033-1038, 1983.

DAWLEY, H.H., CARROL, S.F., and MORRISON, J.E. The discouragement of smoking in a hospital setting: The importance of modeled behavior. *Int. J. Addict.* 16(5): 905-910, 1981.

DAWLEY, H.H., MORRISON, J., and CARROL, S. Compliance behavior in a hospital setting: Employee and patients' reaction to no-smoking signs. *Addict. Behav.* 5: 329-331, 1980.

DAWLEY, H.H., MORRISON, J.E., and CARROL, S.F. The effect of differently worded no-smoking signs on smoking behavior. *Int. J. Addict.* 16(8): 1467-1471, 1981.

GALLUP OPINION INDEX. *Report No. 108*, June 1974.

GLAD, W.R., and ADESSOR, V.J. The relative importance of socially induced tension and behavioral contagion for smoking behavior. *J. Abnorm. Psychol.* 85(1): 119-121, 1976.

HOUPT, J.L., ORLEANS, C.S., GEORGE, L., and BRODIE, H.K.H. *The Importance of Mental Health Services to General Health Care.* Cambridge, MA: Ballinger, 1979.

NATIONAL INTERAGENCY COUNCIL ON SMOKING AND HEALTH. *Smoking and the Workplace: National Interagency Council on Smoking and Health Business Survey,* January 1980. (Available from the Council at 291 Broadway, Suite 1005, New York, NY 10007.)

RIFFER, J. Hospitals challenged to restrict smoking. *Hospitals*, March 16, 1982, pp. 20-24.

RUSSELL, C. Experts put smoking's cost to nation in the billions. *Washington Star*, November 7, 1977, pp. A1 and A10.

RUSSELL, M.A.A., COLE, P.U., and BROWN, E. Absorption by nonsmokers of carbon monoxide from air-polluted tobacco smoke. *Lancet* 1(3): 576-579, 1973.

STERLING, J.D., and WEINKHAM, P.S. Smoking characteristics by type of employment. *J. Occupat. Med.* 18: 73-75, 1976.

SURGEON GENERAL. *The Surgeon General's Report on Health Promotion and Disease Prevention.* DHEW (PHS) Publ. No. 79-55071. Washington, DC: U.S. Government Printing Office, 1974.

The International Journal of the Addictions, 19(3), 335–353, 1984

The "Urge to Classify" the Narcotic Addict: A Review of Psychiatric Classification. II.

Arie Cohen, PhD

School of Education
Bar-Ilan University
Ramat-Gan, Israel

Abstract

Attempts to classify drug addicts are divided into three main groups: (1) psychiatric classifications, (2) psychosocial classifications, and (3) classifications by pattern of abuse. An extensive literature review of the psychiatric classifications of narcotic addicts suggests that there is no one diagnosis that fits all narcotic addicts and that the importance of psychopathology in drug addiction has been exaggerated. It is concluded that theoretical psychiatric classifications of narcotic addicts have failed to stimulate empirical research and that empirical classifications have not demonstrated their utility for treatment and prognosis.

The first part of the present article (Cohen, 1982) reviewed psychiatric classifications of narcotic addicts. These classifications included theoretical as well as empirical classifications which have been divided into "early attempts," "psychoanalytic orientations," and studies based on the *Diagnostic and Statistical Manual* (DSM) classification system. The present article continues the review of psychometric alternatives as well as other attempts at psychiatric classification of narcotic addicts and finally discusses the issues involved in this approach.

 0020-773X/84/1903-0335$3.50/0

PSYCHOMETRIC ALTERNATIVES

Among the psychometric alternatives to the diagnostic interview, the Minnesota Multiphasic Personality Inventory (MMPI) is undoubtedly the most prevalent and most studied instrument. Nevertheless, although the number of MMPI studies on drug addicts runs over a hundred, relatively few investigators attempted to delineate the MMPI diagnosis of narcotic addicts.

The first report of MMPI profiles of narcotic addicts is that of Hill, Haertzen, and Glaser (1960). In their study, Hill et al. employed the two highest coding systems (Hathaway, 1947) in classifying 200 male narcotic addicts at Lexington Hospital. They developed their diagnostic system of MMPI codes on the basis of clinical experience and experimental work, as well as the underlying assumption that psychopathy is the cause of narcotic addiction. Hill et al.'s four-category classification included the normal addict, the conduct disorder psychopathic addict, the conduct disorder neurotic addict, and the conduct disorder schizoid addict. (The distribution of Hill et al.'s classification appears in Table 1, along with the classifications to be discussed later.) On the basis of their findings, Hill et al. have concluded that psychopathy has a considerable significance in the etiology of addiction.

Olson (1964) employed Hill et al.'s MMPI classification in comparing male and female drug addicts. The distribution of the diagnoses in the male sample was almost identical to that of Hill et al., while the female addicts were classified more than the males as psychopaths and less as neurotics and schizoids.

Sutker (1971) compared the MMPI diagnoses of addicts in treatment and nonaddicted prisoners. The comparison of the two samples indicated that addicts were more likely to be diagnosed as psychopaths and less as normal individuals than the prisoners. These findings led Sutker to conclude that a more refined conceptualization of sociopathy is needed in identifying the manifestation of antisocial behaviors (cf. Gendreau and Gendreau, 1973; Penk and Robinowitz, 1976; Sheppard, Ricca, Fracchia, and Merlis, 1973b; Sutker, 1974; and Sutker and Allain, 1973).

Sheppard, Fracchia, Ricca, and Merlis employed MMPI classification in a sample of drug addicts committed to treatment by court order (1972) and in a sample of suburban addicts applying for treatment (Sheppard, Ricca, Fracchia, and Merlis, 1973a). A comparison of the MMPI diagnoses between the two samples indicated that the suburban addicts, who came from a higher socioeconomic background than the committed addicts, were more disturbed and less sociopathic than the committed addicts. This finding led Sheppard et al. (1973a) to assume that as youth in our society became more experienced and better informed about drug effects, they became more aware of their dangers, and therefore only those who were more psychologically disturbed would venture into extended drug use. Another demonstration of the high variability of psychiatric diagnosis among narcotic addicts may be found in two samples of addicts from the military. Hampton and Vogel (1973) and Black (1975) obtained the MMPI diagnoses of two samples of Vietnam returnees who used heroin. Although the addicts in both samples came to treatment in the same period and had a similar military experience in Vietnam, Black's sample (1975) had twice as many psychotics and only half the number of "normals" as that of Hampton and Vogel (1973). Ludenia (1973) collected 759 MMPI profiles of "drug addicts" from a wide variety of agencies in 23 states, mostly in the Midwest. In this heterogeneous sample, Ludenia found that only 17% of the valid profiles were diagnosed as sociopaths. The reasons for the low proportion of sociopathy may be ascribed to the low rate of heroin abuse in the sample and to the high proportion (34%) of profiles from academic counseling centers. Schooff and Keegan (1975) employed Goldberg's classification method (1972) in a comparison of "streetwise" polydrug abusers (28% primarily heroin abusers) to "prescription medication abusers" and found the streetwise addicts to have a higher rate of sociopathy than the prescription abusers. Koslowsky and Deren (1975) employed an actuarial approach based on the Sixteen Personality Factor Questionnaire (16PF; Cattell, 1970a) in order to obtain the psychiatric diagnosis of narcotic addicts. They correlated (*Rp* correlation) each individual 16PF profile to the mean profiles of normal, criminal, neurotic, and psychotic samples, and then assigned each individual profile to the group which correlated significantly with that profile. The distribution of the classified profiles (29% of the sample) among the four clinical groups was almost even.

Table 1 summarizes the psychiatric diagnoses of the aforementioned clinical studies. The high variability among the studies within each category is immediately apparent. One source for this variability, which is common in any comparison of psychiatric classification, is the variability in the sample's characteristics. Indeed, how can we compare "situational" addicts in the military (cf. Robins, 1974) who have been prescreened for serious mental problems to suburban addicts for whom addiction may be only the presenting problem. However, an additional source of variability across the studies may be attributed to the manner in which the MMPI was used as a diagnostic tool. The first cause for this kind of variability lies in the manner in which the invalid cases were handled. In some studies only valid cases were included in the sample; in others, they were reported but not counted as part of the sample; and in still another group of studies, the invalid cases were included in the sample. Furthermore, a confusion exists as to the method of selecting valid cases. Another cause for the variability of the diagnoses across the studies is the use of different procedures for categorizing the MMPI profiles (cf. Glueck and Stroebel, 1969). In the 10 clinical studies reported in Table 1, six different classification procedures were used.

Table 1

MMPI Diagnoses of Narcotic Addicts

Study	Sample	Classification method	No. invalid cases	% unclassified	% normal	% sociopath	% neurosis	% psychosis/ schizoid
			Clinical Studies					
Black (1975)	100 enlisted men, heroin users	Meehl (1956)	10	26	21	21	9	23
Hampton and Vogel (1973)	101 enlisted men, heroin users	Meehl (1956)	10	23	39	26	1	11
Hill et al. (1960)	200 male narcotic addicts at Lexington	Authors' classification	21	15	6	43	19	17
Koslowsky and Deren (1975)	2,179 narcotic addicts in treatment	16PF *Rp* correlations		71	6	8	8	7
Ludenia (1973)	759 drug abusers from various agencies	Author's classification	111	27	13	17	6	37
Olson (1964)	60 males, mostly narcotic addicts	Hill et al. (1960)		12	8	38	22	20
	60 female addicts in treatment	Hill et al. (1960)		13	8	50	17	12
Schooff and Keegan (1975)[a]	81 "streetwise" polydrug abusers in treatment	Goldberg (1972)		–	13	37	14	31
Sheppard et al. (1972)	336 male narcotic addicts committed to treatment	Gilberstadt and Duker (1965); Marks and Seeman (1963)		2[b]	6	38	16	38

Sheppard et al. (1973b)	74 "suburban" narcotic addicts	Dahlstrom and Welsh (1960)	–	–	23	7	70
Sutker (1971)	40 male narcotic addicts in treatment	Meehl (1956)	–	12	50	15	23
	40 male nonaddicts, prisoners		–	42	30	5	23
		Analytic Studies[c]					
Berzins et al. (1974)	750 male narcotic addicts at Lexington	Cluster analysis	62	–	9	–	29[d]
	750 female narcotic addicts at Lexington	Cluster analysis	57	–	43	–	–
Collins et al. (1976)	59 male narcotic addicts in a VA hospital	Q-type factor analysis	38	26	15	–	21
Die (1974)	209 male narcotic addicts at Lexington	Cluster analysis	51	–	14	–	34[d]
Hill et al. (1962)	594 male alcoholics, narcotic addicts, and prisoners	Rectangular factor analysis	24	11	41	13	11

[a] 5% of the sample is unaccounted for.
[b] Organic involvement.
[c] Categories assigned by Goldberg procedure (1972).
[d] *T* score of *L* Scale was not available; assumed to be $\geqslant 47$.

One more problem unique to the use of MMPI among drug addicts in treatment was identified by Henriques, Cutter, Arsenian, and Samaraweera (1972). Henriques and his colleagues found some confusion among their subjects regarding the manner in which the MMPI items should have been answered. Some subjects answered the items on the basis of recalling their psychological state under the influence of drugs, others considered their state prior to their drug use, and some responded according to their state as rehabilitated, drug-free individuals. Finally, the psychopathic deviate scale (*Pd*) is especially biased against the addict. Visible street addicts are likely to be arrested, to be in discord with their families, and to have unsteady employment records, simply because of their addiction. All these issues will cause an unfavorable *Pd* score. In view of these factors, it seems that clear guidelines and even modified instructions for the use of MMPI among addicts are needed.

All in all, it may be concluded that so far the use of the MMPI as an alternative to the psychiatric interview has failed to give a clear description of the psychopathologies to be found among narcotic addicts.

While the aforementioned studies attempted to classify drug addicts into categories which had been defined a priori, other investigators attempted to delineate via MMPI profiles "natural" groups of drug addicts (cf. Lorr, 1976).

Hill, Haertzen, and Davis (1962) reported the first study in which this approach was applied. They submitted MMPI profiles of addicts, alcoholics, and prisoners to a rectangular factor analysis and obtained five factors. By assigning each individual profile to one of the first three valid factors they obtained five different types of subjects. Through the observation of the averaged profile of each type they identified the different types as (1) undifferentiated psychopath, (2) primary psychopath, (3) neurotic psychopath (depressed), (4) neurotic psychopath (hypomanic), and (5) schizoid psychopath (nonhypomanic). Nevertheless, when Hill et al.'s (1962) labels for their types are compared to the diagnosis of these types according to the Goldberg (1972) method for classifying MMPI profiles, it seems that Hill et al.'s labels are biased and based on a preconceived notion that all drug addicts are psychopaths (see Table 1: Analytical Studies). Berzins, Ross, English, and Haley (1974) applied cluster anlaysis to 1,500 MMPI profiles of narcotic addicts and obtained two homogeneous and replicable clusters and a group of unclustered profiles. Their first cluster was characterized by distress, nonconformity, and disturbed thinking. The second type presented themselves as "adequate," poised, untroubled, and outgoing. Berzins et al. demonstrated the internal validity of their types by comparing them on an additional set of psychometric measures. Die (1974) replicated Berzins et al.'s study by employing two different clustering techniques in another sample of narcotic addicts with similar findings. Collins, Burger, and Taylor (1976) submitted 59 MMPI profiles to a Q-type factor analysis and obtained eight types, of which three were valid.

It is of interest to note that in spite of the high variability in the samples' characteristics and statistical techniques, as well as the fact that not all the MMPI scales were used in all studies, the profiles of the comparable clusters were highly similar. (The median Pearson correlation among the MMPI profiles of the "healthy" types is .79 [$p < .01$], and among the "sick" types it is .87 [$p < .01$]).

The findings of the analytic studies further support the concept that different clinical groups exist among narcotic addicts. Nevertheless, some issues should be considered in further use of these techniques. In regard to Q-type factor analysis, it may be argued (Cattell, 1970b, p. 41) that it generates pure dimensions rather than groupings of people. Furthermore, factor analysis of MMPI profiles is affected by item overlap, namely the use of one item in more than one scale (Farley and Cohen, 1974; Shure and Rogers, 1965). Another concern in the use of cluster analysis is that it generates low-coverage classifications (Blashfield and Draguns, 1976), so that large portions of the samples remain unclassified (see Table 1: Analytic Studies). It is quite possible that the use of fewer MMPI scales will generate distinct groups with a smaller portion of unclassified subjects (cf. Sines, 1976). Furthermore, the comparison of the clusters on additional variables, such as pattern of substance abuse and life histories, may be useful in understanding the underlying nature of the types.

OTHER ATTEMPTS

This section reviews additional classifications that do not fit any of the previous categories.

The first study in this group is that of Keup (1972), who focused on the interaction of psychosis and drug addiction. On the basis of psychiatric data on 160 drug addicts, Keup classified addicts into five major groups. His first group included addicts whose main symptom was addiction without any trace of endogeneous psychosis, while addicts in the second group had few negligible psychotic symptoms. For these two groups of addicts, Keup suggested treatment only for the addiction. The third group, on the other hand, included patients in whom both addiction and psychosis were present, and both conditions required treatment. The fourth group was characterized by addiction as a symptom for underlying psychosis. For this group of addicts, Keup recommended antipsychotic treatment with gradual introduction of treatment for addiction. The last group included patients with florid psychosis and addiction. Keup argued that the addicts in this group did not (or not yet) fit addiction treatment and that the psychosis should be treated first. The finding that 46% of Keup's sample belonged to one of the last three categories may suggest that about half of drug addicts in general suffer from psychosis. Nevertheless, while most of Keup's patients had some experience with narcotics, very few of them were actually narcotic addicts.

Another approach to the documentation of psychopathology among drug addicts is to identify their psychiatric symptoms without making a formal psychiatric diagnosis. Such an approach, which may be utilized in treatment planning and treatment evaluation, has been employed by Schooff and Keegan (1975), who used the Symptom Checklist 90 (SCL-90: Derogatis, Lipman, and Covi, 1973).

Very few psychiatric classifications of drug addicts have been reported outside of the United States. In Sweden, Holmberg and Jansson (1968) classified 114 addicts (13% narcotic addicts) as asthenic addicts, addicts with schizothymic attitude, addicts with hysteroid attitude, and addicts with psychoinfantile attitude. In Australia, B.J. Phillips, I.F. Phillips, and Davidson (1975) compared 30 adolescent female delinquent drug users to a comparable group of nonuser delinquents. The psychiatric categories included projection tendencies, ruminative traits, schizoid traits, and sociopathic traits. All these characteristics differentiated significantly between the drug user and nonuser samples.

In France, Seibel (1976) classified a sample of 29 drug addicts as psychopaths, psychotics, neurotics, and addicts without definite diagnosis. It is of interest to note that 65% of the 20 narcotic addicts in the sample were diagnosed as psychopaths.

OVERVIEW

One Diagnosis for All Narcotic Addicts?

Table 2 summarizes the psychiatric diagnoses reported by the studies which are reviewed here. The various diagnoses were grouped into four major categories: normal personality, personality disorders, neurosis, and psychosis. Diagnoses which did not fit into any of these categories were placed under "others," with a footnote to indicate the specific nature of the group. The reader should note that the grouping of such varied psychiatric conditions is bound to be somewhat subjective. In addition, the reader should keep in mind that, while all the samples in Table 2 relate to narcotic addicts, most of the investigators have used the term "narcotic addict" rather loosely and without giving clear definitions or detailed criteria for this term.

The first noticeable finding in Table 2 is that the frequencies of the various diagnoses vary dramatically among the studies. This variability may be attributed to the following factors: (1) variability in the samples' characteristics, as well as intentional and unintentional preselection processes; (2) differences among the studies in the categories which have been used in the various classification systems, as well as the less-than-ideal reliability of the psychiatric diagnosis in general; (3) differences among investigators in their biases toward the narcotic addict (Clausen, 1957, p. 45); (4) historical changes in the public attitude toward addiction, as well as fluctuations in the availability of heroin; (5) possible historical changes in the manifestations of psychopathology across generations (cf. Schimel, Salzman, Chodoff, Grinker, and Will, 1973).

In spite of the high variability among studies, some general conclusions may still be drawn from Table 2. The most obvious conclusion is that there is no single psychiatric diagnosis that fits all narcotic addicts. Nevertheless, character disorders, especially in the area of antisocial behavior, are found in almost all the studies and in high frequencies (range = 0-93%; median = 57%; semi-interquartile range [Q] = 22). However, it should be noted that these high frequencies indicate merely a co-occurrence of addiction and antisocial behavior rather than a cause-and-effect relation. Thus, some narcotic addicts may develop antisocial characteristics during their course of addiction, others may be criminals who have become addicted to heroin because of its high availability in the underworld circles (cf. Greenberg and Adler, 1974), while still others may be individuals who express their antisocial characteristics by being addicts. In addition, it should be noted that this diagnosis has the highest dispersion across studies, possibly indicating the wide variability of investigator bias on the relationship between addiction and antisocial behavior.

Psychoses, most often schizophrenia, is the second most frequent diagnosis (range = 0-48%; median = 7.5%; Q = 9.2). In general, this diagnosis is frequently reported by investigators with psychoanalytic orientation (Chein, Gerard, Lee, and Rosenfeld, 1964; Gerard and Kornetsky, 1955; Kaufman, 1974) and among adolescents and individuals from high socioeconomic backgrounds. Furthermore, there is a negative correlation between the sample size and its percentage of psychoses, indicating that as the number of cases in the sample decreases, the percentage of psychoses in the sample tends to increase. Thus it is possible that a high percentage of psychoses in a sample may reflect a sample bias or an investigator bias. It is of interest to note that the prevalence of psychoses among addicts at Lexington has been almost constantly reported as 2% (Pescor, 1939; Pfeffer and Ruble, 1946; Vogel, 1951); although this is somewhat higher than the rate of psychosis in the general population (cf. Babigian, 1975; Gruenberg and Turns, 1975), it is still low. In addition, Vaillant (1966) noticed that although 7% of his sample of addicts were diagnosed as schizophrenic at some time in their past and an additional 14% were diagnosed as schizoids, only 1% of his sample appeared to fulfill the diagnostic criteria of schizophrenia at a 12-year follow-up. This, as well as other findings, led Vaillant to conclude that the "apparent relationship between schizophrenia and addiction was evanescent" (p. 605). Another point of interest is that among narcotic addicts schizophrenia is more prevalent among individuals with high socioeconomic status than among those with low socioeconomic status, while the opposite is true in the general population (Lewis, 1978).

Table 2

Psychiatric Diagnoses of Narcotic Addicts

Study	Sample characteristics	% normal	% others	% character disorder	% neurosis	% psychosis
Chambers et al. (1970)	54 White female narcotic addicts at Lexington Hospital	–	2	85	4	9
	37 Black female narcotic addicts at Lexington Hospital	–	–	92	–	8
Chein et al. (1964)	20 adolescent female narcotic addicts at Riverside Hospital	–	–	60	–	40
Gerard and Kornetsky (1955)	30 adolescent male narcotic addicts at Lexington Hospital	–	–	53	–	47
	23 adolescent males, control group	43	–	9	26	22
Hekimian and Gershon (1968)	22 narcotic addicts at Bellevue Hospital	–	–	73	14[a]	14
Kaufman (1974)	23 high and middle SES opiate users in private treatment	9	–	26	17	48
	94 drug abusers referred for diagnosis	40	–	24	10	25
	705 low SES methadone patients	89[b]	2[c]	3	3	3
Kolb (1925)	230 male (?) narcotic addicts from all over U.S.	14	22[c]	51	14	–
Ling et al. (1973)	60 male veterans in treatment for narcotic addiction	53	32[c,d,e]	30	–	–

Messinger and Zitrin (1965)	6,039 narcotic addicts convicted of a major crime	0.65	55.10[f]	44.70	0.03	–
	16,236 nonaddicts convicted of a major crime	7.40	73.70[f]	14.40	0.70	2.50
Pescor (1939)	1,036 male narcotic addicts at Lexington	4	22[c]	66	6	2
Shultz (1930)	318 male narcotic addicts at Bellevue Hospital	13	6[e]	80	–	0.3
Smith et al. (1966)	100 narcotic addicts at Lexington	4	1	90	3	2
Weissman (1970)	26 male narcotic addicts in treatment	–	46[g]	54	–	–
Wieland and Tislow (1971)	126 narcotic addicts in a methadone clinic	49	33[h]	–	–	18
Willis (1969)	58 British narcotic addicts in treatment	–	–	93	–	7
	49 American narcotic addicts in treatment	–	–	90	–	10

[a] Including "depression and others."
[b] Including 87% not referred for psychiatric diagnosis.
[c] Alcoholism and other non-narcotic drug dependencies.
[d] Including 8% for whom no diagnosis was made; the total in this study is more than 100% due to multiple diagnosis.
[e] Homosexualism.
[f] Including "minor character disorders" and mental deficiency.
[g] Depression–unspecified.
[h] Borderline state.

The category of "no psychiatric diagnosis" or "normal" is quite infrequent in Table 2 (range = 0-89%; median = 4%; Q = 13.4), and in almost half of the studies its frequency is null. Therefore it is of interest to note that the second highest percentage in this category (53%) was reported by the only study (Ling, Holmes, Post, and Litaker, 1973) in which a reliable diagnostic mechanism (Feighner, Robins, Guze, Woodruff, Winokur, and Munoz, 1972) was used. Nevertheless, it is not clear whether this high proportion of normal addicts is the result of the diagnostic mechanism or the sample characteristics.

Neurosis is the least frequent diagnosis among narcotic addicts (range = 0-26%; median = 1.6%; Q = 4), and its frequencies across studies are the least dispersed.

Another point of interest is the differences between Table 1 and Table 2. Such a comparison indicates that in contrast to psychiatric evaluation, the MMPI-based diagnosis is less likely to implicate sociopathy and more likely to implicate psychosis, neurosis, and normal personality.

Is the Narcotic Addict "Different"?

The only study that compared the psychiatric diagnosis of narcotic addicts and nonaddicted controls is that of Gerard and Kornetsky (1955). They found that the adolescent narcotic abuser is more likely to have a psychiatric diagnosis than his non-heroin-abusing counterpart. Although these findings cannot be generalized because of the study's methodological limitations (Lindesmith, 1968; pp. 164-166), the data in Table 2 tend to support the impression that there are more disturbed people among narcotic addicts than in the general population. However, this impression is probably exaggerated for several reasons. First, epidemiological studies indicate that even in the general population, only about 18% are diagnosed as "well" or symptom-free (Leighton, Harding, Macklin, Macmillan, and Leighton, 1963; Srole, Langner, Michael, Opler, and Rennie, 1962). Second, all the diagnostic studies which are reviewed here are limited as to a special kind of addict, namely the institutionalized addict. Third, when the addict appears for his psychiatric evaluation, it can be assumed that his style and level of functioning leave much to be desired for him. Fourth, an addict in treatment is likely to exaggerate his emotional problems in order to obtain sympathy or other benefits, and in order to rationalize to the psychiatrist, as well as to himself, why he has become an addict. Fifth, even after his physiological withdrawal is over, the addict in treatment has to readjust to normal daily living, a state he has not experienced in several years. Naturally, this process of readjustment may involve some emotional stress that may affect the addict's diagnostic process—the labeling criteria and conclusions. Thus, it is quite possible that from a psychiatric point of view, once the addict readjusts to a drug-free life-style he is not so different from the average person. A strong statement on this issue was made by a previous director of the National Institute of Mental Health who claimed that "it had become clear that conventional concepts of normality and abnormality in relation to personality characteristics did not appear to apply to addicts, at least not without considerable qualification" (Felix, 1978, p. 8).

Nevertheless, even if the impression that the addict is more disturbed than the "average person" is accepted as valid, what does it mean? Lindesmith (1968) discusses this issue by using an analogy. Suppose, argues Lindesmith, in studying the personality types of individuals with venereal disease one finds that in this group, personality types are distributed differently than in the general population. In this case, continues Lindesmith, "one does not speak of a predisposing personality type as a cause of venereal disease, but it would certainly be relevant in a consideration of exposure to the disease. Personality influences may well operate in a similar selective manner in the case of exposure to addiction" (p. 172). The reader should keep in mind that one doesn't realistically suffer exposure to addiction; the exposure is or may be to specific drugs, drug use, or a drug-oriented life-style. Thus, it seems that psychopathology may be at best only one factor, among many others, in the etiology of addiction or drug use.

The Use of Psychiatric Diagnosis

The two most important uses of psychiatric diagnosis are for planning treatment and predicting outcomes. Thus, it is surprising how little attention has been given to these issues in studies of the psychiatric diagnosis of narcotic addicts. An extensive literature search on the use of psychiatric classification in prediction of treatment for narcotic addiction has failed to identify any study on the subject. The only reference on this issue is Winick's observation (1957) that "the psychiatric classification of the addict does not determine the progress of his addiction. A patient with a severe character disorder may recover from an addiction in a short time, while a patient with a mild neurosis may be unable to stop taking drugs" (p. 20). Thus, it seems that existing research has failed to demonstrate the utility of psychiatric diagnosis in the treatment of the narcotic addict. Furthermore, some investigators even argue that the mere labeling of the addict is not only useless but may be harmful (cf. Szasz, 1961; J.R. Williams, 1976). Undoubtedly, extensive research on the use of psychiatric diagnosis among narcotic addicts is urgently needed. Such research, however, should avoid the common pitfalls in addiction research (cf. Nathan and Lansky, 1975; Sadava, 1975).

One possible way to respond to some of the criticism against the psychiatric classification of narcotic addicts is by developing a meta-classification of narcotic addicts in which the use of psychiatric classification is restricted to a specific group of addicts.

This model—which follows some concepts of R.H. Williams (1953) and Keup (1972) as well as the multiaxial scheme of the current *Diagnostic and Statistical Manual of Mental Disorders* (American Psychiatric Association, 1978)—suggests that addicts should be classified first on the basis of the interdependency of addiction and psychopathology. Thus, it is possible to categorize narcotic addicts into three major groups: (1) normal individuals who happened to become addicted to narcotics; (2) emotionally or mentally disturbed individuals who happened to become addicts, but for whom addiction and psychopathology are two independent entities that happened to occur in the same individual; (3) finally, individuals whose addiction and psychopathology are interwoven with one another and with one reinforcing the other. While further theoretical formulations of this model, as well as the operational definitions of the groups, are beyond the scope of this article, the model has direct implications for further classifications of addicts and their treatment. Thus, addicts whose addiction is independent of psychopathology (Groups 1 and 2) may be classified further on the basis of their cultural, ideological, social, and personal characteristics (cf. Bejerot, 1972; Braucht, 1973; Brotman and Freedman, 1968; Cohen, 1977; Flanzer and Aprill, 1977; Nurco and Lerner, 1974; Stimson, 1973, and Zinberg, 1967), while the emotionally handicapped addicts (Group 3) may be classified on the basis of their psychiatric diagnosis. Similarly, treatment for the psychopathology-free addiction may be different from treatment for the psychopathology-dependent addiction.

The preceding model has several implications for policy planning, treatment sites, and staff training. Thus, a drug user who applies for treatment should receive a thorough evaluation on his medical, psychiatric, psychological, and social status. Such an evaluation may take place in a central intake facility and should include a medical and psychiatric examination, a personality assessment, an evaluation of the applicant's social network, his coping skills, his educational and vocational needs, his work habits, the nature and extent of his involvement in illegal activities, and his previous treatment experience as well as evaluations on many other aspects of his life. On the basis of such an evaluation the applicant may then be referred to a psychiatric ward in a general hospital, a psychiatric hospital, an outpatient methadone maintenance clinic (with or without psychotherapy), to a rehabilitation center or a therapeutic community, or to any other public or private, inpatient or outpatient treatment program which is suitable to his therapeutic needs. Thus, the evaluation process, including psychiatric diagnosis, will determine if the applicant needs an available treatment and how likely he is to use it effectively. Needless to say, such a variety of treatment facilities and treatment needs requires a staff from various disciplines and with high diversity of training and backgrounds.

CONCLUSION

A thorough review of the literature on psychiatric classification of narcotic addicts indicates that the theoretical psychiatric classifications have not stimulated empirical research. Empirical psychiatric classifications, on the other hand, seem to be used as an end to themselves or as a means for the diagnostician to justify his preconceived notions on narcotic addicts. Furthermore, psychiatric classification by its very nature tends to focus on pathology rather than helping us to better understand who the addict is as a person, what his relevant support systems and social networks are, and what his therapeutic needs are. In addition, rarely have psychiatric classifications been used for treatment planning, collecting baseline data, or for the development of treatment techniques or criteria for treatment success and failure. Thus it seems that the empirical psychiatric classifications have not, as yet, made any significant practical or theoretical contributions to the substance abuse research.

Menninger (1963), in his discussion on the "urge to classify," describes a little girl playing in one of the many dry river beds in central Arizona, classifying and reclassifying the many attractive pebbles around her. Investigators who insist on a mere psychiatric classification of narcotic addicts with no regard to its therapeutic implications or to the addicts' psychosocial characteristics, are, just like Menninger's little girl, playing the classification game.

ACKNOWLEDGMENTS

The preparation of this paper was supported by National Institute on Drug Abuse grant number 1 H81 DA 01864 under the directorship of Harriet L. Barr at Eagleville Hospital and Rehabilitation Center, Eagleville, Pennsylvania. The author gratefully acknowledges the assistance of M. Dichter Harrison in the preparation of this manuscript and the skillful typing of Aileen Q. Wietstruk, as well as the cooperation of many librarians in the Greater Philadelphia area.

REFERENCES

AMERICAN PSYCHIATRIC ASSOCIATION. Task Force on Nomenclature and Statistics. *Diagnostic and Statistical Manual of Mental Disorders (DSM-III Draft)*, first printing. Washington, DC: Author, 1978.

BABIGIAN, H.M. Schizophrenia: Epidemiology. In A.M. Freedman, H.I. Kaplan, and B.J. Sadock (eds.), *Comprehensive Textbook of Psychiatry. II*, Vol. 1, 2nd ed. Baltimore: Williams and Wilkins, 1975.

BEJEROT, N. *Addiction: An Artificially Induced Drive.* Springfield, IL: C.C. Thomas, 1972.

BERZINS, J.I., ROSS, W.F., ENGLISH, G.E., and HALEY, J.V. Subgroups among opiate addicts: A typological investigation. *J. Abnorm. Psychol.* 83: 65-73, 1974.

BLACK, W.F. Personality characteristics of Viet Nam veterans identified as heroin abusers. *Am. J. Psychiatry* 132: 748-749, 1975.

BLASHFIELD, R.K., and DRAGUNS, J.G. Evaluative criteria for psychiatric classification. *J. Abnorm. Psychol.* 85: 140-150, 1976.

BRAUCHT, G.N. A psychosocial typology of adolescent alcohol and drug users. In M.E. Cafetz (ed.), *Alcoholism: A Multilevel Problem. Treatment, Organization and Management.* Proceedings of the Third Annual Alcoholism Conference of the National Institute on Alcohol and Alcoholism. Rockville, MD: National Institute on Alcohol Abuse and Alcoholism, 1973, pp. 129-144.

BROTMAN, R., and FREEDMAN, A. *A Community Mental Health Approach to Drug Addiction* (Office of Juvenile Delinquency and Youth Development, J.D. Publ. No. 9005). Washington, DC: United States Government Printing Office, 1968.

CATTELL, R.B. *Handbook for the Sixteen Personality Factor Questionnaire.* Champaign, IL: Institute For Personality and Ability Testing, 1970(a).

CATTELL, R.B. The integration of functional and psychometric requirements in a quantitative and computerized diagnostic system. In A.R. Mahrer (ed.), *New Approaches to Personality Classification.* New York: Columbia University Press, 1970(b).

CHAMBERS, C.D., HINESLEY, R.K., and MOLDESTAD, M. Narcotic addiction in females: A race comparison. *Int. J. Addict.* 5: 257-278, 1970.

CHEIN, I., GERARD, D.L., LEE, R.S., and ROSENFELD, E. *The Road to H.* New York: Basic Books, 1964.

CLAUSEN, J.A. Social and psychological factors in narcotics addiction. *Law Contemp. Probl.* 22: 34-51, 1957.

COHEN, A. *A psychosocial typology of drug addicts.* Paper presented at the National Drug Abuse Conference, San Francisco, May 1977.

COHEN, A. The "Urge to Classify" the narcotic addict: A review of psychiatric classification. I. *Int. J. Addict.* 17: 213-225, 1982.

COLLINS, H.A., BURGER, G.K., and TAYLOR, G.A. An empirical typology of heroin abusers. *J. Clin. Psychol.* 32: 473-476, 1976.

DAHLSTROM, W.G., and WELSH, G.S. *An MMPI Handbook: A Guide to Use in Clinical Practice and Research.* Minneapolis: University of Minnesota Press, 1960.

DEROGATIS, L.R., LIPMAN, R.S., and COVI, L. SCL-90: An outpatient psychiatric rating scale–Preliminary report. *Psychopharmacol. Bull.* 9: 13-17, 1973.

DIE, J.G. The application of cluster analysis to the development of a typology of narcotic addicts (Doctoral Dissertation, University of Houston, 1973). *Diss. Abstr. Int.* 34: 4037B, 1974 (University Microfilms No. 74-2872).

FARLEY, F.H., and COHEN, A. Common-item effects and the smallest space analysis of structure. *Psychol. Bull.* 81: 766-772, 1974.

FEIGHNER, J.P., ROBINS, E., GUZE, S.B., WOODRUFF, R.A. Jr., WINOKUR, G., and MUNOZ, R. Diagnostic criteria for use in psychiatric research. *Arch. Gen. Psychiatry* 26: 57-63, 1972.

FELIX, R.H. Psychiatric, psychological, and epidemiological aspects of drug dependence: Status prior to 1944. In W.R. Martin and H. Isbell (eds.), *Drug Addiction and the U.S. Public Health Service.* Rockville, MD: National Institute on Drug Abuse, U.S. Department of Health, Education, and Welfare, 1978.

FLANZER, J.P., and APRILL, F.A. A diagnostic-treatment model for effective group treatment of drug abusers. *J. Psychedelic Drugs* 9: 143-150, 1977.

GENDREAU, P., and GENDREAU, L.P. A theoretical note on personality characteristics of heroin addicts. *J. Abnorm. Psychol.* 82: 139-140, 1973.

GERARD, D.L., and KORNETSKY, C. Adolescent opiate addiction: A study of control and addict subjects. *Psychiatr. Q.* 29: 457-486, 1955.

GILBERSTADT, H., and DUKER, J. *A Handbook for Clinical and Actuarial MMPI Interpretation.* Philadelphia: W.B. Saunders, 1965.

GLUECK, B.C. Jr., and STROEBEL, C.F. The computer and clinical decision process. II. *Am. J. Psychiatry* 125: Suppl., 2-7, 1969.

GOLDBERG, L.R. Man versus mean: The exploitation of group profiles for the construction of diagnostic classification system. *J. Abnorm. Psychol.* 79: 121-131, 1972.

GREENBERG, S.W., and ADLER, F. Crime and addiction: An empirical analysis of the literature, 1920-1973. *Contemp. Drug Probl.* 3: 221-270, 1974.

GRUENBERG, E.M., and TURNS, D.M. Epidemology. In A.M. Freedman, H.I. Kaplan, and B.J. Sadock (eds.), *Comprehensive Textbook of Psychiatry. II.*, Vol. 1, 2nd ed. Baltimore: Williams and Wilkins, 1975.

HAMPTON, P.T., and VOGEL, D.B. Personality characteristics of servicemen returned from Viet Nam identified as heroin abusers. *Am. J. Psychiatry* 130: 1031-1032, 1973.

HATHAWAY, S.R. A coding system for MMPI profiles. *J. Consult. Psychol.* 11: 334-337, 1947.

HEKIMIAN, L.J., and GERSHON, S. Characteristics of drug abusers admitted to a psychiatric hospital. *J. Am. Med. Assoc.* 205: 125-130, 1968.

HENRIQUES, E., CUTTER, H., ARSENIAN, J., and SAMARAWEERA, A.B. Personality characteristics and drugs of choice. *Int. J. Addict.* 7: 73-76, 1972.

HILL, H.E., HAERTZEN, C.A., and DAVIS, H. An MMPI factor analytic study of alcoholics, narcotic addicts and criminals. *Q. J. Stud. Alcohol* 23: 411-431, 1962.

HILL, H.E., HAERTZEN, C.A., and GLASER, R. Personality characteristics of narcotic addicts as indicated by the MMPI. *J. Gen. Psychol.* 62: 127-139, 1960.

HOLMBERG, M.B., and JANSSON, B. Experiences from an out-patient department for drug addicts in Göteborg. *Acta Psychiatr. Scand.* 44: 172-189, 1968.

KAUFMAN, E. The psychodynamics of opiate dependence: A new look. *Am. J. Drug Alcohol Abuse* 1: 349-370, 1974.

KEUP, W. Differences in therapy for drug users according to their motive for abuse. In W. Keup (ed.), *Drug Abuse: Current Concepts and Research.* Springfield, IL: C.C. Thomas, 1972.

KOLB, L. Types and characteristics of drug addicts. *Ment. Hyg.* 9: 300-313, 1925.

KOSLOWSKY, M., and DEREN, S. A comparison of three procedures for classifying addicts (extended report). *J. Consult. Clin. Psychol.* 43: 433, 1975.

LEIGHTON, D.C., HARDING, J.S., MACKLIN, D., MACMILLAN, A.M., and LEIGHTON, A.H. *The Character of Danger: Psychiatric Symptoms in Selected Communities*, Vol. 3: *The Sterling County Study of Psychiatric Disorder and Socio-Cultural Environment.* New York: Basic Books, 1963.

LEWIS, M.S. Nearest neighbor analysis of epidemiological and community variables. *Psychol. Bull.* 85: 1302-1308, 1978.

LINDESMITH, A.R. *Addiction and Opiates.* Chicago: Aldine, 1968.

LING, W., HOLMES, E.D., POST, G.R., and LITAKER, M.B. A systematic psychiatric study of the heroin addicts. In *Proceedings of the 5th National Conference on Methadone Treatment*, 1973, pp. 429-432.

LORR, M. Cluster and typological analysis. In P.M. Bentler, D.J. Lettieri, and G.A. Austin (eds.), *Data Analysis Strategies and Designs for Substance Abuse Research* (NIDA Research Isseus No. 13, Stock No. 017-024-00562-2). Washington, DC: U.S. Government Printing Office, 1976.

LUDENIA, K. Personality characteristics of drug abusers (Doctoral Dissertation, University of Missouri-Columbia, 1972). *Diss. Abstr. Int.* 33: 6063B, 1973. (University Microfilms No. 73-7056).

MARKS, P.A., and SEEMAN, W. *An Atlas for Use with the MMPI: Actuarial Description of Abnormal Personality.* Baltimore: Williams and Wilkins, 1963.

MEEHL, P.E. Profile analysis of the MMPI in differential diagnosis. In G.S. Welsh and W.G. Dahlstrom (eds.), *Basic Readings on the MMPI in Psychology and Medicine.* Minneapolis: University of Minnesota Press, 1956.

MENNINGER, K., with MAYMAN, M., and PRUYSER, P. *The Vital Balance: The Life Process in Mental Health and Illness.* New York: Viking Press, 1963.

MESSINGER, E., and ZITRIN, A. A statistical study of criminal drug addicts. *Crime Delinquency* 11: 283-292, 1965.

NATHAN, P.E., and LANSKY, D. Common methodological problems in research on the addictions. *J. Consult. Clin. Psychol.* 46: 713-726, 1975.

NURCO, D.N., and LERNER, M. Occupational skills and life-styles of narcotic addicts. In C. Winick (ed.), *Sociological Aspects of Drug Dependence.* Cleveland: CRC Press, 1974.

OLSON, R.W. MMPI sex differences in narcotic addicts. *J. Gen. Psychol.* 71: 257-266, 1964.

PENK, W.E., and ROBINOWITZ, R. Personality differences of volunteer and nonvolunteer heroin and nonheroin drug users. *J. Abnorm. Psychol.* 85: 91-100, 1976.

PESCOR, M.J. The Kolb classification of drug addicts. *Public Health Rep.* Suppl. No. 155: 1-10, 1939.

PFEFFER, A.Z., and RUBLE, D.C. Chronic psychoses and addiction to morphine. *Arch. Neurol. Psychiatry* 56: 665-672, 1946.

PHILLIPS, B.J., PHILLIPS, I.F., and DAVIDSON, E.C. Juvenile delinquent drug abuse in females: A clinical study. *Aust. N. Z. J. Psychiatry* 9: 281-286, 1975.

ROBINS, L. *The Viet Nam Drug User Returns* (Special Action Office Monogr. Ser. A, No. 2). Washington, DC: U.S. Government Printing Office, 1974.

SADAVA, S.W. Research approaches to illicit drug use: A critical review. *Genet. Psychol. Monogr.* 91: 3-59, 1975.

SCHIMEL, J.L., SALZMAN, L., CHODOFF, D., GRINKER, R.R. Sr., and WILL, O.A. Jr. Changing styles in psychiatric syndromes: A symposium. *Am. J. Psychiatry* 130: 146-155, 1973.

SCHOOFF, K.G., and KEEGAN, J.F. *Profiles of prescription medication abusers.* Report to the Committee on Problems of Drug Dependence, National Academy of Sciences, May 21, 1975.

SEIBEL, S.D. Quelques aspects psychiatriques des toxicomanies modernes. *Ann. Med. Psychol.* 134 II: 300-309, 1976.

SHEPPARD, C., FRACCHIA, J., RICCA, E., and MERLIS, S. Indications of psychopathology in male narcotic abusers, their effects and relation to treatment effectiveness. *J. Psychol.* 81: 351-360, 1972.

SHEPPARD, C., RICCA, E., FRACCHIA, J., and MERLIS, S. Indications of psychopathology in applicants to a county methadone maintenance program. *Psychol. Rep.* 33: 535-540, 1973(a).

SHEPPARD, C., RICCA, E., FRACCHIA, J., and MERLIS, S. Personality characteristics of urban and suburban heroin abusers: More data and another reply to Sutker and Allain (1973). *Psychol. Rep.* 33: 999-1008, 1973(b).

SHULTZ, C. The work done in the narcotic ward at Bellevue Hospital, May 28, 1928 to May 16, 1929. *Am. J. Psychiatry* 10: 465-538, 1930.

SHURE, G.H., and ROGERS, M.S. A note of caution on the factor analysis of the MMPI. *Psychol. Bull.* 63: 14-18, 1965.

SINES, J.O. Actuarial prediction. In P.M. Bentler, D.J. Lettieri, and G.A. Austin (eds.), *Data Analysis Strategies and Designs for Substance Abuse Research* (NIDA Res. Iss. No. 13, Stock No. 017-024-00562-2). Wahsington, DC: U.S. Government Printing Office, 1976.

SMITH, W.G., ELLINWOOD, E.H. Jr., and VAILLANT, G.E. Narcotic addicts in the mid-1960's. *Public Health Rep.* 81: 403-412, 1966.

SROLE, L., LANGNER, T.S., MICHAEL, S.T., OPLER, M.K., and RENNIE, T.A.C. *Mental Health in the Metropolis*, Vol. 1: *The Midtown Manhattan Study.* New York: McGraw-Hill, 1962.

STIMSON, G.V. *Heron and Behavior: Diversity among Addicts Attending London Clinics.* New York: Wiley, 1973.

SUTKER, P.B. Personality differences and sociopathy in heroin addicts and non-addict prisoners. *J. Abnorm. Psychol.* 78: 247-251, 1971.

SUTKER, P.B. Personality characteristics of heroin addicts: A response to Gendreau and Gendreau. *J. Abnorm. Psychol.* 83: 463-464, 1974.

SUTKER, P.B., and ALLAIN, A.N. Incarcerated and street heroin addicts: A personality comparison. *Psychol. Rep.* 32: 243-246, 1973.

SZASZ, T.S. *The Myth of Mental Illness.* New York: Harper and Row, 1961.

VAILLANT, G.E. A 12-year follow-up of New York narcotic addicts. III. Some social and psychiatric characteristics. *Arch. Gen. Psychiatry* 15: 599-608, 1966.

VOGEL, V.H. Discussion. In R.G. Knight and C.T. Prout, A study of results in hospital treatment of drug addictions. *Am. J. Psychiatry* 108: 303-308, 1951.

WIELAND, W.F., and TISLOW, R.F. *Incidence and treatment of psychiatric symptoms in patients on a methadone maintenance program.* Report to the Committee on Problems of Drug Dependence, National Academy of Sciences, February 17, 1971.

WEISSMAN, S. The significance of diagnosis in the treatment of narcotics addicts. *Int. J. Addict.* 5: 717-730, 1970.

WILLIAMS, J.R. *Effects of Labeling the "Drug-Abuser": An Inquiry* (NIDA Res. Monogr. No. 6, DHEW Publ. ADM (76-320). Rockville, MD: National Institute on Drug Abuse, 1976 (NTIS No. PB 249 092).

WILLIAMS, R.H. A frame of reference of the analysis of drug behavior. In *Conferences on Drug Addiction among Adolescents.* New York: Blakiston, 1953.

WILLIS, J.H. Drug dependence: Some demographic and psychiatric aspects in U.K. and U.S. subjects. *Br. J. Addict.* 64: 135-145, 1969.

WINICK, G. Narcotic addiction and its treatment. *Law Contemp. Probl.* 22: 9-33, 1957.

ZINBERG, N.E. Facts and fancies about drug addiction. *Public Interest* 6: 75-90, 1967.

The International Journal of the Addictions, 19(3), 355–366, 1984

Note

Drug Misuse/Abuse Intervention: A Schematic Tool for Decision Making and Planning

Stanley Einstein,* PhD

Middle Eastern Summer Institute on Drug Use

Abstract

A catalytic conceptual tool is presented to facilitate the concerned reader's decision making with regard to personally developing and/or participating in more effective drug misuse/abuse intervention efforts. The reader is asked to consider and select the interface between 16 areas of potential intervention, 4 sources of drug abuse typologies, and 6 foci for intervention which is most suitable to his/her roles, skills, interests, and concerns.

Much of today's feelings of apathy, hopelessness, and ritualistic responsiveness about the growing drug problem arises from our less than clear interpretation of what the issues are. More and more people are getting used to the notion that effective combatting of drug abuse means offering viable alternatives to drug abuse. Treatment, law enforcement, and education are the primary ideologies, processes, and strategies which are currently being used.

Unfortunately, only these alternatives are being used because policymakers continue to misunderstand that there are many possible options and areas to intervention. Indeed, the use of treatment and education presumes that we have only limited ideological alternatives for the active drug user, as well as to prevent

*Address correspondence to the author at 113/41 East Talpiot, Jerusalem, Israel.

 0020-773X/84/1903-0355$3.50/0

such behavior. This is related to and reinforces the myth that there are only two types of people: drug users and nonusers.

Notwithstanding the experiences in treatment and prevention, many people continue to feel overwhelmed by the contemporary drug problem and continue to hope that the experts will take care of it. This is not because there aren't any viable solutions. More than likely the sense of not knowing what to do arises from the very framing of the question: *What are the alternatives to drug abuse?* This question is so huge in what it actually and potentially encompasses that the immediate reaction to it may be that of feeling overwhelmed. We need not, and should not succumb to this feeling.

Possible planned efforts to combat drug abuse—and the roles that we can play as professionals and citizens in these alternatives—become more obvious when we begin to pinpoint what drug abuse is or may be.

SOURCES OF TYPOLOGIES

Drug abuse is not a single entity nor a unitary concept. Indeed there are at least four sources of definitions for drug abuse. There are:

1. *Abusing drug laws and rituals*: the breaking of drug-related laws, mores, and rituals by using particular drugs in particular ways and for particular reasons
2. *Self-abuse*: the direct or indirect consequences to the person taking drugs, resulting from their use for other than medically and/or socially approved reasons, irrespective of the consequences to others in the drug user's life space
3. *Abuse of others*: the direct or indirect consequences to the people other than the drug misuser (born, unborn), resulting from the use of drugs for other than medically and/or socially approved reasons, irrespective of the consequences for the user
4. *Abuse of the ecology/environment*: the direct or indirect consequences to the macrosystem(s) in which the drug user acts/interacts, resulting from the use of drugs for approved or disapproved reasons (medically approved and/or socially approved reasons), irrespective of the consequences for the user (i.e., effects on the macrosystem's quality of life, styles of life, physical state, etc.)

Developing meaningful and workable alternatives to drug abuse begins to be possible if we note the type of drug abuse that we are considering at a given point in time.

FOCUS OF INTERVENTION

Having decided the type of drug abuse we are concerned about, the next step in developing plans and policies is to decide who is the focus of intervention. As long as we remain caught up in the stereotyped outlook that the focus of our efforts must remain with the visible drug user, his unique characteristics and behavior, and certain drugs, our plans will result in ongoing ritualized reactions. We have the choice of focusing our efforts on:

1. Drugs themselves, licit as well as illicit ones
2. Abstainers, be they individals who have never misused or used drugs, or those who have ceased their misuse
3. Active drug misusers
4. Intervention agents, be they individuals doing treatment, teachers, clergy, law enforcement representatives, parents, peers, etc.
5. The general community
6. Systems/networks

AREAS OF INTERVENTION

The next decision facing us has to do with the area of possible intervention. Now that we have decided the type of drug abuse we wish to affect, and what our primary focus is to be, we can come to terms with the direction of our efforts. Acknowledging that the directions or areas that we select are arbitrary ones, we nevertheless should consider the following potential areas:

1. Scientific knowledge
2. Personal attitudes and values
3. Cultural values
4. Semantics of drug use/abstinence
5. Treatment
6. Education
7. Law enforcement
8. Research
9. Genetics
10. Social pharmacology
11. Public policy
12. Politics
13. Economics
14. Philosophy
15. Religion
16. Media

These areas have been noted time and time again as being crucial factors in understanding drug use behavior. Unfortunately, our efforts generally start and stop with law enforcement, treatment, and education, and we pay lip service to all the others (see Table 1). It should be equally obvious that in any given community, other facets could be added.

Table 1

Drug Use: Critical Issues and Factors

Drug Use
- Type
- Frequency
- Amount
- Pattern
- Manner
- Meaning
- Place of use
- Availability
- Drug potency
- Function(s)

Characteristics of Users
- Age
- Sex
- Ethnicity/race
- Religion
- Status:
  - Educational
  - Vocational
  - Occupational
  - Marital
  - Socioeconomic
  - Medical
  - Psychological
  - Intelligence

Behavior of Users
- Physical
- Psychological
- Social functions and dysfunctions
- Conventional, deviant, and drug-oriented social involvement

Semantics of Drug Use/Abstinence
- Definitions:
  - Medical
  - Legal
  - Social
  - Religious
  - Scientific
- Street semantics
- Professional semantics
- Concepts
- Issues
- Problems

Attitudes and Values
- Drug user stereotypes
- Drug stereotypes
- Attitudes about:
  - Drug use
  - Medicines
  - Illness
  - Health
  - Treatment
  - Abstinence

Law Enforcement
- Drug-related laws
- Medication-related laws
- Social substance-related laws
- Behavior-related laws
- Control mechanisms/systems

Scientific Knowledge
- Theories about:
  - Drug use
  - Drug action
  - Treatment
  - Communication
  - Pain
  - Illness-health
  - Deviance
  - Risk taking
  - Decision making
  - Control
  - Compliance
  - Research
  - Prevention
  - Coping
  - Adaptation
  - Behavior
- Classification of:
  - Drug users
  - Drug use
  - Drugs
  - Treatment
  - Prevention
  - Research
  - Intervention agents
  - Control mechanisms

(continued)

Table 1 (continued)

Treatment
Why treat?
Site of treatment
Evaluation-screening
Goals
Treatment techniques
Strategies
Policies and procedures
Treatment roles
Ongoing evaluation
Follow-up
Early case finding
Prevention
Criteria–success/failure
Needed support system
Invervention agent
issues and patterns

Economics
Illegal facets
Legal facets
Individual factors
System factors

Public Policy
Laws
Policies
Procedures
Politics

Cultural Values
Drug related
People related
Activity related
Life-style related

Education
Non-drug-related alternatives to living
Drug-related alternatives to living
Coping/adaptational skills
Decision making
Reality-oriented life-style(s)
"Alternative" life-style(s)
Respect for:
- People
- Chemicals
- Feelings

The education agent
Community roles and
responsibilities

Genetic Aspects
Lethal/nonlethal
Drugs
Medicines
Social substances
Environmental chemicals
Individual/group

Mass Media
People-oriented patterns of living
Object-oriented patterns of living

Social Pharmacology
Substance:
- Use
- Meaning
- Distribution

Use:
- Support/inhibition factors
- Individual–future personal chemistry

Altered States of Consciousness
Drug related
Non-drug related
Individual
Group

Evaluation
Criteria
Goals
Techniques
Strategies
Utilization
Individuals
Systems
Policies

Philosophy and Religion
Non-drug-related rituals
Drug-related social rituals
Ethics

Research
Defining the problem/issue
Data:
- Collection
- Analysis
- Availability
- Utilization

Table 2

A Schema for Intervention Decision Making

Areas of intervention (I-XVI)	Focus of intervention (a-f)	Sources of drug abuse			
		Drug-related laws, mores, rituals (A)	Self-abuse (B)	Abuse of others (C)	Abuse of the ecology/environment (D)
I. Treatment (including early case finding and prevention)	a. Drugs b. Abstainers c. Drug users d. Intervention agents e. Community[a] f. Systems/networks				
II. Education	a. Drugs b. Abstainers c. Drug users d. Intervention agents e. Community f. Systems/networks				
III. Attitudes	a. Drugs b. Abstainers c. Drug users d. Intervention agents e. Community f. Systems/networks				
IV. Media	a. Drugs b. Abstainers				

	c. Drug users d. Intervention agents e. Community f. Systems/networks				
V. Culture	a. Drugs b. Abstainers c. Drug users d. Intervention agents e. Community f. Systems/networks				
VI. Religion	a. Drugs b. Abstainers c. Drug users d. Intervention agents e. Community f. Systems/networks				
VII. Laws	a. Drugs b. Abstainers c. Drug users d. Intervention agents e. Community f. Systems/networks				
VIII. Politics	a. Drugs b. Abstainers c. Drug users d. Intervention agents e. Community f. Systems/networks				

(continued)

Table 2 (continued)

Areas of intervention (I-XVI)	Focus of intervention (a-f)	Sources of drug abuse			
		Drug-related laws, mores, rituals (A)	Self-abuse (B)	Abuse of others (C)	Abuse of the ecology/environment (D)
IX. Semantics of drug use/abstinence	a. Drugs b. Abstainers c. Drug users d. Intervention agents e. Community f. Systems/networks				
X. Scientific knowledge	a. Drugs b. Abstainers c. Drug users d. Intervention agents e. Community f. Systems/networks				
XI. Research	a. Drugs b. Abstainers c. Drug users d. Intervention agents e. Community f. Systems/networks				
XII. Genetics	a. Drugs b. Abstainers c. Drug users d. Intervention agents e. Community f. Systems/networks				

XIII. Social pharmacology	a. Drugs b. Abstainers c. Drug users d. Intervention agents e. Community f. Systems/networks				
XIV. Public policies and procedures	a. Drugs b. Abstainers c. Drug users d. Intervention agents e. Community f. Systems/networks				
XV. Economics	a. Drugs b. Abstainers c. Drug users d. Intervention agents e. Community f. Systems/networks				
XVI. Philosophy	a. Drugs b. Abstainers c. Drug users d. Intervention agents e. Community f. Systems/networks				

[a] "Community" is a concept which includes the following broad range of theoretical and/or actual constituents: territorial-geographical communities, functional communities, organizational communities, belief system communities, familial communities, political communities, economic communities, mutual interdependence communities, common destiny communities, symbolic communities, and self-perception communities. The reader is asked to sharply delineate according to his/her own world view between general communities and systems/networks under the rubric of Focus of Intervention in this schema.

A conceptual tool, Table 2, was developed (based upon the factors listed in Table 1 and their implications) to enable you the reader to consider what you can and can't do, what your responsibilities and limitations are/will be for potential intervention in each derived cell. This visual schema permits us to consider how to plan effectively without becoming bogged down by the enormity of the personal task which awaits us and challenges us, and which demands a reasonable response.

This schema also clearly reminds us and points out that within a potential context of 16 areas for intervention × 6 foci of intervention × 4 sources of drug abuse, there are 384 unique cells for intervention efforts. Surely there is one cell which is suitable to each person's unique strengths, limitations, interests, available time, etc. From this perspective, drug abuse intervention can no longer be perceived as being the rightful domain of the drug abuse expert—whoever he or she is.

An analysis of the table allows us to acknowledge that *treatment, laws*, and *education* are only three of the possible options open to us as we seek to create meaningful alternatives to drug abuse. Choosing any of them is as arbitrary a decision as any other that we might make. The point is that once we have chosen a particular area based on careful thought, rather than as a panacea or total solution, we should have better results with it than has been our general experience.

For example, what alternatives are available if our concern is to use *treatment* to intervene in the *breaking of drug laws* and we focus upon *drugs*? Obviously one possibility might be to offer substitute drugs in a particular way (i.e., methadone maintenance). This increasingly acceptable treatment, hopefully, should reduce the incidence of drug-related arrests. Theoretically it can also reinforce the appropriate use of medicines and the inappropriate use of drugs, thereby possibly affecting the other two types of drug abuse, *self-abuse* and *abuse of others*.

But what if our interest or concern is to focus upon *systems/networks* in order to affect (prevent, minimize) the abuse of the ecology/environment? Our immediate and priority *areas for intervention* need not be treatment, law enforcement, and education. Indeed they should more likely be politics, religion, philosophy, or the media.

If our concern is effective intervention regarding *self-abuse* for abstainers, active drug users, or intervention agents (i.e., burn out), *personal attitudes and values, cultural values*, and *philosophy or religion* are more likely to result in desirable planned outcomes than is the individually or systemically oriented treatment process, whatever its ideological underpinnings or utilizable technologies.

Table 3

Checklist for Planning Drug Abuse Intervention Efforts

I. Selected area of intervention: ____________________

II. Selected focus of intervention: ____________________

	Types/sources of drug abuse			
Selected intervention factors	Laws, mores, rituals	Self-abuse	Abuse of others	Abuse of the ecology/ environment
1. Screening				
Needed knowledge				
Strategies				
Process				
Techniques				
Site(s)				
Staff				
2. Goals				
Initial				
Ongoing				
Termination				
Outcome				
3. Budget				
4. Policies				
5. Techniques				
Individual oriented				
System oriented				
Concept oriented				
6. Staff				
Skills				
Characteristics				
Expectations				
7. Roles				
Rights				
Responsibilities				
Obligations				
Tasks				
Activity levels				
8. Sites				
9. Temporal factors				
10. Ongoing evaluation				
Data to be collected				
Strategies				
Techniques				
Policies				
Utilization				
11. Outcome				
Criteria:				
Success				
Failure				
Data				
Temporal orientation				
Strategies				
Techniques				
Staff				
Policies				
Utilization				

If there aren't any alternatives that we and our colleagues and neighbors can come up with at a given point in time, then we can move on to areas, or cells, which permit us to effectively utilize our expertise, time, energy, and money. This type of analysis of alternatives to drug abuse is no more than a suggested approach. It is not a guide to the "dos and don'ts" of drug abuse intervention. It offers each of us a framework that we can add to or delete from, while permitting us to decide what role we can play and may choose to play in a contemporary problem area which continues to be colored by ambiguities and hysteria.

Given this type of framework it would be useful to remember that a number of important references should be utilized as we go about developing programs and policies. The notion of viable alternatives to drug abuse assumes that our efforts will meet the basic criteria of being meaningful, achievable, acceptable, and flexible. The selection of alternatives that do not meet these basic criteria dooms our efforts to failure.

Table 3 is designed as a checklist to be used by you the reader, as you go about planning a theoretical and/or practical model program for drug abuse intervention. The factors listed in this table are only the very minimal ones which demand your attention and innovativeness. Your own interests, commitments, world views, and skills will no doubt result in your adding other factors.

It would be most helpful if you would take the time to consider what you feel are some of the meaningful and achievable alternatives to drug abuse, using this kind of framework. The guiding philosophy can be "If you are not part of the solution, then you are part of the problem."

INFORMATION FOR AUTHORS SUBMITTING MANUSCRIPTS

Send a clear double-spaced typewritten original and one duplicate to Ms. Nancy Reid-Rappolt, Editorial Assistant, *International Journal of the Addictions*, c/o Winch, Smith, Ostermann and Mates, MD's, 4141 Geary, Suite 326, San Francisco, California 94118. Also send one duplicate to the Chief Editor, Dr. Stanley Einstein, Building 113/41, East Talpiot, Jerusalem, Israel. DOUBLE-SPACE the entire manuscript; do not use single spacing anywhere, including references.

Include authors' academic degrees and present affiliation. If applicable, cite auspices under which work being reported was done. Specify address to which requests for reprints should be sent.

Begin your TITLE with a word useful in indexing. A 75- to 100-word ABSTRACT should be provided, which precedes each article. A summary is then not necessary. Major and minor headings may be used in the text; indicate major headings by typing in capitals.

Use METRIC UNITS of measure. If measurements were made in English units, give metric equivalents.

Cite all TABLES and FIGURES in the text. Tables should have titles, and figures should have brief legends. In tables, give each column a heading. Indicate units of measure in parentheses in the heading for each column. Do not use vertical rules. Do not use horizontal rules other than those in the heading and at the bottom. Submit PHOTOGRAPHS as glossy prints, untrimmed and unmounted; identify each with pencil lightly on the back and indicate top.

ARTWORK will not be returned unless specifically requested, and will be disposed of three months after publication.

REFERENCES in the text should be enclosed in parentheses and include the author's surname and the date of the item cited. Keep footnotes to a minimum. Footnotes should be collected at the end of the manuscript in their numerical order of appearance.

The BIBLIOGRAPHY (double-spaced) should be given at the end of the article in alphabetical order. Journal references should include authors, title, name of journal abbreviated according to *Chemical Abstracts List of Periodicals*, inclusive page numbers, and date. Book references should include authors, title, place of publication, publisher, and date.

AUTHOR RESPONSIBILITY: It is the sole responsibility of the author(s) to obtain written permission from the author(s), publisher(s), etc. for figures, tables, or any other information excerpted from previously published works which are used in the manuscript(s) considered for publication. It is understood that the manuscript(s) considered for publication in the *International Journal of the Addictions* have not been previously published nor are they under simultaneous publication consideration elsewhere.

Statements and opinions expressed in the articles and communications herein are those of the author(s) and do not necessarily express those of the Editor or publisher.

THE INTERNATIONAL JOURNAL OF THE ADDICTIONS

Volume 19 Number 3 1984

CONTENTS

Editorial: Drug Use Intervention and Control Mechanisms: S. Einstein . . . iii

Paraprofessional Versus Professional Drug Abuse Counselors: Attitudes and Expectations of the Counselors and Their Clients: L. LoSciuto, L. S. Aiken, M. A. Ausetts, and B. S. Brown 233

Drug Taking by Nigerian Students in American Universities: Prevalences for Four Commonly Used Drugs: O. E. Achalu and D. F. Duncan . . . 253

An Empirical Examination of the Social Bond Theory of Drug Use: R. T. Dull 265

Conditioned Abstinence in Alcoholics: A Controlled Experiment: L. Eriksen and K. G. Götestam 287

The Phenomenological Structure of Drug-Induced Ego States. II. Barbiturates and Sedative-Hypnotics: Phenomenology and Implications: J. V. Spotts and F. C. Shontz 295

Smoking Cessation with Hospital Employees: An Example of Worksite Smoking Cessation: H. H. Dawley, Jr., B. J. Fleischer, and L. T. Dawley 327

The "Urge to Classify" the Narcotic Addict: A Review of Psychiatric Classification. II: A. Cohen 335

Note

Drug Misuse/Abuse Intervention: A Schematic Tool for Decision Making and Planning: S. Einstein 355

MARCEL DEKKER, INC., New York and Basel

CODEN: INJABN 19(4) i-vi, 367-478 (1984)
ISSN: 0020-773X

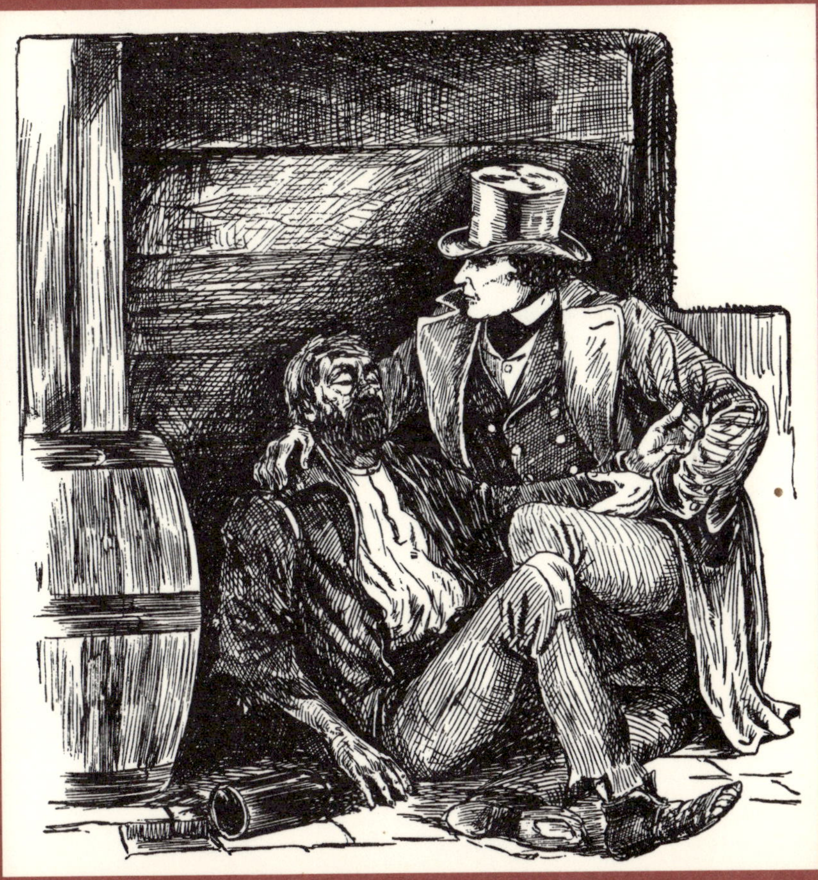

THE INTERNATIONAL JOURNAL OF THE Addictions

Volume 19 Number 4 1984

THE INTERNATIONAL JOURNAL OF THE ADDICTIONS

July 1984

Aims and Scope. This journal is a comprehensive medium for worldwide communication among both concerned laymen and professionals in research, training, and treatment in the field of addiction and substance misuse.

Indexing and Abstracting Services. Articles published in *The International Journal of the Addictions* are selectively indexed or abstracted in:

• Adolescent Mental Health Abstracts • ASCA • Bibliographic Index of Health Education Periodicals (BIHEP) • BioSciences Information Service of Biological Abstracts (BIOSIS) • Classified Abstract Archive of the Alcohol Literature • Current Contents/Clinical Practice • Excerpta Medica • Index Medicus • International Pharmaceutical Abstracts • ISI/BIOMED • Journal of Abstracts of the All-Union Institute of Scientific and Technical Information of the USSR • Psychological Abstracts • Science Citation Index • Selected List of Tables of Contents of Psychiatric Periodicals • Social Sciences Citation Index • State Central Scientific Medical Library/International Book Exchange–USSR

Articles published in *The International Journal of the Addictions* are listed in Selected List of Tables of Contents of Psychiatric Periodicals.

Manuscript Preparation and Submission. See end of issue.

Subscription Information. *The International Journal of the Addictions* (ISSN: 0020-773X) is published eight times annually in February, April, May, July, August, September, November, and December by Marcel Dekker, Inc., 270 Madison Avenue, New York, New York 10016. The subscription rate for Volume 19 (1984), containing eight numbers, is $225.00 per volume (prepaid). The special discounted rate for individual professionals and students is $112.50 per volume. To secure this special rate, your order must be prepaid by personal check. Add $20.00 for surface postage outside the United States. For airmail to Europe, add $32.48; to Asia, add $40.48.

Mailing Address. *Please mail payment with order to:* Marcel Dekker Journals, P. O. Box 11305, Church Street Station, New York, New York 10249.

Contributions to this journal are published free of charge. Second-class postage paid at New York, New York and additional mailing offices. POSTMASTER: Send address changes to *The International Journal of the Addictions*, P. O. Box 5005, Cimarron Road, Monticello, New York 12701.

Library of Congress Catalog Card Number 66-9896

Cover illustration entitled: *The Good Samaritan*, courtesy of the Picture Collection, The Branch Libraries, New York Public Library.

THE INTERNATIONAL JOURNAL OF THE Addictions

The International Journal of the Addictions, 19(4), iii–vi, 1984

Editorial

Preventing Change through Current Substance Use Intervention: A Role Analysis

It has become increasingly more obvious, and acceptable, to believe that effective intervention regarding abstinence, proper uses of available substances/chemicals, and substance misuse should/must by necessity include cooperative efforts by a variety of individuals as well as agencies and systems. Such a view assumes that intervention planning and efforts demand the attention and appropriate involvement of a broad spectrum of participants. Among the available and potential ones are:

- Professional disciplines
- Paraprofessionals, including former users
- Volunteers
- Treatment agencies
- Service agencies
- Control agencies
- Communities
- Networks/systems (familial, social, etc.)

It is the contention of this note that all too often such multifactorial efforts prevent the planned and/or anticipated change(s) from occurring or from being maintained.

Figure 1 schematizes the possible scenario for "planned failure." The reader is asked to consider those factors or elements which s/he would place in each quadrant in order to develop and maintain a particular state of drug use or abstinence. Who are the preferred individuals, types of intervention agents and agencies, and needed communities and systems/networks which are basic to achieving an agreed upon and defined success? Once these are selected, the reader is asked to consider the following issues for each intervention factor in each quadrant.

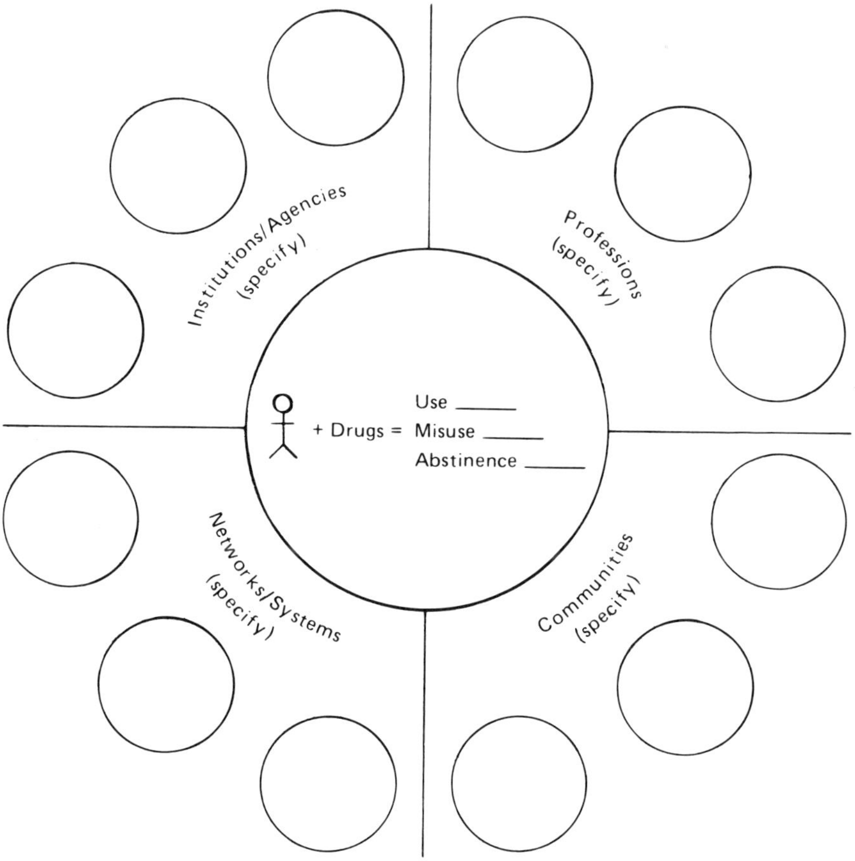

Selected factors in the intervention process	Participants in the intervention environment			
	Institutions/ agencies	Professions/ paraprofessions	Communities	Systems/ networks
Critical concepts				
Issues				
Problems				
Goals/objectives				
Techniques				
Strategies				
Policies				
Sites				
Planned outcome				

Fig. 1.

1. Critical concepts and traditions
2. Issues related to abstinence from drug use (types of drugs, patterns of use, etc.)
3. Problems related to abstinence or drug use
4. Intervention goals (short and long term)
5. Intervention techniques
6. Intervention strategies
7. Intervention policies
8. Intervention staff
9. Preferred site(s) of intervention
10. Planned outcome criteria (success and failure)

As the reader defines and peruses each factor, singly and in relation to one another, s/he should be asking: *Is there basic agreement between each segment of the intervention effort/process in regard to each of these 10 factors?*

If there is agreement, one should be able to assume that the achievement of the predicted outcome(s) will be greatly facilitated. Under such circumstances each intervening factor–individuals, institutions, communities, networks–is most likely to achieve those goals and objectives which are unique and an integral part of its own responsibility. In addition, each one is, or should be, able to facilitate, or not interfere with, the effective functioning of the other intervention components.

What happens when the needed agreement or balance between the segments in the intervention process does not exist? This is all too often the case, for many reasons. A basic source of disagreement stems from the reality that each intervention component brings with it, to each planned or reflexive effort, a set of factors: specific traditions; critical concepts; a determination of what (and/or who) is an issue or problem; a goal or goal system; techniques, strategies, and policies; and preferred sites for intervention and preferred staff; as well as its own desired outcome(s).

Planned failure is the result when there is lack of a basic agreement between *all of the components* of an intervention plan/program; failure for some if not for many of the participants in the process. Published evaluation studies, which continue basically to focus primarily upon the drug user and his/her behavior, all too often miss this simple reality. Intervention occurs in a complex, dynamic environment with many participants.

Our failure to take this fact into consideration, or to develop and maintain the minimal desirable conditions which are needed for effective intervention, may have relatively little to do with drug use, drug action, or the variety of drug users. Rather it more likely has to do with the interface (current/actual as well as potential) between intervention models, the needed components of intervention, and their necessary interacting roles.

Figure 1 is designed to be used as a catalytic tool to prevent, or at the very least to minimize, the continuation of planned failure. "Play" with it and determine who is needed (or not needed) to do what, with selected others in specific types of roles in order to achieve defined short- and long-term outcome(s). You may add to the schema or delete as you decide what type of "game" you wish to play in our growing "field."

S. Einstein, PhD
Jerusalem, Israel

The International Journal of the Addictions, 19(4), 367–381, 1984

Alcohol and Marijuana Use in Adolescents' Daily Lives: A Random Sample of Experiences

Reed Larson,* PhD

Laboratory for the Study of Adolescence
Department of Psychiatry
Michael Reese Hospital and Medical Center
Chicago, Illinois 60616

Mihaly Csikszentmihalyi, PhD

Mark Freeman, MA

Committee on Human Development
Department of Behavioral Sciences
The University of Chicago
Chicago, Illinois 60637

Abstract

High school students filled out reports on their experiences at random times during their daily lives, including 48 occasions when they were using alcohol or marijuana. Alcohol use was reported primarily in the context of Friday and Saturday night social gatherings and was associated with a happy and gregarious subjective state. Marijuana use was reported across a wider range of situations and was associated with an average state that differed much less from ordinary experience.

*To whom requests for reprints should be sent at 2959 S. Cottage Grove, Chicago, Illinois 60616.

 0020-773X/84/1904-0367$3.50/0

INTRODUCTION

Most researchers would agree that use of alcohol and marijuana, particularly by adolescents, must be understood in terms of the social and psychological context in which these drugs are taken. Pharmacologists have concluded that "set and setting" play a decisive role in shaping drug experiences (Jones 1971a, 1971b; Weil, 1972; Weil, Zinberg, and Nelson, 1968). Sociologists have described how effects of these drugs are related to the milieu in which they are used (Becker, 1963; Orcutt, 1972). There can be little question that social and contextual factors influence when these drugs will be taken and how they will be experienced. It is astonishing, then, how little is known about the actual circumstances surrounding their use.

A primary constraint on knowledge about the circumstances surrounding drug use has been methodological. Nearly all attempts at gaining systematic information have relied upon survey methods, despite recognized problems with this approach. Surveys typically gather information from people in settings far removed from the actual contexts of drug use; hence they depend upon people's ability to remember and accurately reconstruct past experiences. Artifacts due to selective forgetting, demand characteristics, and response sets can be substantial (Eichberg, 1975; Goodstadt, Cook, and Gruson, 1978; Hochhauser, 1979). This was dramatically illustrated in a study of adult alcoholics in which the experience of intoxication was remembered as exactly opposite from what had been reported at the time (Tamerin, Weiner, and Mendelson, 1970). Survey methods may be useful for studying rates of use and how these relate to well-established sociological and psychological variables (e.g., Kandel, 1978). But, in order to learn how drug use is embedded within ongoing lives it is necessary to have more direct information.

This paper reports on the use of a new technique to study adolescent drug use. Called the "Experience Sampling Method" (ESM), it involves having people carry electronic pagers (the kind doctors sometimes carry) for a week and filling out self-reports when they receive randomly scheduled signals (Larson and Csikszentmihalyi, 1983). By this means participants provide 30 to 60 self-reports on random moments in their daily lives. Because they report on experience as it occurs, the information is not dependent on recall. Because the signals are scheduled randomly across all hours of the day, reports approximate a representative sample of daily lives, including drug use. This paper is based on research with a randomly selected sample of 75 adolescents, many of whom reported alcohol and marijuana use as a part of their daily activity. The data allow examination of this drug use in relation to the rest of their lives.

A first concern is with external circumstances of adolescent alcohol and marijuana use. Survey research has linked adolescent drug use to peer association (Gorsuch and Butler, 1976; Jessor, Jessor, and Finney, 1973; Kandel, 1973,

1978), suggesting that much drug use takes place with friends. But information is lacking about the time of day, the environment, and the social composition of gatherings at which these drugs are taken. The ESM provides a means for obtaining this kind of data.

A second concern is with the subjective, internal side of adolescent alcohol and marijuana experience. It is generally held that these drugs have a "recreational" purpose, that they bring about a more favorable psychological state (Blum, 1969; Forslund, 1978; Shick and Freedman, 1975) or alleviate a negative one (Braucht, Brakarsh, and Fellingstad, 1973; Paton, Kessler, and Kandel, 1977). However, little evidence exists as to how regularly alcohol and marijuana actually have these effects. An extraordinary range of phenomenological effects have been attributed to marijuana (Grinspoon, 1977; Tart, 1971), but little is known about the frequency with which each is experienced, or even how often the drug is experienced as positive versus negative. The ESM procedure offers a means for obtaining this kind of data by securing reports on subjective states during daily drug use. It allows consideration of drugs states in relation to the baseline of daily states in people's lives.

METHOD

The data set used in this report is a subset from an experience sampling study of 75 White adolescents, conducted in 1977 (Larson, 1979; Larson, Csikszentmihalyi, and Graef, 1980). These teenagers were selected from the student body of a large and diverse suburban high school bordering the city of Chicago. Sampling followed a stratified random procedure, designed to obtain equal numbers of boys and girls; equal numbers of 9th, 10th, 11th, and 12th graders; and equal numbers of students from lower-middle-class census tracts (having an average family income of $14,000) and upper-middle-class census tracts (having an average family income of $25,000). The final sample included 69% of the girls and 45% of the boys initially invited to take part.

Participants in the study carried pagers for 1 week and filled out self-reports in response to signals they received. The signals, sent by a radio transmitter with a 60-mile radius, were scheduled randomly within every 2-hour block of time from 7:30 A.M. until 10:30 P.M. on weekdays and until 1:30 A.M. on Friday and Saturday night. Participants were asked to fill out self-report forms in response to each signal, with the understanding that they retained the right not to respond. Sixty-nine percent of the signals were followed by self-reports, providing a total of 4,489 time samples. Missed self-reports were due to mechanical failure of the pager, to respondents going to bed (in which case they were told to turn off the pager), to respondents unintentionally leaving the pager at home or deciding they wished not to be disturbed, and to a range of other reasons. In a debriefing interview, the students reported lower response rates when with friends and on Friday and Saturday nights.

The data considered here are from the 19 of these 75 students who indicated use of alcohol or marijuana on at least one self-report form. It should be noted that the self-report form did not ask about drug use; rather this information was volunteered in response to questions about activity at the time of the signal. Therefore it is probable that some instances of drug use, particularly those occurring in the intervals between self-reports, went undetected.

These 19 teenagers reported 25 occasions of alcohol use, 19 occasions of marijuana use, and 4 instances when both drugs were being used at the same time. Alcohol use was reported by 17 of the students (11 boys and 6 girls); marijuana, by 7 (3 boys and 4 girls). The average age of these students was 17.1 (SD = .9). Nine were from lower-middle-class census tracts, and 10 were from upper-middle-class census tracts. Because the research was not initially designed to investigate drug use, no information was obtained on these students' prior drug experiences.

The information obtained on the self-report form includes where students were and who was with them at the time of the signal. It also includes ratings of their subjective state, made on a series of standard psychometric scales. Among these are semantic differential ratings of mood, scaled self-assessments of cognitive state, and ratings of motivation and the social situation at the time of the signal. In addition, students were asked about their thoughts at the time of the signal and were provided space for additional comment.

RESULTS

The Objective Circumstances of Alcohol and Marijuana Use

The sample of ESM self-reports made during alcohol and marijuana consumption provides an opportunity to determine the "objective" context under which these drugs are typically used. Figure 1 shows that all but 4 of the 29 instances of alcohol use occurred on weekends, and nearly all of these on weekend evenings. There were no instances of drinking during the school day. Marijuana use, in contrast, was reported across all parts of the week, including school hours. One student reported herself to be "smoking a joint" at 8:00 A.M. before going to school in the morning. On two other occasions students reported marijuana use during lunch time.

There are corresponding differences in where students reported using the two drugs (Table 1). Alcohol was used primarily at friends' homes; it was used 5 times in a public restaurant or bar (the legal drinking age at the time of the study was 18) and only 3 times at home. In contrast, virtually all of the

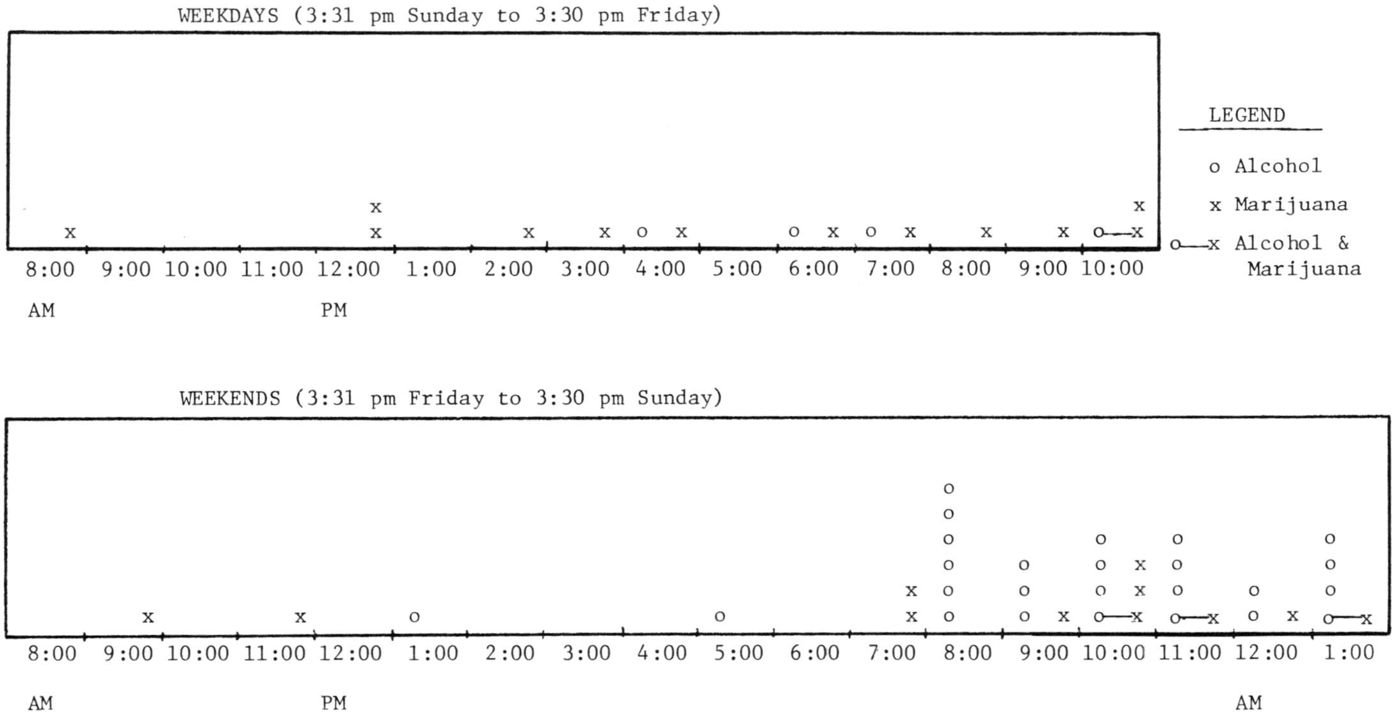

Fig. 1. Times of reported drug use.

Table 1

Locations in Which Drug Use Was Reported[a]

Location	% of time teens spend in this location[b]	Number of occasions: Alcohol	Marijuana	Both
Home	40	2	7	1
Friend's home	5	15	1	3
School	33	0	1	0
Public place	22	8	10	0
Total	100	25	19	4

[a]Significance test for comparison of alcohol and marijuana columns: $\chi^2 = 15.4$, $p = .0015$.
[b]Estimates based on ESM data for the entire sample of 75 adolescents.

marijuana use was reported either at home or in noncommercial public settings: while walking (2 instances), in a car (3 instances), or in a park (1 instance).

A further difference in context involves the number of companions. For the great majority of times, students were with friends when using either substance. However, the two drugs differed substantially in the number of friends involved. Table 2 shows that alcohol was usually consumed in groups of 4 or more people, whereas marijuana use typically took place with only 1 other person.

To summarize, alcohol use was reported primarily on Friday and Saturday evenings, at friends' homes, with large groups of people; in other words, in the context of "parties." Marijuana use, in contrast, was reported over a broader range of contexts, occurring at all times during the week and in multiple environments. Whereas alcohol was clearly associated with social gatherings, marijuana use appeared associated with intimate interactions among one or two friends.

Table 2

Number of Companions Reported during Drug Use[a]

Number of companions	Number of occasions: Alcohol	Marijuana	Both
0	0	2	0
1	5	10	2
2-3	2	3	1
4-6	3	1	0
7+	11	0	1
Total	21[b]	16[b]	4

[a]Significance test for comparison of alcohol and marijuana: Kendall τ B = .60, $p = .0001$.
[b]Subjects failed to report number of friends for several occasions.

Subjective States during Alcohol and Marijuana Use

The sample of self-reports also provides a record of adolescents' subjective experiences at the time of alcohol and marijuana use. To compare these ratings to the rest of daily experience, they were converted to *z* scores, for which a value of 0.0 corresponds to each individual's mean rating for that item across all of his or her self-reports. An interval of 1.0 corresponds to an individual's standard deviation. Table 3 shows the average reported states when using alcohol and marijuana, as compared to the overall average state, or baseline, of 0.0.

It is apparent from Table 3 that the experiences associated with alcohol use are substantially different from the normal state. For nearly all the mood items the students indicated feeling significantly more positive than usual, with the largest deviations on the dimensions Excited, Sociable, Free, and Open. The mood items dealing with activation (Alert, Strong, and Active) show the least elevation. On the cognitive state items, students reported levels below average when using alcohol. Concentration and Control of Actions were rated significantly lower than baseline, with Control nearly a full standard deviation below normal. Lastly, on the item dealing with motivation ("Do you wish you were doing something else?"), the students reported being favorably disposed to the situation they were in.

During marijuana use, changes in experiential state were not as evident. Whereas reported moods during alcohol use were clearly positive, during marijuana use the averages for several items were actually in a negative direction. Only two mood items, Excited and Free, showed significantly positive levels. Reported cognitive states were lower than baseline; however, only Control of Actions differed significantly from the mean.

Across all items, changes in state associated with marijuana appeared to be weaker than those associated with alcohol; it is striking then that, on the one motivation item, students reported a stronger wish to be doing what they were doing during marijuana use. This drug is not markedly associated with positive moods; nonetheless the students indicated positive motivation when they were using it.

Case Study: A Heavy Marijuana User

In order to examine more closely the pattern of drug experience among adolescents, it will be useful to look at the reports of one individual. Rick Marelli (pseudonym) was a high school senior of average intelligence, the youngest of four in a suburban middle-class family. Figure 2 shows the moods he reported during a follow-up conducted 2 years after the original study. The mood scale used in the graph is based on the first 10 semantic differential items from Table 3. Alongside these values is a summary of the situations he reported

Table 3

Reported State When Drug Use Was Reported[a]

Self-report item	Mean z score: Alcohol (N = 25)	Marijuana (N = 19)	Both (N = 4)
Mood items			
Affect			
Happy (vs sad)	.61***	.37	1.09
Cheerful (vs irritable)	.52**	.19	1.22**
Friendly (vs angry)	.56**	.09	1.13**
Sociable (vs lonely)	.76**	.29	1.30**
Activation			
Alert (vs drowsy)	.01	–.38	0.08
Strong (vs weak)	.22	–.27	0.40
Active (vs passive)	.42*	–.20	0.05
Other			
Involved (vs detached)	.56**	.20	0.52
Excited (vs bored)	.91***	.57*	1.46**
Free (vs constrained)	.71**	.55**	0.73
Open (vs closed)	.70**	.27	0.57
Clear (vs confused)	–.06	–.40	0.21
Cognitive and Motivational States			
Cognitive			
Concentration	–.45*	–.31	0.15
Ease of Concentration	.03	–.29	–0.75
Self-consciousness	–.26	–.16	0.43
Motivational			
Control of Actions	–.87**	–.76**	–1.61*
Do you wish you were doing something else?	–.40*	–.64**	–0.96
Social Interaction			
Is talk joking (vs serious)?	.79***	.27	0.49
Are the goals of others the same as yours (vs different)?	.18	.47*	0.32
Do you expect to receive positive feedback (vs negative feedback)?	.44*	.32	0.50

[a] Significance tests of deviation from zero: $*p < .05$, $**p < .01$, $***p < .001$.

for each pager signal. In total Rick provided 46 random self-reports; 15 of these (1 out of every 3) involved consumption of either alcohol or marijuana, or both.

Rick received the first signal at 12:45 P.M. on a Monday, when walking home from school with a couple of friends. His mood was relatively positive, but it was substantially lower when he filled out a report later, 6:42 P.M. In the debriefing interview, he said he and his friends had been carrying some beers, which they drank in the afternoon, and the alcohol, he felt, had had a depressing effect on his mood. On the 6:42 P.M. pager sheet he added the comment: "Should not have got so buzzed. Delays school work." His mood recovered later, but there was no indication that he got to the school work. At 8:40 P.M. he reported listening to the radio and tapping with drumsticks on a backgammon set. ("There was nothing better to do.") And at 10:24 P.M. he was cooking popcorn and drinking beer with his father.

On Tuesday Rick reported no alcohol or marijuana use, and his moods were as positive as any other day. In English class feelings were low, but in Biology they were better, partly because he was thinking about girls. At 12:45 P.M. he was riding a motorcycle with friends, and at 7:35 he was playing basketball and reported the highest moods of the week. It appears he was able to have a good time without drugs.

Nonetheless, when the pager signaled on Wednesday morning at 10:30 A.M., he reported taking a break from school with friends and that they had "just finished getting high" and were walking down the street listening to the Grateful Dead. Feelings were positive, but it is not clear whether this was because of the drug, the music, or the reprieve from school. He also reported feeling less in control than usual and was concerned about getting caught.

For the rest of the day his mood appeared to be dominated by pain from dental braces, inflicted during his visit to the orthodontist at noon. The marijuana in the morning did not keep him from feeling low. When signaled at 4:24 P.M., he was playing softball and smoking more marijuana, which temporarily lifted his mood. But during the next two reports that day, Rick was alone, walking in the rain with a low mood and sore teeth.

Thursday evening at 6:00 P.M. his mouth was still sore, but he was attempting to overcome the pain with improvised meditation techniques. He got stoned, put on "Jesus Christ Superstar," and (as he described it later in the interview) was "trying to absorb energy from the situation." On the self-report form he reported very high Concentration and very high Control. However, Concentration, Control, and positive mood all deteriorated by 7:05 when he was eating supper with his parents. And they were still low at 10:00 P.M. when he was watching TV and again getting high.

Friday turned out to be a day of extensive alcohol and marijuana use. About noon a group of friends started drinking beer and smoking pot. When Rick was signaled at 3:20 P.M. he was feeling quite good. But then he and his friends separated for awhile, and at 3:40 P.M. he described himself as "dulled out." He was watching TV alone and drinking another beer. Later in the afternoon, at 5:00, he was again with friends, was selling some joints, and his mood was up slightly. In the debriefing interview he described it as what might be called a "do or die" situation: "You gotta keep partying. If not, you're just going to get tired." He was trying to get a "second wind" but instead was

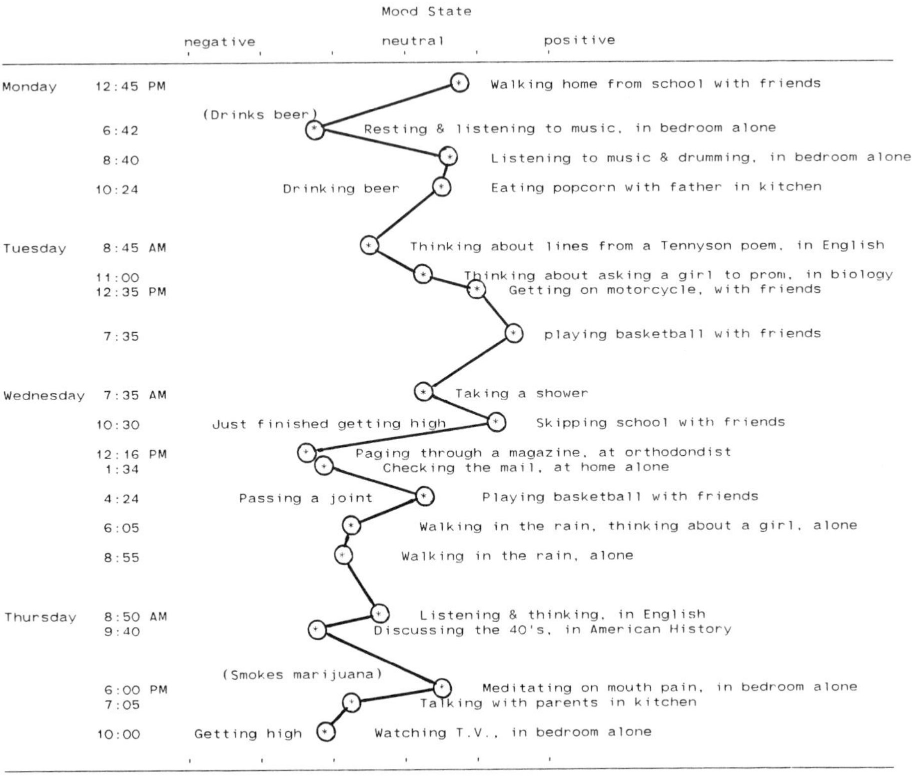

Fig. 2. Moods and activities reported by Rick Marelli. Information in parentheses was obtained from the interview afterward; everything else comes from the reports made at the time.

crashing. As the evening continued he and his friends continued to drink beer, smoke marijuana, and go from place to place looking for a good party; but on the self-report form he wrote, in an increasingly scrawling hand, that he felt very out of control as well as "weak," "passive," and "bored." For he and his friends, the party spirit had devolved into aimless driving around. The last report of the day (at 1:10 A.M.) showed him talking amicably with his mother about "how rotten the night was." In the interview Rick explained that he had not had fun; he "just got drunk." The pattern of Rick's partying is one we found common among these adolescents (Csikszentmihalyi and Larson, 1984).

The following morning at breakfast he was still thinking about what a "rotten time" he had had and was feeling low. His mood had risen a little at 11:30 when he was smoking a bong of hashish while watching "Robin Hood" on

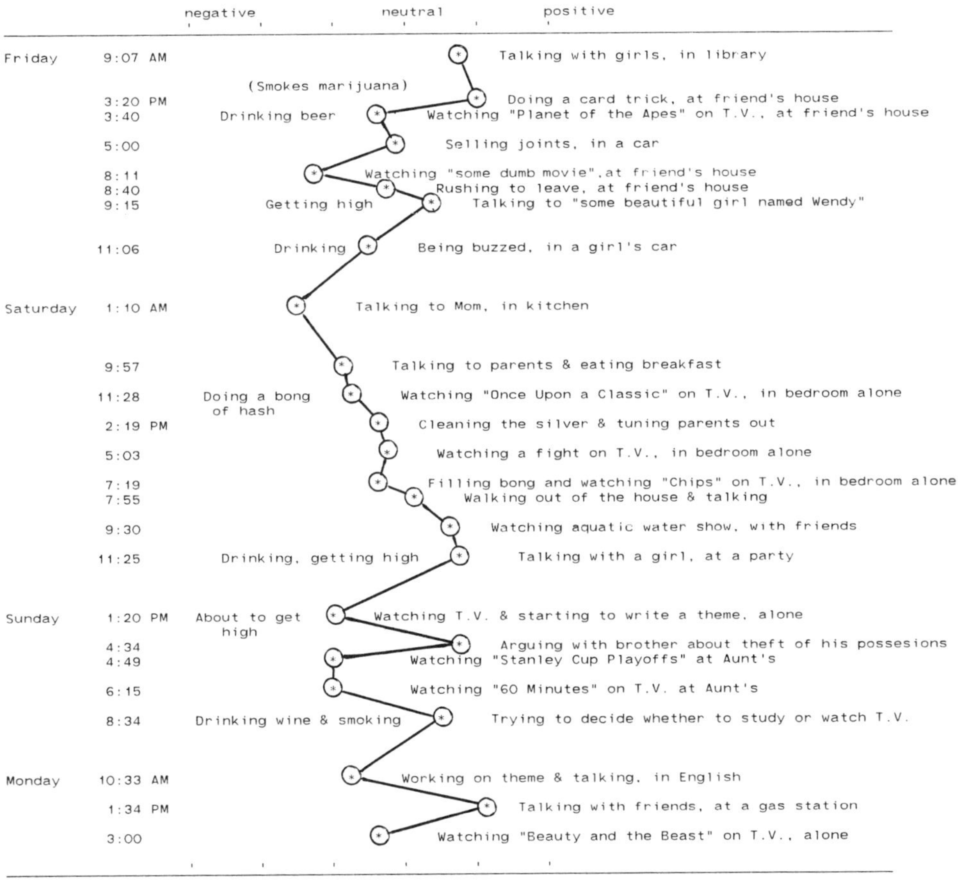

Fig. 2. (continued)

TV. Bored in spite of the hashish, he said in the interview, "I'd rather be high and bored than not high and bored." Marijuana and hashish were not necessarily elevating for Rick, yet he persisted in their intake.

Most of Saturday afternoon was spent cleaning silverware in preparation for his aunt's visit. Resentful of the work and the hypocrisy he saw in these special preparations, he wrote a string of obscenities on the self-report form. To deal with the situation, he smoked more marijuana, which evidently helped him to feel free. In the evening he did some more bongs, watched "Chips" on TV, and again became angry about his obligations. Later he went out with friends, reported drinking and smoking again, but indicated having a much better time than the night before.

But Sunday was Mother's Day, which brought more conflict with his family. At 1:20 P.M. he reported he was getting high in order to write a theme. Later he had a fight with his brother and then got trapped at his aunt's house where all he could do was watch TV.

This narrative account suggests how drug use fits into Rick's life. The reports show him smoking marijuana to enjoy times with friends and times by himself. He used it in attempts to kill pain, cope with his family, and do homework. It appeared to be a part of nearly all social occasions, as well as something to do while alone. Yet there is no clear suggestion in these data that it had a positive influence on his mood; as often as not it left him feeling out of control. Alcohol appeared to be consumed in a narrower range of circumstances and appeared to be related to a more consistent change in state. Except for the miserable experiences on Friday, drinking alcohol was nearly always associated with a positve mood. Clearly Rick is an example of a heavy drug user; nonetheless his experiences during the week exemplify the pattern for the entire group.

DISCUSSION

The findings of this study are of a preliminary nature, but they do suggest basic patterns in how use of alcohol and marijuana fits into adolescents' daily experience. For this sample, alcohol was clearly a social drug, used almost entirely in a specific social context: Friday and Saturday night parties. The associated subjective state was one of high gregariousness, including feelings of cheerfulness, openness, and joviality. Alcohol and this sociable mood appeared to be an almost inseparable part of this social context. Rick Marelli's self-reports provided several examples of how alcohol use occurred as a normative part of such gatherings.

Marijuana, in contrast, appeared to be more of a private drug, most often used with one or two friends. Whereas alcohol use was reported by many individuals in a specific social context, marijuana use was reported by fewer individuals but across a wider range of contexts. It was reported at large social gatherings and solitary occasions, at home and in public, and across all hours of the week. In contrast to alcohol, marijuana use was associated with few changes in emotional or cognitive state. Notably, it was not related to positive affect, a finding that contradicts information from survey and laboratory research indicating positive or even "euphoric" moods as a frequent product of marijuana (Grinspoon, 1977). This suggests that adolescents' memories of drug use, as reported afterward, may be much more positive than is actually the case in immediate experience.

If only minimal emotional or cognitive benefits are being derived from marijuana, it becomes essential to examine other, perhaps more subtle, motivating factors related to its use. In addition to the variety of social and symbolic factors described by others (e.g., Dembo et al., 1976; Kandel, 1978), it seems important• to consider the particular ends that marijuana use may serve in relation to other routine tasks and activities. It is striking to us that the pattern of states reported during marijuana use is exactly opposite to that reported by these same adolescents during school classes. Whereas marjuana use is characterized by significantly high feelings of excitement, freedom, and wishing to be doing what one is doing, the experience of class is characterized by significantly high boredom, constraint, and wishing to be doing something else (Csikszentmihalyi and Larson, 1984). This pattern suggests that the drug serves as a response tofeelings of boredom and constraint induced by the school experience. Rick Marelli certainly appeared to be using it as an antidote to school as well as the oppression he experienced at home on Saturday and Sunday.

A related way of understanding the function of alcohol and marijuana use is to see them as examples of a broader range of habits that people adopt to structure their experiences, habits that in another context were described as "micro-flow" activities (Csikszentmihalyi, 1975). These include regular actions like smoking, snacking, gesturing, pacing, and watching television. The direct impact of these activities on experience is not necessareily positive, but by focusing attention on familiar routines, they exclude threatening material from awareness. Thus the use of alcohol and marijuana might be motivated less by the positive state they produce and more by the fact that they keep in abeyance the sense of constraint and boredom that might otherwise permeate teenagers' consciousness (Creason and Goldman, 1981).

The contribution of the Experience Sampling Method to the study of substance abuse lies in its capacity to obtain detailed information about how drug use fits into daily lives. In addition to the study of adolescents, it would seem to have potential for investigation of amphetamine use among housewives, alcohol use among businesspersons, and stimulant use among college students. The depth of information obtainable is illustrated by a study of bulimia in which we were able to identify the sequence of experiences prior to, during, and subsequent to the symptomatic bingeing and purging behavior (Johnson and Larson, 1982). This kind of contextual analysis of drug taking could provide detailed knowledge about the daily conditions eliciting use, knowledge that might be extremely valuable to efforts at treatment and prevention.

The success of investigations using this method depends on establishment with participants of the "research alliance," a working understanding about the procedures and purposes of the research (Offer and Sabshin, 1967). It is essential that participants not feel they are being coerced into disclosing what they consider private information. In addition, thorough precautions need to be taken to protect the confidentiality of their responses.

Perhaps the greatest constraint on the method relates to sampling: the sampling both of persons and experiences. There can be little doubt that certain categories of heavy users would be unwilling to participate in this kind of study—although Rogers and Layton (1979) have shown remarkable success in getting herion addicts to provide reports on their experiences. One can also imagine that certain drug states, like an LSD "trip" or heavy alcohol intoxication, might prevent a person from filling out a form or take away the motivation for doing so. For example, in the study reported here, we have little idea of what types of drug experiences might have been systematically missed.

Such methodological problems, however, are not insurmountable. With a thorough prescreening of the subject pool it would be possible to assess subject attrition, and a rigorous debriefing interview following the week of study would allow evaluation of the sample of drug experiences. Use of heart rate monitors in conjunction with the ESM procedure might aid in assessing the accuracy of reports on drug intake for drugs having known cardiovascular effects (Hoover, 1984). The relatively limited information considered in this study could be enhanced with self-report questions designed to obtain information about dosage levels, timing of drug use, and other pertinent situational contingencies. The findings presented here about adolescent drug experiences represent but a small indication of what might be found.

REFERENCES

BECKER, H. *The Outsiders: Studies in the Sociology of Deviance.* New York: Free Press, 1963.

BLUM, R. *Drugs.* San Francisco: Jossey-Bass, 1969.

BRAUCHT, G., BRAKARSH, D., and FELLINGSTAD, D. Deviant drug use in adolescence. *Psychol. Bull.* 79: 92-106, 1973.

CREASON, C., and GOLDMAN, M. Varying levels of marijuana use by adolescents and the amotivation syndrome. *Psychol. Rep.* 48: 447-454, 1981.

CSIKSZENTMIHALYI, M. *Beyond Boredom and Anxiety.* San Francisco: Jossey-Bass, 1975.

CSIKSZENTMIHALYI, M., and LARSON, R. *Being Adolescent.* New York: Basic Books, 1984.

DEMBO, R., SCHMEIDLER, J., and KOVAL, M. Demographic, value and behavioral correlates of marijuana use among middle-class youth. *J. Health Soc. Behav.* 17: 177-187, 1976.

EICHBERG, R. Some words of caution on subjective concepts. In J. Elinson and D. Nurco (eds.), *Operational Definitions in Socio-behavioral Drug Use Research.* National Institute on Drug Abuse, 1975.

FORSLUND, M. Functions of drinking for native American and white youth. *J. Youth Adolescence* 7: 327-, 1978.

GOODSTADT, M., COOK, G., and GRUSON, V. The validity of reported drug use: The randomized response technique. *Int. J. Addict.* 13: 359-367, 1978.

GORSUCH, R., and BUTLER, M. Initial drug abuse: A review of predisposing social-psychological factors. *Psychol. Bull.* 83: 120-137, 1976.

GRINSPOON, L. *Marijuana Reconsidered.* Cambridge, MA: Harvard University Press, 1977.

HOCHHAUSER, M. Bias in drug abuse survey research. *Int. J. Addict.* 14: 675-687, 1979.

HOOVER, M. *An exploration of the relationships among moods, activities, heart rate, and gross motor activity in the daily lives of eight people.* PhD dissertation in progress, University of Chicago, 1984.

JESSOR, R., JESSOR, S., and FINNEY, J. A social psychology of marijuana use: Longitudinal studies of high school and college youth. *J. Pers. Soc. Psychol.* 26: 1-15, 1973.

JOHNSON, C., and LARSON, R. Bulimia: An analysis of moods and behavior. *Psychosom. Med.* 44: 341-351, 1982.

JONES, R. Marijuana-induced "high": Influences of expectation, setting and previous drug experience. *Pharmacol. Rev.* 23: 359-367, 1971a.

JONES, R. Tetrahydrocannabinol and the marijuana-induced social "high", or the effects of the mind on marijuana. *Ann. N.Y. Acad. Sci.* 191: 155-165, 1971b.

KANDEL, D. Adolescent marijuana use: Role of parents and peers. *Science* 181: 1067-1070, 1973.

KANDEL, D. *Longitudinal Research on Drug Use; Empirical Findings and Methodological Issues.* Somerset, NJ: Halsted, 1978.

LARSON, R. *The significance of solitude in adolescents' lives.* Unpublished PhD dissertation, University of Chicago, 1979.

LARSON, R., and CSIKSZENTMIHALYI, M. The experience sampling method. In H. Reis (ed.), *New Directions for Naturalistic Methods in the Behavioral Sciences.* San Francisco: Jossey-Bass, 1983.

LARSON, R., CSIKSZENTMIHALYI, M., and GRAEF, R. Mood variability and the psychosocial adjustment of adolescents. *J. Youth Adolescence* 9: 469-490, 1980.

OFFER, D., and SABSHIN, M. Research alliance versus therapeutic alliance: A comparison. *Am. J. Psychiatry* 123: 1519-1526, 1967.

ORCUTT, J. Toward a sociological theory of drug effects: A comparison of marijuana and alcohol. *Sociol. Soc. Res.* 56: 242-253, 1972.

PATON, S., KESSLER, R., and KANDEL, D. Depressive mood and adolescent illicit drug use: A longitudinal analysis. *J. Genetic Psychol.* 131: 267-289, 1977.

ROGERS, H., and LAYTON, B. Two methods of predicting drug taking. *Int. J. Addict.* 14: 299-310, 1979.

SHICK, J., DORUS, W., and HUGHES, P. Adolescent drug using groups in Chicago parks. *Drug Alcohol Depend.* 3: 199-210, 1978.

SHICK, J., and FREEDMAN, D. Research in nonnarcotic drug abuse. In S. Arieti (ed.), *American Handbook of Psychiatry,* 2nd ed., Vol. 6. New York: Basic Books, 1975.

TAMERIN, J., WEINER, S., and MENDELSON, J. Alcoholics' expectancies and recall of experiences during intoxication. *Am. J. Psychiatry* 126: 1697-1704, 1970.

TART, C. *On Being Stoned: A Psychological Study of Marijuana Intoxication.* Palo Alto, CA: Science and Behavior Books, 1971.

WEIL, A. *The Natural Mind.* Boston: Houghton Mifflin, 1972.

WEIL, A., ZINBERG, N., and NELSON, J. Clinical and psychological effects of marijuana in man. *Science* 162: 1234-1242, 1968.

The International Journal of the Addictions, 19(4), 383–401, 1984

Paraprofessional Versus Professional Drug Counselors: The Progress of Clients in Treatment

Leona S. Aiken,* PhD

Leonard A. LoSciuto, PhD

Mary Ann Ausetts, MA

Institute for Survey Research, and
Psychology Department
Temple University
Philadelphia, Pennsylvania 19122

Barry S. Brown, PhD

National Institute on Drug Abuse
Rockville, Maryland 20857

Abstract

The progress in treatment of 302 methadone maintenance and drug-free outpatient clients was examined as a function of the background of their 82 counselors. Counselors were either ex-addict paraprofessionals (EXAs), non-ex-addict paraprofessionals (NEAs), or degreed professional counselors (PROs). Client progress was assessed in five areas: drug use, criminality, educational activities, employment, and life quality. In the first four areas, status at treatment entry contrasted with that at two subsequent measurement points: the first interview and a

*To whom requests for reprints should be sent at the Institute for Survey Research, Temple University, Philadelphia, Pennsylvania 19122.

 0020-773X/84/1904-0383$3.50/0

4-month follow-up. In no area of evaluation were outcomes substantially more favorable for clients of one counselor group over another. It was concluded that the three counselor groups were equally effective.

The concern of the present study is the progress through treatment of clients of three types of counselors: (1) professional counselors who hold at least a bachelor's degree and who do not have addict backgrounds (PROs), (2) ex-addict paraprofessional counselors who do not hold a bachelor's degree (EXAs), and (3) non-ex-addict paraprofessionals who neither hold a bachelor's degree nor have a history of drug addiction (NEAs). While there has been consensual agreement that counseling by the indigenous paraprofessional—here, the ex-addict—is advantageous for clients, there is a dearth of literature which examines differential effectiveness of ex-addicts versus other counselor groups (Ottomanelli, 1978).

Four recent considerations of differential effectiveness are confined to the methadone maintenance modality. Brown and Thompson (1976), in the most extensive of the four studies, compared the functioning of 52 addict-clients assigned to 29 nonaddict counselors with that of 84 addict-clients assigned to 30 ex-addict counselors. One-year evaluations of client status based on measures of percentages of clients retained or completing treatment, mean number of months in treatment, percentage of clients arrested and mean number of arrests, and percentage of retained clients who were employed yielded no significant differences between clients of the two counselor groups. While counselors in this study were not dichotomized according to educational level, as they were in the present study, the nonaddict counselors had more education and more counseling experience than the ex-addict counselors; the latter were hired on the basis of intelligence and sensitivity.

More recently, Longwell, Miller, and Nichols (1978) and Connett (1980) have compared the drug use (via urinalysis) of clients of paraprofessional and professional counselors. Longwell et al. compared clients of 10 ex-addict paraprofessionals with those of 16 non-ex-addict counselors, of whom 13 held at least a bachelor's degree; they found no differences in percentage of clean urines among client groups assigned to treatment by ex-addicts, non-ex-addicts, or both types of counselors. Connett, comparing clients assigned to four paraprofessional counselors versus five professional counselors, also reported no difference in percentage of clean urines across groups after 6 months in treatment. However, this lack of difference at posttest was difficult to interpret, since clients of professionals had initially higher levels of polydrug use than those of paraprofesssionals. The study also does not clearly speak to the matter of the ex-addict status of counselors, since drug use history of counselors was not discussed.

In a single study of the modification of personality traits through drug treatment, Ottomanelli (1978) compared changes in MMPI and *Pyp* (Haertzen and Panton, 1967) scores of clients assigned to four professional counselors with master's degrees in psychology or social work versus three paraprofessional ex-heroin addict counselors still maintained on methadone. While significant decreases in the MMPI Depression (*D*) and Schizophrenia (*Sc*) scales were found for clients of professionals, no analogous change was noted in clients of paraprofessionals.

The four studies together give little, if any, evidence of differential effectiveness of professional versus paraprofessional counselors. However, with perhaps the exception of the study by Brown and Thompson (1976), these studies have been questioned by their own authors on grounds of ungeneralizability of any results whatever derived from small numbers of counselors. Such a limitation is certainly not confined to considerations within the drug abuse field. The far broader literature on paraprofessional effectiveness within the mental health field is subject to these same limitations (Durlak, 1979; Nietzel and Fisher, 1981). In this regard it is noteworthy that Connett (1980), Longwell et al. (1978), and Ottomanelli (1978) themselves indicate the desirability of far more extensive investigations with larger numbers of clients.

The present study is an extensive investigation of differential counselor effectiveness, and it surpasses previous investigations in a number of ways. First, numbers of clients and counselors exceed those of prior studies and provide adequate power for statistical contrasts of groups. Second, for the first time two groups of paraprofessionals (EXAs and NEAs) are contrasted with one another, and both groups are further contrasted with professional counselors (PROs). Third, the present study involves the drug-free outpatient as well as the methadone maintenance modality, the latter being the only modality examined in previous investigations.

The present study also has the advantage that consideration has been given to the job functions, and particularly the counseling activities, of the three counselor groups. Aiken, LoSciuto, Ausetts, and Brown (1984) reported marked similarity among counseling activities of the three groups. This is particularly important in that the internal validity of this study requires that differences among counselor groups in counseling activities or treatment provided should not be confounded with counselor group differences on critical counselor variables (Luborsky, Singer, and Luborsky, 1975; Nietzel and Fisher, 1981)—here, educational level and drug use background. Outcome criteria in this study go beyond drug use to include employment, education, and criminality; and in addition, information about life-style, including social relationships and daily activities during the course of treatment. Finally, in order to increase confidence in measured outcomes based on client reports, both clients and their counselors were interviewed concerning client progress, to provide converging assessments of the same dimensions of treatment. This check on validity is responsive to recent questioning of the validity of drug research survey data (Hochhauser, 1979) and in keeping with attempts to assess the validity of clients' self-reports (e.g., Amsel, Mandell, Matthias, Mason, and Hockerman, 1976; Bale, 1979).

Rather than being a one-shot investigation of client progress, part of the present study was a 4-month follow-up of initially interviewed clients. A cross-section of current clients were initially interviewed, and their status was later reassessed. Thus, individual clients varied in the length of time in treatment prior to the evaluation points.

METHOD

Programs and Respondents

Counselors were included in this study only if they were full-time workers with a caseload of 25 or more clients for whom they had primary responsibility for the treatment regimen. Depending on staff size, interviews were conducted with either all or a random sample of counselors in a program, and usually with two top administrators per program. Four clients of each participating counselor, randomly selected from all clients who had been with the counselor at least 1 month, were also interviewed. The topics covered in all interviews were more extensive than described here; they include job description and attitudinal data reported by counselors and clients, and are summarized in Aiken et al. (1984) and LoSciuto et al. (1984). In all, 82 counselors, 302 clients, and 29 administrators participated. Demographic characteristics of counselors and clients are summarized in Table 1.

Respondents were from nine methadone maintenance (MM) and six drug-free outpatient (DF) programs within five major cities or surrounding areas: New York, Washington, DC, Chicago, Los Angeles, and San Francisco. A sixteenth program had both a methadone and a drug-free unit. Where possible, programs were chosen which had all three types of counselors, so as to avoid confounding program differences in terms of treatment regimen and client population with counselor group differences. In only two programs was a counselor group missing. The data were collected in 1977.

Procedure: Initial Study

Face-to-face interviews were conducted with all respondents at the program site. Data gathered from clients reflected upon aspects of their lives prior to treatment entry: demographic information, drug use history, treatment history, educational history, employment history, and criminal history. Questions were specifically asked about the year before entry into the current treatment program and the 30 days just before treatment entry. With regard to client progress in treatment up to the interview, clients were asked about their drug use,

Table 1

Demographic Characteristics of Counselors and Clients of the Three Groups

	Counselor group			Significance of difference
	PRO	NEA	EXA	
Counselors				
Sample size	31	20	31	
Sex (% male)	48.4	60.0	80.6	$p < .05$
Ethnic identity (%)				
Black	25.8	70.0	71.0	
White	67.7	20.0	22.6	$p < .01$
Other	6.5	10.0	6.4	
Mean age (yr)	29.9	36.5	39.4	$p < .001$
Clients				
Sample size	116	71	115	
Sex (% male)	61.2	64.8	63.5	$p > .20$
Ethnic identity (%)				
Black	43.6	52.9	49.6	
White	35.5	32.9	36.3	$p > .20$
Spanish-American	20.9	14.3	14.2	
Mean age (yr)	28.7	31.9	30.4	$p < .05$

education, employment, and criminality in the whole time since entry into treatment and also in the 30 days prior to the interview. In addition, in a self-administered questionnaire, they were asked about their life-styles in an assessment of the quality of their lives.

As previously indicated, data about each client were gathered also from counselors. Counselors reported specifically on the drug use, education, employment, and criminality of clients during the first criterion period of the study (i.e., the 30 days prior to the interview) in order to corroborate client responses for this same period. In addition, counselors reported on counseling input to each client during the course of the current treatment episode. Prior and/or concurrent input from counselors, other than the current primary counselor, was noted; the counselor group (PRO, NEA, EXA) and duration of input from each other counselor were determined.

Finally, administrators commented on any differences they saw in the caseloads of the three client groups.

Procedure: 4-Month Follow-up

The follow-up occurred 4 months after the initial interviewing. Each counselor in the study who was still working at the same program was asked to document the progress of each of the clients who had been interviewed previously, whether or not the client remained in treatment. Data were gathered about those clients who had remained with their primary counselors between the first and second data collection periods. If the counselor in question had left the program since the first interview, his clients were omitted from follow-up. If a client in question had switched to another primary counselor in the time between the first and second data collection episodes, then the data of this client were omitted from follow-up.

Counselors completed mail follow-up forms for each of their clients in the study. They reported on the current treatment status (in or out of treatment) of each client. For clients who had left treatment, counselors reported on the time and reason for each client's leaving, as well as the drug use, employment, education, and criminality of these clients in their last 30 days of treatment. For those clients who remained in treatment, counselors were asked about the same areas but with reference to the 30 days just prior to the follow-up. Follow-up data were collected concerning 257 of the original 302 clients (86%), of whom 186 remained in treatment, 68 had left treatment, and 3 had transferred to new programs.

RESULTS

The results are organized into six sections. The first reports any differences among the three client groups at the outset of treatment which might confound the interpretation of differences among these groups in treatment outcomes. This section is followed by a brief section on the convergence of clients' self-reports with counselors' reports of the same outcomes, to provide some measure of the validity of outcomes. The next sections consider patient progress in three aspects of their lives: drug use, productive activities including education and employment, and criminality. Data are presented councerning three points in time: the 30 days prior to treatment, the 30 days prior to the first interview, and the point of follow-up. In a final section, the more subjective psychological dimension of quality of life is examined.

In the presentation of results, percentages of members of the three client groups falling in certain categories are often reported. These percentages are always reported in the group order PRO, NEA, EXA.

Initial Differences among Client Groups

As seen from Table 1, client groups did not differ at all markedly in demographic characteristics, with only the relatively small age difference reaching significance. Five areas of client background, in addition to demographics, were explored in client interviews: drug use and treatment, educational, employment, and criminal history during the time periods of the whole year prior to treatment entry and the 30 days just prior to treatment entry. Across the five areas, client groups were contrasted on 94 measures, with only three differences, about the number expected by chance, reaching significance. (The 94 measures, plus a description of the three significant differences, are given in Aiken et al. [1984].) Descriptions by administrators of typical caseloads of the counselor groups corroborated the lack of difference evidenced in client self-reports, with 75% of administrators reporting equivalent numbers of heavy heroin users across groups; 75%, equivalent criminal records; and 71%, equivalent chance for success in treatment.

As previously explained, clients were interviewed not at entry into treatment but rather at some time during the course of treatment. In neither modality was there a difference in length of stay in treatment ($F < 1$) prior to the first interview; methadone clients had been in treatment on the average 21 months; drug-free clients, 7 months.

Client groups did not differ in the extent of input from other primary counselors prior to their current counselors, in the distribution of counselor group membership of previous counselors, or in the extent of or counselor group distribution of input from counselors other than the primary counselor at the time of the study. In the methadone maintenance modality, clients had spent on average 80% of their treatment time with current counselors; in the drug-free modality, 86% of their time. In sum, based on explorations of demographics, dimensions of treatment evaluation, and prior and current treatment input, there was little, if any, evidence of differences among clients in the three counselor groups, which differences would serve to distort analyses of client progress as a function of the counselor group of the clients' primary counselors.

Agreement between Client and Counselor Reports

In order to corroborate client self-reports of the 30 days prior to the first interview, the same questions were asked of counselors and clients concerning drug use in 12 drug categories, criminality, and employment status. In turn, to corroborate counselor follow-up reports, a subset of clients corroborated counselor responses. Percentage agreement on drug use versus nonuse across all categories was 87%. Agreement on employment status was 87%; on having been arrested, 96%; and on having been jailed, 95%. The substantial agreement provided confidence in both client and counselor reports, upon which initial and follow-up analyses, respectively, were based.

Drug Use

Drug Use Following Entry into Treatment: First Interview

Clients at the first interview estimated their frequency of use of 12 drugs or categories of drugs during two 30-day periods: (1) the 30 days prior to treatment entry and (2) the 30 days prior to the interview. The drugs and drug groups were marijuana/hashish, drug store items containing drugs, inhalants, hallucinogens, amphetamines, barbiturates, sedatives, cocaine, heroin, illegal methadone, other opiates, and alcohol to excess. For analysis, the 12 drug groups were considered separately, rather than combining use of all drugs into one drug involvement index, due to the substantial problem of interpretation of composite measures of drug use (Douglass and Khavari, 1982). The one exception was the construction of an Opiate Index as an overall measure of the use of heroin, illegal methadone, and/or any other opiate which leads to methadone eligibility. This index was simply the greatest frequency of use among the categories of opiates involved.

Drug use in the 30 days prior to the interview was low overall in most categories: inhalants, 0%; drug store items, 1%; amphetamines, 1%; hallucinogens, 2%; illegal methadone, 3%; other opiates and synthetics with morphine-like effects, 5%; alcohol to excess, 8%; barbiturates, 9%; and cocaine, 11%. In no case in either modality was there an association between the percentage of clients using any of these drugs and the counselor group ($p \geqslant .15$ in all cases by χ^2 test).

In the remaining three categories—that is, marijuana/hashish (52%), sedatives and tranquilizers (21%), and heroin (21%), as well as in the composite Opiate Index (24%)—percentages of clients using these drugs were sufficient in the 30 days prior to the interview to warrant more complete analysis. (See Table 2 for percentages of use by client group and modality.) Estimates of change in frequency of use from the 30 days prior to treatment entry to the 30 days prior to the first interview as a function of client groups were examined in analyses of covariance in which four covariates were employed: (1) the pretest level of use in the 30 days prior to treatment entry to adjust for any small pretest level differences among groups, and (2)-(4) the number of months the client had spent with previous primary counselors in each of the three counselor groups. These latter three covariates were employed to control for any possible differential counselor effects due to previous counseling.

In the methadone maintenance modality, there were no counselor group effects for any of the three drug categories or for the Opiate Index. In the drug-free modality, the only effect of client group was that for the use of marijuana/hashish, $F(2, 89) = 3.60$, $p < .05$, with clients of EXAs over and above others showing a decrease in use frequency. Percentages of clients who used any marijuana/hashish, however frequently, were 65, 40, and 59 by clients of PROs, NEAs, and EXAs, respectively, in the 30 days prior to treatment entry; and 63, 38, and 48 in the 30 days prior to the first interview.

Drug Use at Follow-up

In the follow-up study, counselors indicated for clients still in treatment how often the clients had used the 12 drug groups in the 30 days prior to

Table 2

Percentages of Any Drug Use during the 30 Days Prior to the First Interview and 30 Days Prior to Treatment Entry, as a Function of Counselor Group and Treatment Modality for Frequently Used Drugs

		Methadone maintenance (%)			Drug-free outpatient (%)			
Drug category	Time[a]	PRO	NEA	EXA	PRO	NEA	EXA	All groups (%)
Marijuana/hashish	Follow-up	49	32	35	50	27	39	39
	Interview	57	53	43	63	38	48	52
	Entry	54	40	41	65	40	59	50
Sedatives and tranquilizers	Follow-up	13	18	17	9	0	6	13
	Interview	17	24	27	28	12	14	21
	Entry	23	25	28	40	6	29[c]	27
Heroin	Follow-up	23	21	23	34	10	19	23
	Interview	15	19	17	39	24	26	21
	Entry	73	73	56	44	41	46	60
Composite Opiate Index[b]	Follow-up	23	26	27	33	10	24	25
	Interview	17	22	21	42	29	26	24
	Entry	80	76	66	50	47	51	65
		No. of cases						
Sample size								
Interview		75	54	71	41	17	44	302
Follow-up		52	49	67	39	13	37	257

[a]For the time variable, "entry" signifies the 30 days prior to treatment entry; "interview," 30 days prior to interview; "follow-up," 30 days prior to follow-up.

[b]The Opiate Index includes heroin, illegal methadone and other opiates, and synthetics with morphine-like effects. These values were not 100% in the methadone maintenance modality due to a number of clients having been transferred from other methadone programs.

[c]Groups differ ($p < .05$) when considered in terms of use versus no use, as tabled, but not when the continuous variable of use frequency is considered.

follow-up; for those clients who had terminated, in the 30 days prior to termination. For drug-free clients, there were no significant differences in the proportion of clients using any category of drugs ($p > .15$ in all cases by χ^2 test). For methadone maintenance clients, differences were noted in three nonopiate categories. First was barbiturates, $\chi^2(2) = 15.48$, $p < .001$, with 2%, 7%, and 26% of clients of PROs, NEAs, and EXAs, respectively, using any barbiturates. Second was amphetamines, $\chi^2 = 6.95, p < .05$, with 4%, 21%, and 10% of clients in the three groups, respectively, with any such use. Third was drugstore items, $\chi^2(2) = 7.17$, $p < .05$, with 17%, 0%, and 8% of clients in the three groups, respectively, with any such use. It should be noted that in each case, a different client group showed the greatest use: EXAs for barbiturates, NEAs for amphetamines, and PROs for drugstore items.

Clients' Views of Aid from Counselors

During the first interview clients were asked, in open-ended fashion, to indicate what their counselors had done to help them become and remain drug-free. About an eighth of all the clients stated that their counselors had done nothing, with such responses made by 20%, 13%, and 9% of clients of PROs, NEAs, and EXA, respectively, $\chi^2(2) = 6.20, p < .05$. These clients often further explained that they believed that they themselves were completely responsible for their own progress and that no one else could help them with their drug problems. Among the clients who indicated that their counselors had helped, the three most frequently mentioned forms of support were constant across groups; in order of frequency, these were: encouragement and help with coping, just talking, and giving insight into the drug problem.

Summary

Associations between drug use levels of clients and type of counselor were almost completely lacking at the point of the first interview. In fact, only one group difference was found: at this measurement point, slight decreases in marijuana use of clients of EXAs (but not NEAs and PROs) in the drug-free modality during treatment. At follow-up, three inconsistent polydrug use differences were found in the methadone maintenance modality, each with a different client group having the highest use. These differences, in some sense, balanced one another out, rather than providing a consistent picture of excessive polydrug use by one over the other client categories.

Productive Activities

Attending school or being employed (including being actively engaged as a homemaker) are two aspects of productive life-style. Both these classes of activities were considered.

Education

In Table 3, the educational activities of clients are given separately for vocational training and then for any schooling other than vocational training. Clients of the three groups did not differ at all in the percentages receiving any educational training, vocational or otherwise, in the 30 days prior to treatment entry (10%, 11%, and 9% for clients of PROs, NEAs, and EXAs, respectively); yet there tended to be an association between counselor group and the percentage of all clients receiving any schooling in the 30 days prior to the first interview (22%, 18%, and 11% for clients of PROs, NEAs, and EXAs, respectively), χ^2 (2) = 5.08, $p < .10$; $p < .05$ for the difference between PROs and EXAs.

At the time of follow-up, approximately equal percentages of each client group were enrolled in vocational school ($p > .20$). However, a substantially higher proportion of clients of PROs (26%) than of either NEAs (11%) or EXAs (9%) were enrolled in academic programs, $\chi^2(2) = 11.74, p < .01$.

An interesting comparison among counselor groups can be made by considering the educational status at follow-up of clients not in school at the time of the first interview. Of clients not initially in school, 23%, 8%, and 9% of clients of PROs, NEAs, and EXAs, respectively, were in school at follow-up, $\chi^2(2) = 8.90, p < .05$.

In order to interpret the finding that clients of PROs had a consistent schooling advantage, the eligibility of clients for further schooling was considered, in terms of the joint distribution of age and previous academic achievement at treatment entry. Clients of PROs, it will be recalled, were the youngest at treatment entry (see Table 1), and this age difference might have been correlated with prior educational achievement in such a way that there were more likely candidates for schooling among PROs. In fact, 18%, 6%, and 12% of clients of PROs, NEAs, and EXAs, respectively, held high school diplomas or GEDs and were also between the ages of 16 and 25, an age range in which college might likely be considered, $\chi^2(2) = 6.18$, $p < .05$ for the difference among the three groups; $z = 2.59$, $p < .01$ for the contrast between PROs and NEAs. For clients between the ages of 12 and 20 who had not completed high school, analogous percentages were 4, 1, and 3, respectively. These differences in percentages of likely school candidates are not large enough to account completely for the advantage to PROs over EXAs in school enrollment, particularly since the larger difference in school eligibility fell to clients of PROs over NEAs, and not PROs over EXAs. In sum, it appeared that some, but not all, of the difference in school attendance by clients of the three groups might be attributable to demographic characteristics.

Employment

Employment status of the groups at the three measurement periods is also summarized in Table 3. Percentages of clients employed at treatment entry

Table 3

Percentage of Clients Engaged in Productive Activities and Indices of Criminality, as a Function of Counselor Group at Three Measurement Points

	30 days prior to treatment entry (%)			30 days prior to first interview (%)			Follow-up measurement (%)		
Client status	PRO	NEA	EXA	PRO	NEA	EXA	PRO	NEA	EXA
Vocational training	4	3	7	9	2	4	13	7	9
Other schooling	7	10	3	15	16	8	26	11	9
Employed	29	30	28	25	34	26	48	55	40
Housewife	46	48	53	67	68	77	—[a]	—	—
Arrested	4	7	9	4	1	6	2	6	6
Any time in jail	7	9	12	3	3	5	2	6	5

[a]Data not collected at follow-up.

were almost identical across groups. Again at the time of the first interview, groups did not differ significantly in percentages employed, $p > .20$. With previous counselor input and number of days employed in the 30 days before treatment entry partialled out, change in number of days employed from 30 days prior to treatment to 30 days prior to the first interview also did not differ across groups. Of clients not employed at entry into treatment, 13%, 22%, and 12% of clients of PROs, NEAs, and EXAs, respectively, were employed in the 30 days prior to the first interview, $p > .20$.

Women's status as housewives was considered as a component of the employment variable. While 49% had been housewives in the 30 days prior to treatment entry, fully 71% were so occupied during the 30 days prior to the first interview, with a relatively uniform increase between these time periods noted in the three counselor groups (see Table 3) and no difference in the percentage of housewives across groups just prior to the interview ($p > .20$).

At follow-up, there was once more no association between employment status and counselor group. A comparison was made across groups of the employment status at follow-up of clients who had been unemployed at the point of the first interview. There was no association between counselor group and these rates. On an encouraging note, in each counselor group there was a significant gain in the employment rate between the first interview and the follow-up, $p = .001$, .001, and .06 for clients of the three groups, respectively.

Clients were questioned about six specific sources of their income during the 30 days prior to the first interview: work, welfare, unemployment compensation, a spouse, parents, and other relatives; in addition to their being asked in open-ended fashion about other income sources. Work was most often mentioned, followed by welfare or food stamps. For only this latter source was there a tendency for association with counselor groups, the source having been mentioned by 38%, 23%, and 35% of clients of PROs, NEAs, and EXAs, respectively, $\chi^2(2) = 5.83$, $p < .10$. For all other sources mentioned, these percentages were very similar across groups, with similarities substantially outweighing the one difference.

On a more subjective note, when clients were asked what their counselors had done to help them find and/or keep jobs, no evidence emerged that any counselor group was more supportive of employment efforts than any other. Clients did, however, see their counselors as supportive of employment-related activities. Of clients unemployed at the time of the first interview, 29%, 37%, and 36% of clients of PROs, NEAs, EXAs, respectively, indicated that their counselor had gotten them job leads, arranged for job interviews, or arranged for clients to meet with people who had access to jobs.

Summary

Participation in some form of schooling was associated with counselor group at the time of both the initial and follow-up interviews, with the advantage accruing to the clients of PROs. In contrast, there was no association between counselor group and employment rates at any measurement point.

Criminality

Client groups were remarkably similar in both measures of criminality (i.e., being arrested or jailed) in the 30 days prior to treatment entry and the 30 days prior to the first interview, as well as during all the time between the first interview and the follow-up measurement point. At no point did any differences in percentages approach conventional significance levels (see Table 3).

Quality of Life

During the initial interview only an attempt was made to assess some dimensions of "quality of life" for clients apart from their drug use, productivity (education and employment), and criminality. Areas of questioning fell into five categories: (1) participation in routine activities, that is, ordinary chores, tasks, and activities in which many nonaddicted individuals regularly indulge; (2) participation in antisocial activities, primarily related to drugs and the street; (3) physical health; (4) social isolation versus nonisolation; and finally (5) clients' perceptions of their physical environment.

Routine Activities

Routine activities included matters of personal hygiene, household chores, spending time with family members and friends, and engaging in entertaining activities such as hobbies and sports. Across 22 such items, there were no differences among client groups in the frequency with which clients engaged in each of these activities in the 30 days prior to the first interview ($p > .20$ in all cases).

Antisocial Behaviors

More central than routine activites for this study were client reports of the frequency with which clients engaged in a number of socially undesirable behaviors. These included using, buying, and selling drugs; and other illicit behaviors such as stealing, pimping, and prostituting. Across 11 such activities, there were no differences among counselor groups in their reported frequencies of engaging in such activities ($p > .20$ in all cases).

Physical Health

Indices of physical health also failed to reveal either differences among counselor groups or evidence for extremely poor health in general. Specifically, clients in all groups reported on average good appetites and no marked difficulty in sleeping, and rated their health as good ($p > .20$ for all three contrasts among client groups).

Social Isolation

Indicators of social interaction show that clients were not, as a whole, isolated. Only 14%, 21%, and 19% of clients of PROs, NEAs, and EXAs, respectively, lived alone in the 30 days prior to the first interview, $\chi^2(2) = 1.87$, $p > .20$ for differences among groups. In terms of steady opposite-sex relationships, there was no contingency between client group and whether a client lived with an opposite-sex partner (55%, 49%, 49%) or had an opposite-sex partner with whom to visit regularly (24%, 23%, 23%), $\chi^2(4) = 2.00$, $p > .20$ for contingency between group and relationship status. Approximately 20% of clients lived with parents, and 40% had their own children living with them; these percentages were also equivalent across groups ($p > .20$ in both cases). Clients who lived with anyone rated themselves as on average satisfied with the people with whom they lived; ratings were constant across groups, $F(2, 250) = 1.44$, $p > .20$.

Physical Environment

In all, 15%, 7%, and 14% of clients of PROs, NEAs, and EXAs, respectively, had changed residences in the 30 days prior to the first interview, $\chi^2(2) = 2.74$, $p > .20$. Asked to rate their satisfaction with their homes and neighborhoods, clients gave ratings which were stable across counselor groups ($F < 1$ in both cases).

Summary

Across five areas of life quality examined, no differences were found among client groups.

DISCUSSION

Considering all outcomes in the present investigation, one is forced to conclude that there is essentially no evidence of differential effectiveness of the three counselor groups, except in the area of stimulating client educational activities. A conclusion of no difference can be taken as meaningful only if two critical research design criteria have been met. First, the design must have had sufficient statistical power that differences could have been detected had they truly existed in the population. Second, the data must be of sufficient stability that the failure to find differences cannot be attributed to the presence of a large amount of error of measurement; such error precludes the detection of meaningful treatment effects. Only in light of a demonstration of sufficient statistical power and adequate measurement can the finding of no difference among groups be interpreted as an accurate representation of a phenomenon under investigation.

The present design was of adequate statistical power; that is, the design was sufficiently sensitive, in terms of number of cases, that any existing differences in the population would have been detected. In this study, differences which even approached significance at $p = .10$ were reported, to increase the possibility of detecting discrepanices among groups. According to the criterion proposed by Cohen (1977), the present design, with one minor exception, provided acceptable statistical power (80%) for all reported comparisons, given moderate effect sizes (true differences) in the population and a Type I error probability of .05. The one exception was the power of tests of difference in drug use at follow-up of the 89 drug-free clients; given a Type I error rate of .05, the power would be 72% (i.e., 72% chance of detecting a true difference instead of the 80% stipulated by Cohen). If a Type I error rate of .10 were employed, as was the case here, the power would reach an acceptable 82%. In all, on the basis of power analysis, it is concluded that had differences existed, they would have been detected in this design.

The issue of adequacy of measurement is a more complicated one and merits discussion of the format for data collection, including consensual and validity checks, as well as the capacity of the questionnaire to detect differences, if they existed.

Client self-reports served as the data for comparison at the time of the first interview. At follow-up, counselor reports were the basic data. At each measurement point, however, data relevant to the same questions were gathered from both counselor and clients. Disagreements between counselor and client reports (e.g., in percentages of clients employed or using a particular drug at a particular level) were typically very small and without bias for one respondent group to present a more favorable picture than the other. Further, with regard to drug use data, counselors had employed information from urine tests during the interview when giving their drug use estimates. This provided, in the case of the most critical outcome measure, not only consensus as evidence of data accuracy but also an outside criterion of validity.

Given evidence for consensus and external criterion validity, a consideration is required of the capacity of the questionnaires themselves to detect differences. At the simplest level, there must be neither ceiling nor floor effects in the data. For data reported in both Tables 2 and 3, such problematic effects do not exist. In addition, stability of measurement is required. The convergence of counselor and client responses provides evidence of interjudge reliability. Moreover, the broad range of responses for the same activity tends to be consistent over time. For example, those clients reporting that they were in vocational training ranged from 5% at the first measurement point (30 days prior to treatment entry), to 6% at the second measurement point (30 days prior to the first interview), and to 10% at follow-up. To take a more frequent self-report as an example, 29% of the clients were employed during the 30 days prior to treatment entry, compared to 27% at point 2 and 46% at follow-up. The preceding results lend credence to the questionnaires' potential sensitivity to any differences, had they existed.

One might argue that the hard criteria used for assessing differences (e.g., whether a client is employed or not, or is using a specific drug or not) do not reflect the full picture of counseling efforts as a function of counselor groups. Aiken et al. (1984), in a job description of activities of the three counselor groups, found that these groups converged in the counseling activities they provided their clients. Yet another picture can be gleaned by asking clients what their counselors actually do to help them. When such questions were asked for drug use and employment, only a few differences emerged. In the case of drug use, clients of PROs were somewhat less willing to say that their counselors had helped them. In the case of employment, no differences were noted. In a similar vein, one might evaluate counselors in terms of their clients' feelings about them. LoSciuto et al. (1984) reported somewhat more favorable feelings of clients of EXAs to their counselors than clients of PROs and NEAs, in terms of knowledgeability about drugs and the street, willingness to bring problems to counselors, and expectations that counselors would help with problems. These differences in favor of clients of EXAs were relatively small, however, and were not associated with differences in outcomes. Since it is ultimately the clients' outcomes with which service providers must be concerned, it was concluded that there was no evidence of a favorability of one counselor group over another in this study (regardless of the criteria adopted).

Given that overall differences are not evident in counselor effectiveness in this study, the question arises as to whether any of the counselors are really engaged in helping the clients. Our previously reported studies show that they are, both by counselors' own self-reported activities and by clients' and administrators' reports and perceptions of their counselors. The wide variety of functions and activities of the counselors was consistent with the literature. Counselors generally exhibited high levels of energy in attempting to better the lives of their clients, and the efforts were recognized by both clients and administrators. Further, there was more variation within than between counselor groups in the extent of participation in all activities (Aiken et al., 1984; LoSciuto et al., 1984).

Examination of Tables 2 and 3 allows us to eliminate still another possible reason for the lack of differential effectiveness among counselor groups. That is, it might be speculated that differences failed to show up because none of the counselor groups was effective, regardless of their efforts to help. While broad ranges of percent responses for each activity were consistent across time, the actual percentages of reported socially desirable activities generally increased during the treatment period. The percentage of those employed, for example, was higher at follow-up than at measurement points 1 and 2. Even more critical are the corresponding figures reported for drug use. Table 2 shows that the overall percentages of those reporting drug use at follow-up are in every case much lower than the percentage reporting such use just prior to treatment entry.

A possible explanation of the lack of difference lies in the convergence among counselor groups in their treatment goals and treatment techniques over time. Regardless of counselor background, the focus of treatment may well narrow; counselors in general may develop into addiction specialists, using relatively few techniques and having narrowly defined outcome goals and criteria of success. All this focus on the specific addiction aspects of the clients' problems may well occur in the face of much more global rehabilitation needs on the part of clients. It would be of interest to study the development of counselors as they work in drug treatment settings; that is, to examine those changes which might occur which transform counselors with a variety of backgrounds and approaches into the relatively homogeneous group described here.

In all, it seems reasonable to conclude that lack of differential effectiveness among counselor groups does not at all mean that the groups are inactive or ineffective. Rather, the lack of group differences may stem from a tendency of counselors to do many of the same things, modified by a rational approach to the employment of the specific talents of individual counselors, regardless of group membership. In any case, the lack of differences seems to be a real effect, rather than a spurious result of inadequate statistical power or insensitive measurement.

ACKNOWLEDGMENT

This research was supported by NIDA contract number 271-76-4410 to the first and second authors.

REFERENCES

AIKEN, L.S., LO SCIUTO, L.A., AUSETTS, M.A., and BROWN, B.S. Paraprofessional versus professional drug counselors: Diverse routes to the same role. *Int. J. Addict.* 19(2): 153-173, 1984.

AMSEL. Z., MANDELL, W., MATTHIAS, L., MASON, C., and HOCKERMAN, I. Reliability and validity of self-reported illegal activities and drug use collected from narcotics addicts. *Int. J. Addict.* 11(2): 325-336, 1976.

BALE, R.N. The validity and reliability of self-reported data from heroin addicts: Mailed questionnaires compared with face-to-face interviews. *Int. J. Addict.* 14(7): 993-1000, 1979.

BROWN, B.S., and THOMPSON, R.F. The effectiveness of formerly addicted and nonaddicted counselors on client functioning. *Drug Forum.* 5(2): 123-129, 1976.

COHEN, J. *Statistical Power Analysis for the Behavioral Sciences.* New York: Academic Press, 1977.

CONNETT, G.E. Comparison of progress of patients with professional and paraprofessional counselors in a methadone maintenance program. *Int. J. Addict.* 15(4): 585-589, 1980.

DOUGLASS, F.M., and KHAVARI, K.A. A major limitation of the percentile index of overall drug use indulgence. *Int. J. Addict.* 17(2): 283-294, 1982.

DURLAK, J.A. Comparative effectiveness of paraprofessional and professional helpers. *Psychol. Bull.* 86(1): 80-92, 1979.

HAERTZEN, C.A., and PANTON, J.H. Development of a "psychopathic" scale for the addiction research center inventory (ARCI). *Int. J. Addict.* 2: 115-127, 1967.

HOCHHAUSER, M. Bias in drug abuse survey research. *Int. J. Addict.* 14(5): 675-687, 1979.

LONGWELL, B., MILLER, J., and NICHOLS, A.W. Counselor effectiveness in a methadone maintenance program. *Int. J. Addict.* 13(2): 307-315, 1978.

LO SCIUTO, L., AIKEN, L.S., AUSETTS, M.A., and BROWN, B.S. Paraprofessional versus professional drug abuse counselors: Attitudes and expectations of the counselors and their clients. *Int. J. Addict.* 19(3): 233-252, 1984.

LUBORSKY, L., SINGER, B., and LUBORSKY, L. Comparative studies of psychotherapies. *Arch. Gen. Psychiatry* 32: 995-1008, 1975.

NIETZEL, M.T., and FISHER, S.G. Effectiveness of professional and paraprofessional helpers: A comment on Durlak. *Psychol. Bull.* 89(3): 555-565, 1981.

OTTOMANELLI, G.A. Patient improvement, measured by the MMPI and *Pyp,* related to paraprofessional and professional counselor assignment. *Int. J. Addict.* 13(3): 503-507, 1978.

The International Journal of the Addictions, 19(4), 403–410, 1984

An Analysis of Alcohol Portrayal on Prime-Time Television

Emily J. Futch,* MA

Stephen A. Lisman,† PhD

Department of Psychology
SUNY–Binghamton
Binghamton, New York 13901

Marilyn I. Geller, PhD

Susquehanna Psychological Affiliates
Binghamton, New York 13905

Abstract

A content and functional analysis of alcohol use was conducted on the 15 most popular prime-time television programs in late 1979. These shows were videotaped and then rated by two independent observers. Interrater agreement, averaged over all code categories, was 91%. Results indicated that alcohol use and verbalizations about alcohol are frequent occurrences on prime-time television. Antecedent conditions to alcohol ingestion were identified. However, no consistent behavioral consequences of alcohol use were observed.

How do children and adolescents come to know about alcohol—for example, settings for appropriate drinking, motives for drinking, and abuses of alcohol?

*Present address: 2421 6th Avenue West, Bradenton, Florida 33505.
†To whom reprint requests should be addressed at the Department of Psychology, SUNY–Binghamton, Binghamton, New York 13901.

0020-773X/84/1904-0403$3.50/0

Obvious answers come readily and have been documented ad nauseum: peers, family, culture, etc. Certainly, it is becoming clear that children and adolescents know much about different aspects of alcohol, often long before they have had much personal experience with the drug. Indeed, Christiansen, Goldman, and Inn (1982) found that young adolescent nondrinkers and older, more experienced drinkers reported many of the same expectancies about alcohol's effects on behavior.

One frequently overlooked source of information about the effects of alcohol is that omnipresent staple of our daily lives—television. Indeed, children are heavy viewers of television. They view approximately 3½ hours a day (Wartella, Alexander, and Lemish, 1979) and report that television is one of their prime sources of information about alcohol and drugs (Frejer, Smart, Whitehead, and Lajorest, 1971). As both Knieveton (1976) and Collins and Marlatt (1981) conclude, since direct experience with and knowledge about alcohol is relatively limited or ambiguous for many children and adolescents, it is quite possible that their learning about and subsequent use of alcohol are heavily influenced by viewing the alcohol use of televised models. Therefore, it seems somewhat surprising that, with the exception of anecdotal reports, little is known about the role of television in influencing drinking in youth. Until recently, even simple descriptive information was lacking on the way that alcohol use is portrayed on television, outside of commercial advertising.

The methodologically most sophisticated investigations of alcohol depiction on television appear to be those of Garlington (1977) and Lowery (1980), both of whom focused on afternoon "soap operas." Garlington found that alcohol-related events appeared during 3 1-minute intervals per program, and that most drinking occurred at home. However, he chose not to present data about and reasons for the drinking that occurred. Lowery also examined alcohol portrayals on "soaps" and found that they occurred 1.5 times per 30 minutes of programming. Further, she reported that 47% of the total recorded incidents were for purposes of social facilitation (i.e., ritualistic or tension reducing), 30% for escape from reality, and 23% for crisis management. Analyses of drinking consequences led her to conclude that 70% of incidents were reinforced (positively or negatively) or had no consequences, while 30% were punished. Although we question Lowery's units of analysis (program scenes, instead of temporal units) and her categorizations of motives for drinking, her study offers a clear advance over most others in its attention to what viewers may be learning about drinking motives and outcomes. Further, both Lowery and Garlington are most systematic in their careful establishment of highly reliable coding systems. However, both of these studies focused on soap operas, which are viewed considerably less frequently by children than are programs at other times of the day (Wartella et al., 1979).

McEwen and Hanneman (1974) conducted one of the first examinations of televised alcohol use during evening "prime time"—typically defined as 8-11

P.M., Monday through Saturday, and Sunday from 7 to 11 P.M. They found that alcohol was by far the most frequently depicted drug, with from 1.3 to 1.6 alcohol-related incidents occurring per hour. In addition, they reported that alcohol was typically portrayed in a positive, social fashion, usually involving at least two people. While their study was a fine first effort to describe televised alcohol portrayal during the time of day when young viewers are plentiful, it was limited by several factors. First, the authors failed to monitor interrater agreement of the rating code throughout the study. They reported good reliability for the rating code as assessed during its preparation and development only. More importantly, in light of subsequent reports (discussed later), we feel that McEwen and Hanneman may have underestimated verbal references to alcohol use, since they recorded only those alcohol incidents that lasted at least a few seconds. Finally, due to the broad drug-oriented scope of their study, they appear to have omitted many potentially relevant categories of alcohol use, thereby constraining the conclusions they could reach.

Despite this noteworthy beginning, our literature review reveals that no subsequent investigations of alcohol portrayal during prime time have attempted to provide more complete analytic information regarding, for example, contexts, motives, or consequences of drinking.* Yet, without such information, it is often difficult to understand the meaning of frequency counts, per se, even if the latter were free of methodological flaws. For example, the *Christian Science Monitor* reported the findings of a study by Dillin (1975), which indicated that portrayal of alcohol use appeared on 80% of prime-time programs. Aside from the problem of evaluating the scientific merit of a research report described in a newspaper, the study offers little meaning beyond these numbers. Fernandez-Collado, Greenberg, Korzenny, and Atkin (1978) and Greenberg, Fernandez-Collado, Graef, Korzenny, and Atkin (1979) found that prime-time and Saturday-morning viewing depict alcohol incidents more than 2 times per hour. However, from their reports, it is not possible to conclude anything about drinking motives, contexts, or consequences. Breed and DeFoe (1978) attempted to interpret their findings that alcohol-drinking acts averaged 4.7 per prime time hour, by including an analysis of the types of drinkers. Yet, their breakdowns in terms of "villains," "weak characters," and "good guys" seem of dubious value.

In the study described here, our purpose is to delineate alcohol-related events on prime-time television, that portion of television heavily viewed by children and adolescents. Our study represents improvements over previous analyses of prime-time programming in the following ways: (1) inclusion of additional coding categories to gather more information; (2) refinement of code

*At press time we found we had overlooked an excellent study by W. Breed and J.R. DeFoe (The portrayal of the drinking process on prime-time television. *J. Commun.* 31: 58-67, 1981). Despite procedural differences, several of their major conclusions are consistent with those of our study reported here.

categories to include, for example, a sex breakdown of the major characters involved in alcohol use; (3) continuous-time recording of alcohol-related events, so that potentially useful data will not be lost; (4) improvement in the assessment of reliability of ratings; (5) addition of a functional analysis to assess antecedents and consequences of alcohol use.

METHOD

Overview

The 15 most popular prime-time programs were selected from the Nielson ratings of November 16, 1979 (see Note 1). An observational code was developed that included a number of variables delineating alcohol use in those same television shows. Relevant code categories were either developed by the present researchers or selected and revised based upon code categories used in three earlier content analyses (Fernandez-Collado et al., 1978; Garlington, 1977; McEwen and Hanneman, 1974) already reported. These 15 shows were then videotaped and rated according to the procedures described in the next section.

Observers and Observational Procedures

Two undergraduates served as independent observers of the videotaped materials. The observers were initially trained in the use of the observational code by (1) demonstrating knowledge of the code definitions via written reproduction and (2) practicing the use of the code and receiving feedback regarding their performance. The observers received approximately 10 hours of training, which was sufficient to bring about a coding interrater agreement of approximately 75%.

The observers independently coded the videotaped materials, and both were informed that reliability would be calculated for all of their observational ratings. One observer viewed and coded all of the videotaped materials, while the second observer provided observational data for interrater reliability. Interrater agreement was computed for 33% of the television programs; these programs were randomly selected. Due to the continuous recording of duration of alcohol use and the nature of the observational categories, the observers were instructed to view each program two times to facilitate accurate recording when and if any alcohol incident occurred.

Our observational code comprised the following categories: duration (of alcohol on camera), frequency of appearance, reference to alcohol (e.g., verbal comment or direct ingestion), length of program, type of beverage, type of program, reason for drinking, characters involved in drinking, place of drinking, and consequences for drinking (Note 2).

RESULTS

Reliability

The average interrater reliability for duration of beverage use, a continuous measure, was 95%. This was calculated by dividing the larger time recording into the smaller of the pair of recordings. Reliability for the dichotomous measures of verbal references, beverage type, reason for drinking, place of drinking, and characters involved in drinking was calculated by dividing the number of agreements on occurrence by the number of agreements and disagreements. Interrater agreement for verbal references was found to be 95%; for beverage type it was 93%; for place of drinking, 89%; and for characters involved in drinking, 90%. Overall interrater reliability was found to be 91%.

Frequency and Duration

Our results reveal that 12 of the 15 television programs demonstrated alcohol-related events; that is, either the actual use of alcohol or a verbal reference. All 15 programs demonstrated the use of nonalcoholic beverages. Although most studies referred to in our literature review expressed their results in terms of frequency per hour of televised programming, the role of alcohol in the construction of a story line may vary considerably depending on whether the writers are allowed 30 minutes or 60 minutes. To maximize our interpretive opportunities, we have provided a breakdown of our data to reflect differences between: (1) 30- versus 60-minute programs; (2) analysis of data on a program versus hourly basis.

Note that 4 of the 15 programs revealed no alcohol use at all, and 1 revealed a single verbal reference. Two hour-long programs from 10 to 11 P.M. were among the most popular of the 60-minute programs, but their late hour might be viewed as an opportunity to more freely portray drinking, as one of many adult themes more likely to be portrayed on television during later hours. Yet our data for "Dallas" and "Trapper John" revealed substantially fewer depictions of alcohol in each category of Table 1.

Table 1 also reveals that calculation of the portrayal of alcohol incidents on an hourly basis yields data that consistently exceed those calculated on a "per program" basis. Clearly, calculation of the portrayal of alcohol on an hourly basis is the preferred statistic, according to its appearance in the literature reviewed. However, Table 1 shows that the largest contribution to the portrayed alcohol incidents is made by verbal references on 30-minute programs.

Although most of the literature reviewed reports alcohol portrayal in terms of frequency (e.g., incidents/time unit), we felt that meaningful interpretation of such data would be facilitated by also determining the total duration of these incidents. Therefore, we summed the duration, in seconds, of all alcohol

Table 1

Mean Frequency of Alcohol Incidents

	Hourly	All programs	30-min programs ($N = 10$)	60-min programs ($N = 5$)
Frequency of appearance	2.20	1.46	1.30	1.80
Verbal references	5.30	3.53	4.80	1.00
Total incidents	7.50	5.00	6.10	2.80

incidents—not including verbal references—and divided that by the number of alcohol incidents in order to derive the average duration of each appearance of alcohol on the screen. We found that the average duration for each appearance of alcohol was 96.9 seconds, or just slightly more than 1.5 minutes each. Multiplying this mean by the mean frequency-of-appearance data in Table 1, we found that, on the average, alcohol appeared for 2.4 minutes per program, or 3.4 minutes per hour.

Antecedents and Consequences

Despite the apparent subjectivity of this category, reasons for drinking were rated with the reliability of .89. Incidents of drinking, not including verbal references, were classified as Hospitality, 25%; Enjoyment, 29%; Celebration, 33%; and Tension Reduction, 13%. To our surprise, only one incident of alcohol use had an observable or readily inferrable consequence attached to it. The one exception was classified as having positive consequences.

Other Descriptive Information

At an agreement level of .93, types of alcohol beverages were observed to be frequently unclassifiable by virtue of vague or overly general depiction, or more often, to consist of wine or beer. Spirits, consumed either straight or in mixed drinks, comprised 18% of the categorizable beverages.

The location where alcohol was consumed was categorized with a reliability of .84, the lowest agreement level attained. Alcohol was depicted being consumed in the home during 42% of the portrayals; in a bar during 17%; in a restaurant, 4%; and in wide range of other settings, 37%.

Finally, there seemed to be few sex differences in the depiction of alcohol incidents—both the drinking of alcohol and the verbal reference to it. With a reliability of .90, alcohol incidents involved a male star on 14 occasions and a female star on 9; a male "regular" was involved on 9 occasions, and likewise, a female "regular" on 9 occasions.

DISCUSSION

Including verbal references, we found that alcohol incidents characterized 80% of programs, a figure exactly comparable to that reported by Dillin (1975). Like Fernandez-Collado et al. (1978) and Greenberg et al. (1979), we found alcohol incidents during prime time more than 2 times per hour. Greenberg et al. (1979) noted that of the alcohol users on prime time, 65% were male and 35% female; we observed a 60:40 ratio for stars and a 50:50 ratio for program "regulars." The comparability of our data to those of Garlington and of Lowery is limited by their respective concentration on "soaps." However, it is notable that Lowery found 1.5 alcohol portrayals (not including verbal references) per 30 minutes of programming, and Garlington reported alcohol-related events during almost 3 1-minute intervals for each half hour of programming. Both sets of results find clearly comparable counterparts in the cells of our Table 1. In sum, although we observed programs televised only during 1 week, our 1 week's observations offer a highly representative sample and, as such, present a valid basis from which to derive the following conclusions and implications.

In short, as we observed them, many of the qualitative aspects of alcohol portrayals on television seemed consistent with appropriate, societally approved forms of consumption. Male and female characters typically drank for pleasure, consumed alcohol at home, and rarely drank "straight" distilled spirits, preferring wine, beer, and mixed drinks.

We agree with Greenberg et al. (1979), who caution against the temptation to overinterpret descriptive data by making assertions about what amount of alcohol portrayal is safe, too much, etc. At the frequency levels we observed, whatever influence televised alcohol incidents may have on youngsters' drinking will likely be due more to the quality and nature of the portrayals than the mere frequency of such portrayals. Lamentably, the effect on youngsters of repeated exposure to portrayals of alcohol consumption (even at low frequencies) is, as yet, undocumented and awaits further study. In addition, we found no portrayal of any consistent consequences attached to drinking episodes. And, even had we observed them, we would not know how—in the context of an entire program—these consequences would be perceived and evaluated by young viewers (cf. Kinder, 1975).

What we wish most emphatically to convey is that understanding the meaning of descriptive data such as ours awaits a next, most important step—plugging these data into experimental studies. Given contemporary sophistication in research design and methodology, the time is surely ripe for alcohol researchers to develop experiments that might parallel those that elucidated the impact of televised aggression on children. We have just completed such a study, designed to examine the influence of some prime-time portrayals of drinking on children's attitudes (and behaviors) toward alcohol (Lisman, Futch, and Geller, 1984). Similar experiments examining the impact of the frequency and duration of such portrayals, and the degree of familiarity of the observing children with alcohol's effects are also warranted. While such studies develop, we would encourage further random sampling of weekly programming using our detailed rating procedures in order to monitor the stability and change of televised alcohol portrayals in response to expressed public concerns.

NOTES

1. The top 15 television shows (excluding "60 Minutes") in mid-November 1979 were: (1) "Taxi," (2) "The Jeffersons," (3) "Dallas," (4) "Alice," (5) "One Day at a Time," (6) "Three's Company," (7) "M.A.S.H.," (8) "Trapper John," (9) "Archie Bunker's Place," (10) "Charlie's Angels," (11) "Angie," (12) "Eight Is Enough," (13) "Happy Days," (14) "WKRP," (15) "Little House on the Prairie."
2. A more detailed description of the code categories will be sent on request.

REFERENCES

BREED, W., and DE FOE, J.R. Drinking on television. *Bottom Line on Alcohol in Society* 2: 28-29, 1978.

CHRISTIANSEN, B.A., GOLDMAN, M.S., and INN, A. Development of alcohol-related expectancies in adolescents: Separating pharmacological from social-learning influences. *J. Consult. Clin. Psychol.* 50: 336-344, 1982.

COLLINS, R.L., and MARLATT, G.A. Social modelling as a determinant of drinking behavior: Implications for prevention and treatment. *Addict. Behav.* 6: 233-239, 1981.

DILLIN, J. TV drinking: How networks pour liquor into your living room. *Christian Science Monitor,* June 30, 1975, pp. 1-6.

FERNANDEZ-COLLADO, C.F., GREENBERG, B.S., KORZENNY, F., and ATKIN, C.K. Sexual intimacy and drug use in TV series. *J. Commun.* 28: 30-37, 1978.

FREJER, D., SMART, R.G., WHITEHEAD, P.C., and LAJOREST, L. Sources of information about drugs among high school students. *Public Opinion Q.* 4: 236-241, 1971.

GARLINGTON, W.K. Drinking on television: A preliminary study with emphasis on method. *J. Stud. Alcohol* 38: 2199-2205, 1977.

GREENBERG, B.S., FERNANDEZ-COLLADO, C., GRAEF, D., KORZENNY, F., and ATKIN, C.K. Trends in use of alcohol and other substances on television. *J. Drug Educ.* 9: 243-253, 1979.

KINDER, B. Attitudes toward alcohol and drug abuse. II. Experimental data, mass media research, and methodological considerations. *Int. J. Addict.* 10: 1035-1054, 1975.

KNIEVETON, B.H. Social learning and imitation in relation to television. In R. Brown (ed.), *Children and Television.* Beverly Hills, CA: Sage, 1976.

LISMAN, S.A., FUTCH, E.J., and GELLER, M.I. *Alcohol and television: What children see and how it affects them.* Presented at the National Council on Alcoholism Forum, Detroit, April 1984.

LOWERY, S.A. Soap and booze in the afternoon: An analysis of the portrayal of alcohol use in daytime serials. *J. Stud. Alcohol* 41: 829-838, 1980.

MC EWEN, W.J., and HANNEMAN, G.J. The depiction of drug use in television programming. *J. Drug Educ.* 4: 281-293, 1974.

WARTELLA, E., ALEXANDER, A., and LEMISH, D. The mass media environment of children. *Am. Behav. Sci.* 23: 33-52, 1979.

The International Journal of the Addictions, 19(4), 411–418, 1984

Alcohol and Drug Use in the Elderly Visited at Home

M. T. Malcolm, MD, MRCPsych

Clatterbridge Hospital
Bebington, Wirral, Merseyside
United Kingdom

Abstract

During a 3 year prospective study, 223 new patients aged 65 and over were seen at their own residences. This setting enabled a detailed record to be made of current medication and alcohol use. The average consumption was 2.9 different drugs daily per patient, but one-third of the patients took 4 or more different preparations. One patient in 10 showed a severe alcohol-related problem. These findings were in a group with an average age of 77, not overtly physically ill, referred for a psychiatric opinion.

INTRODUCTION

An elderly person referred to a hospital doctor usually has several problems. The medical, psychiatric, social, and environmental aspects and their interactions have to be assessed. While direct hospital admission can enable various professions to assess and treat the individual, this is an unreal and unfamiliar setting. More may be achieved by an initial visit to the patient's home, where practical difficulties can be considered in their true setting. Neighbors and relatives can be interviewed, the facilities of the home observed, and the drink cupboard and pill cabinet examined.

0020-773X/84/1904-0411$3.50/0

METHODS

Between September 1978 and September 1981 a prospective study was made of all patients over 65 referred to the author for a domiciliary visit. Domicile was taken to include own home, sheltered accommodation, or old folks' home. A full history was taken including the opinion of the general practitioner and views of the family. A detailed examination was made of all available medicaments, and all currently taken preparations were listed. Alcohol consumption was assessed as best as possible from history, accounts from others, and polite inspection. Recent care from physicians or geriatricians was noted.

RESULTS

Two hundred and fifty-one patients aged over 65 were referred. This constituted 50% of all referrals, though only 15% of the population served is in this age group. Of the 251, 28 were repeat visits, leaving a study group of 223 new patients. The average age was 77.3 years; 82 were aged over 80 and 7 were over 90. One hundred and sixty-six (74%) were female, giving a female:male ratio of 3:1. Though interaction of diagnoses was common, the major presenting problem/diagnosis is shown in Table 1. Eighty patients, 36%, had recently been seen by a physician or geriatrician. Most patients, 179, were still living in their own homes. Sixteen were in sheltered accommodation, with a warden. The remaining 28 lived in old folks' homes.

Each patient took on average 2.9 different preparations each day. Only 23 patients took no medication. More than one-third took 4 or more different preparations each day. Table 2 shows the distribution in detail. Table 3 shows

Table 1

Main Presenting Problem/Diagnosis

	No. of patients	%
Senile dementia	101	45
Depression	46	21
Paranoia	25	11
Alcohol problem	20[a]	9
Toxic state	10	5
Social problem	9	4
Anxiety	8	4
Hypomania	4	2
Total	223	

[a]A further patient had an alcohol problem as a secondary diagnosis.

Table 2

Number of Different Preparations

No. of preparations	No. of patients	%
0	23	10
1	41	18
2	39	17
3	42	19
4	26	12
5	26	12
6	17	8
7	4	2
8	1	0.5
9	3	1.5
10	1	0.5
Total	223	

the most commonly used drugs; those taken by fewer than 3 patients are excluded. These figures refer to drugs currently taken; most patients had additional, often large, supplies of other medicaments. Not all were necessarily toxic; one old lady living alone had accumulated 700 pints of milk in a few weeks! Phenothiazines, 37%, were the most widely used. Thirty-five percent of patients were on benzodiazepines, 9% taking them day and night. In 2, possibly 3, cases which were admitted, the true quantity of benzodiazepines being used at home was underestimated, resulting in physical withdrawal states, as described by Petursson and Lader (1981). Three patients were on depot injections, 2 fluphenazine and 1 flupenthixol.

Surprisingly, ony 77 patients (35%) admitted any alcohol consumption. Seventeen drank beer or stout; 28, wine or sherry; and 54, spirits. It was difficult to assess "occasional" or even "regular" consumption. More easy to judge was "problem" drinking, which typically led to ataxia or collapse due to alcohol, regular drunkenness, alcoholic paranoia, brain damage, or arrest for drunk and disorderly behavior. In these terms 21 patients had a real alcohol problem. Four of these patients abused beer; 7, wine; and 16, spirits, some abusing more than one beverage. In 11 of the 21 cases the family doctor was fully aware of the situation and diagnosis. Eleven patients had started to drink to excess in recent years, in response to isolation, medical illness, or family problems; these may be termed a reactive group. The other 10 had merely continued heavy drinking into old age. Nine patients were female and 12 were male, giving a female:male ratio of 1:1.3. The average age of the females was 78; of the males, 74.

Table 3

Medications in Current Use

	No. of patients	%
Phenothiazines	83	37
Benzodiazepines (night)	62	28
Aperients	59	26
Diuretics	43	19
Analgesics	39	17
Benzodiazepines (day)	34	15
Antidepressants (tricyclic)	31	14
Digoxin	19	9
Potassium	18	8
Vitamins	17	8
Chlormethiazole	17	8
Antirheumatics	15	7
CVS dilators	14	6
Anti-Parkinsonian	12	5
Tonics	12	5
Antacids	10	4
Antibiotics	10	4
Steroids	10	4
Iron	9	4
Antidepressants (tetracyclic)	9	4
RS dilators	8	4
Barbiturates	7	3
Antidiabetic	7	3
Beta-blockers	6	3
Thyroxine	4	2
GTN	4	2
Quinine	3	1.5
Phenytoin	3	1.5
MAOI	3	1.5
Other medications	<3	–

DISCUSSION

The assessment of elderly patients in their own homes, in close conjunction with family doctors and physicians when necessary, has proven valuable over a 3-year period. This view has been endorsed by Arcand and Williamson (1981). The average of just under 3 medications a day might not seem excessive, but it is the 37% of patients on 4 or more that causes concern, in terms of compliance, interaction, and side effects occurring in a group of people with an average age of 77. Sometimes when relief of symptoms is not obtained by medication, new preparations are added rather than old ones stopped or exchanged. This is also well known in hospital wards.

It is not surprising that phenothiazines should be so widely prescribed. Sedation, often in the absence of more appropriate facilities, is important. Benzodiazepines, with their long half-lives, are regrettably a close second among the present patients in spite of repeated warnings about their use in the elderly (Committee on Review of Medicines, 1980). Skegg, Doll, and Perry (1977) in reviewing patients' prescriptions, found increasing consumption with age, especially of psychotropics. The widespread use of drugs for physical illness emphasizes the interaction of diagnoses in this age group. It has been suggested that 23% of the population over 65 regularly use analgesics (Office of Population Censuses and Surveys, 1979). While there are differences in survey techniques, it may be that the lower figure of 17% in the present group reflects denial of use; alcohol use may be similarly denied. Analgesics, like aperients, are usually self-prescribed and thus beyond doctors' direct control. Of the 7 patients on barbiturates, only 1 was epileptic. It is still necessary to urge reductions in barbiturate use. Antihypertensives, apart from diuretics or beta-blockers, were rarely used. Though 25 patients were suffering from "paranoia" (late-onset schizophrenia, paraphrenia, paranoid states) and presumably not very cooperative, it was surprising that only 3 were on depot injections of major tranquilizers. The widespread use of legally prescribed and legally purchased drugs in the general elderly population has been reviewed by Petersen et al. (1979).

Twenty-one patients, 10%, had clear-cut alcohol abuse problems, and there may have been other patients whose excessive drinking was overlooked. With increasing numbers both of elderly and alcoholics it is hardly surprising that there are many elderly alcoholics. In the absence of a florid picture the elderly alcoholic may be missed unless the possibility is considered. Mishara and Kastenbaum (1980), in their informative book, reported heavy drinking in 6% of the general elderly population but admitted denial of use to be relevant. In 1964, when alcohol abuse was less prevalent, Droller (1964) found 7 alcoholics in 404 old people seen at home; 5 of the alcoholics were unknown to the family doctor. Incidence and recognition have increased.

Rosin and Glatt (1971) described both an inveterate (remote-onset) group, who have merely continued heavy drinking into old age, and a reactive group precipitated by loneliness and infirmity. They agree with Droller (1964) in describing pressure put upon relatives to provide alcohol as blackmail. This situation was found in the present study even in housebound patients and those living in old folks' homes. The latter has been described by Blose (1978). The causes of reactive alcoholism in the present patients and the outcome have been discussed elsewhere (Malcolm, 1984). Social pressures and loneliness as a cause of alcohol abuse in the elderly have been reviewed by Peck (1979). Edwards et al. (1973), in a classic survey which included elderly alcoholics, found a female to male ratio of 1:1.3, identical to the present work.

CONCLUSION

Old people may be visited by a wide range of health care professionals, and it is important that alcohol-related problems be borne in mind by these visitors. As is suggested in this paper, the home visit gives a far better opportunity for a full assessment than a patient's attendance at hospital. The elderly, including those who have no alcohol problems, may deny even occasional use of alcohol, reflecting an old-fashioned attitude to any form of drinking. It seems unlikely that 65% of the present group were the abstainers they claimed to be. The home help, social worker, or doctor must know that alcohol problems in the aged are common. Regrettably, only half the present cases were recognized by the family doctor. Physicians, who had seen 36% of the present patients, are increasingly aware of the problem. Surgeons, who treat fractured hips or skulls, must consider alcohol in the causation, postoperative management, and subsequent prevention of falls. The siting of psychiatric units in general hospitals helps spread information between disciplines by cross-referrals. Increasing contact with the community (e.g., by hospital-based community psychiatric nurses) also assists in education and in the recognition and follow-up of elderly alcoholics. We need to show friends, relatives, and professional visitors that to supply alcohol to an old person, when there exists a clear alcohol-related problem, is not kindness.

The aims of treatment for the two categories of drinkers, the remote and recent onset, are different. If a person has been drinking most of his life, and has consequent problems, then abstinence must be the goal though hopefully giving compensatory expansion in other fields. If recent drinking problems are a result of loneliness, pain, immobility, grief, or rejection, then clearly other management plans are appropriate. A carefully arranged move to an old folks' home, a new start in a different home, treatment for a painful hip, day clubs and centers, all can help. In these cases resumption of moderate drinking, which may have been a lifetime pattern, can be an aim and indeed a help in socialization. As full a life as possible should be available to the elderly so that they do not resort to alcohol or sedatives for relief of boredom, loneliness, or frustration. We must ask relatives and friends to give their own time and show involvement, not just bring a bottle, even when demanded. The opinions and ideas of elderly people should be listened to, not merely tolerated.

Society, too, must offer more than sedation to the elderly. A day or night sedative may be an immediate response, but does it last, and solve the problem? It may add to the difficulties. Slow metabolism in the elderly and long half-life of drugs easily lead to confusion. Development of dependence is not unknown. Relief of symptoms demands more than increasing medication. Some patients might be better with no medication (drug holidays), though withdrawal problems and psychological dependence must, of course, be remembered. Drugs are often used as an economical way of preventing "wandering" by old people. The patient may see his action as quite purposeful; he is going for a walk or seeking something. Sufficient staff and facilities are required to satisfy the patient's needs. Replacing 19th-century mechanical restraint with 20th-century pharmaceutical methods is not progress.

Natural sleep, which may be shorter in duration in the aged, and which should follow an active day, is not the same as long periods of drug-induced unconsciousness. The latter, which may be cheaper than providing caring staff at night in institutions, or may be more convenient for the family, can lead to many problems. "Depression" is often to be treated by an attack on the cause, not by suppression of symptoms by antidepressant drugs.

In general, reduced dosage, frequency, and number of preparations are advisable in the elderly, together with regular review. We all hope to be elderly one day, and we all must aim for a higher quality of life for elderly people. The abuse of alcohol and drugs show deficiencies in society's provision.

ACKNOWLEDGMENTS

My thanks for observation and discussion to Dr. J.S. Madden, Regional Alcohol and Addiction Unit, Chester, England; and Dr. J.A. Aitken, Department of Medicine for the Elderly, Clatterbridge, Wirral, England.

REFERENCES

ARCAND, M., and WILLIAMSON, J. An evaluation of home visiting of patients by physicians in geriatric medicine. *Br. Med. J.* 283: 718-720, 1981.

BLOSE, I.L. The relationship of alcohol to aging and the elderly. *Alcohol Clin. Exp. Res.* 2: 17-21, 1978.

COMMITTEE ON THE REVIEW OF MEDICINES. Systematic review of the benzodiazepines. *Br. Med. J.* 280: 910-912, 1980.

DROLLER, H. Some aspects of alcoholism in the elderly. *Lancet* 2: 137-139, 1964.

EDWARDS, G., HAWKER, A., HENSMAN. C., PETO, J., and WILLIAMSON, V. Alcoholics known or unknown to agencies: Epidemiological studies in a London Suburb. *Br. J. Psychiatry* 123: 169-183, 1973.

MALCOLM, M.T. Problem drinking in the elderly. In *Alcohol-Related Problems.* Chichester, Sussex: Wiley, 1984, pp. 139-146.

MISHARA, B.L., and KASTENBAUM, R. *Alcohol and Old Age.* New York: Grune and Stratton, 1980.

OFFICE OF POPULATION CENSUSES AND SURVEYS. *The General Household Survey 1977.* London: H.M.S.O., 1979, p. 152.

PECK, D.G. Alcohol abuse and the elderly: Social control and conformity. *J. Drug. Issues* 9(1): 63-71, 1979.

PETERSEN, D.M., WHITTINGTON, F.J., and BEER, E.T. Drug use and misuse among the elderly. *J. Drug Issues* 9(1): 5-26, 1979.

PETURSSON, H., and LADER, M.H. Benzodiazepine dependence. *Br. J. Addict.* 76: 133-145, 1981.

ROSIN, A.J., and GLATT, M.M. Alcohol excess in the elderly. *Q. J. Stud. Alcohol* 32: 53-59, 1971.

SLEGG, D.C.G., DOLL, R., and PERRY, J. The use of medicines in general practice. *Br. Med. J.* 1: 1561-1563, 1977.

The International Journal of the Addictions, 19(4), 419–430, 1984

Evaluation of a Substance Abuse Prevention Program for Junior High School Students

Joel M. Moskowitz,* PhD

Eric Schaps, PhD

Gary A. Schaeffer, PhD

Janet H. Malvin, PhD

Pacific Institute for Research and Evaluation
Napa, California 94558

Abstract

Seventh-grade students in the experimental school received two primary prevention strategies. One strategy, Effective Classroom Management, was an unstructured affective approach provided by the students' classroom teachers. The other strategy was Drug Education, a mini-course taught directly to students by a specialist. The seventh-grade students from another school served as a comparison group. Both process and outcome evaluation data were collected. Results indicated positive program effects for females on drug knowledge, cigarette smoking, and perceptions of their peers' attitudes toward and use of drugs. No effects attributable to the intervention were found for males. The discussion is in terms of problems inherent in unstructured affective strategies and the need for further research on drug education.

*To whom requests for reprints should be sent at the Prevention Research Center, Pacific Institute for Research and Evaluation, 2532 Durant Avenue, Berkeley, California 94704.

 0020-773X/84/1904-0419$3.50/0

The focus of drug abuse prevention has moved away from the "scare tactics" of the past. Instead, primary prevention has adopted the notion that personal satisfaction with self and institutions will inhibit the tendency to abuse substances. This strategy has largely been based on correlational studies that found an association between self-attitudes and values, and drug abuse (e.g., Ahlgren and Norem-Hebeisen, 1979; Smith and Fogg, 1978).

Prevention programs for schools have generally followed the lead of "humanistic" educators in their emphasis on affective development. The combination of two such programs is evaluated in the present study. The first program, Effective Classroom Management (ECM), was aimed at fine-tuning teachers' sensitivity to the cognitive and affective needs of students. In-service training was provided to increase the interpersonal skills of teachers.

The second program, Drug Education, was a course delivered directly to students. This course provided an opportunity for the development of self-understanding, decision-making skills, and resistance to peer pressure. Although some drug information was provided, the focus of the course was on affective awareness and social competencies. This should be contrasted with previous drug education courses which have featured factual information and have yielded negligible or mixed results (see reviews by Blum, 1976; Goodstadt, 1973; Schaps et al., 1981).

The present study examined the combined effects of these two strategies on the mediating dispositions of drug use and actual drug involvement. As a result of exposure to "affectively" trained teachers, students were expected to report an improved classroom climate, to have better attitudes toward school, and to have more positive self-esteem and fewer discipline problems. Because of direct skill building received in Drug Education, students were expected to know more about the consequences of substance use and to perceive greater costs and fewer benefits (i.e., negative and positive consequences) of substance use. Positive changes in students' attitudes toward substance use and perceptions of their peers' attitudes toward the use of substances were also hypothesized. The course was considered somewhat less likely to influence personal involvement in substance use, because the brief interval between the completion of the course and posttest was considered insufficient time to achieve behavioral change (see Note 1). Finally, the course was considered least likely to affect students' attitudes toward or use of "hard" drugs, because students at this grade level are typically opposed to these drugs.

METHOD

Design

The study employed a nonequivalent control group design with a pretest and posttest. One of two junior high schools (grades 7-9) from a middle-class, suburban public school system in northern California was assigned to the experimental condition and the other school to the control condition. All teachers in the experimental school were offered ECM in-service training (for 2 years including the year prior to this study), and all grade 7 students participated in Drug Education. The control school received neither program.

Subjects

The experimental and control groups consisted of all grade 7 teachers and students from the experimental and control schools (Note 2). Of the 31 grade 7 teachers in the experimental school, eight (26%) completed ECM in-service training only in the year prior to the study, four (13%) completed training only in the study year, and eight (26%) completed both years of training. There were no significant differences between the participants in the training and the 11 nonparticipants in terms of sex, prior teaching experience, or academic department. There were also no significant differences between experimental participants and control teachers on these variables. Experimental teachers averaged 13.85 (SD = 6.49) years of teaching experience; control teachers averaged 14.10 (SD = 5.70). Of the experimental teachers, 62% were females; of the controls, 75% were females.

At the beginning of the study, the experimental group consisted of 419 students and the control group consisted of 268 students. Seventy-two students (17%) from the experimental group and 47 students (18%) from the control group were excluded from the analysis due to attrition or lack of parental permission for testing. In addition, 12 experimental group students and four control group students were excluded because they reported using a fictitious drug.

The analysis included 335 students in the experimental group (53% male and 96% White) and 217 students in the control group (47% male and 87% White). Mexican-Americans (3%) comprised the largest minority group.

Procedures

ECM

ECM training in the study year consisted of seven 2-hour sessions held weekly after school, followed by two "reunion" sessions of 2 hours each (Adams, Slimmon, and Schaps, 1982). The participating teachers were paid $200 and were offered postgraduate credit.

Experimental teachers were trained in one or both of two versions of ECM. In the year prior to this study, participating teachers received 24 hours of training in communication, problem solving, and self-esteem enhancement. In the year of the study, participating teachers were taught techniques in communication, classroom management, and self-esteem enhancement (see Table 1).

Table 1

Skills Taught in ECM In-Service Training

Communication
I-messages (Gordon, 1974)
Clarifying responses (Raths, Harmin, and Simon, 1966)
Reflecting feelings (Gordon, 1974)
Reflecting content (Gordon, 1974)
Classroom management (Dreikurs and Cassel, 1972; Glasser, 1969)
Positive and negative verbal feedback
Positive and negative nonverbal cues
Tangible reinforcers
Time out
Self-esteem enhancement (Canfield and Wells, 1976)

The training sessions followed a standard format. First, a self-concept enhancement technique or activity was introduced. Then the skills taught in prior sessions were reviewed and the teachers' experiences using the skills were discussed. After this, new skills were introduced and practiced.

One of two trainers observed the teachers in their classrooms at least three times during the school year. After each visit, the trainer met briefly with the teacher to provide feedback on the teacher's classroom behavior.

Drug Education

The drug education course consisted of 12 weekly, 45-minute sessions conducted from February through May 1980, during regular class time in 14 social studies classes (Tuck and Schaps, 1982). The course was taught by a specialist in health education.

In the first three sessions, a model of human motivation (based on Maslow, 1980) and a model of systematic decision making were taught. In session four, students selected individual projects based on personal goals (e.g., weight loss). As homework, students kept journals documenting their progress toward reaching their goals over the next 8 weeks. In the fifth and sixth sessions, different styles of group decision making were examined. Also, the influence of advertising on behavior was discussed. In the seventh and eighth sessions, assertiveness training was taught. In session nine a film ("Drugs, Alcohol or Alternatives"; Note 3) was presented that analyzed reasons for using drugs and alternatives to drug use. Session 10 was a discussion of student questions about tobacco and alcohol use. Session 11 was a discussion of student questions about marijuana and other substances. In the final session, students prepared class "newspapers" summarizing their personal projects.

Measures

Process Evaluation

Teacher implementation of ECM was assessed by surveys of teachers after each training session and at the end of the school year. Students completed course evaluations of Drug Education after the fifth, eighth, and final sesssions.

Student Self-Report

Two questionnaires, the Student Questionnaire (SQ) and the Drug and Alcohol Survey (DAS), were administered to all students (Note 4). The SQ measures students' perceptions of themselves and their relationships with their peers, their teachers, and their school. This instrument also measures the belief in one's own control over intellectual or academic performance (locus of control). The SQ assesses affective teaching climate, locus of control for success, locus of control for failure, academic self-esteem, social self-esteem, attitudes toward school, and perceived peer attitudes toward school. The scale reliabilities (coefficient alpha) range from .61 to .89 (Mdn = .80). The DAS assesses drug knowledge; general drug attitudes; perceived benefits (i.e., positive consequences) and costs (i.e., negative consequences) of alcohol, marijuana, and "pill" use (Note 5); attitudes toward "soft" and "hard" drug use (Note 6); perceived peer attitudes toward, and perceived peer use of, soft and hard drugs; and personal involvement in use of each of 10 substances (Note 7). The scale reliabilities ranged from .70 to .96 (Mdn = .88) except for drug knowledge (.40), where guessing probably attenuated the reliability.

The pretest was administered in October 1979 and the posttest in May 1980 during two class sessions. The SQ was administered during the first session, and the DAS was administered during the second session. Makeup sessions were held for students who were absent for the original sessions.

Questionnaires were prelabled with student names on the cover sheet and student identification numbers on page 1. The administrators stressed the confidentiality of the survey and, for added emphasis, instructed students to remove their names from the DAS.

Archival Records

Students discipline records for 4 months in the spring of 1980 were obtained from both schools. Indices were constructed for drug-related problems including use, possession, or sale of tobacco, alcohol, marijuana, and other drugs; and for general behavior problems including all other types of student misbehavior. It was found that due to differences in the two schools' discipline policies, the discipline records were not comparable. Therefore, these data were not used in the between-school comparisons. In addition, drug problems were not analyzed because there were only eight incidences among 552 students.

Other records obtained from the school district were the number of unexcused absences for 1979-1980 and grade point averages for each semester (Note 8).

An index of exposure to ECM-trained teachers was created for students in the experimental school. This index equaled the number of courses in which the student was enrolled that were taught by teachers trained in ECM.

Data Analysis

Two approaches were employed in the data analysis. In the first approach experimental versus control group differences were examined. This approach included analysis of the pretest data to explore biases attributable to initial nonequivalence and attrition. Then, posttest data were subjected to analysis of covariance controlling for some initial differences. This analysis examined the combined effects of ECM and Drug Education. The second approach examined students within the experimental school in order to determine whether posttest changes were related to students' amount of exposure to ECM-trained teachers. As all students had Drug Education, this analysis examined the effects of ECM. Type I error was set at .01 to control for experimentwise error, and separate analyses were conducted for males and females due to heterogeneity of variance in many measures (Note 9).

RESULTS

Process Evaluation

The teachers who participated in the ECM in-service training found it interesting, enjoyable, and well organized. They reported that they had mastered most of the skills covered in the training and found them to be useful in the classroom. Daily use of the different communication skills was reported by 11% (clarifying responses) to 26% (reflecting feelings, reflecting content) of the teachers, and daily use of the various discipline skills was reported by 0% (tangible reinforcers, time out) to 61% (positive nonverbal cues) of the teachers. The self-concept enhancement activities were used daily by 6% of the teachers.

Students reported that Drug Education was interesting, enjoyable, useful, and well organized. Although the individual classes differed substantially in how they rated the first five sessions of the course, all classes rated the subsequent sessions highly.

Outcome Evaluation

Initial Equivalence and Attrition

Analyses were conducted to determine (1) whether students in the experimental and control groups were equivalent on the pretest measures and (2) whether the experimental and control groups were affected differentially by attrition. A two-way analysis of variance was performed on each pretest measure with condition (experimental vs control) and attrition status (attrited vs non-attrited) as the factors. A main effect for condition would suggest initial nonequivalence, and hence would limit both internal and external validity. A main effect for attrition status would limit external validity, and the interaction between condition and attrition status would limit both internal and external validity.

For males, significant main effects for condition were obtained on 2 of 25 pretest meausres, GPA, $F\ (1, 291) = 17.82, p < .001$; and hard drug attitudes, $F\ (1, 295) = 7.19, p < .01$. As compared to the control students, experimental males were initially lower on GPA and more opposed to hard drug use. A significant main effect for attrition status was obtained on one variable, GPA, $F\ (1, 291) = 11.13, p < .001$. As compared to attrited students, nonattrited students had higher GPA. A significant condition × attrition interaction was obtained on drug knowledge, $F\ (1, 297) = 9.08, p < .01$. For the experimental group, attrited students has less drug knowledge; whereas for the control group, attrited students had more knowledge.

For females, significant main effects for condition were obtained on three measures, locus of control for success, $F\ (1, 292) = 7.20, p < .01$; locus of control for failure, $F\ (1, 295) = 13.13, p < .001$; and social self-esteem, $F\ (1, 297) = 6.96, p < .01$. Compared to control females, experimental females were initially higher on these affective variables. No significant main effects for attrition status or attrition status × condition interactions were found.

In sum, initial differences occurred primarily for females on affective variables. These differences favoring the experimental students may bias the posttest analyses of related affective measures toward finding positive treatment effects (Reichardt, 1979). Attrition status differences were found only for males on both types of variables limiting the generalizability of the posttest results. The only significant interaction occurred for males on drug knowledge. A treatment effect obtained on this variable would be confounded with the alternative explanation of differential attrition.

Experimental Versus Control Differences

A one-way analysis of covariance was conducted on each posttest measure with condition (experimental vs control) as the factor and the corresponding pretest as the covariate (Note 10). As unexcused absences were not measured at pretest, analysis of variance was conducted on this variable. Treatment effect sizes are presented in the metric of the posttest control group standard deviation.

The results of the posttest analyses are summarized in Table 2. For males, positive effects were obtained on 2 of the 25 variables, unexcused absences (.32 SD) and drug knowledge (.41 SD). For females, six positive effects were found. Positive effect sizes were obtained on drug knowledge (.42 SD), soft

Table 2

Summary of Results of Covariance Analyses[a]

	Males		Females	
Posttest measures	*B*	*F*	*B*	*F*
Affective climate	.61	<1	.67	2.03
Attitudes toward school	.70	<1	.63	<1
Social self-esteem	.68	<1	.61	3.39
Academic self-esteem	.64	<1	.68	5.62
Peer attitudes toward school	.45	1.01	.54	3.31
Locus of control for success	.37	<1	.54	<1
Locus of control for failure	.61	3.50	.54	1.15
GPA	.88	<1	.98	<1
Unexcused absences	–	6.80*	–	<1
Drug knowledge	.37	9.67*	.40	10.40**
General drug attitudes	.70	<1	.71	1.31
Soft drug attitudes	.57	1.50	.63	1.19
Alcohol benefits	.51	2.16	.61	3.62
Pot benefits	.64	<1	.61	1.14
Alcohol costs	.49	2.20	.52	<1
Pot costs	.53	<1	.53	<1
Soft peer attitudes	.50	<1	.32	12.97**
Soft peer use	.42	1.62	.43	13.92**
Alcohol involvement	.76	2.20	.76	<1
Cigarette involvement	.88	<1	.78	9.82*
Pot involvement	.95	<1	.89	1.44
Hard drug attitudes	.44	<1	.41	1.68
Pill benefits	.45	<1	.51	2.82
Pill costs	.53	<1	.46	<1
Hard peer attitudes	.46	3.95	.27	14.73**
Hard peer use	.38	3.12	.36	15.27**

[a]The error *df* ranged from 221 to 277 for males and from 237 to 271 for females. *B* refers to the unstandardized regression coefficient. Analysis of variance was performed on unexcused absences.

*$p < .01$.

**$p < .001$.

peer attitudes (.41 SD), soft peer use (.45 SD), hard peer attitudes (.43 SD), hard peer use (.48 SD), and cigarette involvement (.27 SD).

Effects of ECM Exposure

Within the experimental school, students were enrolled in from 1 to 11 classes taught by ECM-trained teachers. The students were categorized into three levels of ECM exposure. The first level contained students who were enrolled in 1 to 4 ECM classes; the second level, 5 to 7 classes; and the third level, 8 to 11 classes.

The relationship between the level of ECM exposure and the 10 school-related posttest measures was hypothesized to be monotonic. The exposure level was coded as two orthogonal components, and each posttest measure was regressed in a stepwise procedure on its corresponding pretest (where available) and on the two components. Either a significant linear component or significant linear and quadratic components could be interpreted as an effect of ECM. If only the quadratic component were significant, an ECM effect would not be implied because the relation would not be monotonic.

In none of the 20 regressions was the linear or the quadratic ECM exposure component significant. Hence, there was no evidence that greater exposure to ECM-trained teachers was associated with more positive student outcomes.

DISCUSSION

The intervention produced a pattern of positive effects for female students that are more likely the result of Drug Education than ECM. Of the six effects, all were hypothesized for Drug Education but none was hypothesized for ECM. Furthermore, amount of exposure to ECM-trained teachers was unrelated to students' outcomes on these variables.

The two isolated effects found for male students in the experimental-control comparisons are readily explained by differential attrition or school differences unrelated to the intervention. Hence, both strategies appear to have been ineffective for males.

ECM apparently failed to equip teachers to overcome school-related factors that predispose students to abuse substances. The technology of ECM largely consists of unstructured verbal and nonverbal behaviors that teachers are expected to integrate into their regular classroom behavior. This technology may have been ineffective for many important reasons, not the least of which is the fact that ECM skill implementation is contingent upon the occurrence of particular student behaviors. That is, students must "give" teachers the opportunity to use the skills. Such opportunities vary considerably from classroom to classroom; thus, the level of treatment any classroom receives is variable. Moreover, there may be little opportunity to apply the skills in many classrooms.

Another problem may have been the teachers themselves. With unstructured affective prevention programs like ECM, teacher effects are unavoidably confounded with program effects. Teachers' classroom styles may be incompatible with the ideology of ECM, and their behavior could undermine program implementation. However, given our sample of teachers who self-selected for training, marked incompatibility with the philosophy of ECM is rather unlikely.

The failure to find positive program effects for ECM might be linked to our training procedures. However, there is no indication in the scant literature on implementation as to what constitutes optimal procedures to promote effective implementation (Scheirer and Rezmovic, 1982). Inasmuch as the ECM teachers volunteered for training, and received 18 to 42 hours of training and at least three follow-up classroom visits by a trainer, it seems reasonable to assume that ECM would be implemented adequately. Nevertheless, the teacher self-reports indicated that most skills were not used daily.

The effects obtained for Drug Education in this study differed from those found in an evaluation of an earlier version of the course (Schaps et al., 1982). Whereas both studies found positive effects for girls on drug knowledge and perceptions of peer attitudes toward "soft" drug use, the present study also found effects on perceived peer attitudes toward "hard" drug use and perceived peer use of "soft" and "hard" drugs. The prior study found positive effects on alcohol and marijuana involvement while the present study revealed a decrease in cigarette involvement.

There is no parsimonious explanation for the different effects obtained in the two evaluations. The reasons are not apparent from examination of the two curricula. Perhaps the efficacy of drug education interacts with characteristics of different school environments or student populations. This possibility might lead to the matching of schools with certain types of programs. One direction for future research is the tailoring of drug education to various populations and settings. This seems particularly warranted given the finding that only girls were positively influenced by the courses.

Overall, this study shows that drug education holds some promise as a substance abuse prevention strategy for seventh-grade girls in a suburban California school. The results also suggest that is is difficult to change the classroom socioemotional environment through in-service training in an unstructured affective strategy. Even if such change were achievable, it remains to be seen whether it would promote more positive self-concepts among students and reduce the risk of substance abuse. In contrast, a drug education course that trains students in intra- and interpersonal competencies appears to have at least some short-term impact on females.

ACKNOWLEDGMENTS

This research was supported by a grant from the Prevention Branch, National Institute on Drug Abuse (DA02147). The opinions stated in this report are those of the authors. We thank John W. Condon for assisting in the data analysis.

NOTES

1. Follow-up data collected 1 year after the posttest have been reported by Moskowitz, Malvin, Schaeffer, and Schaps (1982).
2. Special education students and teachers in both schools were not included in this study.
3. Film is available from Barr Films, P.O. Box 5667, Pasadena, CA 91107.
4. The details of the scaling procedures and results have been reported by Moskowitz, Condon, Brewer, Schaps, and Malvin (1979); and by Moskowitz, Schaeffer, Condon, Schaps, and Malvin (1981).
5. Operationalized as "pep pills, sleeping pills, uppers, downers, soapers."
6. The "soft" substances included alcohol, cigarettes, and marijuana; the "hard" substances included seven drugs: inhalants, barbiturates or tranquilizers, amphetamines or stimulants, cocaine, PCP, LSD or psychedelics, and heroin or morphine.
7. The involvement scales consisted of items assessing current use, lifetime use, and intentions to use, for the following substances: alcohol, cigarettes, marijuana or hashish, inhalants, barbiturates or tranquilizers, amphetamines or stimulants, cocaine, PCP, LSD or psychedelics, and heroin or morphine. "Street" names were provided for most substances. Current use was operationalized as "during the last 4 weeks," and intentions to use was operationalized as "during the next year."
8. The "pretest" measure of GPA is not truly a pretest because it was obtained after the treatment began and may have been affected by ECM.
9. Due to nonnormality and heterogeneity of variance, $\log(X + 1)$ transformations were performed on the following variables: unexcused absences, general behavior problems, hard drug attitudes, and hard peer use.
10. Additional analyses of covariance employed the corresponding pretest and pretest-treatment interaction as covariates. The latter term allows for different regression slopes in the two conditions. In one of the 50 analyses the pretest-treatment interaction term was significant. These results did not affect the interpretation of the results from the ANCOVA employing only the pretest as a covariate. Thus, there was no evidence that the effectiveness of the treatment was related to the students' initial status.

REFERENCES

ADAMS, S., SLIMMON, L., and SCHAPS, E. *Effective Classroom Management II–Junior High Documentation–Year 02.* Napa, CA: Pacific Institute for Research and Evaluation, 1982.

AHLGREN, A., and NOREM-HEBEISEN, A. Self-esteem patterns distinctive of groups of drug-abusing and other dysfunctional adolescents. *Int. J. Addict.* 14: 759-777, 1979.

BLUM, R.G. *Drug Education: Results and Recommendations.* Lexington, MA: Lexington Books, 1979.

CANFIELD, J., and WELLS, H. *100 Ways to Enhance Self-Concept in the Classroom: A Handbook for Teachers and Parents.* Englewood Cliffs, NJ: Prentice-Hall, 1976.

DREIKURS, R., and CASSEL, P. *Discipline Without Tears.* New York: Hawthorne Books, 1972.

GLASSER, W. *Schools Without Failure.* New York: Harper and Row, 1969.

GOODSTADT, M.S. Myths and methodology in drug education: A critical review of the research evidence. In M.S. Goodstadt (ed.), *Research on Methods and Programs of Drug Education.* Toronto: Alcoholism and Drug Addiction Reserach Foundation of Ontario, 1973, pp. 113-145.

GORDON, T. (with N. Burch). *T.E.T.: Teacher Effectiveness Training.* New York: Peter H. Wyden, 1974.

MASLOW, A. *Motivation and Personality.* New York: Harper and Row, 1980.

MOSKOWITZ, J., CONDON, J., BREWER, M., SCHAPS, E., and MALVIN, J. *The Napa Project: Scaling of student self-report instruments* (ERIC Document Reproduction Service No. ED 205 530). Napa, CA: Pacific Institute for Research and Evaluation, 1979.

MOSKOWITZ, J., MALVIN, J., SCHAEFFER, G., and SCHAPS, E. Evaluation of a junior high school primary prevention program. *Addict Behav.* 8: 393-401, 1983.

MOSKOWITZ, J., SCHAEFFER, G., CONDON, J., SCHAPS, E., and MALVIN, J. *Psychometric properties of the "Drug and Alcohol Survey"* (ERIC Document Reproduction No. ED 212 678). Napa, CA: Pacific Institute for Research and Evaluation, 1981.

RATHS, L., HARMIN, M., and SIMON, S. *Values and Teaching.* Columbus, OH: C.E. Merrill, 1966.

REICHARDT, C. The statistical analysis of data from nonequivalent group designs. In T. Cook and D. Campbell (eds.), *Quasi-Experimentation: Design and Analysis Issues for Field Settings.* Chicago: Rand McNally, 1979, pp. 147-205.

SCHAPS, E., DI BARTOLO, R., MOSKOWITZ, J., PALLEY, C., and CHURGIN, S.A. A review of 127 prevention program evaluations. *J. Drug Issues* 11: 17-44, 1981.

SCHAPS, E., MOSKOWITZ, J., CONDON, J., and MALVIN, J. Process and outcome evaluation of a drug education course. *J. Drug Educ.* 12: 353-364, 1982.

SCHEIRER, M., and REZMOVIC, E. *Measuring the implementation of innovations.* Annandale, VA: American Research Institute, 1982.

SMITH, G., and FOGG, C. Psychological predictors of early use, late use and nonuse of marijuana among teenage students. In D. Kandel (ed.), *Longitudinal Research on Drug Use.* Washington, DC: Hemisphere, 1978.

TUCK, P., and SCHAPS, E. *Process documentation–Drug Education II: 1979-1980 school year.* Napa, CA: Pacific Institute for Research and Evaluation, 1980.

The International Journal of the Addictions, 19(4), 431-439, 1984

Human Smoking Patterns and Smoke Deliveries

Philip M. Moody,* PhD

Department of Behavioral Science
University of Kentucky
Lexington, Kentucky 40536-0086

Abstract

This study, based on a sample (N = 517) of adult medical patients at a southeastern medical center who were current users of cigarettes, reports the interrelationships among the puff characteristics of cigarette smoking behavior and smoke deliveries of tar and nicotine. Average puff duration, average puff volume, and the number of puffs were found to be significantly positively correlated with daily tar and nicotine intake. Intervals between puffs and total time smoking were not correlated with nicotine and tar intake. It was concluded that "how" a person smokes affects "how much" this person is exposed to tar and nicotine.

This paper focuses on the effect of smoking patterns on smoke delivery of tar and nicotine of adult medical patients at a southeastern medical center. Such information would be useful to health professionals who are concerned about the factors contributing to the maintenance of cigarette smoking.

A number of research programs have been concerned with the study of smoking patterns (Creighton and Lewis, 1978a; Graham et al., 1968; Hilding, 1956; Moody, 1980) but only a few studies have focused on the effect of smoking patterns on smoke deliveries (Ashton and Watson, 1970; Creighton and Lewis, 1978b). Ashton and Watson (1970) did a study of puffing frequency and

*Address reprint requests to the author: Associate Professor, Department of Behavioral Science, Room 105, College of Medicine Office Building, University of Kentucky, Lexington, Kentucky 40536-0086.

0020-773X/84/1904-0431$3.50/0

nicotine intake in volunteer cigarette smokers. A total of 36 volunteer healthy subjects were studied, 15 women (42%) and 21 men (58%), with an age range from 19 to 35 years. All were smokers and their normal daily cigarette consumption ranged from 3 to 30. The subjects participated in an experiment for 60 minutes; during this time the number of puffs for each cigarette smoked was recorded by an observer. The cigarette stubs were analyzed for nicotine content. These researchers found that smokers of low-nicotine cigarettes had a higher puff frequency and drew into their mouths nearly the same amount of nicotine as smokers of high-nicotine cigarettes. Ashton and Watson (1970, p. 681) concluded that "these findings are thus consistent with the possibility that there exists an 'optimum' nicotine dose for a given activity and that smokers unconsciously modify their smoking patterns in an attempt to obtain this dose."

Creighton and Lewis (1978a) conducted a study in which a panel of smokers of a medium-delivery cigarette (about 1.4 mg nicotine) were monitored for a period of about 1 month and then asked to smoke, for a similar period, a brand with a substantially different nicotine delivery (about 1.0 mg for half of the panel and about 1.8 mg for the other half of the panel). The sample consisted of 8 male and 8 female volunteers. The smoking data (puff volume, puff duration, interval between puffs, and the number of puffs) were recorded on a smoking analyzer and data logger. Representative smoking patterns of each subject were duplicated by machine to measure deliveries of tar, nicotine, and carbon monoxide.

Creighton and Lewis summarized their findings as follows:

> Analyses of these data showed that on the average, smokers increased the intensity with which they smoked the lower delivery brand and decreased the intensity of smoking the high delivery brand when compared with the control brand. . . . The amounts of tar, nicotine and carbon monoxide taken from the medium and high delivery brands by the smokers were similar. . . . Although they smoked the low delivery brand more intensely, the smokers did not equalize the deliveries taken from the high and medium delivery brands. (1978a, p. 299)

Finally Creighton and Lewis (1978b) studied the effect of smoking patterns on smoke deliveries utilizing a puff duplicator machine. They varied the puff volumes and interval between puffs to cover the range typically observed when human smokers are studied. Their study results indicated "that the actual deliveries of smoke components and the ratios of the deliveries of smoke components are not primarily dependent on a single factor such as the volume of smoke drawn, the interval between puffs or the shape of the puff. . . . All three factors have their own influence on the deliveries and ratios of deliveries as well as having an interaction effect" (Creighton and Lewis, 1978b, p. 310).

These authors concluded that it is not possible to predict with accuracy the deliveries of a cigarette simply from a knowledge of the volume of smoke drawn by a human smoker.

The present study is an attempt to shed some light on the relationships of human smoking patterns and smoke deliveries, but it utilizes data from human smoking patterns and analysis of the actual deliveries of nicotine and tar based on the cigarette butts returned for analysis.

A means of measuring puff volume, duration, and interval, and the nicotine and tar delivery per cigarette was reported in a paper entitled "Procedures for Characterizing Human Smoking Behavior" (Griffith et al., 1972).

The equipment for determining how a person smokes consists of an airflow-measuring cigarette holder, a high-speed recorder for determining the flow characteristics during the course of a puff, and a slow-speed recorder to determine total smoking time and intervals between puffs. The puff volume was calculated from the analog recording by the high-speed recorder. Tar and nicotine delivery per cigarette was determined by analyzing the nicotine content of the filter and, on the basis of the known filtration properties of the filter, calculating the tar and nicotine delivery per cigarette. To obtain the necessary calibration data in order to ascertain tar and nicotine delivery for each brand of cigarettes, a representative sample of every case for each brand of cigarettes was pooled. Then analyses for tar and nicotine in the filter tip for various numbers of puffs were made. A plot was constructed of nicotine deposited in the filter tip versus tar and nicotine delivered. Using this information, the tar and nicotine delivered to a smoker can be calculated from the analysis of the nicotine deposited in the filter tips of subjects' cigarettes during normal smoking (Griffith et al., 1972). This value multiplied by the number of cigarettes smoked per day gives the total daily exposure to nicotine and tar.

In conducting a test on a subject, a cigarette of the brand currently smoked by the person was placed in the cigarette holder and the individual was asked to light the cigarette. With the lighting of the cigarette the smoking regime was considered to be initiated, and it was completed when the subject finished smoking the cigarette. After the test subjects were given 1-week supplies of their regular brands of cigarettes and asked to save their cigarette butts daily. The butts from 7 consecutive days were returned to the laboratory for butt analysis of tar and nicotine delivery.

METHOD

The sample ($N = 517$) consisted of patients admitted to the adult medical floor at a southeastern medical center from July 1971 through June 1973 and who were current users of cigarettes. These subjects were volunteers who were allowed by their attending physicians to participate in the study. Data were obtained on all patients admitted to the adult medical floors over a 2-year period; however, only 305 of the 517 patients returned the cigarette butts from 7 consecutive days for butt analysis of tar and nicotine delivery. Comparisons of race, sex, and age produced no appreciable differences between the sample and other patients.

The sample of patients ranged from 21 to 75 years old, with the mean age of 39.1. Eighty-two percent were White and 18% non-White, and 51% were males and 49% were females.

The method previously described for measuring smoking characteristics was used (Griffith et al., 1972). Subjects utilized the smoker characterization equipment only one time. A previous study of 100 subjects who each utilized the smoker characterization equipment twice over a week period revealed that there were no significant differences at Time 1 versus Time 2 for any of the smoking parameters except for average butt length from cigarettes returned for analysis (Griffith and Moody, 1976). Also, in comparing experimental and field observations of human smoking characteristics, it was found that the average puff intervals are shorter and the total smoking times are less in the laboratory observations than those noted by field observations (Moody, 1980).

RESULTS

A description of the sample according to smoking patterns and smoke deliveries is contained in Table 1. Also included in this table are the values from other studies. As can be seen from Table 1, the sample utilized in the current study is much larger than in the other research reports, with the exception of the Schultz and Seehofer study (1978).

The present study sample had the lowest average puff number (9.3), compared to highs of 15-19, 14, and 11 in the Schultz and Seehofer (1978) study. The average puff duration, 2.12 seconds, falls within the range of 1.34-2.44 seconds. The average puff volume of the sample, 43.5 mL, falls within the middle of the range 33.0-60.0 mL. The average puff interval was 25.8 seconds for the study population, compared to the range of 30-43.6 found in other studies. Thus, the total time smoked (232 seconds) for the present sample was much less than in Creighton and Lewis (1978a) and Comer and Creighton (1978) study populations. Furthermore, the average butt length of the current study sample was longer (35.8 mm) than the other study results (range, 31.4-29.2 mm).

The interrelationships among the puff characteristics of cigarette smoking behavior and smoke deliveries are reported in Table 2. Puff duration is positively correlated with tar intake ($r = .306; p < .001$) and with nicotine intake ($r = .315$; $p < .001$). Intervals between puffs and total time smoking are not significantly correlated with either tar or nicotine intake. Puff volume is positively correlated with tar ($r = .157; p < .01$) and nicotine ($r = .166; p < .01$) intake as well as the

Table 1

A Comparison of Values for Various Smoking Parameters Reported by Others with Those Reported in the Present Study

	Average no. puffs	Average puff volume (mL)	Average puff duration (sec)	Average puff interval (sec)	Total smoking time (sec)	Average butt length (mm)
Comer and Creighton (1978)						
Laboratory smoking (N = 32)	12.0	33.4	2.16	39.7	426.5	29.2
Rawbone et al. (1978)						
Low-tar smokers (N = 5)	9.8		1.74	43.6		
Middle-tar smokers (N = 7)	10.9		1.92	38.8		
Schultz and Seehofer (1978)						
Observations 1971 (N = 100)	10.5		1.41	50.3		
Observations 1974 (N = 218)	11.8		1.34	41.5		
Profile recordings						
1970	15-19	50	1.8	30		
1971	14	60	1.7	35		
1977	11	55	–	–		
Creighton and Lewis (1978a) (N = 16)						
Higher-delivery cigarettes	13.0	43.8	2.27	38.5	468	31.4
Lower-delivery cigarettes	12.6	46.1	2.44	36.5	467	31.2
Present study (N = 517)	9.3	43.5	2.12	25.8	232	35.8

Table 2

Correlation among the Puff Characteristics of Cigarette Smoking Behavior and Smoke Deliveries for Study Sample (N = 305)

	Tar intake (mg/day)	Nicotine intake (mg/day)
Puff duration (sec)	.306*	.315*
Interval between puffs (sec)	–.044	–.039
Puff volume (mL)	.157**	.166**
Number of puffs	.204*	.204*
Total smoking time (min)	.112	.115

*$p < .001$.
**$p < .01$.

number of puffs (with tar intake, $r = .204$; $p < .001$; and with nicotine intake, $r = .204$; $p < .001$).

DISCUSSION

This study focuses on the effect of smoking patterns on smoke deliveries of a hospital population at a southeastern medical center. Total smoking time and average puff interval were not found to significantly correlate with tar and nicotine intake. It was found that puff duration, puff volume, and the number of puffs are positively associated with tar and nicotine intake. These significant correlations between these puff parameters and smoke deliveries were relatively small. However, it is reasonable to tentatively conclude that "how" a person smokes–in regards to puff duration and volume, and the number of puffs–affects "how much" this person is exposed to tar and nicotine.

The data from the present study provide some insights into the relationships of puff parameters and smoke deliveries of cigarettes. The study is not without weaknesses, in that this investigation has studied human smoking patterns and smoke deliveries among hospital patients. The study of the use pattern(s) of any substance (drugs, medications, social substances, and food) may be related to the available role demands in a variety of types of environments. Therefore, research on "healthy" subjects in differing types of social environments is needed.

Another possible weakness of the present investigation is that the method for ascertaining smoke deliveries may have erred. For example, Creighton and Lewis (1978b) state:

> The most common way of estimating actual deliveries of nicotine and some particular matter components for human smokers is to analyze filter tips from their discarded butts. This method has the disadvantage of assuming a constant filtration efficiency based on standard machine

> smoking which may lead to systematic as well as random errors in delivery estimates. (p. 311)

Also, this conclusion must be tempered by the fact that smoke velocity or intensity of drawing a puff greatly influences tar and nicotine deposition in the cigarette butt (cf. Creighton and Lewis, 1978b; Rawbone et al., 1978). Perhaps more meaningful data might be generated by correlating smoking behavior with the amount of smoke absorbed by the smoker, as determined by blood serum levels of carboxyhemoglobin and nicotine (cf. Russell, 1979).

However, in a recent publication by Rawbone et al. (1978) in which analyses of smoking parameters and cigarette smoke absorption were discussed, it was noted that:

> There is a significant correlation between the amount of smoke absorbed by the smoker and the smoke exposure index derived from the volume and time periods of inhalation following the puffing of a cigarette. (p. 192)

Thus, the present investigation does give some insight into human smoking profile patterns (rather than smoking machine patterns) and their relationship with smoke deliveries. Obviously, more detailed research is needed in this important area of research.

One possible research design for studying the relationship of "how" people smoke to "how much" would be:

1. From an appropriate number of adult smokers, selected at random, obtain, on a machine, their smoking patterns for their particular brands of cigarettes.
2. Provide these smokers with their brands of cigarettes, which have varying amounts of tar and nicotine.
3. Again measure their smoking patterns over time and analyze the data to see if any changes have taken place (i.e., did the puff duration and volume increase for those subjects utilizing lower-tar and/or -nicotine cigarettes?).

There are implications of this and related studies for the development of intervention programs toward smoking. Some people are advocating a lower-tar and lower-nicotine approach to the making of cigarettes. Without knowledge of "how" and "how much" people smoke, such an approach of "low-tar and low-nicotine" cigarettes may not do anything to decrease the cigarette dependency of smokers. Russell (1977), in an article on smoking problems, stated:

> I believe that the reason why it has been relatively easy to bring smokers down to the [presently low-tar and low-nicotine cigarettes] is

> because it had not really required them to reduce their tar and nicotine intake. They have simply adjusted by taking larger puffs, one or two more puffs, a few more cigarettes and inhaling more deeply and this has been relatively painless, and largely unconscious. (p. 29)

Finally, the findings of this study imply that it might be possible to decrease the dependency on cigarettes by altering the patterns of how people smoke. Perhaps, through behavioral modification techniques, smokers might be taught how to decrease their number of puffs, puff duration, and volume for each smoked cigarette, while at the same time encouraging them to smoke only the same number of cigarettes per day.

ACKNOWLEDGMENT

This study was supported by a project grant from the Tobacco and Health Research Institute, University of Kentucky.

REFERENCES

ASHTON, H., and WATSON, D.W. Puffing frequency and nicotine intake in cigarette smokers. *Br. Med. J.* 3: 679-681, 1970.

COMER, A.K., and CREIGHTON, D.E. The effect of experimental conditions on smoking behavior. In R.E. Thornton (ed.), *Smoking Behavior.* London: Churchill-Livingstone, 1978, pp. 76-86.

CREIGHTON, D.E., and LEWIS, P.H. The effect of different cigarettes on human smoking patterns. In R.E. Thornton (ed.), *Smoking Behavior.* London: Churchill-Livingstone, 1978a, pp. 289-300.

CREIGHTON, D.E., and LEWIS, P.H. The effect of smoking patterns on smoke deliveries. In R.E. Thornton (ed.), *Smoking Behavior.* London: Churchill-Livingstone, 1978b. pp. 301-314.

GRAHAM, S., GROUCH, S., LEVIN, M.L., and BOCK, F.G. Variations in amounts of tobacco tar retrieved from selected models of smoking behavior simulated by smoking machines. *Cancer Res.* 21: 523-530, 1968.

GRIFFITH, R.B., BENNER, J.F. and REINHARDT, B. Procedures for characterizing human smoking behavior. In *Proceedings of the University of Kentucky Tobacco and Health Research Institute.* Lexington: Tobacco and Health Research Institute, January 11-13, 1972, pp. 19-30.

GRIFFITH, R.B., and MOODY, P. *Quantitative smoking behavior: 1. Precision and reliability of measurements.* Unpublished paper, 1976.

HILDING, A.C. On cigarette smoking, bronchial carcinoma and cilliary action: Smoking habits and measurements of smoke intake. *N. Engl. J. Med.* 254: 775-786, 1956.

MOODY, P. The relationships of quantified human smoking behavior and demographic variables. *Soc. Sci. Med.* 14A: 49-54, 1980.

RAWBONE, R.G., MURPHY, K., TATE, M.E., and KANE, S.J. The analysis of smoking parameters: Inhalation and absorption of tobacco smoke in studies of human smoking behavior. In R.E. Thornton (ed.), *Smoking Behavior.* London: Churchill-Livingstone, 1978, pp. 171-194.

RUSSELL, M.A.H. Smoking problems: An overview. In *NIDA Research Monograph 17.* Washington, DC: DHEW, PHS, December 1977, pp. 13-33.

RUSSELL, M.A.H. Tobacco dependence: Is nicotine rewarding or adversive? In N.A. Krasnegor (ed.), *Cigarette Smoking as a Dependence Process* (NIDA Research Monograph 23). Washington, DC: DHEW, PHS, 1979, pp. 100-122.

SCHULTZ, W., and SEEHOFER, F. Smoking behavior in Germany–The analysis of cigarette butts (KIPA). In R.E. Thornton (ed.), *Smoking Behavior.* London: Churchill-Livingstone, 1978, pp. 259-276.

The International Journal of the Addictions, 19(4), 441–451, 1984

An Ecological Analysis of the Interrelationships among Drug Abuse and Other Indices of Social Pathology

David N. Nurco,* DSW

Department of Psychiatry
University of Maryland
School of Medicine
Baltimore, Maryland

John W. Shaffer, PhD

The Johns Hopkins University
School of Medicine
Baltimore, Maryland

Ira H. Cisin, PhD

George Washington University
Washington, DC

Abstract

In a study of the interrelationships among 12 separate indices of social pathology, including drug abuse, in which census tracts were the units of analysis, moderate to high intercorrelations among all indices were observed. A subsequent components-types factor analysis revealed only a single eigenvalue greater than unity, suggesting that the interrelationships among the several indices may be most parsimoniously explained

*To whom inquiries should be sent at 1229 W. Mt. Royal Avenue, Baltimore, Maryland 21217.

0020-773X/84/1904-0441$3.50/0

in terms of a single underlying construct–*generalized social pathology*. Exact factor scores on this construct were computed for each tract, and those may be viewed as estimates of the degree of social upheaval present.

INTRODUCTION

To what extent is narcotic drug abuse related to other forms of social pathology? Although there is widespread agreement among social scientists that drug abuse is merely a symptom of a more general syndrome of social malaise, relatively few investigations have sought to answer this question directly. Exceptions to this statement include the pioneering research of Chein, Gerard, Lee, and Rosenfeld (1964), and the more recent study by Nurco (1972). Both investigations, despite differences in location, scope, and methodology, concluded that narcotic addiction is most prevalent in those geographic areas characterized by deprivation and crime as well as by other indices of social and personal upheaval.

Actually, the question concerning relationships among various indices of social pathology can be addressed at two distinct levels: the individual and the ecological. The corresponding units of analysis are the individual subject and the geographic subarea. If the individual is chosen as the unit of analysis, the research question takes the following form: Are persons who are involved in one form of socially disapproved behavior also likely to be involved in other forms of socially disapproved behaviors? On the other hand, if the geographic subarea is chosen as the unit of analysis, the research question may be phrased as follows: Do areas with high rates of one form of social pathology also tend to have high rates of other forms of social pathology? These two questions, although undoubtedly related, differ in research focus and are by no means identical. Moreover, it is conceivable that somewhat different answers could be given to each, and it is certainly true that speculations regarding causal mechanisms might well differ depending on which of the two research strategies is pursued. In either case, it should be clear that both represent cross-sectional approaches which can, at best, establish correlation only, and that ultimate questions concerning cause cannot be definitively answered on the basis of the data collected.

BACKGROUND OF THE PRESENT STUDY

Investigation of the question as to whether social pathology can best be viewed as a single construct or as a collection of relatively unrelated indices was pursued within the context of a larger-scale research project whose primary focus was on drug abuse in Baltimore during the period 1945-1982. Among other things, this project was designed to (1) develop profiles of narcotic addicts in terms of variables such as age, race, sex, and place of residence; (2) develop special profiles of female narcotic addicts for several different time cohorts; (3) determine the specific geographic areas within Baltimore City where narcotic addicts tend to congregate; and (4) provide, using the methods of street ethnography (Weppner, 1977), a descriptive history of changes in addict characteristics and patterns of narcotic distribution from the late 1940s to the present. In the course of this research, recent census tract data pertaining to a variety of social indices became available, thus affording the opportunity to address the issue of generality versus specificity with respect to several different indicators of social pathology.

METHOD

As already indicated, the ready availability of census tract data dictated an analysis in terms of geographic area rather than individual subject. Thus the research question, operationally stated, becomes: Are indices (i.e., rates) of social pathology, especially prevalence of narcotic abuse, highly correlated within census tracts, or are they relatively separate and statistically independent measures? If substantial intercorrelations are found to exist, this would suggest the presence of an underlying communality that could perhaps best be expressed as a weighted combination of the separate measures. Moreover, on a more theoretical level, it would suggest that the various indices of social pathology are most parsimoniously regarded as different expressions of the same underlying source or cause. While such a chain of reasoning is not without flaws, it does represent a model widely employed in the social and behavioral sciences (Jackson and Borgatta, 1981; Rummel, 1970).

Although it is clear that the census tract corresponds only roughly to the sociological concept of *neighborhood,* the former is the unit for which data are available and represents the standard unit of analysis for many federal, state, and municipal purposes. Moreover, since census tracts are typically larger and therefore likely to be more heterogeneous than neighborhoods, one might anticipate that interrelationships among indices based on the former are likely to be attenuated. Hence, any findings concerning the magnitude of such interrelationships are likely to be underestimates of those that would have been obtained if neighborhood data had been available.

For the 201 noninstitutional census tracts in Baltimore City, the following indices, each expressed as a rate per 100 or per 100,000, were recorded: number of arrests for narcotic violations, number of arrests for other drug violations, percent unmarried, percent non-White, number receiving aid to families with dependent children (AFDC), number receiving general public assistance (GPA), number receiving food stamps, number of arrests for all causes other than narcotic or other drug violations, number of illegitimate births, number of homicides, number of cases of venereal disease reported, and number of dwellings averaging more than one person per room (see Note 1).

Statistical Analysis. Means, standard deviations, and ranges on each of these 12 variables were computed, and the intercorrelation matrix (Pearson product-moment *r*) was formed. Afterward, this matrix was factor analyzed using the method of principal components with unities in the main diagonal (communalities of 1.00). Only components having eigenvalues greater than 1.00 (i.e., variances in excess of those associated with the individual standardized variables) were retained for further analysis (Nunnally, 1978; Rummel, 1970).

RESULTS

The means, standard deviations, and ranges of the 12 variables over all 201 census tracts are presented in Table 1. It will be noted that considerable variation across tracts is the rule, and that this is especially the case with regard to narcotic and nonnarcotic drug arrests.

The intercorrelation matrix of the 12 indices was next formed; this is presented in Table 2. In absolute magnitude, the correlations range from a low of .44 (between homicide deaths and nonnarcotic drug arrests) to a high of .89 (between aid to families with dependent children and the number of persons per room). Even the smallest of these correlations is substantial, and all are statistically significant beyond the .001 level (Note 2). Thus it is clear from even a casual inspection of the matrix that the 12 indices have a great deal in common, in that a particular census tract's standing on one index is substantially predictable from its standing on another.

The degree to which the 12 indices reflect a common, underlying source (or sources) may be more formally, mathematically addressed using the methods of factor analysis. According to Kim and Mueller (1978), this technique is based on the assumption that some underlying factors (sources of variance), which are smaller in number than the observed variables, are responsible for the covariation among the latter. Thus, the observed variables are viewed as imperfect or compounded expressions of the underlying "causes" or sources of variance (i.e., the factors). Although several different factor-analytic methods exist, the one used here is the most widely employed and rests on the firmest mathematical base (Nunnally, 1978). Moreover, most of the different methods yield highly comparable results.

Application of the method of principal components to the correlation matrix shown in Table 2 yielded only a single component (factor) with an eigenvalue in excess of 1.00, thus indicating that the interrelationships among the 12 indices, as well as their total variation, may most parsimoniously be explained in terms of a single underlying source. The eigenvalue associated with this single factor (first prinicipal component) was 8.71, or 72.6% of the trace

Table 1

Means, Standard Deviations, and Ranges of 12 Social Indices for Baltimore Census Tracts (N = 201)

Social index[a]	Mean	SD	Range
1. Narcotic arrests	102.69	111.53	0-570
2. Nonnarcotic drug arrests	489.40	303.89	0-1403
3. Percent unmarried	69.09	11.24	41.73-92.50
4. Percent non-White	52.37	40.84	0.03-99.85
5. Aid to families with dependent children	5525.91	4132.31	0-16463
6. General public assistance	2025.83	1833.32	0-9758
7. Food stamps	3392.54	2637.84	0-14344
8. Non-drug-related arrests	5931.96	3980.76	106-20882
9. Illegitimate births	51.11	27.57	0-95.45
10. Homicides	59.18	56.78	0-242
11. Total venereal disease	2198.13	1894.40	0-8491
12. Percent of dwellings with average number of persons per room ⩾ 1	5.48	4.35	0-26.07

[a] All indices expressed as number of cases per 100,000, except Indices 3, 4, 9, and 12.

Table 2

Product-Moment Intercorrelations among 12 Social Indices for Baltimore Census Tracts (N = 201)

	Index											
Index[a]	1	2	3	4	5	6	7	8	9	10	11	12
1. Narcotic arrests												
2. Nonnarcotic drug arrests	.71											
3. Percent unmarried	.69	.62										
4. Percent non-White	.63	.53	.76									
5. Aid to families with dependent children	.67	.69	.84	.72								
6. General public assistance	.62	.66	.73	.57	.75							
7. Food stamps	.61	.60	.80	.57	.77	.79						
8. Non-drug-related arrests	.65	.74	.82	.56	.84	.86	.81					
9. Illegitimate births	.69	.68	.87	.86	.86	.74	.74	.79				
10. Homicides	.46	.44	.56	.59	.56	.56	.47	.55	.61			
11. Total venereal disease	.79	.74	.87	.84	.82	.71	.74	.77	.88	.57		
12. Percent of dwellings with average number of persons per room ⩾ 1	.63	.60	.76	.67	.89	.55	.59	.74	.77	.50	.78	

[a] All indices expressed as number of cases per 100,000, except Indices 3, 4, 9, and 12.

Table 3

Factor Loadings (Product-Moment Correlations) of 12 Social Indices on First Principal Component (Generalized Social Pathology Factor)

Index[a]	Factor loading
1. Narcotic arrests	.80
2. Nonnarcotic drug arrests	.79
3. Percent unmarried	.92
4. Percent non-White	.81
5. Aid to families with dependent children	.93
6. General public assistance	.84
7. Food stamps	.84
8. Non-drug-related arrests	.90
9. Illegitimate births	.93
10. Homicides	.66
11. Total venereal disease	.93
12. Percent of dwellings with average number of persons per room ⩾ 1	.84

[a] All indices expressed as number of cases per 100,000, except Indices 3, 4, 9, and 12.

(total variance represented in the matrix). Thus, 72.6% of the total variation represented by the 12 separate indices is "captured" by this single underlying source (Note 3).

The degree to which each index reflects the underlying source variable is measured by its "factor loading." Factor loadings are the product-moment correlations between the factor and each of the separate indices, and these are presented in Table 3.

It will be noted from Table 3 that the underlying source factor (which, for lack of a better term, will be labeled *generalized social pathology*) is primarily reflected in total cases of venereal disease (r = .93), illegitimate birth rate (r = .93), aid to families with dependent children (r = .93), percent nonmarried (r = .92), and non-drug-related arrests (r = .90). The smallest loading, which is still quite substantial, is that associated with homicide rate (r = .66). Narcotic and nonnarcotic arrest rates have intermediate loadings (r = .80 and .79, respectively). Percent non-White, which is not an index of social pathology per se, nevertheless has a substantial loading of .81 that reflects the tendency for social pathology to be concentrated in tracts with predominantly non-White populations.

On the basis of the analyses performed, it is possible to compute an exact score for each census tract on the Generalized Social Pathology (GSP) factor. Such scores probably represent the most precise estimates available of the degree of overall social malaise or upheaval present within a particular tract. The GSP scores for each of the 201 census tracts are presented in Table 4 in rank order

Table 4

Rank Order and Factor Score on Generalized Social Pathology for 201 Noninstitutional Census Tracts in Baltimore City: 1980

Rank	Census Tract	Factor Score	Rank	Census Tract	Factor Score	Rank	Census Tract	Factor Score	Rank	Census Tract	Factor Score	Rank	Census Tract	Factor Score
1	1004	73.1	41	1512	59.4	81	2502.03	52.1	121	2719	44.7	161	2404	40.1
2	1205	71.4	42	1503	59.3	82	1509	51.9	122	2403	44.4	162	1202	40.0
3	1901	70.6	43	2718.02	59.3	83	2803.02	51.9	123	0903	44.2	163	2720.01	39.9
4	1204	70.5	44	0907	59.3	84	2007.01	51.7	124	2005	44.2	164	2708.03	39.9
5	1001	69.9	45	1513	59.1	85	0905	51.6	125	2707.01	44.2	165	2501.02	39.8
6	1603	69.6	46	2506	58.6	86	0702	51.2	126	2201	44.1	166	2703.01	39.6
7	1002	69.3	47	0605	58.5	87	2503.01	51.2	127	2607	44.1	167	0102	39.6
8	2503.02	68.1	48	1304	58.4	88	1206	51.0	128	2606.02	44.0	168	2702	39.4
9	1801	67.7	49	0603	58.4	89	2502.02	50.9	129	0103	44.0	169	2501.01	39.3
10	0402	67.4	50	2101	58.3	90	2604.03	50.8	130	2709.02	43.8	170	1307	39.1
11	1703	67.3	51	0906	58.1	91	2710.02	50.8	131	2303	43.8	171	2804.03	39.1
12	1501	67.2	52	1506	57.9	92	2804.02	50.7	132	2602.01	43.7	172	2503.03	39.0
13	1802	66.4	53	1606	57.8	93	2804.04	50.6	133	2505	43.7	173	2703.02	38.7
14	0804	66.3	54	2716	57.4	94	1102	50.5	134	0104	43.7	174	2401	38.7
15	1602	66.3	55	1301	57.3	95	2606.01	50.4	135	2604.04	43.6	175	2720.03	38.6
16	1303	65.8	56	2002	57.2	96	0201	50.1	136	0601	43.5	176	2605	38.5
17	0807	65.6	57	1803	57.1	97	1507.02	49.9	137	2008	43.4	177	2601.01	38.4
18	0808	65.3	58	1903	56.9	98	2604.02	49.9	138	2708.05	43.4	178	1308.03	38.3
19	1302	65.3	59	1504	56.9	99	0901	49.6	139	1308.01	42.8	179	2603.01	38.2
20	2502.04	65.1	60	1203	56.9	100	0401	49.4	140	2801.01	42.4	180	2708.01	37.9
21	0909	64.7	61	2603.03	55.5	101	1101	49.4	141	2602.02	42.3	181	2701.01	37.8
22	0501	64.2	62	1508.02	55.3	102	2802	49.3	142	0701	42.2	182	0801.01	37.7
23	1702	64.2	63	2710.01	54.7	103	2102	49.3	143	2608	42.1	183	2715.01	37.6
24	0301	64.1	64	1608.02	54.3	104	0105	49.1	144	1306	42.0	184	2704.01	37.6
25	0802	63.9	65	1701	54.0	105	2801.02	48.9	145	2604.01	42.0	185	2704.02	37.5
26	1403	63.9	66	1902	53.8	106	2803.01	48.2	146	1308.04	42.0	186	2701.02	37.5
27	1604	63.1	67	2717	53.7	107	2006	48.2	147	2504.01	41.4	187	2708.04	37.4
28	0704	63.0	68	2301	53.6	108	1507.01	48.1	148	1305	41.2	188	2711.02	37.3
29	1402	62.9	69	1607	53.5	109	1207	48.0	149	0902	41.2	189	2603.02	37.2
30	1502	62.1	70	2003	53.5	110	0801.02	47.6	150	2708.02	40.9	190	2706	37.0
31	1601	62.1	71	0904	53.5	111	0202	47.4	151	2402	40.7	191	2601.02	36.8
32	0908	61.7	72	2718.01	53.4	112	1511	47.3	152	2610	40.6	192	2501.03	36.6
33	0805	61.6	73	2007.02	53.2	113	0203	46.6	153	2609	40.5	193	2705.01	36.6
34	0703	61.5	74	1510	53.2	114	2709.01	46.5	154	2711.01	40.4	194	1201	36.2
35	0302	61.5	75	1508.01	53.1	115	2602.03	46.5	155	2804.01	40.4	195	2707.03	36.1
36	0803.01	61.5	76	1605	53.0	116	1401	46.3	156	0101	40.4	196	2713	36.0
37	0604	61.3	77	1505	52.9	117	0602	45.3	157	2502.06	40.3	197	2714	35.9
38	0806	60.6	78	0803.02	52.3	118	2504.02	45.1	158	2707.02	40.2	198	2712	35.4
39	2004	60.5	79	1608.01	52.2	119	2709.03	44.9	159	2611	40.2	199	2705.02	35.3
40	2001	60.0	80	2502.01	52.0	120	2302	44.8	160	2502.05	40.2	200	2715.03	35.0
												201	2720.02	34.3

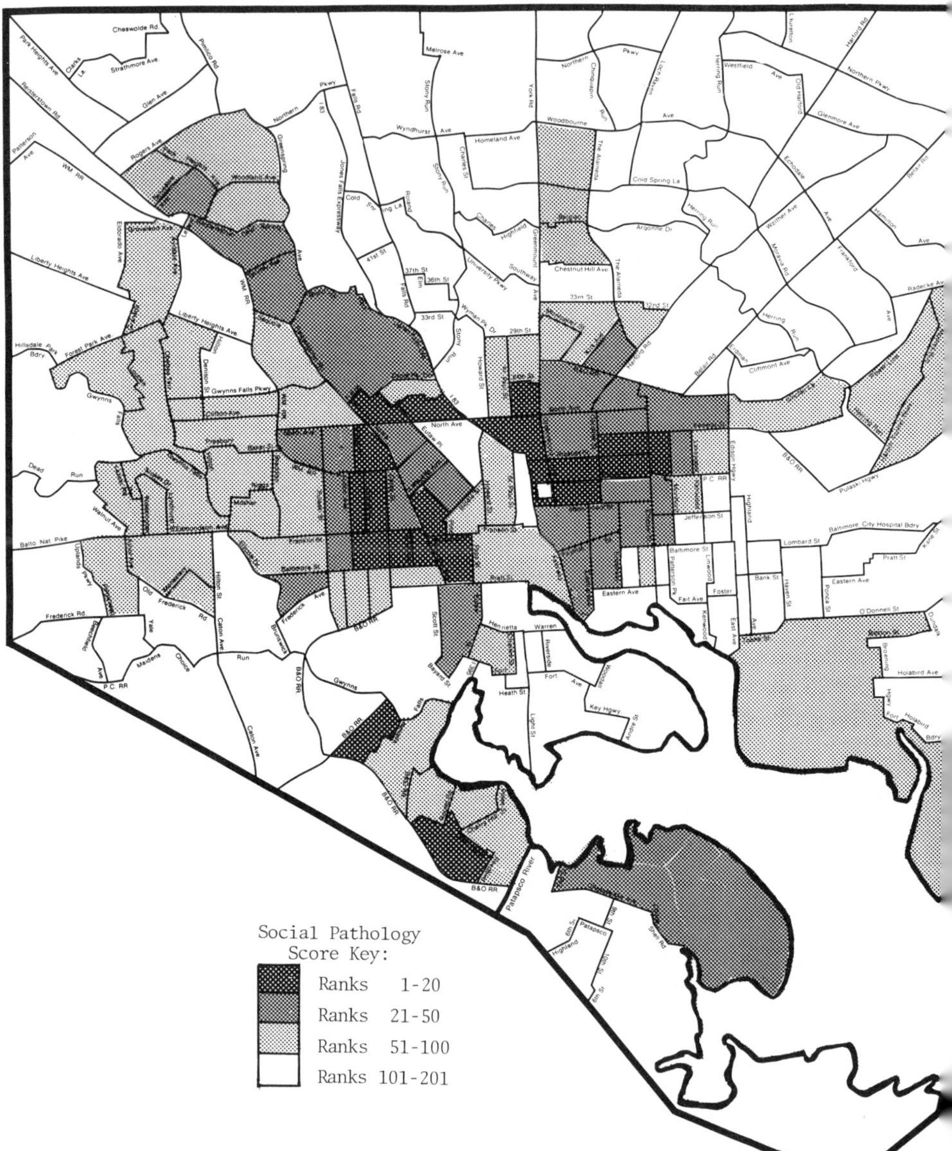

Fig. 1. Baltimore City census tracts with relative standings on generalized social pathology score: 1980.

of magnitude. These scores, which have been rounded to one decimal place, are in standardized form, with an overall mean of 50 and a standard deviation of 10.

Tracts with GSP scores above the median are shown in Fig. 1, with the more darkly shaded tracts having the highest scores. Those tracts with the very highest scores tend to cluster around the recently revitalized "Metro Center" of the city, which includes the central business district. This central area has been substantially rehabilitated and is no longer characterized by high rates on the various indices of social upheaval. Other substantially rehabilitated areas, in comparison with their standing in an earlier report (Nurco, 1972), include, for example, Tracts 103, 104, 401, and 2201. Apparently, the city's effort to improve these areas has been successful.

Those tracts with very high GSP scores tend to be characterized by high rates of poverty and high population densities. In addition to the ones surrounding "Metro Center," such tracts include Lower Park Heights, Cherry Hill, Westport, and Curtis Bay. Moreover, there appears to be a tendency for social pathology to be spreading along the northwest corridor radiating out from the city's center, although other areas are involved as well.

DISCUSSION

It should again be emphasized that the present series of analyses are based on "ecological correlations," that is, correlations among rates using aggregates (census tracts) as the units of analysis. All conclusions, therefore, must be restricted to the aggregate, sociological level, rather than to the individual or personal level.

With this caution clearly in mind, it is obvious that those census tracts having a high degree of prevalence of one form of social pathology are likely to have a high prevalence of other forms as well. In other words, this research provides strong evidence for both the existence and explanatory power of a concept of "generalized social pathology" that can be measured and used to describe geographic subareas. All of the variables included in the present analyses proved to be highly related to this general concept, especially illegitimate birth rate, prevalence of venereal disease, and percent of population unmarried. It is interesting to note that each of these indices, together with the prevalence of aid to families with dependent children, reflects a breakdown in traditional values and mores with respect to sexual behavior and the integrity of the family. Whether or not such a breakdown is the cause or merely one of the many symptoms or correlates of societal deterioration is, of course, beyond the scope of cross-sectional studies such as this.

All of the foregoing notwithstanding, it is important to note that the concept of generalized social pathology is one which we attribute to a given geographic area based on an evaluation of the behaviors of individuals endogenous to that area. While this evaluation undoubtedly reflects the values and orientation of the society at large, it is unlikely to reflect the attitudes and values of the persons engaging in such societally disapproved behaviors. Indeed, the behaviors endorsed by the dominant culture may be regarded as undesirable or even self-defeating by those considered to be "socially deviant." Due concern for such "existential realities" would be essential to the success of any planned interventions designed to alter the behaviors in question.

Strictly speaking, the present findings apply only to a single metropolitan area, although it seems reasonable to expect that they are likely to generalize to other geographic areas as well. In our opinion, future research of this type could be meaningfully extended in two major directions. First, the patterns of covariation among the societally defined indices of social pathology used in the present study could be investigated in other cultural (i.e., European and non-European) contexts. In other cultures, it is conceivable that more than one dimension of variation would be found. Second, it would seem important to develop additional measures of social pathology more suited to affluent areas, in that the more gross indices employed herein may have insufficient incidence/prevalence to permit reliable and valid measurement. More suitable measures might include divorce rates, incidence of civil suits, and extent of utilization of private mental health services. The development and validation of these and other indices could provide the basis for a more objective evaluation of "quality of life" or "social well-being" across a wide range of cultures with varying degrees of material affluence.

ACKNOWLEDGMENTS

Research such as this can be accomplished only with the help and cooperation of many individuals and agencies. These include the Baltimore City Police Department: Commissioner Frank J. Battaglia, Lt. Joseph Newman, and Sgt. Emory Starry; the Baltimore City Health Department: Dr. John B. DeHoff and Mr. Sheldon Baylin; the Baltimore Planning Department: Mr. George Becker and Mr. Ray Schreiner; and the Baltimore City Department of Social Services: Mrs. Roberta Hennick. This research was supported by contract number 271-79-3614 of the Addiction Research Center, National Institute on Drug Abuse, to Chesapeake Physicians, Inc. All funds were administered by Friends Medical Science Research Center, Inc. We wish to thank Mr. Grenville Whitman, Ms. Janis Duncan, Mr. Timothy Kinlock, and Mrs. Vera Stover for their advice and assistance.

NOTES

1. Percent unmarried, percent non-White, and number of dwellings averaging more than one person per room were obtained from 1980 census data. All arrest indices pertain to calender year 1980 and were obtained from the Baltimore City Police Department. AFDC, GPA, and food stamp indices refer to all active cases on October 31, 1980, as determined by the Baltimore City Department of Social Services. Number of homicides pertain to calendar years 1979 and 1980, while number of illegitimate births and number of cases of venereal disease pertain to 1980. These latter three indices were obtained from data provided by the Baltimore City Health Department.
2. Since the entire population of tracts is involved, the issue of statistical significance may seem irrelevant. However, we agree with the position of Winch and Campbell (1969) to the effect that such an analysis provides evidence for the existence of nontrivial, nonrandom phenomena.
3. In an effort to determine the extent to which these findings were dependent on the specific distributions of the variables studied, tracts were rank ordered on each of the 12 rate variables, and the entire analysis was repeated using the matrix of rank-order correlations. This reanalysis resulted in no diminution in the clarity of the resulting pattern, and the overall conclusions remain unchanged.

REFERENCES

CHEIN, I., GERARD, D.L., LEE, R.S., and ROSENFELD, E. *The Road to H.* New York: Basic Books, 1964.

JACKSON, D.J., and BORGATTA, E.F. (eds.). *Factor Analysis and Measurement in Sociological Research.* Beverly Hills, CA: Sage Publications, 1981.

KIM, J.O., and MUELLER, C.W. *Introduction to Factor Analysis.* Beverly Hills, CA: Sage Publications, 1978.

NUNNALLY, J.C. *Psychometric Theory* (2nd ed.). New York: McGraw-Hill, 1978.

NURCO, D.N. An ecological analysis of narcotic addicts in Baltimore. *Int. J. Addict.* 7: 341-353, 1972.

RUMMEL, R.J. *Applied Factor Analysis.* Evanston, IL: Northwestern University Press, 1970.

WEPPNER, R.S. *Street Ethnography.* Beverly Hills, CA: Sage Publications, 1977.

WINCH, R.F., and CAMPBELL, D.T. Proof? No. Evidence? Yes. The significance of tests of significance. *Am. Sociol.,* May 1969, pp. 140-143.

The International Journal of the Addictions, 19(4), 453–458, 1984

Research Note

Glue Sniffing: A Pilot Study of the Cognitive Effects of Long-Term Use

W. M. Allison, BSc

National Children's Home
Pitlochry PH16 5JW
Scotland

D. W. A. Jerrom, BA, MPhil

Department of Psychology
University of Stirling
Stirling FK9 4LA
Scotland

Abstract

A psychological test battery briefly assessing memory, intelligence, and attention was administered to 10 delinquent solvent inhalers and 10 matched controls. The solvent abuse group showed significant impairment in tests of memory, nonverbal intelligence, and attention and concentration. The implications for future research are discussed.

There is increasing evidence in the solvent abuse literature of cortical damage resulting from the long-term abuse of toxic inhalents. King et al. (1981) report 19 cases of encephalopathy resulting from toluene abuse, and McAllister et al. (1981) report a case of solvent intoxication leading to the onset of ideopathic epilepsy. Altenkirch and Schulze (1979) report 25 cases of clinically severe toxic polyneuropathy among abusers addicted to inhaling glue containing methylethylketone solvents. Grabski (1961) describes a case of cerebellar degeneration in a chronic toluene inhaler. Toluene is also implicated in the report by Escobar and Aruffo (1980) of an inhaler addicted to toluene substances for 12 years; on postmortem examination the patient had diffuse cerebral and cerebellar atrophy and axonopathy.

 0020-773X/84/1904-0453$3.50/0

Table 1

Neuropsychological Investigations of the Effects of Solvent Abuse

Dodds and Santostefano (1964)	Bigler (1979)
Subjects	Subjects
a. 12 males	a. 10 psychiatric patients with history of chronic abuse
b. Mean age, 13.8	b. Aged 16-20 years
c. Of mainly Spanish-American descent	c. 3 control groups of psychiatric noninhaling subjects
d. Arrested for public intoxication	Solvents
e. Matched control group of non-solvent users	Various
Solvents	Measures
Glue; type not specified	Wechsler Adult Intelligence Scale, Halstead-Reitan Battery
Measures	Findings
Nonstandardized test battery to measure cognitive functioning	Generalized neuropsychological deficits in chronic inhalers
Findings	Limitations of study
No difference between groups	Subjects used multisubstances
Limitatons of study	Not specified if experimental subjects suffered from other psychiatric conditions
Nonstandardized test instruments	
Short-term glue sniffers included in experimental group	

This evidence of cortical damage would suggest that chronic abusers should also show signs of impairment on neuropsychological tests. There are two published investigations in this area, which have produced contradictory results; Table 1 gives details of these.

This paper reports a pilot study investigating the incidence of psychological impairment following chronic solvent abuse.

METHOD

This study forms part of a wider investigation of the prevalence of solvent abuse in a population of 65 male adolescent offenders currently inmates in three List D schools in the west of Scotland. Each youth participated in a structured interview with the first author; the interview established whether or not the subject had inhaled glue or other toxic substances and if there was a history of abuse, and gathered various types of information about the drug habit. Eighty percent of the population had inhaled solvents at least once; the detailed results of this survey will be published elsewhere.

The 10 subjects with the most serious history of solvent inhaling were selected for inclusion in the experimental group. The most popular substance inhaled was the glue "Evostick," the toxic component in this being toluene/

acetone. Five subjects reported subjective physical or pychological symptoms as a result of their long-term abuse, the commonest being chest pain, rapid fatigue with exertion, and impaired memory and concentration. The 10 control subjects were youths from the original survey who had never inhaled solvents, matched to the experimental group for age, educational level, and reading age as assessed by the educational psychologists in the institution. Each experimental subject was matched to a control subject from the same institution. Care was taken to exclude from both groups any subjects with a history of head injury or illness which might produce psychological impairment. Table 2 presents background data on the subjects.

Prior to both interviewing and testing it was explained to the subject that the interviewer had no authority or connection with the institution, and a guarantee was made of the confidentiality of all results.

Five psychological tests were used; these were always given in the same order. The tests were selected to briefly assess three aspects of cognitive functioning: intelligence, memory, and attention. All of the tests selected were also those which have been demonstrated to be sensitive to cognitive impairment as a result of trauma or alcohol-related brain damage. The WISC vocabulary test was used as a short-form measure of verbal IQ. Performance on this test has been shown to be reliable and relatively resistant to neuropsychological disturbance (Blatt and Allison, 1968). The WISC Block Design Test was used as a

Table 2

Background Characteristics

	Mean		Standard deviation		Range	
	E group	C group	E group	C group	E group	C group
1. Age (yr)	15.45	15.43	0.25	0.26	15.1-15.9	15.0-15.9
2. Length of solvent abuse (yr)	4.6	–	1.79	–	3-8.5	–
3. Other drug/ alcohol use	NIL	NIL	–	–	–	–
4. Frequency of use when inhaling most	Daily	–	–	–	–	–
5. Type of family	Low socioeconomic status; frequent parental alcoholism and discord					
6. Religion	Christian					
7. Educational status	Below average attainment; 10 years state education–frequent truancy					
8. Nationality/ ethnicity	Native west of Scotland (U.K.)					

measure of nonverbal intelligence. The Wechsler Memory Scale (WMS) was used as a standard measure of memory functioning; the test contains seven subtests tapping various facets of memory. Two of the seven subtests of the WMS, Visual Reproduction and Logical Memory, were readministered following a 10-minute delay as a test of long-term memory. Last, the Paced Auditory Serial Addiction Task (PASAT) test was used as a measure of attention and concentration. In this test the subject is presented with a series of 21 digits with a 4-second gap between each number. The subject is asked to add each digit to the one immediately preceding it and give the answer aloud prior to the next digit; the percentage of correct responses is the test score (Gronwall and Wrightsen, 1975).

RESULTS

The 10 solvent inhalers scored at a statistically significantly lower level compared to the control group on the WISC Block Design Test, the WMS memory quotient, and the PASAT. The mean scores, standard deviations, and significance levels for these test results are presented in Table 3.

Inspection of Table 3 shows that the control group scored higher on Block Design than on Vocabulary, the results usually found in a delinquent population (Sattler, 1974). However, in the inhaler group this effect is reversed, the mean Vocabulary score being 1 scale point higher than the mean Block Design score.

Table 4 presents mean scores on the seven subtests of the WMS. The inhalers have a lower mean score on all but two of the subtests, these being Information and Orientation. Logical Memory and Visual Reproduction were retested after 10 minutes as a measure of long-term memory; a percentage-forgotten score for the retests was computed to weight for the amount of initial recall by subtracting the delayed recall score from initial recall and then dividing by initial recall.

Table 3

Summary of Test Results per Group

	Test			
	Block Design	Vocabulary	PASAT	WMS
Solvent group				
Mean	5.3	6.5	65%	81.4
SD	1.56	1.4	30.44	8.11
Control group				
Mean	9.5	7.5	90%	93.7
SD	1.7	1.11	12.51	9.16
t value	5.72	0.26	2.21	3.18
2-tailed prob. value	0.001	NS	0.05	0.01
df	18	18	18	18

Table 4

Mean Group Scores per Weschler Memory Subtest

Subtest	Solvent group Mean	Solvent group SD	Control group Mean	Control group SD
Information	4.8	1.5	4.4	0.96
Orientation	5	0	5	0
Mental control	6	1.94	7.1	1.44
Digit span	9.2	1.03	12.2	2.14
Associate learning	15.15	3.56	16.25	3.1
Logical memory				
1st test	3.8	2.77	6.45	2.1
% forgotten on retest	20	22	13.27	7.6
Visual reproduction				
1st test	6.2	2.25	9.3	1.76
% forgotten on retest	29	26.85	8	15.44

Table 4 also presents the initial and delayed recall scores for these two tests and the percentage-forgotten scores. Inhalers forgot significantly more on the Visual Reproduction test ($t = 2.14$, $p < .5$), but there was no significant difference in forgetting between the two groups on the Logical Memory test.

On the PASAT, inhalers obtained a mean score of 65%, in comparison to 90% scored by the control group. This 25% difference between the two groups was statistically significant ($t = 2.21, p < .05$).

DISCUSSION

The results of this pilot study show evidence of psychological impairment as a result of long-term solvent abuse. Inhalers displayed impaired function across a wide range of cognitive functions, attention, verbal and visual memory, and visuospatial problem solving. Overall they scored at a statistically significantly lower level on all but four of the tests used; these four tests all measured aspects of verbal ability.

This study is open to two criticisms regarding design. First, the psychologist was not blind to the experimental condition of the subject. However, great care was taken to conform to the correct test administration procedures, and the tests employed are both reliable and in widespread clinical and research use in the United Kingdom and the United States. The second shortcoming in design concerns how much time had elapsed since the experimental group last inhaled glue. All subjects were asked when they had last inhaled: The times given ranged from 6 weeks to 10 days; however, obviously if the subjects were using solvents in the institution they would be most unlikely to admit to doing so. It is thus possible that the overall performance of the inhalers was caused by their having been recently intoxicated, rather than by a permanent functional impairment. However, Dodds and Santostefano (1964) failed to find any evidence of psychological impairment in a group of inhalers tested only 14 hours after being arrested for public intoxication. We do not, therefore, consider our results to be an artifact of the effects of recent solvent use, but obviously future research should attempt to control for this by using physical tests of the presence or absence of the relevant toxins in the blood of subjects (viz., Lush et al., 1980, pp. 304-313).

Future investigations of the neuropsychological effects of solvent abuse should include two other improvements in design. First, subjects should be tested longitudinally to test for possible recovery or further deterioration. Second, neurological investigations, such as the EEG, brain scan, and neurological examination, should be used to seek confirmation or to refute the presence of organic changes.

REFERENCES

ALTENKIRCH, H., and SCHULZE, H. Glue sniffing and sniffing neuropathy. *Nervenarzt* 50(1): 21-27, 1979.

BIGLER, E.D. Neuropsychological evaluation of adolescent patients hospitalised with chronic inhalant abuse. *Clin. Neuropsychol.* 1(1): 8-12, 1979.

BLATT, S.J., and ALLISON, J. *Psychological Tests.* New York: Harper and Row, 1968.

DODDS, J., and SANTOSTEFANO, S. A comparison of the cognitive functioning of glue sniffers and non sniffers. *J. Pediatr.* 64(4): 565-570, 1964.

ESCOBAR, A., and ARUFFO, C. Chronic thinner intoxication: Clinico-pathologic report of a human case. *J. Neurol. Neurosurg. Psychiatry* 43: 986-994, 1980.

GRABSKI, D.H. Toluene sniffing producing cerebellar degeneration. *Am. J. Psychiatry* 118: 461-462, 1961.

GRONWALL, D., and WRIGHTSEN, P. Cumulative effect of concussion. *Lancet* 22: 995-997, 1975.

KING, M.E., DAY, R.E., OLIVER, J.S., LUSH, M., and WATSON, J.M. Solvent encephalopathy. *Br. Med. J.* 283: 663-665, 1981.

LUSH, M., OLIVER, J.S., and WATSON, J.M. *Forensic Toxicology.* London: Croom Helm, 1980.

MC ALLISTER, C., LUSH, M., OLIVER, J.S., and WATSON, J.M. Status epilepticus caused by solvent abuse. *Br. Med. J.* 283: 1156, 1981.

SATTLER, J.M. *Assessment of Children's Intelligence.* London: Saunders, 1974.

The International Journal of the Addictions, 19(4), 459-468, 1984

Note

An Examination of the Drug Abuse Scale of the Mill on Clinical Multiaxial Inventory

Patrick M. Flynn, PhD

Robert C. McMahon,* PhD

University of Miami
Coral Gables, Florida 33124

Abstract

The Millon Clinical Multiaxial Inventory, which includes a drug abuse scale, was administered to a group of known drug abusers several times during the course of treatment. The scoring characteristics of the drug abusers in this sample were found to be consistent with those of drug abusers used in the MCMI standardization sample. Group scores obtained in the present sample on the MCMI drug abuse scale at intake and after 1 and 3 months of treatment show considerable consistency. The results suggest that this drug abuse scale may be measuring relatively enduring characteristics, uninfluenced by treatment, at least in the short term.

Presently, there does not exist an adequately validated and established drug abuse scale which is embodied in a widely used clinical diagnostic instrument. Cavior, Kurtzberg, and Lipton (1967) developed a heroin addiction scale using the MMPI which was subsequently supported in a cross-validation study (Sheppard, Rica, Fracchia, Rosenberg, and Merlis, 1972).

*To whom correspondence and requests for reprints should be addressed: Associate Professor of Counseling Psychology, Department of Educational Psychology, University of Miami, P.O. Box 248065, Coral Gables, Florida 33124.

 0020-773X/84/1904-0459$3.50/0

Although promising, it is narrow in scope, addressing only one type of drug use (heroin), and it has not achieved clinical popularity as a diagnostic scale. Another shortcoming was recently reported by Lachar, Berman, Grisell, and Schooff (1979), who found that the heroin addiction scale could not separate heroin addicts and psychiatric controls.

A recently published clinical diagnostic instrument, the Millon Clinical Multiaxial Inventory (MCMI), is becoming popular in the clinical community and has a specifically constructed Drug Abuse Scale. The MCMI is a relatively short (175 true/false items) diagnostic instrument consisting of 20 clinical scales which measure syndromes derived from a comprehensive theory of personality and psychopathology (Millon, 1977). It fills the obvious need in clinical settings for a diagnostic instrument which not only provides information regarding personality styles, pathological personality syndromes, and symptom disorders, but also assesses characteristics related to the probability of repeated or recent drug abuse. As a screening device, the MCMI may be used to identify individuals in need of further evaluation, such as those exhibiting severe psychopathology and unable to function, thus requiring residential treatment. The instrument may also be a useful tool in the treatment planning process as it provides information regarding chronic and acute psychopathology which when identified may be treated with appropriate therapeutic techniques. A brief description of the MCMI scales is provided in Table 1.

The primary purpose of this study is to determine the scoring characteristics on the Drug Abuse Scale of a known drug-abusing group and to compare the known group scores to those of the sample used in the standardization of the MCMI. A secondary purpose is to examine consistency or change in group Drug Abuse Scale scores during the first 3 months of treatment.

METHOD

Data were collected during a research project conducted in Broward and Dade Counties, in Florida, between May 1, 1981, and October 31, 1981. The sample in the study consisted of drug treatment patients who participated in the Treatment Outcome Prospective Study (TOPS). TOPS involved a national survey of drug abusers receiving treatment conducted by the Research Triangle Institute under contract with the National Institute on Drug Abuse. As part of TOPS, program researchers administered three survey forms and the MCMI. The survey forms were developed by the Research Triangle Institute to collect background information on drug abusers, including behavioral, socioeconomic, and demographic data (Research Triangle Institute, 1980). These survey instruments were administered at the time of a client's intake into treatment, and then again 1 month and 3 months after initiation of treatment. The subjects were given a small monetary incentive for participation upon completion of the instruments.

Table 1

MCMI Scale Descriptions and Corresponding DSM-III Diagnostic Syndromes[a]

Scale	MCMI classifications	DSM-III classifications	Characteristics
1	Schizoid-asocial	Schizoid	Displays emotional blandness, weak affectional needs, and limited enthusiasm for and involvement in interpersonal relationships
2	Avoidant	Avoidant	Experiences dysphoric mood, disturbing ideation, interpersonal hypersensitivity, social isolation, and rejection
3	Dependent-submissive	Dependent	Socially passive and interpersonally submissive; has little initiative and perceives self as fragile and ineffectual
4	Histrionic-gregarious	Histrionic	Characterized by gregarious and seductive interpersonal style, emotional lability, and poor cognitive integration of experiences
5	Narcissistic	Narcissistic	Inflated self-image; is exploitive in interpersonal situations; displays undisciplined cognitive expansiveness and social imperturbability
6	Antisocial-aggressive	Antisocial	Hostile, suspicious, and vindictive in interpersonal relationships; views self as independent, hard headed, and fearless
7	Compulsive-conforming	Compulsive	Emotionally restrained, socially conforming, and may be disposed to a highly structured and repetitive life pattern
8	P. aggressive-negativistic	Passive aggressive	Unstable emotionality and an ambivalent behavioral style; typically discontented with self and others and disillusioned with life

(continued)

Table 1 (continued)

Scale	MCMI classifications	DSM-III classifications	Characteristics
S	Schizotypal-schizoid	Schizotypal	Social detachment; behavioral peculiarities; irrelevant, tangential, and dissociated thinking; may be anxious and apprehensive or show emotional blandness and general deficiencies in activation
C	Borderline-cycloid	Borderline	Experiences intense but labile emotionality and dysregulated activation; may be preoccupied with maintaining emotional supports but has conflicting ambivalent feelings toward others and self-punitive conscience
P	Paranoid	Paranoid	Fiercely independent and mistrustful, defensive, and provocative in interpersonal relations; may be disposed to distorted cognitions and delusions of grandure and/or persecution
A	Anxiety	Anxiety disorder: panic, phobic and obsessive types	Experiences restlessness, apprehension, and various somatic complaints related to physiological overarousal; symptoms may be related to phobic stimuli or experienced in a more generalized manner
H	Somatoform	Somatoform disorder: somatization pain and hypochondriacal types	Expresses psychological difficulties through somatic channels, characterized by fatigue and weakness, and may be preoccupied with a variety of dramatic but nonspecific pains in unrelated parts of the body
N	Hypomanic	Manic disorder; moderate	Labile emotionality, restlessness, irritability, overactivity, distractability, and impulsivity

(continued)

Table 1 (continued)

Scale	MCMI classifications	DSM-III classifications	Characteristics
D	Dysthymic	Dysthymia	Although able to meet daily responsibilities, experiences behavioral apathy, feelings of discouragement, and self-deprecatory cognitions and guilt
B	Alcohol abuse	Alcohol abuse	Probable history of alcoholism with distress and disruptions in social and occupational functioning; possible past attempts to overcome problem
T	Drug abuse	Drug abuse	Has a likely recurrent or recent pattern of drug abuse with related difficulty in impulse control and social conformity
SS	Psychotic thinking	Schizophrenic disorder	Periodically exhibits disorganized, confused, and regressive behavior with associated inappropriate affect, delusions, and hallucinations
CC	Psychotic depression	Major depression	Severely depressed mood, pervasive pessimism, hopeless resignation, and associated symptoms, including psychomotor retardation and/or agitation; usually incapable of normal daily functioning
PP	Psychotic delusion	Paranoid disorders	Expresses interrelated delusions of a persecutory or grandiose nature and may manifest periodic belligerence

[a]Adapted from Millon (1982, p. 35).

The drug treatment modalities represented in this study included two residential components, two outpatient drug-free components, and one outpatient methadone program.

Table 2

Summary of Demographics for Subjects

Demographic variable	Sample of subjects for this study		MCMI standardization sample	
	N	%	*N*	%
Age				
18-25	41	28	218	14
26-35	89	62	416	26
36-45	11	8	443	28
46-55	3	2	373	23
56+	0	0	141	9
Sex				
Male	92	64	922	58
Female	52	36	669	42
Race				
White		66		81
Black		23		14
Latino		9		3
Oriental		1		1
Other/mixed		1		1
Total *N*	144		1,591	

The subjects in this study consisted of adult (18 and over) clients willing to participate in TOPS. Clients with low reading levels (below sixth grade), and also those who did not speak fluent English, were not included in the study. Of 185 eligible subjects, 144 chose to participate. One hundred and thirty-nine MCMI protocols were determined to be usable. Demographic data for both the present sample and the MCMI standardization sample are shown in Table 2. Drug use information is provided in Table 3.

RESULTS

The MCMI was constructed in such a manner that individual baserate scores of 75 and above indicate a "presence" of the clinical characteristics measured by the scale, and baserate scores of 85 and above indicate a "prominence" of the clinical characteristics. The data from the present study reveal that, as a group, the drug abusers who were receiving treatment exhibited baserate scores on the Drug Abuse Scale indicative of the "presence" of drug abuse. Also, as a group, the subjects' scores on the Drug Abuse Scale were not significantly different between administrations at intake and 1 month and 3 months into treatment for drug abuse. Descriptive statistics, regarding scores on the MCMI Drug Abuse Scale for the present sample of the drug abusers, are shown

Table 3

Types of Drugs Used, Age of Initial Drug Use, and Years Since First Drug Use (%)

	Marijuana	Inhalants	Hallucinogens	Cocaine	Heroin	Street methadone
Ever used	97.9	34.0	69.4	96.5	75.7	38.9
Age of initial use						
6-10	4.9	0.7	0.0	0.0	1.4	0.0
11-15	47.9	19.4	20.1	11.8	11.8	4.9
16-20	39.6	10.4	37.5	50.0	45.8	12.5
21-25	4.9	3.5	8.3	25.0	14.6	9.7
26-30	0.7	0.0	3.5	6.3	2.1	7.6
31-35	0.0	0.0	0.0	3.5	0.0	2.8
36-40	0.0	0.0	0.0	0.0	0.0	0.7
41-45	0.0	0.0	0.0	0.0	0.0	0.0
46-50	0.0	0.0	0.0	0.0	0.0	0.0
N/A[a]	2.1	66.0	30.6	3.5	24.3	61.8
Years since first use[b]						
0-1	0.0	0.0	0.0	0.7	0.0	1.4
1-3	1.4	2.1	4.2	11.1	3.5	6.9
4-6	4.2	3.5	8.3	20.1	5.6	8.3
7-9	16.7	2.8	9.0	21.5	18.8	6.9
10-12	18.8	9.0	22.9	20.8	22.2	10.4
13-15	25.7	8.3	18.1	15.3	13.2	4.2
16-18	18.1	6.3	5.6	4.2	6.9	0.0
19-21	7.6	2.1	1.4	2.1	2.8	0.0
22-24	2.8	0.0	0.0	0.0	0.0	0.0
25-27	0.7	0.0	0.0	0.7	0.7	0.0
28-30	1.4	0.0	0.0	0.0	0.7	0.0
Over 30	0.0	0.0	0.0	0.0	0.0	0.0
N/A	2.8	66.0	30.7	3.5	25.8	61.9

(continued)

Table 3 (continued)

	Other opiates	Minor tranquilizers	Major tranquilizers	Barbiturates	Sedatives and hypnotics	Amphetamines
Ever used	77.8	77.8	24.3	7.36	7.57	66.0
Age of initial use						
6-10	0.7	0.7	0.0	0.7	0.7	0.7
11-15	11.1	10.4	2.8	14.6	9.0	12.5
16-20	39.6	39.6	12.5	43.1	40.3	40.3
21-25	12.5	16.0	6.3	9.7	14.6	7.6
26-30	9.0	8.3	1.4	4.9	4.9	4.9
31-35	2.8	1.4	1.4	0.7	4.2	0.0
36-40	1.4	0.0	0.0	0.0	0.7	0.0
41-45	0.7	0.0	0.0	0.0	0.7	0.0
46-50	0.0	0.0	0.0	0.0	0.7	0.0
N/A[a]	22.2	23.6	75.7	26.4	24.3	34.0
Years since first use[b]						
0-1	0.7	0.0	0.7	0.0	0.7	0.0
1-3	18.8	9.0	1.4	5.6	14.6	5.6
4-6	10.4	14.6	6.3	8.3	12.5	7.6
7-9	12.5	19.4	6.9	12.5	20.1	10.4
10-12	15.3	17.4	5.6	20.8	16.7	19.4
13-15	10.4	7.6	2.8	13.2	6.9	12.5
16-18	5.6	5.6	0.7	9.0	2.1	6.9
19-21	1.4	1.4	0.0	1.4	0.7	2.1
22-24	0.0	0.7	0.0	1.4	0.7	1.4
25-27	0.7	0.0	0.0	0.0	0.0	0.0
28-30	0.7	0.0	0.0	0.7	0.7	0.0
Over 30	0.7	0.7	0.0	0.7	0.0	0.0
N/A	23.1	23.8	75.7	26.5	24.5	34.1

[a] N/A (not applicable), includes missing data.
[b] Present age minus age at first use.

Table 4

Descriptive Statistics for MCMI Drug Misuse Scale

	Mean	Range	Min.	Max.	SD	*N*
First MCMI	83.0863	80	35	115	15.8802	139

Table 5

MCMI Results for Repeated Measures Analysis of Variance

	Intake mean	1-month mean	3-month mean	*F* ratio	*F* prob.
I, 1, and 3 group	80.72222	76.38889	77.25000	.49	.6124

in Table 4. The results from a repeated measures analysis of variance, for the baserate scores from the group who completed an MCMI at intake, 1 month, and 3 months, are shown in Table 5.

In conclusion, the scoring characteristics of known drug abusers on the Drug Abuse Scale in this study are comprable to those found in Millon's standardization group. The average baserate scores of both drug-abusing groups far exceed those reported for normals in the standardization group. Further, the consistency of group scores from intake to 1 and 3 months after intake into treatment suggests that the Drug Abuse Scale for this group measures fairly enduring characteristics not significantly influenced by standard treatment efforts, at least in the short term.

ACKNOWLEDGMENTS

Data for the present study were collected during a substudy which was part of a national project sponsored by the National Institute on Drug Abuse. We wish to thank both the TOPS project officer, Harold M. Ginzburg, MD, who is Chief of NIDA's Clinical/Behavioral Branch; and Dr. Robert L. Hubbard, Associate Project Director for the TOPS program at RTI, for their cooperation and for making the substudy possible. The article and its conclusions are the sole responsibility of the authors and may not reflect the views of anyone at NIDA or RTI.

REFERENCES

CAVIOR, N., KURTZBERG, R., and LIPTON, D. The development and validation of a heroin addiction scale with the MMPI. *Int. J. Addict.* 2(1): 129-137, 1967.

LACHAR, D., BERMAN, W., GRISELL, J., and SHOOFF, K. A heroin addiction scale for the MMPI: Effectiveness in differential diagnosis in a psychiatric setting. *Int. J. Addict.* 14(1): 135-142, 1979.

MILLON, T. *Millon Multiaxial Clinical Inventory Manual.* Minneapolis: National Computer Systems, 1977.

MILLON, T. *Millon Clinical Multiaxial Inventory Manual* (2nd ed.). Minneapolis: National Computer Systems, 1982.

RESEARCH TRIANGLE INSTITUTE. *Treatment Outcome Prospective Study (TOPS): Overview.* Research Triangle Park, NC: Author, 1980.

SHEPPARD, C., RICCA, E., FRACCHIA, J., ROSENBERG, N., and MERLIS, S. Cross-validation of a heroin addiction scale from the Minnesota Multiphasic Personality Inventory. *J. Psychol.* 81: 263-268, 1972.

The International Journal of the Addictions, 19(4), 469–473, 1984

Note

Drug Use Intervention and Individual/Group Adaptation: Facilitation of Coping in Potential Worlds of Adaptation

Stanley Einstein,* PhD

Middle Eastern Summer Institute on Drug Use

Abstract

A schema is presented designed to help intervention agents and agencies plan and carry out programs which focus on helping individuals, groups, and systems to better "cope"/"adapt" in a variety of selected worlds of adaptation.

The continued confusion over what type(s) of goal(s) to select for drug use intervention—abstinence and/or other types of goals—has led to a misfocusing of our attention and efforts. A productive way of looking at intervention is in terms of *adaptation* or *coping*. From this perspective one assumes that healthy adaptation or coping for the individual, or the group, occurs in various actual or potential worlds which everyone must somehow come to terms with. Table 1 schematizes a selected number of such types of adaptational worlds. Each culture, and each period of historical time, has defined each of these "worlds" and has selected criteria which are used to define successful or unsuccessful adaptation. In the past as well as now, a person (or a group) who visibly did not adapt well within and to these "worlds" was an outcast, a deviant. What was visible was behavior or a life-style. What was reacted to was an evaluation or interpretation of the *meaning* and or *implications* of such behavior or life-style.

*Address correspondence to the author at 113/41 East Talpiot, Jerusalem, Israel.

 0020-773X/84/1904-0469$3.50/0

Table 1

A Schematic Framework for Developing Drug Use/Misuse Intervention Programs

	Needed area of intervention	Process	Focus of intervention behavior				A checklist for planning
Potential worlds of adaptation	Knowledge Planning Decision making Carry out integration	Explore Organize Analysis Obtain feedback	Prevention	Cessation	Maintenance	Development Promotion	Selected world of adaptation:
Biochemical							Planning factors
Psychological							Screening:
Perceptions/sensory stimuli							Goals:
Imagination/images							Budget:
Knowledge/language/ concepts							Policies:
Social							Techniques:
Environmental (internal/external)							Instruments:
Objects (drugs/nondrugs)							Staff:
Temporal (chronological/ nonchronological)							Roles:
							Sites:
							Temporal factors:

Systems/networks							Ongoing evaluation:
Institutions							Outcome:
Values							Utilization:
Cultural							Changes/cessation:
Rituals (secular, religious)							Quality factors:
Ethics							
Events							
Experiences							
Vocational/economic							
Leisure							
Community (organized/ unorganized)							
Explainable/unexplainable							
Unknown (knowable/ unknowable)							
Other: specify							
______ ______							

Effective intervention assumes activities in at least five areas: adequate knowledge, comprehensive planning, relevant decision making, appropriate carrying out, and integration of the results. Each of these areas is a dynamic process and not a static event. Prior to, or as a result of, being involved in each of these intervention areas, and their associated processes, one should define the program goals. If we don't, whatever the outcome, it will be the result of a "happening" and not because of planned intervention.

Table 1 defines the focus of potential intervention goals in terms of four broad generic categories: *prevention, cessation, maintenance,* and *development-promotion.*

The same goals have been selected for both behavior and life-style. The reader can change the goal categories for either behavior or life-style, or both. What is important, for drug use intervention planning, is to know where we are coming from, where we are going, and how we are going to get there. Many current efforts are designed as a travel guide's nightmare.

This table simply provides a framework for planning and for organizing what we are doing and the resulting outcome for evaluation. If, for example, an individual's biochemical world—his *soma*—is our initial "world" of concern for intervention, what do the areas of intervention demand of us? What knowledge do we have; do we need; is available or unavailable? What achievable plans are possible? What desirable plans are impossible or upon reevaluation are even irrelevant? What decisions need to be made; can be made? Who makes these decisions? Who or what is likely to help with these decisions; interfere with them; or even totally block them? Under what circumstances can the needed knowledge be collected; organized meaningfully; understood and then acted upon? Once the intervention has been carried out, what can we learn from it and how do we learn from it? Which usable processes are available to us? What new processes need to be developed? Which processes, having been used, should be discarded? Answers to all of these questions must be related to the *focus of intervention:* behavior and/or *life-style.*

In order to achieve a state of healthy biochemical (physical) adaptation for the individual and by the individual who is taking drugs or abstaining from them, what must be:

1. Prevented?
2. Stopped?
3. Maintained?
4. Developed or promoted?

Theoretically we should be focusing upon all four possible goals at once, both for behavior and for life-style. Reality will most likely demand that we set priorities so that each goal will be more relevant for a particular stage of intervention. Obviously a set of behaviors result in a type of life-style. And a life-style can't exist unrelated to various behaviors. But for intervention planning we can choose to focus our attentions and energies on only one of them and not on both of them.

Once the goals are selected, and well defined, we will need to determine the appropriate technique(s) to be used, who will use them, where they can be used most efficiently and effectively, and when intervention is to cease. Such planning will need to be done and carried out in a variety of "worlds" if the desired outcome is to be healthy adaptation-coping for the individual. It may sound complicated. Perhaps it is until we feel, and are, comfortable with a model of drug use intervention which doesn't pay too much attention to drugs or to drug use.

This model is based upon a simplistic assumption. Every living human being somehow or other adapts or maladapts differentially to the various worlds that s/he was born with or into, or which s/he becomes part of. If we are concerned about drug use as well as the behavior and/or life-style of the drug user, we will have to stop seeing the world from an either/or perspective: drug affected/non-drug affected; drug use related/non-drug use related; populated by drug users or abstainers.

Intervention which is based upon adaptation or coping raises questions regarding *quality, meaning, purpose, structure, survival,* and *existence* in a complex system of relating and interrelated worlds which all of us are a part of and play a role in.

And since all of us have to adapt in the best way we can, to all of these worlds, an adaptation model may be more suitable or preferable for us. In a sense this model permits us to focus upon ourselves and our needs. Drug use can be affected, and visible drug users will benefit tangentially because they exist in our world(s)—as we exist in theirs.

The International Journal of the Addictions, 19(4), 475–477, 1984

Note

An Experiential Model for Drug Use Intervention

Stanley Einstein,* PhD

Middle Eastern Summer Institute on Drug Use

Abstract

A schema is presented designed to help intervention agents and agencies plan and carry out programs which focus upon a broad but selected range of human (individual and systemic) experiences.

The term *experiential* plays an important role in drug use. The effects of drug use are generally described in positive experiential terms. Former drug users (the well-known ex-addict) are hired to treat active drug users or for drug education programs because of their *experiences* in the drug user world as well as because of what they experienced there. The conventional world has concluded and maintains the position that drug use is a *maladaptive experience.* Drug users, as a defensive posture, are often heard to say "If you didn't try it [drugs], if you haven't experienced drugs, don't knock it."

Theoreticians in the field describe types of drug users as *sensation seekers,* and the world in which we live as an emotionally *numbing* one, *agitating* one, *anxiety-provoking* one, *depressing* one, etc. Drug use or self-medication, from this perspective, becomes an individual's way of creating an experience of balance.

Since experiencing oneself, others, and life itself is critical to adaptation and coping, there is utility in developing drug use intervention programs based upon experiential models.

Table 1 lists a selected number of experiences which are or can be part of the life-style of the individual or of groups/systems/networks. An assumption

*Address correspondence to the author at 113/41 East Talpiot, Jerusalem, Israel.

 0020-773X/84/1904-0475$3.50/0

Table 1

A Schematic Framework for Planning an Experiential Model for Drug Use Intervention

	Selected Intervention Factors										
Type of experience	Program initiator (why)	Type of program (what)	Program focus (who)	Techniques Equipment (how)	Intervention agent (who)	Site (where)	Appropriate time (when/ how long)	Needed cooperation (others)	Roles	Policies Decisions Rules	Criteria (success/ failure)
Physical											
Sensory											
Emotional											
Interpersonal											
Social[a]											
Political											
Intellectual											
Creative/aesthetic											
Philosophical											
Spiritual/mystical											
Other: specify ______											

[a]Including sociocultural and environmental.

is made that satisfying experiences within any of these areas, or combinations of them, should prevent drug use, minimize it, or even "cause" drug use to be stopped. If I am feeling good from non-drug-related activities, which have personal meaning to me, there should be less need to seek out drugs and drug users or to be involved with and/or identify with drug use.

This table is designed to remind the reader that a selected number of intervention factors must be considered in order to help an individual (or group) achieve a satisfying non-drug-based experience within a broad range of potentially adaptive experiences.

The types of experiences which we make possible as individuals, families, peer groups, neighborhoods, communities, etc., may be the best medicine for preventing a variety of unacceptable drug-use-related experiences, behavior, and life-styles.

An experiential drug use intervention model assumes that:

1. The decision(s) to initiate a program is (are) suitable for an experiential model generally, and specifically suited to the selected type of experience.
2. The type of program (event) which we develop or plan to create is suitable to achieving a specific type of experience.
3. The program foci—the participants—are capable of experiencing what the program is designed to achieve, are in need of such experiences, and can utilize them as part of their individual and/or group life-styles.
4. The selected techniques are safe and are suitable for a selected type of experience, with a particular individual (and/or group) who is living in a certain way; and there are qualified, responsible intervention agents as well as suitable sites for intervention.
5. The temporal aspects of needed experiential intervention (short term, long term, unlimited time) have been adequately considered in terms of the program's structure as well as the actual and potential participants.
6. The agencies, formal and informal ones, which are needed to develop and carry out such a program exist and relate to one another in a manner which is supportive of effective intervention.
7. The needed roles and policies for such a program have been defined, agreed upon, and carried out, and are sufficiently flexible to make needed changes.
8. Criteria have been selected by which to evaluate success and/or failure for the program totally, as well as for critical factors (components) in the program, for all those who are involved in it. This demands the development of an efficient feedback system.

When issues such as these are adequately planned for, carried out, and reevaluated, and changes are made, when needed, there is a great likelihood for success to be experienced by all people who are sufficiently concerned to be involved in such an effort.

THE AMERICAN JOURNAL OF DRUG AND ALCOHOL ABUSE

Volume 10, Number 1, 1984

CONTENTS

Nontherapeutic Opiate Addiction in Health Professionals: A New Form of Impairment 1
W. E. McAuliffe

Treatment Outcomes of Substance-Abusing Physicians 23
K. N. Vogtsberger

The Black Female Addict's Career Options: A Typology and Theory 39
B. L. Kail and I. F. Lukoff

Characteristics of Physician Addicts 53
H. Wallot and J. Lambert

Heroin Use in the Barrio: Solving the Problem of Relapse or Keeping the Tecato Gusano Asleep 63
J. S. Jorquez

The Psychiatrically Severe Drug Abuse Patient: Methadone Maintenance or Therapeutic Community 77
A. T. McLellan, A. R. Childress, J. Griffith, and G. E. Woody

Client Types in Drug-Free and Methadone Treatment: Comparison of Personality Traits 97
P. A. Mider

Motivation for Drinkers and Treatment Outcome: A Study of Personal and Nonpersonal Effects Drinkers 113
D. Brissett, R. Asher, and J. Spicer

A Pragmatic Alcoholism Treatment Outcome Scale 125
M. A. Schuckit, C. R. Morrison, and E. O. Gold

Books Received 133

MARCEL DEKKER, INC.

270 MADISON AVENUE, NEW YORK, N.Y. 10016

(212) 696-9000

INFORMATION FOR AUTHORS SUBMITTING MANUSCRIPTS

Send a clear double-spaced typewritten original and one duplicate to Ms. Nancy Reid-Rappolt, Editorial Assistant, *International Journal of the Addictions,* c/o Winch, Smith, Ostermann and Mates, MD's, 4141 Geary, Suite 326, San Francisco, California 94118. Also send one duplicate to the Chief Editor, Dr. Stanley Einstein, Building 113/41, East Talpiot, Jerusalem, Israel. DOUBLE-SPACE the entire manuscript; do not use single spacing anywhere, including references.

Include authors' academic degrees and present affiliation. If applicable, cite auspices under which work being reported was done. Specify address to which requests for reprints should be sent.

Begin your TITLE with a word useful in indexing. A 75- to 100-word ABSTRACT should be provided, which precedes each article. A summary is then not necessary. Major and minor headings may be used in the text; indicate major headings by typing in capitals.

Use METRIC UNITS of measure. If measurements were made in English units, give metric equivalents.

Cite all TABLES and FIGURES in the text. Tables should have titles, and figures should have brief legends. In tables, give each column a heading. Indicate units of measure in parentheses in the heading for each column. Do not use vertical rules. Do not use horizontal rules other than those in the heading and at the bottom. Submit PHOTOGRAPHS as glossy prints, untrimmed and unmounted; identify each with pencil lightly on the back and indicate top.

ARTWORK will not be returned unless specifically requested, and will be disposed of three months after publication.

REFERENCES in the text should be enclosed in parentheses and include the author's surname and the date of the item cited. Keep footnotes to a minimum. Footnotes should be collected at the end of the manuscript in their numerical order of appearance.

The BIBLIOGRAPHY (double-spaced) should be given at the end of the article in alphabetical order. Journal references should include authors, title, name of journal abbreviated according to *Chemical Abstracts List of Periodicals*, inclusive page numbers, and date. Book references should include authors, title, place of publication, publisher, and date.

AUTHOR RESPONSIBILITY: It is the sole responsibility of the author(s) to obtain written permission from the author(s), publisher(s), etc. for figures, tables, or any other information excerpted from previously published works which are used in the manuscript(s) considered for publication. It is understood that the manuscript(s) considered for publication in the *International Journal of the Addictions* have not been previously published nor are they under simultaneous publication consideration elsewhere.

Statements and opinions expressed in the articles and communications herein are those of the author(s) and do not necessarily express those of the Editor or publisher.

THE INTERNATIONAL JOURNAL OF THE ADDICTIONS

Volume 19 Number 4 1984

CONTENTS

Editorial: Preventing Change through Current Substance Use Intervention: A Role Analysis: S. Einstein iii

Alcohol and Marijuana Use in Adolescents' Daily Lives: A Random Sample of Experiences: R. Larson, M. Csikszentmihalyi, and M. Freeman 367

Paraprofessional Versus Professional Drug Counselors: The Progress of Clients in Treatment: L. S. Aiken, L. A. LoSciuto, M. A. Ausetts, and B. S. Brown 383

An Analysis of Alcohol Portrayal on Prime-Time Television: E. J. Futch, S. A. Lisman, and M. I. Geller 403

Alcohol and Drug Use in the Elderly Visited at Home: M. T. Malcolm 411

Evaluation of a Substance Abuse Prevention Program for Junior High School Students: J. M. Moskowitz, E. Schaps, G. A. Schaeffer, and J. H. Malvin 419

Human Smoking Patterns and Smoke Deliveries: P. M. Moody 431

An Ecological Analysis of the Interrelationships among Drug Abuse and Other Indices of Social Pathology: D. N. Nurco, J. W. Shaffer, and I. H. Cisin 441

Research Note

Glue Sniffing: A Pilot Study of the Cognitive Effects of Long-Term Use: W. M. Allison and D. W. A. Jerrom 453

Notes

An Examination of the Drug Abuse Scale of the Millon Clinical Multiaxial Inventory: P. M. Flynn and R. C. McMahon 459

Drug Use Intervention and Individual/Group Adaptation: Facilitation of Coping in Potential Worlds of Adaptation: S. Einstein 469

An Experiential Model for Drug Use Intervention: S. Einstein 475

MARCEL DEKKER, INC., New York and Basel

CODEN: INJABN 19(5) i-ii, 479-600 (1984)
ISSN: 0020-773X

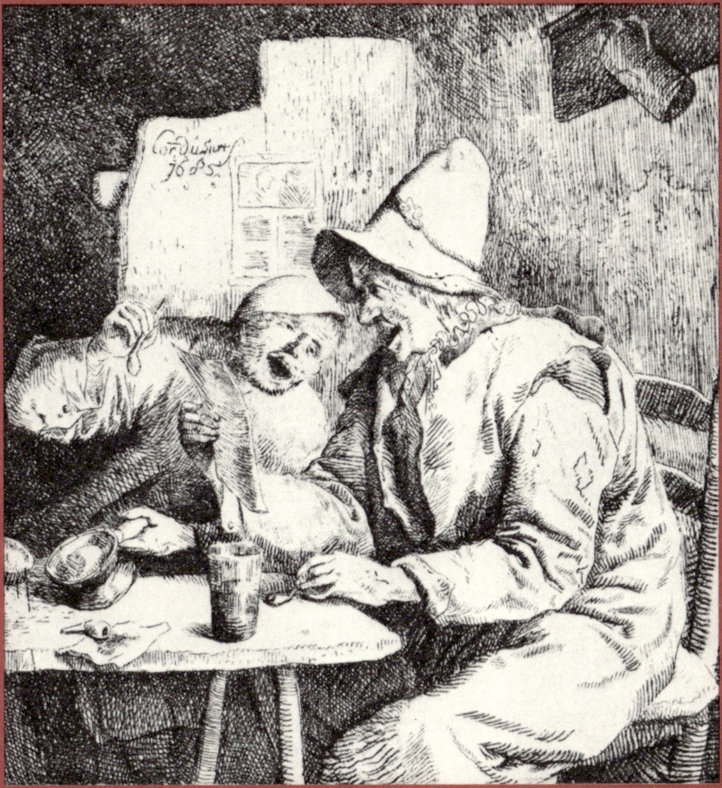

THE INTERNATIONAL JOURNAL OF THE Addictions

Volume 19 Number 5 1984

**THE INTERNATIONAL JOURNAL
OF THE ADDICTIONS**

August 1984

Aims and Scope. This journal is a comprehensive medium for worldwide communication among both concerned laymen and professionals in research, training, and treatment in the field of addiction and substance misuse.

Indexing and Abstracting Services. Articles published in *The International Journal of the Addictions* are selectively indexed or abstracted in:

• Adolescent Mental Health Abstracts • ASCA • Bibliographic Index of Health Education Periodicals (BIHEP) • BioSciences Information Service of Biological Abstracts (BIOSIS) • Classified Abstract Archive of the Alcohol Literature • Current Contents/Clinical Practice • Excerpta Medica • Index Medicus • International Pharmaceutical Abstracts • ISI/BIOMED • Journal of Abstracts of the All-Union Institute of Scientific and Technical Information of the USSR • Psychological Abstracts • Science Citation Index • Selected List of Tables of Contents of Psychiatric Periodicals • Social Sciences Citation Index • State Central Scientific Medical Library/International Book Exchange–USSR

Articles published in *The International Journal of the Addictions* are listed in Selected List of Tables of Contents of Psychiatric Periodicals.

Manuscript Preparation and Submission. See end of issue.

Subscription Information. *The International Journal of the Addictions* (ISSN: 0020-773X) is published eight times annually in February, April, May, July, August, September, November, and December by Marcel Dekker, Inc., 270 Madison Avenue, New York, New York 10016. The subscription rate for Volume 19 (1984), containing eight numbers, is $225.00 per volume (prepaid). The special discounted rate for individual professionals and students is $112.50 per volume. To secure this special rate, your order must be prepaid by personal check. Add $20.00 for surface postage outside the United States. For airmail to Europe, add $32.48; to Asia, add $40.48.

Mailing Address. *Please mail payment with order to:* Marcel Dekker Journals, P. O. Box 11305, Church Street Station, New York, New York 10249.

Contributions to this journal are published free of charge. Second-class postage paid at New York, New York and additional mailing offices. POSTMASTER: Send address changes to *The International Journal of the Addictions*, P. O. Box 5005, Cimarron Road, Monticello, New York 12701.

Library of Congress Catalog Card Number 66-9896

Cover illustration entitled: *The Singing Smokers*, courtesy of the Picture Collection, The Branch Libraries, New York Public Library.

THE INTERNATIONAL JOURNAL OF THE Addictions

The International Journal of the Addictions, 19(5), 479-502, 1984

Outcome Evaluations in Substance Abuse: A Comparison of Alcoholism, Drug Abuse, and Other Mental Health Interventions

Michael S. Goldstein, PhD

Monica Surber, MA

Daniel M. Wilner, PhD

School of Public Health
University of California, Los Angeles
Los Angeles, California 90024

Abstract

Outcome evaluation studies in the areas of alcohol and drug abuse have suffered from design problems. The lack of control groups, prospective designs, adequate outcome measures, and sufficient follow-up has presented the major difficulties. This study reviews all such studies reported in 50 major journals between 1969 and 1979 and compares them to outcome evaluations on other mental health topics reported in the same journals. We find that significant problems remain in each of these areas. In general, drug abuse studies employ the least adequate methodologies. Alcohol evaluations are approximately as rigorous as other mental health evaluations. A major finding is the lack of rigor found in all types of outcome evaluations. Attention must be paid to these issues if outcome evaluations are to remain credible and able to secure continued support.

 0020-773X/84/1905-0479$3.50/0

The assessment of therapeutic outcomes in a broad mental health field represents a challenge to social science theory, methodology, and technique. The most serious problems reside in the issues of *measurement*—both the criteria employed to determine outcome and the data-gathering procedures actually employed. Problems of a different sort, but no less complex, reside in the issues surrounding *study design* framework embodying the logic that permits drawing of conclusions regarding the outcome process.

The crtical issue is, of course, success of outcome; that is, the extent to which therapeutic endeavors result in gain for the patient or client such that there is improvement of underlying disorder, relief of symptoms, and/or restoration of normally adaptive behavior and other mechanisms permitting coping with the psychological rigors of life.

As alcoholism and drug abuse have come to be seen as major public health problems with significant impact on individuals, families, and the fabric of social life, attempts at treatment have proliferated. Currently there are more than 9,000 drug abuse and alcoholism treatment programs of some stability in the United States, with additional individual substance abuse treatment available in nonspecialty community hospitals and from private practitioners (Wilner, Walkley, and O'Neill, 1978).

Systematic substance abuse interventions are notably hard to undertake and accomplish. Alcohol abusers tend to have chronic histories, are notorious repeaters, and are "unpopular" patients with psychiatrists and psychologists. Drug abusers—particularly with heroin involvement—also often suffer from chronic conditions for which no adequate treatment exists and for which they face serious legal vulnerability. As treatments and programs have grown, so have attempts to evaluate them. Such evaluation efforts are not unique to the substance abuse field. They are a response to efforts aimed at rationalizing the delivery of health and human services as well as the legislative mandates concerned with reducing the costs of such services. Attempts to review this proliferating literature on the evaluation of substance abuse programs have focused on four major methodological issues which have limited the value and generalizability of the research.

METHODOLOGICAL ISSUES

The Use of Randomized or Matching Control Groups

The use of inadequate research designs in evaluations of drug and alcohol abuse treatment programs is a major concern to methodologists. A review of 49 alcohol treatment studies done between 1951 and 1963 found that only three randomly assigned subjects to treatment and control groups (Hill and Blane, 1967). A similar review of 40 studies done between 1968 and 1971 found eight with random assignment (Crawford, Chalupsky, and Hurley, 1973). A more inclusive review of 384 studies done between 1951 and 1973 found only 72 that had used randomized or matched control and treatment groups (Emrick, 1975). Similar findings have been reported in the drug abuse field (Callner, 1975; Smart, 1976). While reviews of the literature often imply that the situation is improving through the citation of outstanding studies and prototype research designs (Maisto and Cooper, 1980; L.C. Sobell, Sobell, and Ward, 1980), the representativeness and influence of these changes are unknown.

The ethical acceptability of random designs has been a significant barrier to their adaption in some settings. Many people feel that random assignment may result in the denial of the most appropriate treatment, or sometimes any treatment at all, to those who might benefit from it. While there are methodologic strategies for dealing with such resistance (the control group can receive the standard treatment or the control, and experimental groups may be switched at some point), it may be that the immediate needs of individual patients as perceived by themselves and clinicians, and the needs of researchers to execute well-designed studies will continue to inhibit the use of randomized control groups.

The Lack of Prospective Research Designs

One reason that so few studies have been able to use proper controls is that studies are often retrospective. Not only does this preclude taking an experimental or quasi-experimental approach, but it also severely limits the researcher's ability to gather valid baseline data on the client's behavioral and personal traits. Research reports often are unable to offer even demographic information on the preattrition client population (Maisto and Cooper, 1980). This is especially important in the substance abuse field, where program attrition is often high and selective. As the impact of different treatments varies for types of clients (Armor, Polich, and Stambul, 1976) the utility of such research for program planning is quite limited. The frequent absence of baseline data has made difficult the application of sophisticated statistical techniques to data already collected (Cronkite and Moos, 1978). Calls to include adequate baseline measures in substance abuse treatment research have been and continue to be regularly voiced by reviewers (Institute of Medicine, 1980).

The Lack of Adequate Outcome Measures

The adequacy, both conceptual and methodological, of outcome measures in the field has repeatedly been questioned. Many studies use single measures of substance abuse, often global categories like "continuing," "improved," and "abstinent," or "addicted" and "drug free." Not only are such outcome measures insensitive to subtle changes, but their essential meaning is difficult to interpret (Boudin, Valentine, Ingrahm et al., 1977; Cohen, Howard, Klein, and Newfield, 1976).

In addition, the technique for collecting the information is often some form of self-report. Self-reports are obviously open to question given the stigmatized and/or illegal nature of the behavior in question as well as the client's desire to "please" the agency and the agency's desire to "please" the evaluator (Amsel, Mandell, Matthias et al., 1976; Ball, 1967; Bonito, Nurco, and Schaffer, 1976). Other techniques for assessing outcomes, such as examining police or clinic records and physiological measures (usually analysis of urine samples), have also proven to be not highly reliable (Amsel et al., 1976; Gottheil, Caddy, and Austin, 1975/1980; Lewis, Pollack, Petersen, and Geiss, 1973; L.C. Sobell, 1978).

Studies that base their conclusions on single outcome measures are highly problematic. For example, use of abstinence as the only criterion of outcome extracts a single (albeit important) behavior from the totality of an individual's life and uses it as the sole index of program impact. Should someone who, through the impact of a program, has regained employment, resumed a marriage, and reported increased self-esteem while maintaining a low level of substance use be rated as "improved" as someone who uses a similar amount of alcohol and/or drugs not accompanied by psychosocial improvement? Clearly more wide-ranging measures of outcome are needed. Use of broad standardized intake forms which are designed to assess the full range of an individual's strengths and weaknesses may offer a baseline from which adequate follow-up data could be generalized.

While eliminating substance use may be the primary and long-term goal of an intervention, other measures may be important short-term indicators of success. Emotional, vocational, physical, interpersonal, and social outcomes are all relevant but often neglected (Pomerleau and Adkins, 1980; L.C. Sobell and Sobell, 1980; M.B. Sobell and Sobell, 1973a, 1973b, 1976, 1978). Recently Maisto and McCollam (1980) reviewed 103 studies which were published between 1960 and 1977 and reported alcoholism treatment outcome data for at least 10 patients on at least two outcome variables. They found that while about 90% reported data on drinking behavior, other important outcomes were employed much less frequently (vocational functioning, 77.7%; social functioning, 61.2%; emotional functioning, 40.8%; physical functioning, 38.8%; use of services, 35.0%; residential status, 17.5%; etc.). At times researchers and administrators may be so pessimistic about the possibility of drug abusers' symptoms, behaviors, or life-styles changing that they omit or disregard such indicators.

The Lack of Adequate Follow-Up Data

The psychological and social character of the population studies, the motivation of clinicians, and the lack of adequate research planning and funding have all contributed to what is generally considered to be poor record in collecting accurate follow-up reports. Most alcoholism treatment programs report follow-up rates below 75% (Hill and Blane, 1967) while reviews of the drug abuse literature have found that follow-up losses vary from 10% to 90% (Callner, 1975; Cohen et al., 1976; Smart, 1976). Of course, individuals who drop out or are difficult to locate may well be less "successful" than others (Baekeland, Lundwall, and Kissin, 1975; Gearing, 1970; Miller, Pokorny, Valles, and Cleveland, 1970; Moos and Bliss, 1978). While there have been recent attempts to devise special techniques for following up substance abusers (Goldstein, Abbott et al., 1977; L.C. Sobell and Sobell, 1980), as yet they are used infrequently.

The Present Study

The present study is an attempt to examine the foregoing issues in two ways. First we review the extent to which the concerns described here are accurate descriptions of outcome studies which have been reported in 50 major journals during the period from 1969 to 1979. (See Appendix A for a journal list.) This is a set of well-known and generally respected journals in the broad mental health/human services field. We assume that research reported in these journals has relevance since they (1) have higher standards for publication and (2) are more widely read and cited. Since these same journals also reported outcomes of other types of mental health and human service interventions, we are able to compare our findings from alcohol and drug abuse studies with findings from a large universe of mental health studies in this same period. Thus we are able to assess the extent to which strengths and weaknesses of research in the field of substance abuse treatment are typical of the broader field of evaluation research. Finally, we are able to use these data to see if the research design strengths and weaknesses are typical of all substance abuse studies or whether they are associated with certain types of interventions or sites of treatment.

Our data are based on a set of exhaustive and systematic abstracts prepared for the Databank of Program Evaluations* and on the underlying articles on which the abstracts are based. Studies were included in the Databank if they dealt with at least 10 patients. The studies were in the main not studies in which there was primary interest in the efficacy of pharmaceuticals in treating illness. Studies of effects of pharmaceuticals were included if accompanied or compared

*Grant No. MH 26477, National Institute of Mental Health.

Table 1

Primary Conditions of Research Articles in the Databank of Program Evaluations (N = 2,231)

Aging	101
Alcohol abuse	182
Criminal justice	49
Marital dysfunction	35
Drug abuse	234
Medical problems	54
Juvenile delinquency	62
Mental retardation	37
Adult behavior problems[a]	196
Psychoses	248
Schizophrenia (only)	137
Personality disorder	23
Sexual variance	34
Sociocultural problems[b]	86
Suicide	28
Unemployment	16
Welfare	19
Child behavior problems	141
Smoking	658
Rape	3
Population problems[c]	113
Life crisis[d]	49
Weight problems	66
Child abuse	5
General/unspecified	189
Total	2,231

[a]Neurosis, anxiety disorders, etc., among adults which do not impede basic functioning.
[b]Personal deficits arising from social and cultural deprivation.
[c]Contraception and abortion counseling.
[d]Problems arising from divorce, job loss, etc., among normal adults.

with some other form of treatment, or were employed as the treatment in alcohol and drug abuse studies.

Of the 2,231 studies in the Databank (Table 1), 182 (18.2%) dealt with alcoholism and 234 (10.5%) with drug abuse; the remaining 1,815 studies (81.4%) dealt with the broad array of conditions and topics normally handled in articles appearing in the journals in question. These included, for example, intervention/outcome studies of psychosis (N = 248), of schizophrenia aside from other psychoses (N = 137), of the aging process and senility (N =101), etc. It is helpful to note that the Databank included only intervention/outcome studies and attempted to apply uniform yardsticks to each, covering measurement and study designs already referred to, but also other information about treatment type, treatment site, patient demographics, etc. We are thus in a position to contrast outcome/intervention substance abuse studies with other studies covering other topics being conducted and reported in the same period. The reader should be reminded that most outcome studies in all areas of mental health focus on the patient or client. There is seldom adequate, if any, consideration of the quality of treatment (suitability and training of the therapist, suitability of the technique, overall quality of the program, etc.) or the potential impact of the program on the community in such areas as cost or the community's ability to reabsorb the patients in an appropriate manner. The research designs are seldom attentive to these issues.

FINDINGS

Research Designs

Study designs used in mental health evaluation and outcome research provide important information about the sophistication of the research effort. The basic questions are: Were controls used–is causal attribution possible? Have statistical tests been used to appraise observed differences? Were follow-ups possible in an effort to judge persistence of effect? These questions need to be asked despite full awareness that ideal or controllable conditions seldom prevail in the mental health field studies of the kind reviewed here.

As is shown in Table 2, the overall situation is not impressive. Slightly over three-quarters of the 2,231 outcome studies reported in these 50 prestigious journals did not use controls of any kind. Over a third used the weakest design, "after intervention only; no controls." While the results from the 182 alcoholism studies were about the same as studies in other mental health areas, almost one-

Table 2

Frequency of Six Study Design Characteristics

	Alcoholism		Drug abuse		Other mental health	
Study designs	*N* (182)	%	*N* (234)	%	*N* (1,815)	%
Controls						
Random assignment	28	1.54	15	6.4	332	18.3
Matching	16	8.8	14	6.0	195	10.7
Other controls	30	16.5	38	16.2	268	14.8
Before and after	60	33.0	57	24.4	758	41.8
After only, no controls	64	35.2	115	49.1	627	34.5
Statistical tests	83	45.6	62	26.5	751	41.5

half of the 234 drug abuse studies were of the weakest design. Alcohol studies employed controls about as frequently as studies in other areas and showed a marked superiority to drug abuser studies. Over 40% of the alcoholism studies used some sort of control group (including 15.4% random; 6.0% matched).

The use and reporting of statistical tests on the data, as opposed to merely reporting descriptive statistics, followed the same pattern. Tests were employed in alcoholism studies somewhat more frequently than in other mental health studies (45% vs 41.5%) but were less frequent (26.5%) in the drug abuse research. This design superiority for alcoholism studies may be related to the greater number of inpatient treatment programs in alcoholism studies (see later discussion). It is probably easier to identify and maintain "controls" and have statistical advice available in inpatient circumstances than in outpatient settings.

Baseline Data for Prospective Designs

The collection and reporting of baseline data on sociodemographic and other variables is a prerequisite for carrying out prospective research and for studying subgroups differentially affected by treatment and attrition, thus making possible better understanding of interactions and allowing for the generalization of results. Many studies reported in the Databank can be faulted for inadequate and imprecise reporting of basic demographic information (Table 3). Thus even crudely defined age ("adult vs youth") and sex data are unspecified in almost a quarter of the studies, and race and income levels are missing in over three-quarters of all studies reported. Drug and alcohol studies are about as good as others in specifying age. However, the data reveal few studies on youth (age 18 and younger) and none on the elderly, which is surprising given the extent of substance abuse problems among these groups and the concern of policy makers. Almost a third of the studies did not specify sex! Alcoholism studies are somewhat better (20.9% unspecified) in this regard. Looking only at the studies that specified sex, it is clear that alcohol studies are primarily concerned with males (49.5% males only), whereas drug abuse studies are somewhat more oriented toward women (20.5% males only) but not as much as studies in other mental health areas (14.0% males only).

The racial and income categories reported in the research are often unclear and inconsistent. Drug studies are considerably better than alcohol or other studies in making some attempts to provide data on race. Clearly there has been some concern with including Blacks (15.9% vs 2.2% of alcohol studies and 2.7% other studies). Income data are missing from the vast majority of all studies. When this information is offered it reveals that middle-class individuals are seldom the subjects of research.

Table 3

Sociodemographic Information Reported in 2,231 Studies

Sociodemographic variable	Alcoholism		Drug abuse		Other mental health	
	N	%	*N*.	%	*N*	%
Age						
Unspecified	35	19.2	53	22.6	330	18.2
Youth (0-18)	0	0.0	10	4.3	329	18.1
Adults	143	78.6	143	61.1	825	45.5
Youth and adults	4	2.2	28	12.0	232	12.8
Elderly	0	0.0	0	0.0	99	5.5
Sex						
Unspecified	38	20.9	66	28.2	589	32.5
Males only	90	49.5	48	20.5	258	14.0
1-25% female	40	22.0	72	30.8	71	3.9
26-75% female	11	6.0	40	17.1	533	29.5
76-99% female	0	0.0	0	0.0	96	5.3
Females only	1	0.5	4	1.7	235	12.9
Race						
Unspecified	128	70.3	109	46.6	1,396	76.9
100% White	7	3.8	2	0.9	22	1.2
⩾ 75% White	26	14.3	26	11.1	130	7.2
Black	4	2.2	36	15.9	72	4.0
Spanish-speaking	0	0.0	7	3.0	20	1.1
Native American	6	3.3	0	0.0	4	0.2
50/50 of any two groups	5	2.7	30	12.8	49	2.7
"Minorities"	1	0.5	19	8.1	21	1.2
Income						
Unspecified	120	65.9	182	77.8	1,407	77.5
Lower	24	13.2	31	13.2	228	12.6
Middle	11	6.0	6	2.6	56	3.1
Upper	0	0.0	1	0.4	2	0.1
Lower & middle	20	11.0	11	4.7	64	3.5
Middle & upper	2	1.1	2	0.9	23	1.3
Lower & upper	1	0.5	0	0.0	2	0.1
"Normal"	4	2.2	1	0.4	33	1.8

The Adequacy of Outcome Measures

The Databank classification scheme allowed for as many as four separate measures of outcome. If a single study employed more than four measures we chose those highlighted by the authors of the studies as well as being guided by the general importance of the criteria. We distinguished two broad categories of outcome, behavioral and psychological, fine tuning these criteria as much as possible. We also noted operational characteristics of measurement and how the data were actually collected. All told we identified 5,955 measures distributed among the 2,231 studies, for a rate of 2.7 measures per study—virtually identical for alcoholism, drug abuse, and other mental health studies.

Measures of alcohol and drug abuse ("addiction") appeared as the sole outcome indicator in well over half the substance abuse studies (Table 4); as might be expected, addiction was rarely used (about 7%) in the remaining studies. Various behavioral indicators (social, interpersonal, school, employment, etc.) were used in about half of the other mental health studies but in only about 30% of the substance abuse studies. As might be expected, measures of illegal behavior are found much more frequently in studies of drug abuse (20.1%) than in alcoholism or other studies (3.3% and 4.5%, respectively). Other types of measures are seldom employed in the substance abuse evaluations relative both to their use in other studies and to what we might expect given their theoretical relevance to substance abuse outcomes. Measures of psychological state are particularly notable in their absence. The single exception to this pattern is the measurement of consumer satisfaction as measured by patient opinions or by retention in the treatment program. It was used twice as often in

Table 4

Types of Outcome Measures Used[a]

	Alcoholism (182)		Drug abuse (234)		Other mental health (1,815)[b]	
Type of measure	*N*	%	*N*	%	*N*	%
Addiction only	114	62.5	127	54.3	132	7.3
Addiction and social behavior	56	30.8	71	30.3	954	52.5
Addiction and illegal behavior	6	3.3	47	20.1	84	4.6
Addiction and use of self-follow-up services	15	8.2	10	4.2	186	10.2
Addiction and psychological state	12	6.6	7	3.0	366	20.2
Addiction and attitudes or values	7	3.8	2	0.1	130	7.2
Addiction and consumer satisfaction	27	14.8	66	28.2	388	21.4
Addiction and "other"	15	8.2	20	8.5	784	43.2

[a]Table totals more than *N* of studies since multiple codes are possible. A study might report addiction, criminal behavior, values, etc.
[b]Figures in this column refer to the use of this type of measure in the study regardless of whether addiction was also measured.

Table 5

Nature of Measurement Instruments Employed (operationalized or not)[a]

	Alcoholism (495)		Drug abuse (653)		Other mental health (4,807)	
	N	%	*N*	%	*N*	%
Operationalized, named measures	72	14.5	48	7.4	716	14.9
Operationalized, unnamed measures	317	64.0	519	79.5	2,832	58.9
Unoperationalized measures	98	19.8	78	11.9	1,183	24.6
Unclassifiable	8	1.6	8	1.2	76	1.6

[a]*N* = total number of measures employed.

drug abuse studies as in alcoholism studies and significantly more often than in other studies.

The next consideration deals with the nature of the measuring instruments used to identify intervention outcomes. Table 5 presents findings (based on 5,955 measures) about the frequency with which substance abuse and other evaluations used outcome measures which were either named instruments, unnamed but operationalized instruments, or unoperationalized kinds of measures. In the current discussion a measure is considered to be operationalized if sufficient information was provided to allow for replication.

Overall more than one-third of the 2,231 (not tabled) studies used operationalized measures—not sufficiently specified to permit replication—with drug abuse studies least in this category, no doubt because of heavy reliance in this group of studies on physiologic measures of drugs in the body. With 5,955 measures (rather than studies) as the base (Table 5) we see that about 15% of all measures used consisted of named instruments, with half that proportion in drug abuse measures. Operationalized but unnamed instruments were used in about 60% of measures employed (79.5% of the measures in drug abuse studies).

The literature reveals a continuing strong interest in procedures for collecting and gathering outcome measures and other data referred to in mental health evaluations. Looked at from the viewpoint of all the studies (data not tabled), more than 40% depended on official records (discharge from or readmission to treatment programs, school, delinquency, or substance abuse records) for one or more measures of outcome. One-third of the studies relied on self-reports, and one-quarter were based upon observations by others (parents, surrogates, social workers, etc.). Therapists' observations—that well-known bugaboo—were used in about 15% of the studies. Interviews, tests, and questionnaires were each used in

Table 6

Data Collection Procedure Employed[a]

	Alcoholism (570)		Drug abuse (699)		Other mental health (5,532)	
	N	%	*N*	%	*N*	%
Therapist observation	30	5.3	15	2.1	591	10.7
Other's observation	98	17.2	41	5.9	913	16.5
Self-report	118	20.7	134	19.2	1,103	19.9
Records	106	18.6	357	51.1	1,290	23.3
Interviews	82	14.4	76	10.9	494	8.9
Named tests	70	12.3	47	6.7	687	12.4
Questionnaire	56	9.8	28	4.0	420	7.6
Other	10	1.8	1	0.1	54	1.0

[a]Percent calculated on data collection methods specific enough to be classified.

10% to 20% of the various study categories. Evidence for the suitability of the particular instruments in terms of the subject's age, sex, SES, cultural background, intelligence, etc., was only occasionally specified.

There were 6,801 specified data collection points (Table 6) for the 5,955 measures cited earlier. Alcoholism studies tended to be similar to other studies but varied considerably from drug abuse studies. The latter employed records much more frequently (51.1% vs about 20%), while the observations of others, tests, and questionnaires were used much less often. About 20% of the measures in each category used self-reports.

Although all data collection techniques have their shortcomings, the use of agency records as a research tool is particularly noteworthy for its limitations. Thus we find again that while alcoholism evaluations approximate the norm for all mental health studies, drug abuse evaluations tend to be based on a methodology known for omission and variability in reporting.

The Use of Follow-Up Data

Table 7 reports how long after the completion of treatment follow-up measures were taken, though unfortunately we do not have the data on attrition rates of the studies in question. As shown in Table 7, almost half of the non-substance-abuse interventions reported in the Databank were without follow-up. While studies of alcoholism are significantly more involved in follow-up (about two-thirds), only one-third of the drug abuse studies fall in this pattern. The percentage of studies using more than 24 months is about the same (12%) for all types of studies. Alcoholim studies specify briefer follow-up periods about as frequently as other mental health studies but much often than drug abuse

Table 7

Time of Last Follow-Up Measure

	Alcoholism (182)		Drug abuse (234)		Other mental health (1,815)	
Time	*N*	%	*N*	%	*N*	%
No follow-up	64	35.2	156	66.7	881	48.5
1 month or less	16	8.8	13	5.6	238	13.1
2-6 months	27	14.8	14	5.9	228	12.6
7-12 months	36	19.8	11	4.7	139	7.7
12-24 months	16	8.3	9	3.8	119	6.6
> 24 months	23	12.6	31	13.2	210	11.6

studies. Again, these figures may reflect the fact that alcoholism research is more likely to take place in inpatient settings where a short-term follow-up is relatively easy to achieve.

However, if we examine only those studies which employed some follow-up, our findings are very different. Thirty-one of the 78 (39.7%) drug abuse studies had follow-ups of at least 24 months. This is about twice the percentage of alcoholism studies (23 of 118 studies = 19.5%) and significantly greater (210 of 934 studies = 22.2%) than other mental health outcome studies. The presence of a long-term follow-up did not seem to be related to the use of any particular treatment such as methadone maintenance.

Variability in Methodological Rigor

To this point we have used the Databank to portray in broad terms the characteristics of evaluation studies on alcoholism and drug abuse, as well as to compare them to studies in other areas. Yet it is possible that our overall findings mask significant variability among alcohol and drug abuse evaluation studies. We are especially concerned with the possibility that the site where the study is being conducted and the specific type of treatment being assessed may be associated with the type of study design employed. It is conceivable that studies carried out in inpatient settings, which allow for much greater control over subjects, are thus more likely to be methodologically rigorous. Similarly, it might be that certain types of treatments or interventions lend themselves to more rigorous evaluation designs.

The alcoholism and drug abuse studies we are reporting on took place in a wide variety of settings (Table 8). Hospitals and other inpatient settings accounted for over three-quarters of the primary sites among the alcoholism studies, while less than half of the drug abuse studies took place in such sites. Of course, many studies took place in more than one site. It was possible to code

Table 8

Primary Research Sites[a]

	Alcohol abuse (182)		Drug abuse (234)		Other conditions (2,185)	
	N	%	*N*	%	*N*	%
Hospitals and other inpatient	137	75.3	115	49.0	1,215	66.9
Clinics and other outpatient	48	26.4	139	59.4	1,342	73.9
Prison	3	1.6	4	1.7	64	3.5
Halfway house	11	6.0	14	6.0	24	1.3
Office	3	1.6	6	2.6	44	2.4
CMHC	7	3.8	7	3.0	81	4.5
Residential	7	3.8	22	9.4	87	4.8
Home	3	1.6	2	0.9	130	7.2
Partial	2	1.1	7	3.0	98	4.9
School for MR	–	–	–	–	17	0.9
School	–	–	3	1.3	121	6.7
Armed services	4	2.2	4	1.7	11	0.6
Hotline	–	–	1	0.4	29	1.6
Nursing home	–	–	–	–	23	1.3
Neighborhood	5	2.7	3	1.3	51	2.8
Occupational	1	0.5	–	–	12	0.7
Campus related	1	0.5	1	0.4	38	2.1
Unspecified	6	3.3	8	3.4	112	6.2

[a]Percent total above 100 due to multiple coding of responses.

four separate sites in the Databank. Table 9 divides the studies into those based upon only inpatient site(s), only outpatient site(s), and those with mixed sites.

The tendency among the alcoholism evaluations studies to be based in inpatient settings does appear to be related to a greater use of randomized control designs. While about 15% of alcohol and other mental health studies done in inpatient settings employed random controls, only a single inpatient drug abuse study did so. Beyond this difference, site seems to have no significant bearing on the type of design employed.

The studies reported an extremely diverse group of treatments which were being evaluated (Table 10). Over 60% of the drug abuse studies dealt with methadone programs. Somewhat under a quarter of the alcoholism programs were concerned with Alcoholics Anonymous. About a quarter of the studies reported on programs which offered detoxification only. However, such programs were always being compared to other sorts of treatments. In general, alcoholism programs were more psychotherapeutically oriented than drug abuse programs and tended to employ directive groups and learning theory based programs. With

Table 9

Research Site and Study Design Characteristics

	Alcoholism		Drug abuse		Other mental health	
	N	%	*N*	%	*N*	%
Inpatient only						
Random controls	16	15.8	1	1.8	97	15.4
Other controls	26	25.7	14	25.7	154	24.5
No controls	59	58.4	40	2.7	378	60.1
	101		55		629	
Outpatient only						
Random controls	3	11.5	8	9.6	124	18.9
Other controls	4	15.4	13	15.7	166	25.3
No controls	19	73.1	62	74.3	366	55.8
	26		83		656	
Mixed sites						
Random controls	9	16.4	6	6.3	111	20.6
Other controls	12	21.8	22	22.9	125	23.1
No controls	34	61.8	68	70.8	294	54.4
	55		96		530	

the possibility that treatment type might interact with study rigor, we grouped (Table 11) the reported treatments as either psychotherapy (individual, group, nondirective, directive, and Alcoholics Anonymous), medical (methadone or any other pharmacologic, shock, or somatic treatment), or "other." Overall, the differences in rigor or research design between alcoholism, drug abuse, and all other studies are not great. In most cases the non-substance-abuse studies report a somewhat larger percentage of studies using randomly selected control groups. Drug abuse studies are more likely to fall into the "no control group" category. Clearly these studies—which look at psychotherapy or "other" types of treatments, as opposed to medical or combinations of medical and other treatments—are most likely to be uncontrolled. Perhaps the most striking finding is the high percentage of studies, regardless of therapeutic modality or type of concern, that do not employ any sort of controls in their research design. This finding is particularly pronounced among drug abuse studies.

SUCCESS OF INTERVENTION

The Databank also collected information on how successful the various interventions were reported to be. Up to seven indicators of success or its lack were recorded for each study. It is very difficult to report on this information

Table 10

Treatments[a]

Treatment	Alcohol abuse (182)		Drug abuse (234)		Other conditions (1,815)	
	N	%	*N*	%	*N*	%
Analytic group	30	16.5	35	15.0	144	7.9
Directive group	59	32.4	45	19.2	372	20.5
Individual analysis	15	8.2	18	7.7	160	8.8
Individual directive	44	24.2	47	20.1	225	12.4
Brief psychotherapy	1	0.5	4	1.7	90	5.0
Learning theory based	56	30.8	16	6.8	510	28.1
Methadone	2	1.1	143	61.1	1	0.1
Alcoholic Anonymous	40	22.0	2	0.9	3	0.2
Community	12	6.6	35	15.0	107	5.9
Job training	15	8.2	17	7.3	111	6.1
Pharmacotherapy	30	16.5	22	9.4	216	11.9
Recreational	7	3.8	3	1.3	111	6.1
Shock treatment	2	1.1	–	–	64	3.5
Aftercare	12	6.6	9	3.8	64	3.5
Family therapy	13	7.1	9	3.8	100	5.5
Educational	25	13.7	6	2.6	153	8.4
Abstinence[b]	9	4.9	16	6.8	1	0.1
Videotape	10	5.5	1	0.4	31	1.7
Psychosurgery	–	–	–	–	9	0.5
Medical-surgical	12	6.6	8	3.4	131	7.2
Somatic therapy	2	1.1	–	–	31	1.7
Psychedelic	6	3.3	–	–	2	0.1
Contractual	7	3.8	2	0.9	27	1.5
Unspecified	23	12.6	12	5.1	180	9.9
Other	39	21.4	41	17.5	540	29.8
Comparison	66	36.3	57	24.4	697	38.4

[a]Percents sum to more than 100 due to multiple coding. Some types of substance abuse treatment categories are absent because they were not included in the overall DOPE coding scheme. For example "self-help groups" were not categorized separately although many of the programs included self-help elements. Likewise, elements of confrontation were used in directive groups, AA, videotape, etc.
[b]The use of moral suasion.

in a meaningful way because often authors will present data only on those variables which yield positive results. In addition, not all the variables reported may be equally important. For example, a drug abuse study may find that addiction and criminal behavior are unaffected by the intervention but that knowledge about drug side effects or program retention has improved significantly. Should this be considered evidence of success? Perhaps the program

Table 11

Treatment Modality and Study Design Characteristics

	Alcoholism (182)		Drug abuse (234)		Other mental health (1,815)	
	N	%	*N*	%	*N*	%
Psychotherapy only						
Random controls	5	11.6	0	0.0	105	20.3
Other controls	5	11.6	4	26.7	100	19.3
No controls	33	76.7	11	73.3	313	60.4
Medical only						
Random controls	3	60.0	5	8.6	10	8.0
Other controls	1	20.0	7	12.1	35	28.0
No controls	1	20.0	46	79.3	80	64.0
"Other" treatments only						
Random controls	2	8.7	1	5.6	50	13.5
Other controls	3	13.0	3	16.7	99	26.8
No controls	18	78.2	14	77.8	221	59.7
Psychotherapy & other nonmedical						
Random controls	10	17.2	1	5.6	50	13.5
Other controls	21	36.2	5	27.8	112	26.6
No controls	27	46.6	12	66.7	188	44.7
Medical & any other						
Random controls	1	3.6	6	6.3	26	10.4
Other controls	8	28.6	20	21.1	59	23.5
No controls	19	67.9	69	72.6	166	66.1
All three types together						
Random controls	7	28.0	2	6.7	20	15.4
Other controls	4	16.0	10	33.3	40	30.8
No controls	14	56.0	18	60.0	70	53.8

administrators feel that retention and knowledge are prerequisite to future abstinence and reductions in illegal activities. Thus we present only data on success for the total number of measures (as opposed to studies) reported. Table 12 pulls together evidence of several kinds. For studies with test and control groups (Table 12-A) at least two kinds of success were noted. The first is the case in which a test group was significantly (at the .05 statistical level) improved over a control group; the second is the case where there is a test-control difference in the expected direction which the authors regard as meaningful but which is either not statistically significant or has not been evaluated by statistical test. For studies without control groups (Table 12-B), reliance is on the differences detected before and after. Here there are three distinct cases. The first is where the difference is significant (at the .05 statistical level). The second is the case where the face difference is large, but not

Table 12

Treatment Success for Outcome Measures[a]

A. Outcome between Groups

	Alcoholism (211)		Drug abuse (211)		Other mental health (2,130)	
	N	%	*N*	%	*N*	%
Statistically significant (0.5)	88	41.7	59	28.0	904	42.4
Not statistically significant but author regards as a meaningful difference	44	20.6	56	26.5	516	24.2
No statistical or meaningful difference	79	37.4	96	45.5	710	33.3

B. Before-and-After Outcomes

	Alcoholism (234)		Drug abuse (322)		Other mental health (3,030)	
	N	%	*N*	%	*N*	%
Statistically significant (0.5)	60	24.7	51	15.8	736	24.3
Not statistically significant but author regards as a meaningful difference	122	50.2	207	64.3	1757	58.0
No statistical or meaningful difference	61	25.1	64	19.9	537	17.7

[a]*N*s refer to the total number of measures on which the authors report findings. These are fewer than the total number of measures used in the studies as some of the measures employed are not reported on, and multiple subscales of certain measures may be reported as separate findings.

statistically significant, and "indicates" success to the authors—or where there are differences in the right direction and the statistical test applied is not conclusive but the author finds the differences meaningful. The third is the absence of a statistical, or "meaningful" difference. Considering outcome "between" groups (Table 12-A) we see that about two-fifths of alcoholism and other mental health measures showed "success" on some behavioral or psychological indicator. In other words, in about 40% of the measures in these studies there was statistical evidence of patient gain: improvement in psychological outlook, improved likelihood of release from institution, etc. Drug abuse studies showed relatively less success on similar measures (28.0%). For all outcome research in which it was possible to gauge test control differences, an additional 20-25% of studies showed leanings in the "success" direction without actually reaching customary acceptable statistical levels.

"Before and after" studies showed analogous but lower levels of success achieved in various measures. For studies of alcoholism and of other mental health conditions, about one-quarter of measures were statistically (.05 level) successful, compared with about one-sixth of measures in the drug abuse studies. In another 50-65% of measures (all conditions) before-after differences were "large" and authors concluded success in outcome.

A more rigorous test of outcome success is provided by examining the alcoholism and drug abuse evaluations in a set of 211 studies from the Databank of Program Evaluations in which there was random assignment to test and control groups. These 211 studies were chosen from among the 2,231 studies in the Databank on the basis of the study design information provided in Table 2, and they include all the random assignment studies with primary conditions in problems of aging, alcoholism, drug abuse, juvenile problems, child and adult behavior and adjustment problems, and psychotic states including schizophrenia. "Success" in this special analysis was identified exculsively by attainment of the .5 level of confidence regarding observed and outcome measure differences between groups. Taking all studies together (not a random sampling of all studies in the Databank) the result, as shown in Table 13, is 305 successes out of 561 outcome measures, or 55% meeting the .05 statistical level criteria. Four conditions (problems of aging, drug abuse, juvenile problems, and child behavior problems) showed outcome measure success rates of 60% and higher. Success of measures used in alcoholism studies (41%) was the lowest. Tables 12 and 13 provide an interesting comparison. Table 12, which is much more inclusive, reports a much higher percentage of measures indicating some degree of "success," statistical or as judged by the authors, among studies of alcoholism than does Table 13. For

Table 13

Treatment Success by Condition Measures in Random Assignment Studies

		Success	
	Total measures	*N*	%
Aging problems	35	21	60
Alcohol abuse	73	30	41
Drug abuse	42	25	60
Juvenile problems	64	42	66
Behavioral & adjustment problems			
Children	110	64	58
Adults	183	93	51
Psychotic status	54	30	56
	561	305	55

example, among all studies, 62.3% of the between-groups alcoholism measures and 74.9% of the before-and-after measures indicated "success." Yet among those studies with the most rigorous designs (Table 13), only 41% of the measures indicated success. This pattern is less clear among drug abuse studies, where 54.5% of all the between-groups measures and 80.1% of all the before-and-after measures indicate "success." Sixty percent of the measures in the drug abuse studies with random assignment show "success." This relatively strong showing for drug abuse studies may be due to methadone treatment. Often such studies use program retention as a major measure of success. The legal and administrative pressures for participants to remain in such programs may be partially responsible for their high degree of "success." We should note that while we, and most of the studies themselves, set clear criteria for success, the standards for failure are considerably more ambiguous. Not achieving statistical success at a preordained level does not necessarily imply failure for program planners, administrators, and clinicians. This is especially important when dealing with difficult problems like chronic substance abuse among a particular population.

DISCUSSION

Our findings, based upon a reading of the leading research journals, can only be considered disappointing. Alcohol and drug abuse evaluation studies continue to suffer from massive design problems. Only a small minority present statistical findings in a manner that can be properly understood, no less replicated. Drug abuse studies are particualy poor. The lack of baseline data on the most basic sociodemographic variables (race, SES, sex, etc.) is disappointing and sharply limits the generalizability and practical utility of many studies. Use of addiction/abstinence as the sole measure of outcome is still far too widespread, and the research reports at times (10-20%) do not present the details of their operationalizations in such a manner as to make replication possible. Long-term (>24 months) follow-ups are unusual (10-15%), and two-thirds of the drug abuse studies did not even specify that there was any follow-up at all. These design difficulties are not the special problem of research conducted in one setting or on a particular class of intervention. On the "positive" side we can note that the field of substance abuse research cannot be singled out as suffering from these inadequacies beyond that of other mental health studies. However, in most cases the drug abuse studies are particularly deficient in subscribing to adequate research design.

There remain a host of problems in the conduct of outcome evaluation studies in the field. Improving outcome research is closely linked to the development and maintenance of treatment programs. An important aspect of such improvement will no doubt be increased emphasis on truly integrating outcome evaluations into treatment programs. Although we have no direct data on this point, our sense is that outcome evaluations often are conceived and/or seen as appendages of treatment programs. Unless evaluation becomes an integral part of the treatment process, both the research and the treatments themselves will be seriously hampered. The current lack of integration may be one reason that so much of the research is inadequate to its tasks. If outcome research is to meet its full potential in the future it will also have to define outcome more broadly than the addictive and/or functional status of individuals at some point after the terminations of treatment. What are the "outcomes" for the treatment agents, the client's significant others, the programs themselves, and the social policies upon which the programs are built? If outcome research is to be more fully utilized, these difficult, but necessary dimensions will need to be attended to in the future. Support for both the interventions and the related research is bound–in the long run–to suffer if the quality of the research, particularly that under investigator control, does not materially improve.

Appendix A: Principal Journals Publishing Outcome Studies (1969-1979)

Acta Psychiatrica Scandinavica
American Journal of Drug and Alcohol Abuse
American Journal of Orthopsychiatry
American Journal of Psychotherapy
American Journal of Psychiatry
American Journal of Public Health
Archives of General Psychiatry
Behavior Research and Therapy
Behavior Therapy
British Journal of Addictions
British Medical Journal
British Journal of Medical Psychology
British Journal of Psychiatry
Canadian Psychiatric Association Journal
Child Welfare
Community Mental Health Journal
Comprehensive Psychiatry
Corrective and Social Psychiatry and Journal of Applied Behavior Therapy
Current Psychiatric Therapies
Diseases of the Nervous System
Evaluation Magazine
The Gerontologist
Hospital and Community Psychiatry

International Journal of the Addictions
International Journal of Group Psychotherapy
International Journal of Social Psychiatry
Journal of Abnormal Psychology
Journal of the American Academy of Child Psychiatry
Journal of the American Medical Association
Journal of Applied Behavior Analysis
Journal of Behavior Therapy and Experimental Psychiatry
Journal of Clinical Psychology
Journal of Community Psychology
Journal of Consulting and Clinical Psychology
Journal of Nervous and Mental Disease
Journal of Psychiatric Nursing and Mental Health Services
Journal of Rehabilitation
Journal of Studies on Alcohol
Lancet
Mental Health Digest
Mental Hygiene
New York State Journal of Medicine
Psychological Reports
Psychosomatic Medicine
Psychiatric Quarterly
Psychotherapy and Psychosomatics
Public Health Reports
Social Psychiatry
Social Work
Studies in Family Planning

REFERENCES

AMSEL, Z., MANDELL, W., MATTHIAS, L., MASON, C., and HOCHERMAN, I. Reliability and validity of self-reported illegal activities and drug use collected from narcotic addicts. *Int. J. Addict.* 11: 325-336, 1976.

ARMOR, D.J., POLICH, J.M., and STAMBUL, H.B. *Alcoholism and Treatment.* Santa Monica, CA: Rand Corporation, 1976.

BAEKELAND, F., LUNDWALL, L., and KISSIN, B. Methods for the treatment of chronic alcoholism: A critical appraisal. In R.J. Gibbins et al. (eds.), *Research Advances in Alcohol and Drug Problems,* Vol. 2 New York: Wiley, 1975.

BALL, J.C. The reliability and validity of interview data obtained from 59 narcotic drug addicts. *Am. J. Sociol.* 72: 650-654, 1967.

BONITO, A.J., NURCO, D.N. and SCHAFFER, J.W. The veridicality of addicts' self-reports in social research. *Int. J. Addict.* 11: 719-724, 1976.

BOUDIN, H.M., VALENTINE, V.E., INGHRAM, R.D., BRANTLEY, J.M., RUIZ, M.R., SMITH, G.G., CATLIN, R.P., and REGAN, E.J. Contingency contracting with drug abusers in the natural environment. *Int. J. Addict.* 12: 1-10, 1977.

CALLNER, D.A. Behavioral treatment approaches to drug abuse: A critical review of the research. *Psychol. Bull.* 82: 143-164, 1975.

COHEN, M., HOWARD, A., KLEIN, D.F., and NEWFIELD, K. Evaluating outcome criteria used in methadone maintenance programs. *Int. J. Addict.* 11: 283-294, 1976.

CRAWFORD, J.J., CHALUPSKY, A.B., and HURLEY, M.M. *The evaluation of psychological approaches to alcoholism treatments: A methodological review.* (American Institute for Research Final Report, AIR-96502-3/73-FR). Palo Alto, CA: The Institute, 1973.

CRONKITE, R.C., and MOOS, R.H. Evaluating alcoholism treatment programs: An integrated approach. *J. Consult. Clin. Psychol.* 46: 1105-1119, 1978.

EMRICK, C.D. A review of psychologically oriented treatment of alcoholism. II. The relative effectiveness of different treatment approaches and the effectiveness of treatment versus no treatment. *J. Stud. Alcohol* 36: 88-108, 1975.

GEARING, F.R. Success and failure in methadone maintenance treatment of heroin addiction in New York City. In *Proceedings of the Third National Conference on Methadone Treatment* (PHS Pub. II 2172). Washington, DC: U.S. Government Printing Office, 1970.

GOLDSTEIN, P.J. ABBOTT, W., PAIGE, W., SOBELL, I., and SOTO, F. Tracking procedures in follow-up studies of drug abusers. *Am. J. Drug Alcohol Abuse* 4: 21-30, 1977.

GOTTHEIL, E., CADDY, G.R., and AUSTIN, D.L. *Clinical significance of urine drug screens.* Paper presented at the Canadian Psychiatric Association Annual Meeting, Banff, Alberta, Canada, September 25, 1975. Cited in Maisto and Cooper, 1980.

HILL, M.J. and BLANE, H.T. Evaluation of psychotherapy with alcoholics: A critical review. *Q. J. Stud. Alcohol* 28: 76-104, 1967.

INSTITUTE OF MEDICINE. *Alcoholism, Alcohol Abuse and Related Problems: Opportunities for Research.* Washington, DC: National Academy Press, 1980.

LEWIS, V.S., POLLACK, S., PETERSEN, D.M., and GEIS, G. Nalline and urine tests in narcotics detection: A critical overview. *Int. J. Addict.* 8: 163-171, 1973.

MAISTO, S.A., and COOPER, A.M. A historical perspective on alcohol and drug treatment research. In L.C. Sobell, M.B. Sobell, and E. Ward (eds.), *Evaluating Alcohol and Drug Abuse Treatment Effectiveness: Recent Advances.* New York: Pergamon Press, 1980.

MAISTO, S.A., and MC COLLAM. J.B. The use of multiple measures of life health to assess alcohol treatment outcome: A review and critique. In L.C. Sobell, M.B. Sobell, and E. Ward (eds.), *Evaluating Alcohol and Drug Abuse Treatment Effectiveness: Recent Advances.* New York: Pergamon Press, 1980.

MILLER, B.A., POKORNY, A.D., VALLES, J., and CLEVELAND, S.E. Biased sampling in alcoholism treatment research. *Q. J. Stud. Alcohol* 31: 97-107, 1970.

MOOS, R., and BLISS, F. Difficulty of follow-up and outcome of alcoholism treatment. *J. Stud. Alcohol* 39: 473-490, 1978.

POMERLEAU, O., and ADKINS, D. Evaluating behavioral and traditional treatment for problem drinkers. In L.C. Sobell, M.B. Sobell, and E. Ward (eds.), *Evaluating Alcohol and Drug Abuse Treatment Effectiveness: Recent Advances.* New York: Pergamon Press, 1980.

SMART, R.G. Outcome studies of therapeutic community and halfway house treatment for addicts. *Int. J. Addict.* 11: 143-159, 1976.

SOBELL, L.C. Critique of alcoholism treatment evaluation. In G.A. Marlatt and P. E. Nathan (eds.), *Behavioral Approaches to Alcoholism.* New Brunswick, NJ: Rutgers Center for Alcohol Studies, 1978.

SOBELL, L.C., and SOBELL, M.B. Convergent validity: An approach to increasing confidence in treatment outcome conclusions with alcohol and drug abusers. In L.C. Sobell, M.B. Sobell, and E. Ward (eds.), *Evaluating Alcohol and Drug Abuse Treatment Effectiveness: Recent Advances.* New York: Pergamon Press, 1980, pp. 177-184.

SOBELL, L.C., SOBELL, M.B., and WARD, E. (eds.), *Evaluating Alcohol and Drug Abuse Treatment Effectiveness: Recent Advances.* New York: Pergamon Press, 1980.

SOBELL, M.B., and SOBELL, L.C. Individualized behavior therapy for alcoholics. *Behav. Ther.* 4: 49-72, 1973(a).

SOBELL, M.B., and SOBELL, L.C. Alcoholics treated by individualized behavior therapy: One year treatment outcome. *Behav. Res. Ther.* 14: 195-215, 1973(b).

SOBELL, M.B., and SOBELL, L.C. Second year treatment outcome of alcoholics treated by individualized behavior therapy: Results. *Behav. Res. Ther.* 14: 195-215, 1976.

SOBELL, M.B., and SOBELL, L.C. *Behavioral Treatment of Alcohol Problems: Individualized Therapy and Controlled Drinking.* New York: Plenum Press, 1978.

WEISS, C. *Evaluation Research.* Englewood Cliffs, NJ: Prentice-Hall, 1972.

WILNER, D.M., WALKLEY, R.P., and O'NEILL, E.J. *Introduction to Public Health,* 7th ed. New York: Macmillan, 1978.

The International Journal of the Addictions, 19(5), 503–519, 1984

Predictors of Adolescents' Intentions to Smoke: Age, Sex, Race, and Regional Differences

Clark C. Presson,* PhD

Laurie Chassin, PhD

University of Missouri
Columbia, Missouri 65211

Steven J. Sherman, PhD

Richard Olshavsky, PhD

Michelle Bensenberg, MA

Eric Corty, MA

Indiana University
Bloomington, Indiana 47405

Abstract

The present study investigated the predictors of smoking intentions among subgroups of adolescent nonsmokers, examining age, sex, ethnic, and regional differences. Both proximal factors specific to smoking and more general, distal factors were successful predictors of intentions to smoke. The similarities in prediction outweighed the differences between demographic subgroups. There were three demographic differences: (1) peer and family smoking levels were more important in predicting intentions for girls than boys; (2) smoking

*To whom requests for reprints should be sent at the Department of Psychology, Arizona State University, Tempe, Arizona 85287.

 0020-773X/84/1905-0503$3.50/0

initiation was more of a way of adopting deviant or problem behavior for midwestern than for southwestern subjects; (3) familial smoking models were more related to the intentions of midwestern than southwestern subjects. The theoretical significance of these results and their practical implications for smoking prevention are discussed.

Cigarette smoking is initiated primarily during the adolescent years (*Adult Use of Tobacco,* 1975), and the disappointing results of smoking cessation programs for adults have led antismoking efforts to focus on primary prevention in adolescence as the most effective clinical intervention (Levitt, 1979). However, despite the need for effective smoking prevention strategies, existing programs have not been founded on a clear understanding of the smoking initiation process (Leventhal and Cleary, 1980). Many previous studies, which have focused on cross-sectional comparisons of smokers and nonsmokers, tell us little about smoking initiation, since the differences between smokers and nonsmokers could have resulted from the smoking behavior itself.

Research is thus needed that will identify current nonsmoking adolescents who are at risk to become smokers, based on comprehensive, theory-based studies of smoking initiation (Sherman et al., 1979). One approach has been to identify factors that predict nonsmoking adolescents' intentions to smoke cigarettes in the future (Chassin et al., 1981a, 1981b; Sherman et al., 1983). Adolescents' intentions have been reported as the best predictor of later smoking status (National Institute of Education, 1979), accounting for 13% of the variance in future smoking status up to 5 years later. Thus, factors that are related to adolescents' intentions to smoke should be important "risk factors" in actual smoking initiation.

Chassin et al. (1981a) compared the ability of proximal and distal variables to predict adolescents' intentions to smoke. Proximal variables referred specifically to cigarette smoking and were subjects' attitudes and normative beliefs about smoking (Ajzen and Fishbein, 1970). Distal variables were more general factors not specific to cigarette smoking and were derived from Jessor and Jessor's problem behavior theory (1977). This theory suggests that general factors can identify "deviance prone" adolescents, who are at risk to engage in various behaviors (e.g., alcohol and marijuana use, sexual behavior), in violation of age norms. Chassin et al. (1981a) found that both proximal and distal variables were successful in prediction, although proximal variables generally acounted for more variance in smoking intentions. Moreover, distal variables added only small amounts of explained variance to prediction based on proximal variables alone. Subjects' health beliefs and number of smoking friends also were correlated significantly with intentions to smoke.

While this study identified factors relevant to the smoking initiation process, the findings cannot be generalized beyond its fairly homogeneous White, middle-class, midwestern sample of adolescents. Little is yet known about whether the process of smoking initiation is similar across different demographic groups.

This failure to consider variations in the process and psychological meaning of smoking initiation represents a major limitation on our understanding and on smoking prevention programs as well. Most antismoking programs are aimed at an imaginary "typical" adolescent without consideration of age, sex, ethnic, or subcultural factors (Evans et al., 1979). In fact, however, smoking initiation might involve very different psychological processes among different social networks or demographic groups of adolescents. If so, prevention efforts might be more effective if they addressed factors important to their particular target audiences.

In order to provide a more complete and differentiated picture of smoking initiation, the current study extended Chassin et al.'s (1981a) approach to two different populations from midwestern and southwestern regions of the United States. Age, sex, ethnic, and regional variations in the dynamics of smoking initiation were examined by using several sets of social psychological variables to predict intentions to smoke among different demographic subgroups.

METHOD

Subjects

Subjects were 5,331 6th- to 12th-graders from two communities. There were 4,345 students from Bloomington, Indiana, a predominantly White (90%), small midwestern community. The midwestern sample is the second year's (1981) data from a longitudinal, cross-sequential study. The first-year data from the population are reported in Chassin et al. (1981a). Bloomington is a university community comprised of 17% rural, 57% suburban, and 26% urban residents (over 75% of parents have a high school degree, and 38% have a bachelor's degree; parental occupations are primarily professional, managerial, and skilled labor). There were 986 students from Peoria, Arizona, a racially mixed (62% White) semirural community outside of Phoenix. The socioeconomic status of the southwestern sample was lower than the midwestern, in terms of both parental occupations and education levels (parental degrees: under 50% high school and under 20% bachelor's degrees). For the purposes of analysis, subjects were divided into a middle school sample (grades 6-8) and high school sample (grades 9-12).

Of the 5,331 subjects, 360 (6.75%) were dropped from the analyses because either their questionnaires were incomplete or they gave inconsistent responses to the behavioral intention items (e.g., claiming to be both very likely to smoke and not to smoke in the near future). One-third of the midwestern sample was randomly selected to serve as a holdout sample for cross-validation of the multiple regression analyses (see Note 1). Smokers and ex-smokers were not considered in the analyses. This left final nonsmoking samples of 2,365 (Midwest) and 743 (Southwest). Nonsmokers were defined as those who indicated that they had never smoked or had smoked a few cigarettes "just to try," but not in the last month.

Procedure

Questionnaires were administered in regular classes by members of the research team. Subjects were assured of confidentiality. To help ensure valid answers to questions about the amount of cigarette smoking, a bogus pipeline procedure was given to all subjects before the questionnaire (Evans, Hansen, and Mittlemark, 1977). In this procedure, a small saliva specimen is collected from each subject, and they are told that chemical analysis of saliva could accurately detect nicotine (and the amount they smoke).

A detailed description of the variables in the questionnaire has been reported in detail elsewhere (Chassin et al., 1981a; Note 2). The questionnaire included both proximal variables, which deal specifically with cigarette smoking, and distal variables, which are more general factors not specific to smoking. Proximal variables included attitudes and normative beliefs about smoking, along with behavioral intentions to smoke (derived from Ajzen and Fishbein, 1970). In addition, we measured amount of smoking in the immediate social environment (among peers, parents, and older siblings), beliefs about the effects of smoking on adolescent health, perceived prevalence of smoking (among boys, girls, men, and women), perceived controllability of smoking, the amount of direct experience with smoking, and causal attributions about whether the subject's own (non)smoking behavior was due to personal or situational factors.

The distal variables were derived from "problem behavior theory" (Jessor and Jessor, 1977; Note 3) and represent more general personality and perceived environment factors. The personality variables include perceived locus of control, general attitudinal tolerance of deviance, and measures of values and expectations of both academic success and independence. In addition, two "disjunction" variables were derived that measured the amount of discrepancy between subjects' values and expectations concerning academic success and independence. The perceived environment variables included parents' and friends' expectations concerning the subjects' academic and general success, and perceived parental and friends' supportiveness and control, as well as perceived agreement between parents, between parents' and friends' values, and between the subjects' and their friends' values.

RESULTS

The main purpose of this paper is to specify the factors that predict adolescents' intentions to smoke, within each demographic subgroup. However, before we address the predictability of smoking intentions within each subgroup, we first briefly summarize demographic differences in mean scores on our predictor variables (Note 4).

Demographic Differences

Midwestern Versus Southwestern Nonsmokers

The southwestern sample consistently represented an environment that viewed smoking as more positive and acceptable. Southwestern nonsmoking adolescents were more positive in their attitudes toward smoking (middle school only), saw smoking as less unhealthy, and perceived less negative normative beliefs about smoking. The midwestern sample was also much less "deviance prone" on the Jessor and Jessor (1977) distal variables (e.g., a higher internal locus of control, a higher value on academic success, higher expectations for academic success, a lower tolerance for deviance for middle school only, higher friends' expectations, more friends' support, more parental support, friends with stricter standards for good behavior, greater agreement between parents, greater agreement between friends and parents, and greater agreement between themselves and their friends).

The social environments of the two groups also differed in acceptability of smoking. Nonsmokers in the Southwest were exposed to more regular and ex-smokers (15.5% and 8.1% of the population, respectively) than were nonsmokers in the Midwest (12.5% and 5.2%, respectively). They also had more friends, parents, older siblings, and boy (girl) friends who smoked than did Midwesterners. There was also far more intermingling of smokers with nonsmokers in the Southwest; correlations between a subject's smoking status and the number of his or her closest friends who smoked were much higher in the Midwest than in the Southwest.

Male Versus Female Nonsmokers

Overall, boy and girl nonsmokers differed on several predictor variables. On the proximal variables, boy nonsmokers had significantly less negative attitudes (Midwest only) and normative beliefs about smoking than did girls. In addition, boys were consistently more "deviance prone" than girls on the distal variables. For example, boys reported greater tolerance for deviance, friends with less strict standards of behavior, less perceived parents' and friends' support, friends with lower expectations, and less agreement with friends. For the midwestern sample only boys also reported a more external locus of control, less perceived parental support, lower value on academics, and less agreement between parents and friends. However, girls did have higher values on independence, higher expectations for achieving independence (Midwest only), and a greater disjunction between their values and expectations for independence (Southwest only).

Thus, boys were more favorable toward smoking in their attitudes and beliefs, and were also more "deviance prone." There were no significant sex differences in actual smoking rates except for the midwestern high school sample, where more girls were smokers (16.1% of boys, 19.3% of girls, $\chi^2(1) = 34.7, p < .05$). However, girls reported being exposed to more smoking in their social networks. Compared to boys, girls reported that more of their five closest friends were smokers and more often that their best friends (Southwest only) and boy (girl) friends smoked.

Middle School Versus High School Nonsmokers

Older subjects had a more positive attitude toward smoking and saw smoking as more controllable. However, younger subjects had more positive normative beliefs about smoking and saw smoking as less of a health hazard. On the distal variables, older subjects had more "deviance prone" scores in having a greater tolerance for deviance, higher expectations for independence, higher values on independence (Midwest only), less perceived parental support (Midwest only), and lower parental expectations (Midwest only). However, younger subjects were more "deviance prone" in scoring more external, reporting less friends' support,. less agreement with their friends, and larger discrepancies between their values and expectations for actually attaining academic success. Finally, older subjects were in a social environment that contained more smokers. They reported more close friends that smoked and estimated a higher prevalence of smoking among boys and girls than did younger subjects.

White Versus Non-White Nonsmokers

Race comparisons were made only within the southwestern sample since the midwestern sample did not contain enough non-White subjects. Non-Whites had more positive attitudes toward smoking and more positive normative beliefs about smoking, and they saw smoking as less of a health hazard. On the Jessor and Jessor (1977) variables, non-Whites had generally more "deviance prone" scores. Finally, in terms of social environment, non-White subjects reported more close friends, best friends, and older brothers who smoked cigarettes.

Predicting Behavioral Intentions

The major focus of the current study was to understand the dynamics and likelihood of smoking initiation in groups of adolescent nonsmokers. First, the general success of prediction across all the subgroups is reported. Next, we examine whether the success of prediction or the relative importance of variables in the prediction varied for the different subgroups. With some important exceptions, the overall patterns of prediction across subgroups showed many more similarities than differences.

General Predictability of Intentions

Both the proximal and distal sets of variables were successsful in predicting behavioral intentions in multiple regression analyses (see Table 1). Ajzen and Fishbein's (1970) proximal variables were consistently the most successful predictors, with multiple *R*s ranging from .63 to .77, accounting for between 40% and 59% of the variance. Both the attitudinal and normative components carried significant weight for all subgroups. The distal variables from Jessor and Jessor (1977) were significant but less successful predictors, with multiple *R*s ranging from .40 to .61, accounting for between 16% and 37% of the variance. A subject's general tolerance for deviance was the single most important distal variable in prediction (Note 5).

In addition to the multivariate models, several other variables were used to predict behavioral intentions. These variables were less successful than the proximal and distal multivariate models. For example, health beliefs showed a moderate but consistent relation to intentions (Pearson *r*s from .30 to .47, accounting for between 9% and 22% of the variance), while perceived control was generally unrelated to intentions.

Prevalence estimates of smoking among boys, girls, men, and women were used to predict intentions in a multiple regression. Prevalence estimates were not consistently successful, with multiple *R*s ranging from .11 to .22, accounting for between 1% and 4% of the variance. Second, the number of five closest friends who smoked was shown by simple correlations to have a generally significant relation to intentions (Pearson *r*s from .10 to .38, accounting for between 1% and 14% of the variance).

Finally, *t* tests were used to assess the impact of smoking among particular smoking models on subject's intentions. The smoking intentions of nonsmoking subjects who had a father (or other model) who smoked were compared with the intentions of those whose father (or other model) did not smoke (Note 6). The presence of all the familial smoking models was associated with significantly stronger intentions to smoke in the midwestern sample only. Having a best friend or boy/girlfriend who smoked was associated with stronger intentions to smoke in both samples.

Table 1

Summary of the Analyses Predicting Behavioral Intentions from Proximal, Distal, and Additional Variables

	Middle school				High school			
	Midwest		Southwest		Midwest		Southwest	
	Boys (*N* = 520)	Girls (*N* = 599)	Boys (*N* = 143)	Girls (*N* = 159)	Boys (*N* = 554)	Girls (*N* = 542)	Boys (*N* = 198)	Girls (*N* = 189)
Proximal Variables								
Multiple *R*	.67***	.63***	.76***	.77***	.67***	.63***	.70***	.66***
Weights of components								
β-Attitudinal	.37***	.53***	.70***	.64***	.46***	.43***	.43***	.56***
β-Normative	.43***	.17***	.12*	.28***	.34***	.33***	.43***	.20***
Distal Variables[a]								
Multiple *R*	.43***	.42***	.53***	.60***	.40***	.45***	.44**	.49***
Weights for variables[b]								
Personality system								
β-Tolerance for deviance	.24***	.24***	.32**	.40***	.19***	.32***	.33***	.36***
β-Locus of control								.26***
β-Value independence			−.31**					
β-Expect independence				.27*				

Perceived environment system								
β-Friends' support	.12*	.12*						
β-Parents' agreement	–.11*					–.13*		
β-Parents' expectations	–.11*							
β-Friends' strictness	–.14*							
Additional Variables								
Prevalence estimates, multiple *R*	.13	.14*	.14	.22	.16**	.20**	.13	.11
Health beliefs (*r*)	–.32**	–.30**	–.44*	–.35**	–.47**	–.40**	–.38**	–.37**
Perceived control (*r*)	.01	.07	–.11	.05	–.08*	.00	–.01	–.15*
Number of friends who smoke (*r*)	.34**	.29**	.10	.38**	.20**	.33**	.12	.20**

[a] In cases with fewer than 170 subjects, the number of distal variables was reduced to maintain at least 10 subjects per variable (Cohen and Cohen, 1975).

[b] Beta weights for distal variables are listed only if significant; other distal variables did not carry significant weight in any predictions.

*$p < .05$.
**$p < .01$.
***$p < .001$.

Regional Differences in Prediction

As reported earlier, smoking was generally more socially acceptable in the Southwest than in the Midwest. We now consider whether that mean difference in social acceptability is reflected in different patterns of prediction for behavioral intentions.

For the proximal variables, the overall level of prediction was quite similar for the two regions. The southwestern sample had relatively greater weight for the attitudinal component than did the midwestern sample (middle school only).

Since smoking was more socially deviant in the midwestern sample, we expected that it would be more of a "problem behavior" in Jessor and Jessor's (1977) sense, and that the distal variables would prove more important to prediction in the midwestern sample than in the southwestern sample. Surprisingly, however, the distal variables showed somewhat higher levels of prediction in the southwestern sample (especially in the middle school).

The predictions described here used the proximal and distal variables separately. We also analyzed the proximal and distal variables together to test their relative importance in each sample. We tested whether the proximal variables alone were sufficient for the prediction of intention or whether the distal variables accounted for unique, additional variance. To do this, hierarchical regressions were performed with the proximal variables entered in the first step, and the distal variables in the second. F tests were used to test the differences between the multiple Rs for the two steps.

The hierarchical regressions showed that the distal variables added modest, but significant amounts of variance above and beyond the proximal variables only for girls in the midwestern sample (middle school girls, $\Delta R^2 = .041, F(17, 550) = 2.1$; high school girls, $\Delta R^2 = .042, F(17, 515) = 1.8; p < .05$ in both cases). In this sense, the distal variables were more important in the midwestern sample than in the southwestern. When the distal variables were considered separately, they did not show better prediction in the Midwest. However, smoking did appear to be more of a "problem behavior" in the Midwest in that the effects of the distal variables were not mediated through the proximal variables. For the southwestern sample, where smoking was a more socially acceptable behavior and less deviant, the distal variables did not add any predictive power to that attained by the proximal variables alone.

There were also regional differences in the predictability of intentions based on the other social variables. First, the prevalence estimates of smoking were moderately successful as predictors of intentions in the midwestern sample but not at all in the southwestern sample. Second, the number of smoking friends was consistently related to intentions in the midwestern sample, but only for girls in the Southwest.

Finally, we examined the effect of smoking by particular family and peer models. Having a family member who smoked was consistently associated with stronger behavioral intentions to smoke only in the midwestern sample. For the family models, there were eight analyses at each age level (father, mother, older brother, and older sister tested for boys and girls). In the Midwest, 6 of the 8 tests were significant in middle school and 3 of the 8 in high school. The effects were stronger for fathers' smoking (4 of 4 cases significant) than for mothers' (1 of 4). In contrast, for the southwestern sample, the smoking of family members was not related to intentions (only 1 of 16 cases significant). However, having a best friend or a boyfriend/girlfriend who smoked was associated with stronger behavioral intentions to smoke in both regional groups.

Sex Differences in Prediction

As already reported, boys appeared more favorable to smoking than were girls in terms of the proximal variables and also more deviance prone on most of the distal variables. However, girls reported more contact with smokers in their social world.

We had expected that interpersonal variables would be generally better predictors of behavioral intentions for girls than for boys, since Jessor et al. (1973) suggested that girls are more influenced by social concerns and peer pressure. This expectation was not borne out for the proximal and distal variables. For the proximal variables, the attitudinal component always had greater weight for girls than did the more socially oriented normative belief component. For boys there was no consistent pattern (see Table 1). For the distal variables we might expect that the perceived environment system would be more important for girls since they have been reported to be more sensitive to interpersonal influences. However, the perceived environment variables contributed little to prediction except for middle school boys in the Midwest.

However, as expected, there was greater predictability of intentions for girls than for boys on two other social variables, number of smoking friends and smoking among particular peers. The number of smoking friends was related to intentions for girls but not for boys in the southwestern sample (in the Midwest, it was related to intentions for both sexes). Similarly, having a boy/girlfriend or a best friend who smoked was related to significantly stronger intentions for girls in all cases, but for boys it was less consistent. For boys, having a best friend who smoked was associated with stronger intentions only in the midwestern sample. Further, for boys there was no impact of having a girlfriend who smoked. There were no sex differences in the effect of family smoking models, nor any consistent cross-sex or same-sex modeling patterns.

Age Differences in Prediction

There were few age differences in the patterns of prediction. For the proximal variables, the two age levels showed very similar patterns of prediction. For the southwestern sample only, the distal variables predicted intentions more strongly at middle school than at high school. The only other factor that showed any age difference in prediction was family smoking models. For the Midwest, having family members who smoked was associated with intentions more in middle school (6 of 8 cases significant) than in high school (3 of 8 cases).

Race Differences in Prediction

The non-White subsample was consistently more deviance prone than the White subsample, based on the mean group differences. However, the two race subsamples showed few differences in the patterns of predictability of behavioral intentions.

The only race difference in prediction concerned the distal variables. For boys, the distal variables had a higher level of prediction for Whites than for non-Whites. The difference was greater at middle school (multiple *R*s of .55 for Whites, .43 for non-Whites) than at high school (multiple *R*s of .54 and .50). However, for girls, we found the reverse; the distal variables had a higher level of prediction for non-Whites than for Whites. Again, this difference was greater at middle school (multiple *R*s of .55 for Whites, .69 for non-Whites) than at high school (multiple *R*s of .49 and .56). This would suggest that smoking is more of a Jessor and Jessor (1977) "problem behavior" among non-White girls than among White girls.

DISCUSSION

The current data are generally similar to the earlier findings reported by Chassin et al. (1981a). For all subgroups, proximal and distal variables were successful in prediction. In each case, the proximal variables accounted for the most variance, and the attitudinal component generally had greater weight than the normative component. Results for the distal variables suggested that adolescent smoking can be viewed as a "problem behavior" in Jessor and Jessor's (1977) sense, and among these variables tolerance for deviance was the single best predictor. Furthermore, like the earlier study, prevalence estimates were only modestly predictive of intentions, while health beliefs and number of smoking friends accounted for between 5% and 20% of the variance in intentions. In neither study did perceived control of smoking account for meaningful variance in intentions. Thus, the current study serves to replicate the findings and conclusions reported by Chassin et al. (1981a) for a prior year's sample from the midwestern population. This replication suggests some stability in the factors predicting smoking intentions at least for the studied group. However, in applying these findings, it is important to recognize that the meaning of and attitudes toward smoking may well change for adolescents over time.

Beyond replicating the earlier data, the present research extended our knowledge of smoking initiation among adolescents by examining distinct populations of nonsmokers. We compared subjects of different sex, age, race, and geographic region on a variety of factors relevant to smoking initiation. These comparisons revealed many demographic differences in terms of mean levels on the predictor variables. However, despite these mean differences, the question remained whether there were different dynamics of smoking initiation within each demographic subgroup. Somewhat surprisingly, the similarities in prediction of behavioral intentions to smoke across the subgroups outweighed the differences. However, before we discuss the similarities, we first note three minor exceptions in which the prediction of smoking intentions varied across subgroups.

First, peer and family smoking was more important to predicting intentions for girls than boys. This finding reflected the mean differences between boys and girls on the predictor variables; this is consistent with previous research on marijuana use (Jessor et al., 1973) that found girls were more vulnerable to social influence than boys. This finding suggests that "peer pressure" oriented approaches to prevention (e.g., Evans, 1976) might be more important (and more successful) with girls than with boys.

Second, smoking appeared to be more of a "problem behavior" in the midwestern sample than in the southwestern sample. Distal variables accounted for unique variance in behavioral intentions only for the midwestern female subjects. In the Southwest, the effects of distal variables were mediated through the proximal variables. This finding is consistent with the fact that smoking was less acceptable and statistically more deviant in the Midwest. Recall that distal variables represent more generalized factors, not specific to cigarette smoking (e.g., general attitudinal tolerance for deviance). For some samples (e.g., midwestern females) it would not be sufficient for a prevention program to focus only on changing adolescents' specific attitudes and beliefs about smoking. For those populations, more comprehensive approaches to prevention are indicated that attempt to change both smoking-related beliefs and broader personality characteristics (for an example of such a program, see Botvin and Eng, 1980).

The third subgroup difference in prediction was that family smoking models (father, mother, older brother, older sister) were related to smoking intentions for the midwestern sample and not for the southwestern sample. Thus, family models were important for intentions only in the environment where smoking was less prevalent and less socially accepted. This suggests several possibilities about how models influence intentions. In an environment where smoking is perceived as more deviant (as in the Midwest), having a family member who smokes may define smoking as a more acceptable, less deviant behavior for those individuals, making them more likely to intend to smoke. Similarly, in an environment where the behavior is less normative, having a family member who smokes may be a highly salient, noticeable event that heightens modeling processes. In contrast, where smoking is more socially accepted and there are more smoking models, the presence of a family member who smokes would be less salient and the effect of family models would be weaker.

With the exception of these three differences, the patterns of prediction were quite similar across the various subgroups. Thus, the current data suggest that the dynamics of smoking initiation are largely similar for adolescents of different age, race, sex, and geographic region. These findings are of theoretical significance in that they suggest that a basic model of smoking initiation in adolescence may have substantial generalizability. Similar findings have been reported for drug use among Black and Puerto Rican adolescents (Dembo, Farrow, Des Jarlais, Burgos, and Schmeidler, 1981). Moreover, we found basic similarities in predictive factors despite the extensive mean differences between groups on the predictor variables. This suggests an additional important point. It is an individual's relative position within his or her group that determines risk to smoke, rather than the individual's absolute level on any factor. For example, boys were more "deviance prone" than girls on the Jessor and Jessor (1977) distal variables. Yet, girls smoked in equal or greater numbers than boys, and the distal variables were equally predictive of intentions for both sexes. Thus, it is a girl's relative position on these factors with respect to other girls that determines her risk to be a smoker. A girl with less "deviance prone" scores than the average male still might be at risk to smoke if her level were high relative to other girls in her reference group. Similarly, it might take a different score to place a younger and an older adolescent "at risk" (see also Clausen, 1978). Thus, in some ways, comparing subgroups on mean levels of risk factors can be misleading, since between-group differences are less important in determining risk than is one's standing relative to one's own group (Note 7).

The results of the current study are of practical significance as well. In one sense smoking prevention programs should also have substantial generalizability. Specifically, adolescents' attitudes and beliefs about cigarette smoking were most important to prediction (and thus to smoking prevention programs) in all subsamples. One set of beliefs which prevention programs might address involves the short-term health consequences of smoking. While many smoking prevention programs have had limited success focusing on long-term health consequences, the current data suggest that messages aimed at short-term consequences may be more relevant for adolescents and thus more effective. Some support for this hypotheses has been reported by Glasgow, McCaul, Freeborn, & O'Neill (1980).

The data also suggest that an important target audience for smoking prevention programs is composed of "deviance prone" adolescents. These adolescents are relatively nonconventional, have a high tolerance for deviant behavior, and are peer oriented. Perhaps the most important form of "tailoring" of prevention programs is not to consider sex, age, race, or geographic region but to consider the characteristics of "deviance prone" adolescents. For example, adults may not be the best people to influence the smoking intentions of these peer-oriented adolescents. Similarly, using conventional "school leaders" as nonsmoking models should be relatively ineffective for this group, who may not see such students as positive models (Newman, 1970). In fact, it is not clear that a school environment is the best setting for influencing these deviance-prone adolescents. Other sorts of mass media campaigns might be considered as alternatives. The values and aspirations of these high-risk adolescents should be investigated in more depth so that suggestions for antismoking campaigns can be formulated.

In summary, the same general factors were important to the smoking intentions of adolescents of different sex, age, race, and geographical region. Thus, these factors are important to prevention programs for all these subgroups. However, the distinct characteristics of the "high-risk" adolescent should be taken into account in tailoring the language, style, and content of prevention programs to influence the smoking intentions of "deviance prone" adolescents.

ACKNOWLEDGMENT

This research was supported by USPHS grant number HD13449.

NOTES

1. For the multiple regression analyses using proximal and distal variables to predict behavioral intentions, two cross-validation procedures were conducted. First, within the midwestern sample, the beta weights derived from the main sample (i.e., two-thirds of the total sample) were used to predict behavioral intentions for the holdout sample (one-third of the total sample). Second, the beta weights derived from the larger midwestern sample were used to predict behavioral intentions for the southwestern sample. Both of these cross-validations were successful in that the level of prediction in the smaller group using the beta weights from the larger group was very similar to the level of prediction obtained using the smaller group data alone.
2. Because of the large number of variables, a complete description of the questionnaire is not included in this paper. A copy is available from the authors upon request.
3. These variables represent only a subset of those included in Jessor and Jessor's (1977) full model.
4. All reported demographic differences in mean scores were significant at least at the .05 level by t tests.
5. On the average, the distal variables together accounted for an additional 8.2% (range from 5% to 14%) of the variance beyond that accounted for by the simple correlation between tolerance for deviance and behavioral intentions.

6. Subjects who reported that they did not have a father (or other model) were eliminated from that analysis.
7. This point may apply even more strongly to the groups with which an individual identifies. In the current study we measured only group membership, not identification.

REFERENCES

Adult Use of Tobacco. Washington, DC: U.S. Department of Health, Education, and Welfare, 1975.

AJZEN, I., and FISHBEIN, M. The prediction of behavior from attitudinal and normative variables *J. Exp. Soc. Psychol.* 6: 466-487, 1970.

BOTVIN, G., and ENG, A. A comprehensive school-based smoking prevention program. *J. School Health* 50: 209-213, 1980.

CHASSIN, L., PRESSON, C., BENSENBERG, M., CORTY, E., OLSHAVSKY, R., and SHERMAN, S.J. Predicting adolescents' intentions to smoke cigarettes. *J. Health Soc. Behav.* 22: 445-455, 1981 (a).

CHASSIN, L., PRESSON, C., SHERMAN, S.J., CORTY, E., and OLSHAVSKY, R. Self-images and cigarette smoking in adolescence. *Pers. Soc. Psychol. Bull.* 7: 670-676, 1981 (b).

COHEN, J., and COHEN, P. *Applied Multiple Regression/Correlation Analysis for the Behavioral Sciences.* Hillsdale, NJ: Erlbaum, 1975.

CLAUSEN, J.A. Longitudinal studies on drug use in high school: Substantive and theoretical issues. In D. Kandel (ed.), *Longitudinal Research on Drug Use: Empirical Findings and Methodological Issues.* New York: Wiley, 1978.

DEMBO, R., FARROW, D., DES JARLAIS, D., BURGOS, W., and SCHMEIDLER, J. Examining a causal model of early drug involvement among inner-city junior high school youths. *Hum. Rel.* 34: 169-193, 1981.

EVANS, R.I. Smoking in children: Developing a social psychological strategy of deterrence. *Prev. Med.* 5: 122-127, 1976.

EVANS, R.I. HANSEN, W.T., and MITTELMARK, M.B. Increasing the validity of self-reports of behavior in a smoking in children investigation. *J. Appl. Psychol.* 62: 521-523, 1977.

EVANS, R.I., HENDERSON, A., HILL, P., and RAINES, B. Smoking in children and adolescents: Psychosocial determinants and prevention strategies. In N.A. Krasnegor (ed.), *The Behavioral Aspects of Smoking* (NIDA Research Monograph 26). Washington, DC: NIDA, 1979.

GLASGOW, R., MC CAUL, K., FREEBORN, V., and O'NEILL, H. *Immediate and long-term health messages in the prevention of adolescent smoking.* Paper presented at the annual meeting of the Society for Behavioral Medicine, New York, 1980.

JESSOR, R., and JESSOR, S.L. *Problem Behavior and Psychosocial Development: A Longitudinal Study of Youth.* New York: Academic Press, 1977.

JESSOR, R., JESSOR, S.L., and FINNEY, J. A social psychology of marijuana use: Longitudinal studies of high school and college youth. *J. Pers. Soc. Psychol.* 26: 1-15, 1973.

LEVENTHAL, H., and CLEARY, P. The smoking problem: A review of the research and theory in behavioral risk modification. *Psychol. Bull.* 88: 370-405, 1980.

LEVITT, E. The case against smoking withdrawal as a major strategy in the extirpation of smoking. In *Proceedings of the Division 23 Program,* 87th Annual Convention of the American Psychological Association. Washington, DC: APA, 1979.

NATIONAL INSTITUTE OF EDUCATION. *Teenage Smoking: Immediate and Long-Term Patterns* (USDHEW Contract No. 400-79-001). Washington, DC: DHEW, 1979.

NEWMAN, L.M. Status configurations and cigarette smoking in a junior high school. *J. School Health* 40: 28-31, 1970.

SHERMAN, S.J., PRESSON, C.C., CHASSIN, L., BENSENBERG, M., CORTY, E., and OLSHAVSKY, R. Smoking intentions in adolescents: Direct experience and predictability. *Pers. Soc. Psychol. Bull.* 8: 376-383, 1982.

SHERMAN, S.J., PRESSON, C.C., CHASSIN, L., CORTY, E., and OLSHAVSKY, R. The false consensus effect in estimates of smoking prevalence: Underlying mechanisms. *Pers. Soc. Psychol. Bull.* 9: 197-207, 1983.

SHERMAN, S.J., PRESSON, C.C., CHASSIN, L., and OLSHAVSKY, R. *Social psychological factors in adolescent cigarette smoking.* Symposium paper presented at the annual meeting of the American Psychological Association, New York, 1979.

The International Journal of the Addictions, 19(5), 521-539, 1984

Professional Psychotherapy and Its Relationship to Compliance in Treatment

Carol Jean Rogalski,* PhD, ABPP

West Side Veterans Administration Medical Center

Department of Psychiatry
College of Medicine
University of Illinois at the Medical Center

Chicago, Illinois 60612

Abstract

Compliance rates over a 21-month period for 57 drug-abusing patients receiving individual professional psychotherapy in addition to paraprofessional counseling were compared to compliance rates for patients not receiving individual professional psychotherapy. Compliance was defined as remaining in the treatment environment for an agreed upon time and neither leaving the hospital against medical advice nor being given a disciplinary discharge for illegal drug use, stealing, or fighting. Patients receiving professional psychotherapy had been assessed as having either higher levels of psychiatric symptoms or a history of a psychiatric diagnosis, or being potential management problems. Patients who received psychotherapy more likely remained stabilized in the treatment environment and in their role as patient. An additional finding was that clarity of the therapist's role in the ward environment affected the patient's stabilization. This study supports recent findings

*Address reprint requests to the author: Staff Psychologist, West Side Veterans Administration Medical Center, 820 South Damen Avenue, Chicago, Illinois 60612.

 0020-773X/84/1905-0521$3.50/0

that professional psychotherapy can be effective for drug abusers. It suggests that individual psychotherapy/consultation with distressed and difficult patients experiencing disequilibrium in the hospital milieu can be an effective means of restoring that equilibrium.

The merits of individual, professional psychotherapy with drug abusers pose an issue not only in the evaluation of the benefits provided to the client, but also in regard to the morale of the treatment personnel. Not only are considerable amounts of money being spent on the health care of drug abusers in both outpatient and inpatient settings, but competent and concerned clinicians who attempt to provide humanizing environments and therapeutic relationships for clients often receive indifference, hostility, and physical and verbal abuse in return for their services. Administrators, physically and emotionally distant from the day-to-day clinical issues, often impose additional burdens and unrealistic demands on clinical staff to execute life-style changes in their patients. Clarifying patient and professional expectations, characterizing a stabilizing and humanizing environment, and defining doctor and patient roles might allow for both economic and human resources to be expended more profitably.

A sample of the literature since the 1960s on medical, surgical, and psychiatric patients finds relationships among drug and alcohol abuse, organicity, singleness, socioeconomic status, ethnicity, and being diagnosed a personality disorder as only a few of the factors related to noncompliance to the treatment regime—defined as either length of time in treatment or adherence to medication schedule, diet, exercise, or life-style change (see Table 1). Sackett and Haynes and their associates (Sackett and Haynes, 1976; Haynes et al., 1979) have reported 245 scientific articles published before 1974, with that figure increasing by geometric proportions since that time. Features intrinsic to the client which are found consistently to be important determinants of increased compliance are (1) status not as a psychiatric, paranoid, or personality-disordered patient; (2) stabilization of symptomatology; and (3) disability. The compliant patient might thus be characterized as stable, symptomless, and not particularly agitated or distressed, and in a dependent position, viewing himself/herself in need of help and trusting that it will be provided. Features extrinsic to the patient are the emotional atmosphere of the environment, the nature of the patient-doctor relationship, and external and family pressures.

This writer's clinical experience suggests that the noncompliant drug-abusing patient appears to have difficulty in emotionally assuming the role of a patient as defined by the treatment personnel, both administrative and clinical; does not wish to adhere to necessary guidelines and rituals; and cannot tolerate the limitations of the hospital environment or the humanness of the treatment personnel. Different standards of personal conduct and emotional relatedness create disharmony. Ambivalences about desiring a professional or a friend are present. On one extreme the treatment personnel are idealized, with contentment, good health, and ultimate happiness viewed as residing in the hands of the doctor and hospital. Disappointment at the failure to meet the illusion leads to an experience of a narcissistic injury, with subsequent termination of a tenuous treatment alliance. The self-system of the person who seeks help from either a dehumanized institution or an idealized person must be open to receiving such help and must acknowledge, or at least adjust to, the desired role, while remaining with feelings of enhancement and personality cohesiveness. For those patients whose problems necessitate the maintenance of a treatment relationship on an outpatient basis in order to either survive or complete necessary life-style changes, the incorporation of a new role, that of outpatient, is necessary. This new role is created while yet living within one's previous environment, with all the lures, cues, symbols, and affective bonds influencing attitudes and subsequent behavior. From the psychological perspective, if one has encountered and internalized positive nurturing experiences and a firm set of moral guidelines, then one returns to the environment from which one came and is able to continue psychological rehabilitation within the environment. From the sociological perspective (Liazos, 1972), "covert institutional violence" is destructive of the individual and his/her ability to discover productive outlets for impulses. Some might suggest that the environments to which the patients return sufficiently damage self-esteem and human dignity and make the task of life-style change impossible.

Experience with drug abusers reveals greater success in the development of ordered environments in which to detoxify clients than in any long-range success on an individual level to form a treatment alliance which supports a life-style change or psychological rehabilitation. This study looks at one aspect of compliance—the ability to remain within the treatment environment—and its relationship to professional psychotherapy.

STUDY

Setting

This study was conducted between February 1981 and October 1982 on a 20-bed detoxification/rehabilitation unit at the Veterans Administration Hospital, Westside, an affiliate of the University of Illinois.

Patient Population

The veterans who applied for detoxification/rehabilitation during this period were primarily Black, unemployed, and single, between the ages of 20 and 65 years. These qualities alone would be predictive of noncompliance with

Table 1

Studies of Noncompliance with Inpatient Treatment

Authors	Year	Population	Method	Findings/conclusions
Lewis, Lorenz, and Calden	1955	200 tuberculosis inpatients at Veterans Administration Hospital	Chart review of 100 regular discharges compared to 100 irregular discharges on age, race, service-connected status, marital status, distance to home, activity of disease, psychiatric classification, previous history of irregular discharge.	1. Age, race, service-connected status, marital status, distance to home, activity of disease, and psychiatric classification did not discriminate regular and irregular discharges. 2. Previous history of irregular discharges for those who left irregularly. 3. Psychiatric classification did not discriminate; personality differences were subtle.
		250 inpatients	Unclear methodology. Compared intrahospital and extrahospital stress for regular and irregular discharges.	4. No difference in amount of stress; differences in perception and coping styles, and ability to ask for assistance. 5. Three stages of hospital adjustment delineated. a. Regression and acceptance of ward family and dependency. b. Somewhat independent functioning, though still dependent on doctor and nurse. c. Leave-taking. 6. Patients who adjust well to a hospital need a normal flexibility of character structure and making and shifting relationships with people. 7. Staff needs to prevent countertransference reactions or overidentification, hostility, or rejection. 8. Patients need to deal with separation anxiety, isolation, ambivalence, weakness and helplessness, regression.
Greenwald and Bartemeier	1963	191 psychiatric patients	All records during a 7-month period were reviewed on the following variables:	1. 35% went AMA. 2. Residents/therapists rated effective by supervisors had fewer AMA discharges.

			age, sex, previous admissions, length of stay, discharge diagnosis, therapist, type of discharge. Therapists given ratings by their supervisors.	3. Age and sex did not discriminate AMA from non-AMA discharges. 4. Those who went AMA spent less time in the hospital. 5. If a patient went AMA before he will likely go AMA in the future. 6. Sociopathic personalities have more AMA discharges.
Daniels, Margolis, and Carson	1963	283 psychiatric inpatients	All records reviewed on the following variables: religion, admission status, MMPI, length of stay, discharge diagnosis, type of discharge. Statistical comparison between 32 AMA and non-AMA patients. Interviews with staff.	1. 11.3% went AMA. 2. Catholic and Jewish patients more likely to go AMA. 3. Patients admitted on an emergency basis more likely to go AMA. 4. A patient leaving AMA goes within the first 10 days. 5. Discharge diagnosis more likely to show suspiciousness, isolation, paranoid, schizoid features, and be more acutely disturbed. The patient shows lack of insight, inability to communicate, motor agitation, isolation of affect and thought. 6. Males and females differed on MMPI scales; men are intropunitive and women extropunitive, though both viewed as hostile. 7. Four dynamic categories seen: inadequate preparation for hospitalization, threatening aspects of ward, difficulties in patient/doctor relationship, interference from family.
Meyer, Margolis, and Daniels	1963	Follow-up of 32 AMA patients of study by Daniels, Margolis, and Carson (1963)	Interviews from patients' point of view looking at process and content.	1. Contact was established with 59%; 25% refused; 16% not able to be located. 2. Four categories from previous study remained the the same. 3. AMA discharges were not total failures from patients' point of view. 4. Factors seen as important are enforced separation, enforced dependency, limitations in freedom.

(continued)

Table 1 (continued)

Authors	Year	Population	Method	Findings/conclusions
Meyer, Martin, and Lange	1967	280 psychiatric inpatients	42 elopement patients compared to matched group of 42 nonelopement patients. Charts were reviewed and statistical comparisons done for sex, religion, race, occupational status, admission and discharge diagnoses, disposition. Interviews with psychotherapists categorized experience under four headings: internal dynamics, threatening ward environment, patient-therapist relationship, interference from family and external factors. MMPI's were compared.	1. Elopement patients were younger, with an interaction with sex. Males elope more, the younger they are; females do not. 2. No major effect of sex, religion, occupational status, race. 3. Elopement patients were more seriously disturbed, along the psychotic dimension. 4. Eventual successful disposition was somewhat less for elopement patients. 5. No difference in admission diagnosis. 6. Internal factors (confusion and poor impulse control) as likely as specific stresses to precipitate elopement. Reactive elopers appeared more organized in object relationships and reality testing.
Atkinson	1971	2,529 adult and adolescent psychiatric inpatients; all first admissions.	Compared AMA and AWOL patients. Factors reviewed were age, length of stay, and diagnosis.	1. Adolescents go AWOL. 2. Personality disorders and those with psychophysiological disorders go AWOL. 3. Those who leave AMA go within the first 5 days.
Raynes and Patch	1971	237 psychiatric inpatients on an open ward.	Records of AMA and AWOL patients compared to non-AMA patients. Statistical analyses done of age, sex,	1. No differences in age or sex. 2. AWOL patients are 50% Black; since Black males were underrepresented in admission, Black females had the highest AMA/AWOL rate.

			race, marital, previous admissions, diagnosis, type of discharge, and therapist.	3. No difference in marital status. 4. No difference for AMA group on previous admissions; AWOL group had significantly more. 5. Both AMA and AWOL had diagnoses of alcoholism and drug abuse. 6. There was a main effect of therapist. 7. The combined rate of AMA and AWOL patients is 16.9%.
Altman, Brown, and Sletten	1972	52,102 persons from 10 in-patient mental health facilities.	Elopers compared to non-elopers. Statistical comparisons relating elopement to sex, race, marital status, religion, DSM II diagnosis, and age. Intra-psychic factors were inferred.	1. 3.6% eloped. 2. Males eloped at higher rates than females. 3. Non-Whites eloped at higher rates than Whites. 4. Singles had highest rate, followed by divorced and separated. 5. Catholic and "other" religions had highest elopement rates; Jewish and "none" had lowest elopement rates. 6. Acute brain syndrome and personality disorder diagnoses had highest elopement rates. 7. Highest age group was 15-19, followed by age group 10-14 and then a gradual decline until age 90. 8. Elopement was seen as: an impulsive act, representing disregard for established rules and regulations, suggesting "acting out" under stress rather than talking about the situation.
Albert and Kornfeld	1973	28 medical in-patients who were referred for psychiatric consultation because they threatened to leave AMA.	Cases reviewed; no control group and no statistical analysis.	1. No pattern to psychiatric diagnoses. 2. Three reasons were cited for wanting to leave AMA; fear and failure to orient to the hospital environment, anger at dependency and loss of control, psychotic reactions including, though not limited to, depression. 3. Emotional signs and other symptoms which occurred prior to the crisis: sleeplessness which is medicated, daytime restlessness, displays of anger and tears.

(continued)

Table 1 (continued)

Authors	Year	Population	Method	Findings/conclusions
Gillum and Barsky	1974	Patients under a physician's care.	Review of the literature of 40 papers.	1. Patient noncompliance is a major therapeutic problem in approximately 50% of all patients. 2. Four major categories: psychological, environmental and social, characteristics of regime, properties of patient-doctor relationship. 3. Psychological: a. 40% never intended to comply. b. Without adequate coping mechanisms they blame staff when they see the extent of their problem. c. Patients can be defensive, arrogant, aggressive, immature, and unreceptive. 4. Environmental and social: a. When poverty and unemployment are factors, compliance declines. b. Adopting new patterns of behavior, family arrangements, assistance, and reinforcement are difficult. c. Patients from families in disharmony or those living alone have the most difficulty. 5. Characteristics of regime: a. Better when simple. b. Profound changes in habits are difficult; complexity promotes noncompliance. 6. Patient-doctor relationship: a. Feelings of not being understood. b. Need good rapport and free communication. c. If formal and rejecting, or expresses flat disagreement. d. Failure to give feedback.

Planansky and Johnston	1976	200 male psychiatric patients.	100 AMA patients compared to 100 non-AMA patients. Global assessment of personality, illness, and personal situation at time of AMA. Statistical comparison on age, marital status, and diagnosis.	1. 5% of population submitted AMA. 2. Younger patients go AMA. 3. More single, separated, and divorced among the AMA. 4. Diagnoses quite diverse; however, impatience, low tolerance for frustration, panic or crises state not viewed as symptomatic of illness by the patients. These features viewed by staff as symptomatic of mental illness. 5. Global assessments: a. Fleeting need for gratification. b. Unwillingness or inability to communicate. c. Unable to accept discipline. d. Denial of illness. e. Aggression at staff and procedures. f. Loss of freedom or autonomy in real life projected onto hospital staff in the transient situation.
Jankowski and Drum	1977	10,600 general hospital patients.	73 AMA patients compared to 175 non-AMA patients drawn from the total population. Charts were reviewed for sex, diagnoses, and reason for leaving.	1. AMA men to women: 2.2:1.0 vs non-AMA men to women: 1:1.3. 2. Alcoholism and drug abuse were factors in AMA patients. Also, personality disorders, though perhaps as correlate to drug abuse. 3. Cited reasons for leaving were personal and family problems, dissatisfaction with staff and hospital, and refusal of further treatment. For those patients with substance abuse, there was a higher incidence of those who gave no reason for leaving.
Blackwell	1979	Patients receiving pharmacotherapy.	Review of 24 articles on drug compliance.	1. Physicians work on the model that order will be followed. 2. Failure to take medication can lead to dramatic ill effects, or represent a statement of not wanting to lead an artificial existence.

(continued)

Table 1 (continued)

Authors	Year	Population	Method	Findings/conclusions
Blackwell (cont'd.)				3. Patients do not tell the truth to their physicians about difficulties in adherence. 4. Previous experience of benefit leads to adherence skepticism, alternate belief systems; and previous failure leads to poor compliance. 5. Some patients want care and not chemicals. They wish attention and concern and prefer the dependent position.
Schlaugh, Reich, and Kelly	1979	21,333 general hospital admissions.	Chart reviews of all patients leaving AMA in a 2-year period. Factors studied were sex, race, socio-economic status, severity of illness, previous admissions, symptoms at time of discharge.	1. 0.7% of patients leave AMA. 2. Of the AMA patients, 58% are substance abusers. 3. Patients who leave AMA tend to be young, Black, and male. AMA tends to be within the first 5 days. Lower socioeconomic status is a factor, though unrelated to race. 4. At time of discharge the patients showed anxiety and agitation. On the surface, anger is noted, though hypothesis that panic and helplessness is the primary experience. There is impaired comprehension, judgment, and control.

Aminoff and Simon	1980	98 patients with status epilepticus admitted to a general hospital.	Review of records.	1. Failure to comply with medication regime through erratic injestion or discontinuance of medication. 2. Three times as many men as women were admitted with a generalized major motor status. 3. Alcoholism was a factor in 20% of the cases.
Harper, Elliott-Harper, Weinerman, Anderson, and Nelson	1982	127 varied psychiatric patients on short-term assessment and treatment unit.	Chart reviews of demographic, history, assessment, and diagnostic variables of AMA and non-AMA patients.	1. Diagnoses of personality disorder and substance abuse differentiate AMA and non-AMA patients. 2. AMA patients have a poorer mental status, though better perception of self in social functioning and are more street-wise. 3. Those who go AMA stress biological rather than psychological factors in their admission. 4. AMA patients do not relate to psychological explanations.
Lipton	1982	Elderly.	Review of sociodemographic characteristics in use of prescription drugs.	1. Failure to comply with medication regime may be due to memory loss, complexity of regime, social isolation, lack of knowledge, high cost of compliance, attitudes toward professionals, and impaired senses.

hospital care. With rare exception, they were street-addicts, living off the streets and injesting opiates, pentazocine, and cocaine as their three main illegal drugs. Alcohol use was also high. The veterans in the group to be studied were drawn from this population. These patients were using chemicals for an average of 18 years, and 70% reported criminal charges for other than possession of drugs or disorderly conduct. Their demographic characteristics are presented in Table 2.

Patients are referred to the Drug Dependency Treatment Unit either directly from Hospital Admissions or by the Psychiatry Admitting Clinic. The primary diagnosis is one or more DSM III drug or alcohol abuse categories. Clinical experience suggests that the majority of patients are character disorders. However, the personality disorders are not classified as to type, nor are those who acknowledge psychic distress as a factor in their motivational pattern differentiated from the antisocial personality who has little concern with how his/her behavior impacts on others within the environment. The life-styles of the individuals appear, at first glance, to share characteristics in common with the antisocial personality, previously termed "psychopath" or "sociopath." A small percentage of patients present symptoms of more traditional psychiatric significance, and patients known to the unit who have a previous diagnosis of schizophrenia or a major affective disorder are admitted. Overtly toxic and functionally psychotic individuals are not admitted to the unit.

Characteristics of the Unit

The Drug Dependency Treatment Unit is composed of inpatient and outpatient sections, and is coordinated by a psychologist. The inpatient section has a physician from the Medical Service as primary physician, with nursing staff, a clinical psychologist, a social worker, and drug counselors providing support services. The inpatient unit admits patients for detoxification for a minimum of 2 weeks and a maximum 1 month. During this period they live on a locked unit, going off the unit for meals, recreational activities, and clinic appointments. While on the unit the patients are expected to remain free from illegal drug use and criminal activities. They are assigned to a "primary counselor" for individual and group counseling. Patients are also provided other medical surgical, dental, legal, and psychiatric services assessed appropriate. They attend various educational groups which provide vocational, nutritional, and psychological information.

Method

In the period February 1981 to October 1982 patients who presented symptomatology of a psychiatric nature, had a previous psychiatric diagnosis, or were seen as a management/assessment problem were assigned by the

Table 2

Demographic Characteristics of Patient Population

N	57
Age (yr)	
Range	24-59
Mean	33.9
Race (%)	
White	8
Black	90
Spanish-American	2
Marital status (%)	
Single	28
Divorced/separated	56
Married/widowed	16
Employment status (%)	
Employed	21
Not employed	79
Education status (yr)	
Range	8-15
Mean	12.4
Legal status (%)[a]	
No criminal record	10
No information	21
Disorderly, other noncriminal offenses	57
Gambling	6
Drug charges	32
Theft, forgery, burglary, etc.	93
Assault, homicide, rape, etc.	26
Drug use	
Age of initial use (yr)	
Range	12-24
Mean	16.1
Length of use (yr)	
Range	7-37
Median	17.9
Type first used (%)	
Alcohol	23
Alcohol and drugs	25
Drugs	52
Lifetime use (%)	
Range	29-72
Mean	50.4

[a]Numbers exceed 100% due to multiple convictions.

administrative coordinator to the clinical psychologist for individual psychotherapy. The therapeutic model and clinical posture taken was that of a participant/observer,* exploring the inner mental life of the patient, providing attention, validation of their experience, structure, and support.

During this 21-month period, a total of 57 patients were seen. They were asked if they wished to engage in individual psychotherapy in addition to counseling and were informed of the nature of the commitment. All of the patients who were assigned agreed to the sessions. They received three sessions of one-half hour each per week.

Compliance data were gathered for the study patients as well as for all patients during this 21-month period. Compliance was defined as remaining for the agreed upon time and neither leaving against medical advice nor being given a disciplinary discharge for stealing, illegal drug use, or violent behavior.

RESULTS

During this period the overall compliance rate measured by AMA (against medical advice), AWOL (absent without leave), and disciplinary discharge status was 54% for the total population; the data are presented in Table 3. The compliance rate for those patients engaged in individual psychotherapy was 60%. These figures are also presented in Table 3. A chi-square test comparing frequencies yields a nonsignificant finding of 1.70. Thus, analyzing the data in this manner would suggest that individual psychotherapy does not significantly affect compliance in treatment. However, graphs of the compliance data (Figs. 1 and 2) suggested that parameters might be operating which do affect compliance.

Figure 1 represents the cumulative frequency of all patients admitted to the Drug Dependency Center between February 1981 and October 1982, as well as the cumulative noncompliance rate for all counselors. Figure 2 represents the cumulative frequency of all psychotherapy patients assigned during the same period, as well as the cumulative noncompliance rate for the professional psychotherapist. Beginning in February 1981 the participant/observer model of brief psychotherapy was attempted. Figure 2 reveals that by June 1981 the compliance rate for those patients engaged in individual psychotherapy was stabilized. Between June 1981 and April 1982 the total compliance rate for psychotherapy patients was 85%, compared to 58% for all counselors during the same period. A chi-square test yields a significant result of 5.52 ($df = 1$; $p < .02$). This suggests that individual psychotherapy does affect compliance, though other parameters must be considered.

*This brief psychotherapy/consultation model of treatment was developed between February and May 1981 with a senior staff member and psychoanalyst from the University of Illinois, Hyman Muslin, MD.

Table 3

Compliance Rates for a 21-Month Period

Group	Parameter		χ^2
All patients	Admissions, *N*	617	
	Compliance, *f*	336	
	Compliance, %	54	
			1.70[a]
Psychotherapy patients	Referrals, *N*	57	
	Compliance, *f*	33	
	Compliance, %	60	

[a] *df* = 1, nonsignificant.

In May of 1982 the noncompliance rate again rose for a short time and then stabilized. This dramatic change is viewed as representing the changes that went on among patient, psychotherapist, and environment. The psychotherapist had been previously assigned half-time for the period February 1981 to May 1982. She was assigned to the Drug Dependency Treatment Center on a full-time basis beginning June 1982. The assignment was to engage only in clinical duties. Prior to February 1981 she had been the full-time administrator of the unit. With her reappointment of full-time status on the unit, the patients were educated to the differences between administrative and clinical functions, and to the fact that clinical psychotherapy engages the individual to act rather than react within an environment. Having completely separated administrative from clinical functions at this time, there was an additional, interesting, anecdotal finding that the patient government was formed at this time, and that six out of six patients assigned between July and September became officers and founding members of the new patient government.

DISCUSSION AND RECOMMENDATIONS

The intent of this study was to look at compliance in a drug abuse detoxification/rehabilitation unit as a function of involvement in professional psychotherapy. The results suggest that professional psychotherapy can be effective in increasing patient compliance for a particularly difficult patient group. Previous studies in compliance suggest that four factors may account for failure to comply: threatening aspects of the ward environment, the nature of the patient-doctor relationship, external factors such as family influences, and internal dynamics. Few external factors, however, necessarily account for the selective perception and internal mechanisms which lead to communication or misunderstanding; to inability to face conflict, individual opinion, and discussion of issues in an emotionally supportive and rational atmosphere; to feelings of

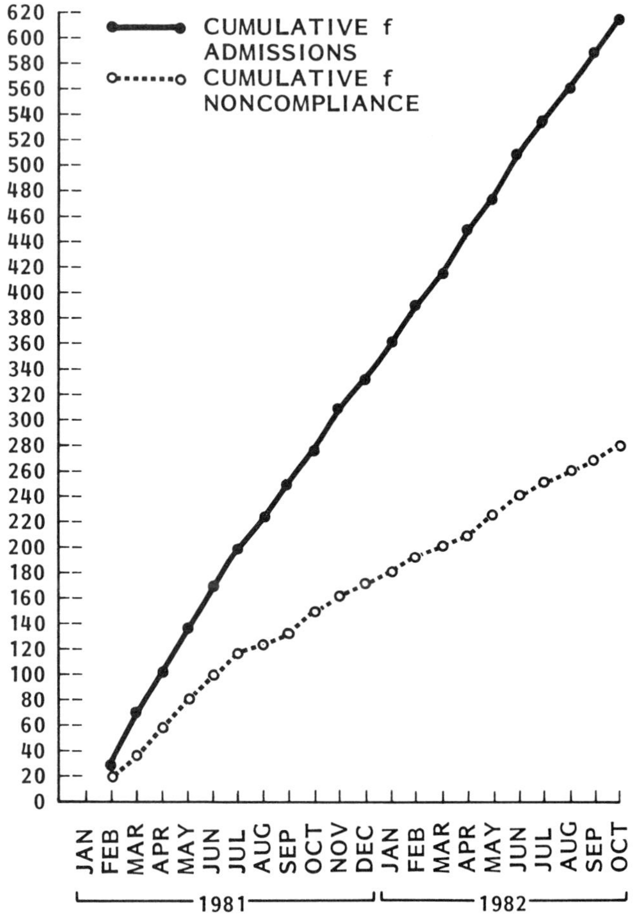

Fig. 1. Cumulative frequency of all patients admitted and cumulative noncompliance between February 1981 and October 1982.

isolation and hopelessness or lack of acceptance within the group; or to increased agitation, restlessness, and symptomatology from unexplainable impulses. The compliance figures between June 1981 and April 1982 suggest that the internal dynamics of the patients were balanced with the three external factors to produce patients who adhered to the treatment regime without elopement. Upon the psychotherapist's return to the unit of a full-time basis, this equilibrium was broken temporarily and then reestablished.

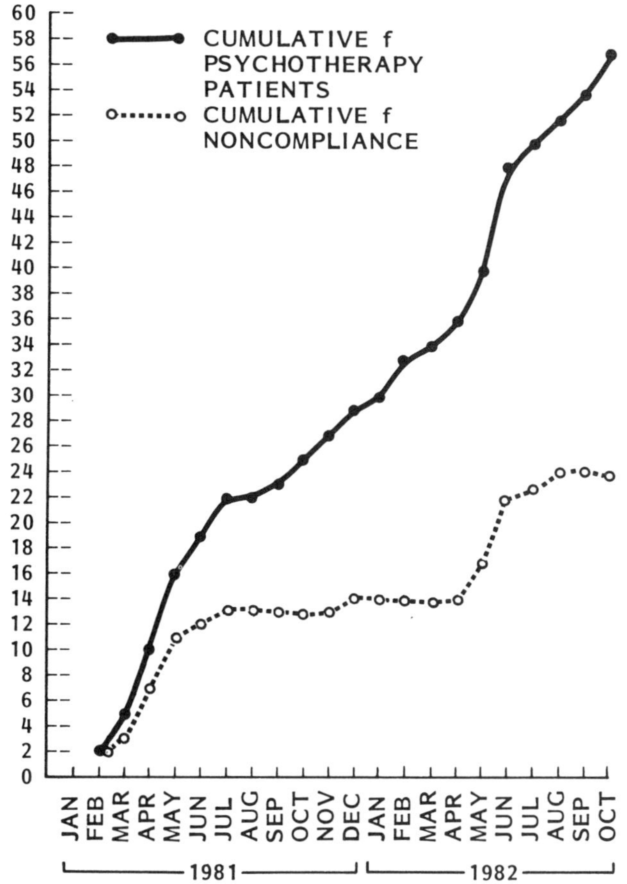

Fig. 2. Cumulative frequency psychotherapy patients and cumulative noncompliance between February 1981 and October 1982.

These findings are consistent with those reported by George Woody and his associates in Philadelphia (Woody, 1982; Woody et al., 1982) that professional psychotherapy in addition to routine paraprofessional counseling services results in greater improvement in patients. This was particularly true for patients who possessed high levels of psychiatric symptoms (McLellan et al., 1983). In the Philadelphia Veterans Administration, administrators paid particular attention to the psychotherapy program and administered it as an integral part of ongoing treatment services. Clinical supervision by senior staff members was provided, and morale issues for the staff members were not ignored but addressed.

Cooperation rather than competition between professional psychotherapists and paraprofessional counselor was stressed, and specific care was taken to define roles and differentiate skills and functions.

Internal politics within an institution have been observed by the experienced clinician to have a great deal to do with the implementation of professionalism within a program. Since environments provided for clients vary dependent on the type of interpersonal interactions which the staff find acceptable for their own self-cohesion, they often serve to maintain the status quo and prevent short-range conflict rather than provide the true nurturance for clients. Separation and individuation of personalities is often discouraged in both client and staff member, and there is hestiancy to provide role models which appear too discrepant from the modal consciousness of the community. Those patients who begin to differentiate themselves from the modal personalities in either the treatment environment or the environments to which they return will find a lack of support from their communities and, in fact, a direct challenge to the emerging self. Compliance with the directive to change their interpersonal milieu and intrapsychic functioning will become a threat to the social, intellectual, and emotional structure of their own communities.

Future directions are recommended for the Westside Drug Dependency Treatment Center, including administrative support for professional psychotherapy, psychological rehabilitation, clinical supervision by senior staff members, encouragement of paraprofessional staff to seek supportive treatment, and assessment research which would correlate objective data with treatment outcome. Thus, treatment energies could be focused on those patients most able to benefit, thus assisting the patients, as well as the treatment personnel, to form mutually enhancing alliances. Under such an organized program, patient satisfaction and staff morale would be improved. In addition, the individual consultation model could potentially operate for all distressed patients who are unable to establish equilibrium in the patient role and could aid in the short-term goal of patient management. Long-term incorporation of internal guidelines for self-care would necessitate continuing research and differentiation of the factors which lead to the development of self-caring individuals and the types of internal mechanisms and external supports necessary to maintain equilibrium.

REFERENCES

ALBERT, H.D., and KORNFELD, D.S. The threat to sign out against medical advice. *Ann. Intern. Med.* 79: 888-891, 1973.

ALTMAN, H., BROWN, M.L., and SLETTEN, I.W. And . . . silently steal away. *Dis. Nerv. Syst.* 33: 52-58, 1972.

AMINOFF, M.J., and SIMON, R.P. Status epilepticus: Causes, clinical features and consequences in 98 patients. *Am. J. Med.* 69: 657-666, 1980.

ATKINSON, R.M. AMA and AWOL discharges: A six-year comparative study. *Hosp. Community Psychiatry* 22: 17-20, 1971.

BLACKWELL, B. Treatment adherence: A contemporary overview. *Psychsomatics* 20: 27-35, 1979.

DANIELS, R.S., MARGOLIS, P.M., and CARSON, R.C. Hospital discharges against medical advice. Part I. Origin and prevention. *Arch. Gen. Psychiatry* 8: 30-40, 1963.

GILLUM, R.F., and BARSKY, A.J. Diagnosis and management of patient noncompliance. *J. Am. Med. Assoc.* 228: 1563-1578, 1974.

GREENWALD, A.F., and BARTEMEIER, L.H. Psychiatric discharges against medical advice. *Arch. Gen. Psychiatry* 28: 117-119, 1963.

HARPER. D.W., ELLIOTT-HARPER, C., WEINERMAN, R., ANDERSON, N.J., and NELSON, T.A. A comparison of AMA and non-AMA patients on a short-term crisis unit. *Hosp. Community Psychiatry* 33: 46-48, 1982.

HAYNES, R.B., TAYLOR, D.W., and SACKETT, D.L. *Compliance in Health Care.* Baltimore: Johns Hopkins University Press, 1979.

JANKOWSKI, C.B., and DRUM, D.E. Diagnostic correlates of discharge against medical advice. *Arch. Gen. Psychiatry* 34: 153-155, 1977.

LEWIS, W.C., LORENZ, T.H., and CALDEN, G. Irregular discharge from tuberculosis hospitals. *Psychosom. Med.* 17: 276-290, 1955.

LIAZOS, A. The poverty of the sociology of deviance: Nuts, sluts, and perverts. *Soc. Probl.* 20: 103-120, 1972.

LIPTON, H.L. The graying of America: Implications for the pharmacist. *Am. J. Hosp. Pharm.* 39: 131-135, 1982.

MC LELLAN, A.T., LUBORSKY, L., WOODY, G.E., O'BRIEN, C.P., and DRULEY, K.A. Predicting response to alcohol and drug abuse treatments: Role of psychiatric severity. *Arch. Gen. Psychiatry* 40: 620-625, 1983.

MEYER, G.G., and MARTIN, J.B., and LANGE, P. Elopement from the open psychiatric unit: A two-year study. *J. Nerv. Ment. Dis.* 144: 297-304, 1967.

MEYER, G.G., MARGOLIS, P.M., and DANIELS, R.S. Hospital discharges against medical advice. Part II. Outcome. *Arch. Gen. Psychiatry* 8: 41-48, 1963.

PLANANSKY, K., and JOHNSTON, R. A survey of patients leaving a mental hospital against medical advice. *Hosp. Community Psychiatry* 27: 865-868, 1976.

RAYNES, A.E., and PATCH, V.D. Distinguishing features of patients who discharge themselves from psychiatric ward. *Comprehensive Psychiatry* 12: 473-479, 1971.

SACKETT, D.L., and HAYNES, R.B. (eds.). *Compliance with Therapeutic Regimens.* Baltimore: Johns Hopkins University Press, 1976.

SCHLAUGH, R.W., REICH, P., and KELLY, M.J. Leaving the hospital against medical advice. *N. Engl. J. Med.* 300: 22-24, 1979.

WOODY, G.E. Personal communication, 1982.

WOODY, G.E., LUBORSKY, L., MC LELLAN, A.T., O'BRIEN, C.P., and BECK, A.T. *Psychotherapy for opiate addicts: Does it help?* NIDA Contract Report, Philadelphia, 1982.

The International Journal of the Addictions, 19(5), 541–549, 1984

Alcohol Use by Juvenile Offenders

Bernard Segal, PhD

Center for Alcohol and Addiction Studies
University of Alaska, Anchorage
Anchorage, Alaska 99508

Steven S. Hobfoll, PhD

Department of Sociology of Health
Ben Gurion University of the Negev
Beersheva, Israel

Fred Cromer, PhD

Mathematical Sciences
University of Alaska, Anchorage
Anchorage, Alaska 99508

Abstract

Reasons for alcohol use were examined in a sample of detained and adjudicated juveniles at a state residential facility. By means of factor analysis, patterns of self-reported reasons for using alcohol were identified. The findings suggest that alcohol appears to have become primarily associated with coping and/or altering mood. The implications of this finding are briefly discussed with respect to treatment and prevention.

INTRODUCTION

This study explores the nature of self-reported reasons for drinking reported by juvenile offenders and seeks to determine if identifiable patterns of use and reasons for use can be found. Recent research (Segal, Huba, and Singer, 1980) has shown that relatively independent and specific factors for use of alcohol can be identified, and that such use needs to be understood in terms of a multidimensional rather than a unidimensional

 0020-773X/84/1905-0541$3.50/0

approach. The present study seeks to extend the work of Segal et al. (1980) to a juvenile population.

Although research (Ellinwood, 1971; Simonds and Kashani, 1979, 1980; Tinklenberg, 1974; Tinklenberg et al., 1981) has begun to focus on substance abuse by delinquent youth, such investigations have generally attempted to determine the nature of the relationship between drug use and criminal offense(s). Other studies have sought to identify personality correlates of drug-using juvenile offenders (Beachy, Petersen and Pearson, 1979; Braught, Brakarsh, Follingstad, and Berry, 1973; Cocketz, 1971; Stayton and Diener, 1979). Blane and Chafetz (1980), however, looked at the relationship between dependency needs and sex-role identity and drinking in delinquent juveniles, and found that while dependency needs were related to alcohol use, sex-role identity was not associated with drinking behavior. It was believed by Blane and Chafetz that the drinking behavior shown by their sample "may be prodomed to alcoholism." The relationship of drinking to the seriousness of the offense was not conclusive. Their findings nevertheless demonstrated that psychological factors, such as a need for autonomy and independence, may be important mediating factors related to the drinking behavior of the juveniles in their study. The present study, while also concerned with the role of psychological factors in youthful drinking behavior, attempts to focus on identifying patterns of reasons for drinking. In this manner we can explore more closely what some of the motives are which contribute to drinking behavior rather than simply focusing on drinking per se. This approach may help to provide more specific knowledge concerning the early precursors or roots of problem drinking.

METHOD

Subjects

A sample population of 92 detained or adjudicated males was obtained from among the residents of the State of Alaska's residential youth facility, the McLaughlin Youth Center, located in Anchorage, Alaska, during the spring of 1979. Table 1 presents a description of some of the background characteristics of the sample. Briefly, ages ranged from 12 to 18, with a mean and median age of 16 years. Eighteen of the participants were Alaska Natives, 59 were White, 1 was Black, and 14 did not indicate ethnicity. The youth housed at the center were from all over the state, with 52 from cities and 40 from smaller, rural communities. Some of the participants were detained awaiting adjudication of offenses, while others were adjudicated as delinquent and remanded to the custody of the Youth Center. Their offenses ranged fom petty theft, such as shoplifting, to assault and murder. The most frequent offense was for breaking

Table 1

Background Characteristics[a]

Age (yr)	N	Predominant charge	N
12	1	Breaking and entering	16
14	8	Burglary	12
15	17	Joy riding	10
16	29	Theft	6
17	28	Alcohol/drug charges	6
18	8	Grand theft auto	5
19	1	Assault/disorderly conduct	5
Mean = 16, SD = 1.2		Runaway	5
		Armed robbery	3
Ethnic group	N	Other charges	19
Alaskan Native	18	Not known	15
Non-Native	59		
Black	1		
Not stated	14		

[a]From Segal et al., 1982a.

and entering, followed by burglary. Other offenses included joy riding, alcohol- or drug-related offenses, and grand theft auto.

All participants volunteered to take part in the study after the research project was explained to them and their anonymity was ensured. The questionnaires were administered in a single setting in groups of 20-30 within each of the cottage units. Only male residents' profiles were used in the study due to the small number of female residents (fewer than 10) who were at the center at the time of the study.

Instruments

Each participant completed a brief assessment battery consisting of the Alcohol-Drug Use Survey (Segal, 1979a), the Interest and Preference Inventory (Segal, 1979b), and the State-Trait Anxiety Scale (Spielberger et al., 1970). In addition to obtaining basic demographic information, the Alcohol-Drug Use Survey is designed to elicit self-reports on the extent, duration, and frequency of use of alcohol and other drugs, together with reasons for such use. The survey contains a total of 25 questions specifically related to reasons for alcohol use. The responses to these items constituted the source of data for this report.

Procedure

Following an analysis of the frequency of responses to the reasons for using alcohol, five reasons were excluded from further analysis due to lack of response.

The remaining 20 reasons were analyzed using a principal components analysis with a varimax rotation. Following the derivation of a seven-factor solution, the factor correlation matrix derived from the seven-factor solution was also subjected to a principal components procedure, with a varimax rotation, to obtain higher- or second-order factors. A three-factor second-order solution was obtained.

RESULTS

Of the 92 completed profiles which were obtained, all 92 respondents, including the younger-age residents (12-16 years), reported drinking alcoholic beverages (beer, wine, or whiskey) prior to their detention. The principal components analysis of the 20 reasons for drinking yielded a seven-factor solution which accounted for 62% of the total variance. This seven-factor solution adequately met the test of significance; that is, it reproduced the correlation matrix ($\chi^2 = 390.2, p < .05$).

Table 2 presents the results of the principal components procedure. Inspection of Factor I reveals a combination of loadings which indicate that persons who score high on this factor tend to use alcohol to help deal or cope with a variety of feelings and problems. High loadings on this factor are for the use of alcohol to relieve sadness, anger, loneliness, and pressure, and to forget one's problems. The modest but negative loading for "makes parties more fun" provides additional support to suggest that this factor represents use of alcohol to transcend problems and/or unwanted feelings. The pattern of loading for this factor closely resembles the first factor extracted by Segal et al. (1980) in their analysis of motives for drinking by youthful college students. Both these factors closely fit what Jessor, Graves, Hanson, and Jessor (1968) described as a personal-effects motive; that is, using alcohol to solve personal problems.

It appears that alcohol has come to be perceived and used as a means of coping with personal needs and problems. The finding by Cahalan, Cisin, and Crossley (1969), from their national survey of drinking practices, that people who were depressed or anxious used alcohol to help with their problems, raises the question of whether "drinking to cope" may be related to a prealcoholic syndrome. Nevertheless, it is apparent that adolescent drinking may be, in large part, related to the perception by adolescents that alcohol provides a means of helping one to deal with problems and unpleasant feelings. This perception, it would appear, may be acquired from the way in which alcohol is used in society as a whole, in which alcohol is portrayed as a socially acceptable beverage which helps one to deal with stress or to resolve problems (Barnes, 1981; Stumphauzer, 1980). It may also be that adolescence is the time when youth begin to differentiate between the social qualities involved in drinking and in the self-medicating use of alcohol. Additionally, since alcohol is not legally available to these minors,

Table 2

Rotated Primary Factor Loadings of Self-Reported Reasons for Alcohol Use

	Factors						
Reasons	I	II	III	IV	V	VI	VII
Feeling sad	.83	–.08	.10	–.03	–.10	–.06	–.11
Personal problems	.78	.05	.09	.14	.03	.03	.05
Because of loneliness	.72	.14	–.24	–.08	–.07	–.30	–.05
Feeling mad	.66	.09	.01	.23	.00	.03	.10
Feeling under pressure	.58	–.18	.00	–.33	.32	.08	.24
Not person want to be	.17	.10	.69	.22	–.18	.13	–.34
Makes parties more fun	–.30	.56	.11	–.04	–.08	.09	.09
To worry less	.07	.72	–.31	.10	.11	–.06	–.20
To get along better	.16	.64	.10	.03	–.03	.30	.28
To feel happier	.10	.31	.41	–.20	.21	.29	–.01
To forget problems	.45	.09	.41	–.16	.25	.17	.09
To relax	.00	.03	.59	.20	.16	–.12	.06
To relieve pain	.18	.06	–.55	.46	.21	–.10	–.02
After hard work	.21	–.02	.00	.71	–.22	.24	.11
Hot weather	–.14	–.01	.21	.70	.28	–.03	–.01
To be sociable	–.01	–.04	–.08	.04	.81	.10	–.18
Nothing else to do	.01	.13	.17	.11	.44	–.48	.31
Just feel like it	.01	–.03	–.01	.10	–.17	–.10	.90
On special occasions	–.03	.09	–.10	.20	.13	.84	–.05

its consumption might tend to be more in line with "coping behavior" than chiefly for social motives.

Factor II shows its highest loading for using alcohol to worry less, followed by loadings for getting along better, to feel better, to feel happier, and to make parties more fun. This factor represents what might be called a "mood change" factor, or using alcohol to change one's subjective affective state. Another way of describing these loadings is using alcohol to reduce personal discomfort by getting high. It is interesting to note that this factor was not found in Segal et al.'s (1980) research with college students.

Factor III has its highest loading for using alcohol because you are not the person you want to be, followed by loadings for using alcohol to feel happier, to forget problems, and to relax. Loading negatively on this factor are use of alcohol to relieve pain and to worry less. This constellation of loadings suggests that this factor represents using alcohol to deal with and/or cope with personal stress and/or tension. Alcohol, as also suggested by Factors I and II, may be serving as a form of self-medication to relieve personal discomfort or stress.

Factor IV's loadings for using alcohol after hard work, in hot weather, and to relieve pain appear to suggest that this factor may reflect the influence of advertising, particularly television commercials for beer, which portray drinking as a reward for hard work or as a means of cooling off, etc. A parallel explanation is that this factor may represent a thirst-quenching factor. The modest inverse loading for feeling under pressure on this factor gives further indication that Factor IV may well represent a "recreational" use factor.

Factor V is represented by a high loading for drinking to be sociable, with accompanying loadings for nothing else to do and, although modest, for feeling under pressure. This factor seems to represents the social aspects of drinking, which are apparently linked to overcoming boredom and to relieving some degree of personal discomfort, particularly in social situations.

Factor VI, with a high loading for drinking on special occasions, together with a moderately high negative loading for drinking because of nothing else to do, would appear to represent a tendency to drink on those special occasions in which alcohol use is sanctioned or institutionalized. This pattern of drinking may represent the beginning of "ritualistic drinking," which is part of our society's drinking behavior.

The last factor, Factor VII, represents drinking because one "just feels like it," and to overcome boredom. This factor, together with Factors V and VI, appears to represent nonproblematic drinking.

The correlations among the primary factors were simplified by extracting three second-order factors using a principal components analysis. The second-order factors were rotated using an oblique procedure. The original variables were then projected onto the second-order factors using the procedure described by Gorsuch (1974). The resulting second-order factor structure did not yield any appreciable loadings on any of the three factors which were derived. Accordingly, there is no indication of any underlying influences among the original seven primary factors. This lack of definable second-order factors indicates that the seven primary factors are relatively independent.

DISCUSSION

The results of the factor analytic procedures indicate that different patterns or factors of reasons for using alcohol exist for the youthful sample of residents of a juvenile detention facility. The seven factors which emerged can be labeled as follows: (1) Personal Problem Solving, (2) Mood Altering, (3) Personal Stress/Tension, (4) Recreational, (5) Social, (6) Ritualistic, and (7) No Special Reason. These findings are consistent with previous research which has identified specific motives or reasons for drinking (Jessor et al., 1968; Segal et al., 1980). Table 3 presents a brief summary of the findings of the factor analysis.

The nature of the factor structure for this sample of youthful males shows quite clearly that alcohol is primarily perceived, at an early age, as something to alter mood and/or to free oneself from conflict or problems. This basic motive

Table 3

Summary of Factors Obtained as Reasons for Drinking

Factor	Summary
I. Personal Problem Solving	Drinking to cope with problems and/or to transcend unwanted feelings.
II. Mood Altering	Drinking to alter mood or to reduce personal discomfort.
III. Personal Stress/Tension	Drinking to reduce stress or tension.
IV. Recreational	Drinking to cool off or to quench a thirst.
V. Social	Drinking related to social situations.
VI. Ritualistic	Drinking on special occasions.
VII. No Special Reason	Drinking because one "just feels like it."

for using alcohol was also found by Van Houten and Golembiewski (1978) in their study of alcohol abuse by juveniles (ages 11-17) who were runaways. Additionally, drinking was reported in their sample as something to do when bored or angry, and when nervous or worried.

This relationship between alcohol and a need to alter one's mood leads us to speculate that adolescent drinking behavior may have more to do with personal needs and stresses than with peer pressure to drink. While peers may help to initiate one to use of alcohol, the subsequent drinking behavior which occurs may be more of a function of personal processes than interpersonal ones. The findings of Huba, Wingard, and Bentler (1979) that adolescents' use of drugs is unrelated to any specialized pattern of interaction with peers or adults, gives added weight to the contention that drinking during adolescence may be more related to attempts to cope than to other reasons.

It appears to be fairly evident from our findings that adolescents have learned to associate alcohol with mood change; that is, as a mood elevator or tranquilizer. Whether this process is related to their modeling of perceptions and actions of the larger society with respect to alcohol, or is related to a modeling of parental drinking attitudes and practices, is in need of further exploration. One would assume, however, that it is an interactive process involving both family and societal attitudes, but it is nevertheless important to begin to understand the contribution of each. Stumphauzer (1980), in a study of adolescents with drinking problems, attributes such drinking to a "complex set of antecedent and consequent events" (p. 281), in which there is no evidence for negative or countercontrols. Part of the reinforcing process, however, was that alcohol did change the way they felt. "Feeling good" was an important and significant effect.

It should be noted that this research is based on exploring the drinking motives of a cohort of delinquent boys, and that these youngsters may be manifesting a pattern of drinking more representative of a group of troubled youth than that of more typical or untroubled adolescents. It would therefore be important to determine if these same factors or motives are present in a more normal or untroubled sample of adolescents. Research, which is currently being pursed by Segal et al. (1982b), has indicated that a major reason for taking/trying drugs, including alcohol, among junior and senior high school students, is to "feel better"; that is, to reduce or relieve stressful emotions. It thus appears, as Barnes (1981) has indicated, that there is evidence to suggest that adolescent drinking behavior may be less of a function of peer influences and more related to the attitudes and behaviors found in the larger adult society, which perceives alcohol as a means of helping to alleviate stress and/or to alter one's mood.

It is apparent that the ways in which attitudes toward alcohol develop in youth need to be examined more precisely, as well as how alcohol becomes associated with coping and/or mood change. The implications for treatment of alcohol misuse and for prevention of alcohol abuse seem clear: The perceptual or attitudinal link between alcohol and mood change or coping needs to be broken. It is important to recognize that adolescents might not simply drink to "feel good," but to "feel better." With respect to treatment or intervention strategies for institutionalized, and seemingly troubled youth, it may well be that in addition to helping them to develop better coping skills, as well as focusing on attempting to relieve the stress which they appear to be experiencing, it may also be helpful to work with these youngsters to achieve more *desirable alternative involvements* which are more rewarding than drug experiences and which are incompatible with reliance on chemicals.

REFERENCES

BEACHY, G.M., PETERSEN, D.M., and PEARSON, F.S. Adolescent drug use and delinquency: A research note. *J. Psychedelic Drugs* 11: 313-316, 1979.

BARNES, G.M. Drinking among adolescents: A subcultural phenomenon or a model of adult behaviors. *Adolescence* 61: 211-229, 1981.

BLANE, H.T., and CHAFETZ, M.E. Dependency conflict and sex-role identity in drinking delinquents. In J.E. Mayer and W.J. Filstead (eds.), *Adolescence and Alcohol.* Cambridge, MA: Ballinger, 1980.

BRAUGHT, G.N., BRAKARSH, D., FOLLINGSTAD, D., and BERRY, K. Deviant drug use in adolescents: A review of psychosocial correlates. *Psychol. Bull.* 79: 92-106, 1973.

CAHALAN, D., CISIN, J.H., and CROSSLEY, H.M. *American Drinking Practices* (Rutgers Center of Alcohol Studies, Monograph No. 6.). New Brunswick, NJ: Rutgers Center of Alcohol Studies, 1969.

COCKETZ, R. *Drug Abuse and Personality in Young Offenders.* New York: Appleton-Century-Crofts, 1971.

ELLINWOOD, E.H., Jr. Assault and homicide associated with amphetamine abuse. *Am. J. Psychiatry* 127: 1170-1176, 1971.

GORSUCH, J.L. *Factor Analysis.* Philadelphia: Saunders, 1974.

HUBA, G.J., WINGARD, J.A. and BENTLER, P.M. Adolescent drug use and peer and adult interaction patterns. *J. Consult. Clin. Psychol.* 47: 265-276, 1979.

JESSOR, R., GRAVES, T., HANSON, R., and JESSOR, S. *Society, Personality and Deviant Behavior* New York: Holt, Rinehart, and Winston, 1968.

SEGAL, B. *Alcohol-Drug Use Survey,* Rev. Unpublished manuscript, University of Alaska, Anchorage, 1979. (a)

SEGAL, B. *Interest and Preference Inventory.* Unpublished manuscript, University of Alaska, Anchorage, 1979. (b)

SEGAL, B., HOBFOLL, S., CROMER, F., and WASSERMAN, P. Patterns of reasons for drug use among detained and adjudicated juveniles. *Int. J. Addict.* 17: 1117-1130, 1982. (a)

SEGAL, B., HUBA, G., and SINGER, J.L. *Drugs, Daydreaming and Personality: A Study of College Youth.* Hillsdale, NJ: Lawrence Erlbaum, 1980.

SEGAL, B., MC KELVY, J., BOWMAN, D., and MALA, T. *Substance taking/trying among high school students.* Unpublished manuscript, University of Alaska, Anchorage, 1982.(b)

SIMONDS, J.F., and KASHANI, J. Drug abuse and criminal behavior in delinquent boys committed to a training school. *Am. J. Psychiatry* 136: 1444-1448, 1979.

SIMONDS, J.F., and KASHANI, J. Specific drug use and violence in delinquent boys. *Am. J. Drug Alcohol Use* 7: 304-322, 1980.

SPIELBERGER, C., GORSUCH, R., and LUSHENE, R. *Manual for the State-Trait Anxiety Inventory.* Palo Alto, CA: Consulting Psychologist Press, 1970.

STAYTON, S.E., and DIENER, R.G. Personality characteristics of juvenile delinquent herion users. *Int. J. Addict.* 14: 585-587, 1979.

STUMPHAUZER, J.S. Learning to drink: Adolescents and alcohol. *Addict. Behav.* 5: 277-283, 1980.

TINKLENBERG, J.R. Drug use among youthful assaultive and sexual offenders. *Res. Nerv. Ment. Dis.* 52: 209-224, 1974.

TINKLENBERG, J.R., MURPHY, P., MURPHY, P.L., and PFEFFERBAUM, A. Drugs and criminal assaults by adolescents: A replicate study. *J. Psychoactive Drugs* 13: 277-287, 1981.

VAN HOUTEN, T., and GOLEMBIEWSKI, G. *Adolescent Life Stress as a Predictor of Alcohol Abuse and/or Runaway Behavior.* Washington, DC: National Youth Alternative Project, 1978.

The International Journal of the Addictions, 19(5), 551-569, 1984

Defining Alcohol Problems as a Repressive Mechanism: Its Formative Phase in Imperial Germany and Its Strength Today*

Irmgard Vogt,† PhD

Abteilung für Sozialwissenschaft
Universität Bochum
West Germany

Abstract

In Germany, in the takeoff years of industrialization, judgments about drinking, drunkenness, and drunken comportment changed drastically. While for centuries drunkenness had been seen as the transitory effect of too much drinking, it now was perceived as a sign of moral weakness which afflicted most strongly the working class. Naming someone a drunkard, then, was as much a label for denouncement as for a sickness, which since then has been called alcoholism. It can be shown that structurally similar processes are in use in today's debate over the changing drinking habits of women in West Germany.

To understand the contemporary German discussion on alcohol consumption, alcohol problems, and alcoholism—with special depiction of so-called problem groups such as women and adolescents—one has to go back in history to

*Prepared for delivery at the 12th International Political Science Association Meeting, Rio de Janeiro, Brazil, August 9-14, 1982.

†Address correspondence to the author: Am Schloss 1, 4815 Schloss Holte, West Germany.

 0020-773X/84/1905-0551$3.50/0

the time when the concepts on drinking and drunkenness were formulated for the first time. Most important in the development of theories on alcohol consumption and alcoholism was the time of imperial Germany (1871-1918), in which all possible problems in connection with alcohol were brought forth in fierce public debates. Innumerable books and pamphlets were published on the issue of drinking, most of them warning against the "devil alcohol" and only a few favoring moderate drinking (cf. Cluss, 1906; Starke, 1906). From the very first beginning of the public debate on alcohol, the drinking habits of the working class stirred up discussion.

In what follows, I concentrate on the formation phase of defining alcohol problems as a repressive mechanism in imperial Germany. With respect to the debate over the drinking habits of women today, the continuities of the concepts on drinking and drunkenness from imperial Germany to the present are sketched out at the end of the paper.

Within West Europe, Germany has been notorious for its licentious drinking styles and habits, and its permissiveness for all possible manifestations of drunkenness. Indeed, there are many testimonies that for centuries, wine and beer were part of everyday meals (Schivelbusch, 1980; Teuteberg and Wiegelmann, 1972) as well as the prerequisites of all festivities and ceremonies which had to be celebrated. Descriptions of all degrees of drunkenness, without much comment on the behavior of the drinker, can easily be found in a multitude of historical documents (e.g., Bassermann-Jordan, 1923; Bauer, 1903; Christoffel, 1957; Hauffen, 1889; Voigt, 1973). Drunken comportment, whether violent, foolish, or otherwise deviant, was not seen as being distasteful or immoral, but was regarded as a natural result of too much drinking.

In the pre- and early industrialization period, hard liquor became the most common alcoholic beverage of the less affluent and the poor because it was easily available and fairly cheap in comparison to beer and wine. The latter, then, became the favorite beverages of the rich and the bourgeoisie, along with fine and expensive liqueurs.

Before showing in detail how the labeling of one's drinking habits as a social problem was used as one of the repressive mechanisms within the class struggles around the turn of the 19th century, let us first have a short look at the production of alcoholic beverages in the 19th century.

In Germany, between 1770 and 1790, it became well known and familiar to use potatoes as the natural agricultural product for the manufacturing of hard liquor. Up until that time, hard liquors were made from wheat, wine, and fruits such as cherries, plums, prunes, and many others. The quantities of hard liquor which could be produced depended on the richness of the yearly yields of the raw products. In years when there was a scarcity of the natural products—because of bad weather in the main harvest seasons, or because of crop destruction in thunderstorms or wars, or because of an epidemic increase of vermin—

there was not much left for the production of hard liquors. The yearly output varied, therefore, according to the harvest figures for the raw products. With the introduction of potatoes as the natural raw material for the production of hard liquor, the situation for the distilleries changed a great deal. They became much more independent of weather conditions and vermin epidemics because there were always enough potatoes, not only to feed people but to produce fairly large quantities of hard liquor as well. This holds especially for Prussia, where an abundance of potatoes were grown. Thus, the production of hard liquor went up by leaps and bounds around the beginning of the 19th century. It increased more steadily during the whole century, making the production of hard liquor from potatoes a profitable enterprise. With the beginning of the 19th century, potato distilleries already outnumbered those working with other raw materials. At the end of the century, most of the hard liquor on the market was made from potatoes (Briefs, 1912; Wassermann, 1909). Some of it was made for industrial use only. Quite some quantities of it were exported to other countries, especially Spain (Briefs, 1912), as well as to the German colonies in Africa (Pan, 1975; Timm, 1982). But most of the spirits produced were consumed by poor people in Germany working in all areas of the industrial and agricultural sectors (for detailed production and consumption data, see Vogt, 1982). Wheat, wine, and fruits as raw materials were used more and more for the production of high-quality liqueurs for the more affluent and rich.

But it was not only the introduction of the potato as a raw material which made the production of spirits go up steeply and steadily; it was also the invention of new machines which helped to increase the output of hard liquor from the same amount of the raw material while the production time decreased constantly. At the same time, the number of workers in the distilleries decreased as well. All these factors helped make it increasingly cheaper to produce large quantities of hard liquors. The production of spirits was one of the first sectors where big industries sprang up, organizing the market according to their own interests.

Of course, this could not be done against the political interests of the state, and indeed the state helped a great deal in the formation phase of the big distilleries. This was accomplished in general by politics in the agricultural sector (Puhle, 1975) and especially by taxation laws for the production and distribution of hard liquors. Within the boundaries of towns, the production of spirits had been taxed for centuries (for details, see Arntz, 1975; Hermbstädt, 1811; Wassermann, 1909), but not in rural areas. Thus, it was much more profitable to set up distilleries in rural areas, instead of towns, even if one had to transport the spirits to the people. With the change from wheat to potatoes as the raw material, quite a few new distilleries sprang up as additional production units in rural areas. Most of the hard liquor on the market, then, was produced in rural areas, and not in towns. According to the new situation the tax laws had to be rearranged and the production of hard liquor had to be taxed regardless of the site of the distillery. This was done at the beginning of the 19th century. In Prussia, in 1810, the taxation laws for hard liquor were expanded from towns to rural areas, and in 1820 the tax was set up according to the supposed productivity of the distilleries. Although the tax was very important as one of the sources of state income, it was fairly low compared with the profits made by the distillers. Besides, with the use of better techniques, which helped make the distillation process go faster with less costs, and with increasing production rates, all at the same time, it was quite possible to go far beyond the supposed productivity of the distillery, which meant making much better profits than was foreseen by the tax laws (Baer, 1878). This holds for the entire 19th century. Increases in taxation, which took place fairly often, had no effect on the quantity produced. On the contrary, the production of hard liquor went up steadily and proved to be a very profitable business for those who managed to expand their distillation capacity. On the other hand, the tax laws had a great impact on the formation of the distillation industry insofar as they favored big industrial setups. Tax increases led to an industrial concentration process. The politics of the state had the effect that in the long run a very strong lobby of big distillers was established which constantly tried to shape the tax laws according to their own interests, and with much success since the second half of the 19th century.

The invention of new production techniques and better machines had a great impact not only on the spirits industry but also on the processing of beer. In some regions of the German-speaking countries, especially in Prussia, beer production decreased heavily between 1750 and 1850, while at the same time the production of spirits shot up. In the second half of the 19th century, breweries slowly recovered from the breakdown of the market brought about by the supply of very cheap hard liquor made possible by the invention of new and cheaper brewing techniques and the establishment of more effective service and selling networks in the centers of industrialization (Biergans, 1959; Knoblauch, 1920; Körner, 1865; Struve, 1899). After 1850 production and consumption rates went up steadily until the First World War. In 1887 the first tax law for the German Reich was implemented, making spirits more expensive than before by raising the production tax, and beer regained quite a number of consumers who formerly preferred to drink spirits. Around 1900 beer could again compete very well with hard liquor; in comparing the amount of pure alcohol consumed by drinking beer and spirits, beer was at least as much accepted by the consumers as spirits. While beer became once more as popular as hard liquor, we can observe a concentration process of breweries similar to that described for distilleries. Thus, the number of small breweries decreased constantly by way of being incorporated into bigger ones, which soon were able to control the regional markets according to their interests.

Wine production did not follow the trend described for hard liquor and beer. During the last century there was no way for wine production to become independent of the yearly harvest. Wine production varied continuously from year to year according to the richness of the harvest. Neither the invention of new machines to make the work easier in the vineyards nor that of new techniques to process the wine was of much influence on the yearly harvest. How much wine could be produced and how good it would be depended on the weather conditions in the last century.

For the problem under discussion, then, hard liquor and beer are of most interest. There are two phases of production and consumption which can be differentiated. In the first half of the century the production and consumption of hard liquor dominated that of all other alcoholic beverages. This holds especially for Prussia. At the end of the century beer was as popular as hard liquor. People were more and more inclined to substitute beer for hard liquor. This does not mean that people were drinking less (Hoffmann, 1965; Vogt, 1981), they just enhanced their drinking habits in using different alcoholic beverages.

The increasing production of alcoholic beverages could be profitable only if there was enough demand for the product. Without a doubt, drugs of all sorts have attracted consumers throughout all centuries more than most other goods on the market because of a variety of effects which go with substances stimulating or depressing the central nervous system. Still, if starving people have the choice of buying either food or alcoholic beverages at a comparable price level, most of them certainly prefer to buy food. There are two ways to drastically influence the choice of consumers. The first is to lower the price of, for example, hard liquor below all levels of food prices; that is, make it as cheap as possible. Although there are no serious historical studies comparing the prices of different consumer goods, including hard liquor and beer, during the first half of the 19th century, there are indications that hard liquor was extremely cheap at that time, making it one of the most alluring goods on the market (Abel, 1981; Böttcher, 1839).

But there were much better ways of selling alcoholic beverages to an increasing number of customers, even at fairly high prices, simply by forcing workers of all professions into the "truck system." The "truck system" refers to a complex exchange modus of goods between employers and workers from which the former profited beyond the usual physical exploitation of the workers during the work hours. The truck system varied according to the setup of the work place. Most common were the following two types: (1) Up to one-half of the payment was given in real goods instead of money, such as very low-quality textiles or unhealthy foodstuff. (2) The workers were forced to buy their necessities of living in grocery stores which were set up by employers, who fixed and controlled the prices. Alcohol was one of the goods which were given to workers as payment instead of money (for details, see e.g., Ritter and Kocka, 1974; Stehr, 1904).

We deal here only with those aspects of the truck system which address themselves to alcoholic beverages. The system itself is not described further here. Even with alcohol, quite a number of different truck systems were in use, and some aspects were superimposed onto others.

For rural workers, the truck system of the 19th century was worse than comparable setups for industrial workers. Rural workers were indeed paid in part with spirits (for an example, see Bismarck, 1834). Since they were totally dependent on their employers, who were in control of their whole lives (Puhle, 1966), they had no choice whatsoever to refuse hard liquor as payment. They could not even trade it for other goods such as food or clothing because they lived in their own quarters, separated from others who might have an interest in hard liquor. The employers did nothing to change the habit; on the contrary, they reinforced it constantly. They preferred to have tipsy workers instead of sober ones, whom they suspected of being more willing to engage in the politics of the trade unions and Social Democratic Party. In the view of the employers, this meant social unrest, if not rebellion. Drunkards seldom engage in politics so long as there is enough to drink, which was guaranteed by quite a number of proprietaries who were at the same time the producers of hard liquor. Alcohol, then, was used not only as a payment, but as a tranquilizer, as well as a means for keeping the suppressed masses of rural workers quiet. Without a doubt, most rural workers became heavy and regular drinkers, and their drinking habits helped a great deal to make the production of spirits a very profitable enterprise.

The truck system with which the industrial workers were exploited differed from that of the rural workers in many respects. Industrial workers fairly rarely received hard liquor as part of their wage payment. Until 1846, however, it was usual to pay the workers in saloons or to make them apply for work there, in places which were under the commission of factory owners and entrepreneurs. The arrangement was deliberately set up in order to make workers drink as much as they could afford. The profit went to the commissionaire and the entrepreneur who installed the saloon for the purpose of making workers drink, even if they desperately needed their money for other goods (Herkner, 1896, 1921; Körner, 1865). The problems which arose from making workers drink close to their work place and in connection with work were so serious that they became a constant object of discussion in the Prussian administration between 1830 and 1850 (Anton, 1953). In 1846, in the Prussian Rhine-Province, the truck system was forbidden by law. Nevertheless, more subtle ways of trucking work, for drink, for example, survived till the end of the century, making it hard for industrial workers to abstain even if they were very willing to renounce alcohol (Stehr, 1904).

Besides, rural workers as well as industrial workers were forced to engage in extremely long work hours by providing them with hard liquor for free. As was well known, people under the influence of alcohol could be made to continue with work beyond their physical resources because, for some hours, they were less sensitive to exhaustion. All in all, then, alcohol helped to exploit workers even further, with the effect of ruining their health fairly quickly. Since there were enough persons in the labor force on the market, for most entrepreneurs it did not matter if they lost workers because of total physical exhaustion due to excessive liquor consumption. Sick and unproductive workers could easily be replaced by new and stronger ones (for a biographical report, see Rehbein, 1911).

In the long years of the pre- and early industrialization period, entrepreneurs and landowners supported their workers' inclination toward alcohol through all means. First of all, they increased the production of hard liquor during these years in enormous quantities (Martius, 1891). They then set up drinking places for hard liquor close to all work places. They used hard liquor as payment and as a surrogate for food and rest. They linked it systematically with hard and heavy work, and they made the workers go beyond all physical signs of exhaustion by giving it out for free. It is no wonder that workers learned to cheer hard liquor more than any other alcoholic beverage and often more than any food. Indeed, workers became heavy drinkers who did not care much about the bad effects of the drink on their health or on their everyday lives. Hard liquor was the stuff they used whenever they could get hold of it during the work hours as well as during the short hours of their leisure time. They had learned by then to alleviate their fate with the help of alcohol.

Drinking and drunkenness became part of everyday life, even of the poor, in the early years of industrialization. This is documented in various publications (cf. Böttcher, 1839; Brühl-Cramer, 1819; Huss 1852). The consequences of excessive and chronic drinking for health were described in clinical terms for the first time and were labeled as "chronic alcoholism." Still, on the whole, it was not a much discussed topic in the first half of the 19th century. The situation changed drastically in the takeoff years of industrialization from 1850 to 1875 (for periodization, see Wehler, 1974a), and drinking as well as chronic alcoholism became a public issue in the second half of the century. The number of publications which dealt with problems arising from eventual and chronic alcohol consumption mushroomed. In all pamphlets and books, much concern was given to the drinking habits of industrial workers but not to those of society in general. Thus, the drinking habits of industrial workers were under constant public scrutiny, but not those of the bourgeoisie and the nobles. For industrial workers, then, there is an abundance of published material on their drinking styles, their motives for drinking, and the negative effects of alcohol on their whole life as it was seen by their more well-to-do contemporaries.

Without a doubt, Engels's (1845) speculations about the motives for drinking of the English working class stirred up a debate which was most fiercely carried on by all enemies of the socialist movement for more than half a century. Even within the socialist movement, the debate became quite passionate around the turn of the century because of widely differing views on the need for alcohol in capitalist society.

Engels was the first to argue that industrial workers were driven to drinking in the first place because of their exhausting work hours as well as their extremely bad living conditions (cf. Reulecke and Weber, 1978), both contributing strongly to a general depression of mood which could be elevated again only by a powerful external stimulant such as alcohol. In his view, alcohol helped them to escape from the bitter realities of their life for a few hours. Industrial workers had become objects of their life circumstances, which were imposed on them by those profiting from capitalism. Yet, they had to pay for the temporary alleviation of their mood by ruining their health even further in the aftermath of alcoholic excesses, thus making them more vulnerable to the diseases which were common in the quarters of the poor during the 19th century, such as tuberculosis, typhus, and cholera.

Engels's arguments were strongly attacked by the broad coalition of those who were in opposition to the social democratic movement (e.g., doctors and psychiatrists, clergymen and the rich). They held that drinking and alcoholism caused the "pauperism" of industrial workers, who could very well make a decent living out of their earnings if only they abstained (cf. Baer, 1878; Baer and Laquer, 1907; Göhre, 1891; Hoppe, 1904; Leixner, 1891). Poverty, then, was not seen as a consequence of the exploitation of industrial workers within a capitalist society but as the result of the behavior of industrial workers who wasted their money on alcohol instead of economizing it for rainy days or spending in on healthy foods. Consumption of alcohol by industrial workers was taken as a symbol and a proof showing that the average wages were high enough not only to guarantee mere physical survival but to allow for extra spending too. Therefore, the life circumstances of the working class in general were not as bad as was constantly repeated by the leaders of the social democratic movement. They were bad only for those who got hooked on alcohol. Baer (1878, p. 330) summarized the position of those opposing Engels's arguments: "If one could stamp alcoholism out of the working class, quite a few of the so-called labor problems (Arbeiterfrage) would be solved."

Two questions arise out of the line of reasoning here: (1) Why do industrial workers spend extra money on alcohol instead of on other and more valuable goods? and (2) How can industrial workers be prevented from spending more money on alcohol?

The first of these questions is intimately tied up with social-Darwinistic and hereditary theories which were virulently expounded in imperial Germany (see, e.g., Chorover, 1979; Wehler, 1974b; Weindling, 1981). As has already been said, the extremely poor (for detailed data, see e.g., Engelsing, 1973) and strenuous life conditions of the working class were not seen as being causally linked to their drinking habits, as was suggested by those who were sympathetic to the social democratic movement (see here, Blocher, 1895; Delbrück, 1901; Grotjahn, 1898). On the contrary, the working class was seen as being inferior to the bourgeoisie and the nobles to begin with because of their hereditary background. Inequality was seen as being naturally built into the human race, differentiating human beings from the very start according to their genes. Those coming from more wealthy and better-educated families had a much better chance of being successful in life because they inherited the aptitudes and the acquired abilities of their fathers and forefathers. The offspring of the lower class had little to expect from their heredity because their fathers had already failed to acquire education and wealth (cf. Ziegler, 1918). Since the biology of heredity was the same for the rich and the poor, the poor had to expect to also inherit the acquired abilities of their ancestors, one of which was their supposed weakness toward alcohol. Different models were in use to explain how the inclination of the lower class toward drinking and drunkenness became hereditary.

Drinking and drunkenness, it was said, causes a general moral weakness of the lower-class male drinker which, on its part, intensifies his need for more alcohol. While his willpower to abstain from alcohol declines more and more, his inner life degenerates because of the constant intoxication of the nerve tissues with alcohol (Morel, 1857). As with acquired abilities, the need for alcohol, the weakening of morality, and the degeneration of inner life could be hereditary in combination or singularly (cf. Baer, 1878; Baer and Laquer, 1907; Hoppe, 1904; Ziegler, 1918). The offspring of drinkers, then, could be born with a general degeneration of the nervous system, or with a weakness of moral strength and willpower, or with a strong disposition toward chronic alcoholism. Morel (1857) constructed a system showing that the descendants of drinkers degenerate progressively within two or three generations. He argued that those born with a general degeneration of the nervous system are feeble human beings who run a high risk of dying in early childhood because of lack of resistance against diseases, or who degenerate later in life by becoming alcoholics themselves, or by attracting severe mental diseases. In his view, they are unable to propagate and die out in the third generation.

In following up Morel's hypothesis, families of drinkers were investigated with great care. It soon became obvious that drinking and drunkenness were often paired not only with feeble health and insanity but with criminality as well. Morel's system had to be expanded beyond its original scope so as to include misconduct of all sorts which could be taken as manifestations of the moral or otherwise degnerated nervous system of the offspring of drinkers. Thus, the sons of drinkers could end up not only as alcoholics, chronically sick persons, or lunatics, but also as criminals. The daughters were said to degenerate in their physical endowment to childbearing, delivering, and nursing (Bunge,

1909); and, in more severe cases, to become prostitutes (cf. Hoppe, 1904). Furthermore, research in genealogies of families of drinkers showed that the families did not die out within three generations but instead bred a high number of socially unfit and criminal descendants (see e.g., Arrivé 1899; Demme, 1891; Grotjahn, 1898, 1906; Hoppe, 1904; Legrain, 1895; Oberdieck, 1897; Wlassak, 1929). Alcoholic ancestors, then, were breeding sick and immoral offspring in successive generations, who, on their part, contributed heavily to a general degeneration of the race.

Psychiatrists took over the concept of degeneration and incorporated it into their own efforts to systematize abnormal and insane behavior. Degeneration was transformed first into the concept of psychopathic abnormalities (cf. Koch, 1891; Moebius, 1900) and later on into that of the psychopathic personality (Birnbaum, 1909; Kraepelin, 1915), which is still in use today (K. Schneider, 1967). From the very start, the idea of the psychopathic personality refers to the description of so-called abnormal behavior within a very broad framework of human behavior including drunkenness and chronic alcoholism. Persons who did not control their drinking in reference to their individual level of physiological compatibility but allowed themselves to get drunk, then, exhibited the first signs of their inner psychopathy. Some psychopathic personalities seem to have a drive toward alcohol which they cannot overcome on their own. Without the stern help of others, they will certainly end up as alcoholics. For others, as a toxicant, alcohol has the effect of lowering their resistance against the repetition of the experience of drunkenness regardless of the consequences. Alcohol as an agent on nerve tissues, then, promotes the development of the inner psychopathy until it is manifested in chronic alcoholism. As in the concept of degeneration, psychopathy is believed to be hereditary. Since the biological transmission of genetical information was unknown, it was assumed that psychopathic personalities suffered from a weak nervous system. This was displayed in immoral and abnormal behavior. Psychopathy cannot be controlled by those suffering from it. They need professional help in order to adjust to normal and moral behavior.

In whichever way one looks at the drinking habits of industrial workers, from the viewpoint of social Darwinism or from that of psychiatry, the motives for drinking can be said to derive from moral weakness as an underlying constant of degeneration as well as psychopathy. Since the writers on drinking and alcoholism often avoided defining moderate drinking, excessive drinking, and sick drinking, or stated the definitions in a way such that barriers between different drinking styles were blurred, the drinking of industrial workers could simply be denounced as a clear sign of moral inferiority.

Here the political impact of the lively discussion in imperial Germany about the drinking habits of industrial workers becomes obvious. The Social Democratic Party, which formed itself as a strong political force between 1869 and 1900, especially during the time when it was forbidden (1878-1890), claimed equal rights for the working class; rights which were already given to the bourgeoisie and, of course, to the nobles. The demand was not restricted to equality of vote. It included challenges concerning the exploitation of the working class within a capitalist society; for example, the socialization of the means of production to guarantee social and political equality for all citizens of the state. From the point of view of the ruling class, the claims of the Social Democratic Party, as the representative of interest for the working class, were extremely dangerous because they demanded an overthrow of the economic and social order for the sake of the poor. To fight the Social Democratic Party, the bourgeoisie and the nobles disputed at all levels of rational and irrational argument. The debate on the unique inclination of the working class toward drink and drunkenness is part of the verbal fight between the classes. By labeling industrial workers as morally weak, something which could be proved scientifically by their drinking habits, the ruling class won one more argument demonstrating their own superiority. Nobody could expect them to share their rights with those who were morally weak and therefore not able to control their behavior. For the sake of the state in general and for the sake of the race, those who were morally strong had to rule over those who were morally weak, to avoid the ruin of society.

In particular, the ruling class had to prevent the working class from drinking and drunkenness. The programs which were under discussion in imperial Germany covered a wide range of measures including, among others, wage problems of the working class, their work and family life conditions, laws to punish drunkenness and to ban alcoholics from public life, and models to diminish the production of alcohol or to make it more expensive and less easily accessible (cf. Baer, 1878; Delbrück, 1901; Grotjahn, 1898, 1923; Hoppe, 1904, Kraepelin, 1915; Stehr, 1904). Only some main points in the debate over wage problems and over criminal law and detention are considered here.

As a number of more or less unsystematic investigations into the household budgets of industrial workers showed, on the average, between 5% and 10% of the yearly income was spent on alcohol. Since alcohol is not necessary for survival, spending money on alcohol was seen as luxurious waste. Some writers held that one had to cut the wages of industrial workers to the minimum level of existence, thus forcing them to give up alcohol in favor of food, which they, then, would need desperately in order to survive. Although the argument had several defenders, it never gained much momentum. Presumably, one of the reasons that it never made it to the front pages can be found in the strong attacks of those writers on alcohol who were in favor of the aims of the Social Democratic Party (cf. Blocher, 1895; Fröhlich, 1904; Laquer, 1913). They were the ones who constantly called to attention how much the working class already suffered from exploitation, making it impossible for them to aspire to higher values. Alcohol was the only means they could afford, from time to time, to escape from their misery for a few short hours. In order to make industrial workers refrain widely from alcohol use, one had to raise their wages so that they would be able not only to feed and clothe their families adequately but to house them sufficiently, and to still have extra money for education and cultural entertainment. The presupposition for temperance, then, was a decent living for the working class, which could take place only through substantial wage increases and a social policy shaped against further exploitation of the working class (for contradicting views, see Kautsky, 1891).

With the foundation of the first asylums for alcoholics (1878 and later; for details, see Martius, 1891; Grotjahn, 1898), new directions were introduced into the discussion. The criminal law of 1871 already contained a paragraph requiring the arrest of those who by drinking handicapped themselves in such a way that they were unable to earn a living (§ 361; abolished in 1969). In the 1890s lowering the restrictions against placing drinkers under legal control was highly debated. It was argued that for the sake of the race, drinkers had to be prevented from reproduction (Ploetz, 1885; Schallmayer, 1903). By making it easier to put drinkers under tutelage and by allowing sterilization of those who were not able to control their drinking, one hoped to eliminate drinkers from propagating, thus avoiding the passing down of a degenerated or psychopathic nervous system. In imperial Germany all the projects for tightening the criminal law against drinking and drunkenness, or for lowering restrictions against legal control (Baer and Laquer, 1907), and putting into effect the idea of systematic channelling of natural selection (Grotjahn 1923), did not come through. It took another 20 years before they were realized during the Third Reich (cf. Binding and Hoche, 1920; Ehrhardt, 1965; Friese and Lemme, 1937; Gütt et al., 1934; Lenz, 1931; Löhr, 1935; Rüdin, 1934).

When we look at the public debate on drinking and drunkenness today, we find several similarities between the situation now and that of imperial Germany.

At the end of the Second World War, the per capita consumption of alcohol had dropped immensely as a byproduct of the food shortages which were triggered by the war. In the years after the war, once again the state–the Federal Republic of Germany (FRG)–did not restrict the production of alcoholic beverages. On the contrary, by subsidizing, directly and indirectly, the agricultural sector, the state helped to set up big distilleries and promoted further concentration of the alcohol industry. Taxation of alcoholic beverages was not increased at the same pace as the purchasing power of the average consumer. Alcohol, then, is fairly inexpensive in West Germany today. The result of state policies can be seen in steep increases in alcohol production and consumption from the end of the war up until the early 1970s, when the yearly per capita consumption stabilized at the high level of 12-13 liters of pure alcohol (for detailed data, see *Statistische Jahrbücher der FRG,* Wiesbaden; and Deutsche Hauptstelle gegen die Suchtgefahren, *Informationsdienst*). The average consumption level is now somewhat higher than in the period around 1900, when per capita consumption is said to have been aroud 9-10 liters of pure alcohol per year.

As we know from recent survey studies, alcohol consumption is typical in all layers of social stratification. The average quantity consumed does not differ systematically with income, education, or the social prestige of a profession. Members of the lower class are as much inclined to drink as members of the middle and upper classes (cf. *Arbeitskreis Alkohol,* 1978; *Der Spiegel*, 1973, 1977, 1981; Prognos, 1979). This holds at least for men. Women, on the other hand, drink less than men on the average, and their willingness to drink might even vary with their position in social stratification (Wieser, 1968, 1973). Lower-class women are said to abstain more often than women from the middle and upper classes, and they seem to abhore drunkenness in public much more strongly than the latter groups. Still, it is not possible to go any further in the description of the different drinking styles and habits of the two sexes, because we desperately lack more sophisticated studies on women's patterns of drinking, drunkenness, and abstinence.

Although we do not know much about the preferred circumstances in which women start to drink or their usual quantity consumed on different occasions, there is a keen discussion on the particularly detrimental effect of alcohol on the female body and psyche. Here again, we find that special subgroups of society are depicted: Today it is women and adolescents (cf. Aktionsprogramm, 1975) whose drinking habits are carefully examined in public, whereas other groups in society, which might drink much more excessively–here, men of all levels of social stratification–go more or less unnoticed. Within the last 10 years, several papers have been published on the special danger women run when they give in to drinking. Most of these are not based on solid empirical research outcomes but repeat virulent prejudices on women's role in highly industrialized Western societies.

Psychiatrists are very much involved in the debate on women's drinking habits. They tend to link women's drinking and drunkenness to women's wish to emancipate themselves from traditional role patterns in favor of more freedom to plan their present and future life. From this point of view, the women's movement is to blame for the increase of alcoholism in women because of its constant "nagging" against traditional female role patterns and its unwillingness to accept the typical women's lot (cf. Frau und Sucht, 1981). Women are said to misunderstand the constitutional guarantee of equal rights in the FRG, and this holds even more for members of the women's movement. It becomes obvious in their quarrels regarding equality in vocational training, in job opportunities, in payment, in sharing family duties, in politics in general, and in jurisdiction. In their wishful thinking, these women deviate more and more from role patterns which–from the point of view of men–proved good for them for centuries, as demonstrated in the relatively small number of women who became alcoholics before 1945 (for contradicting evidence, see Grotjahn, 1898; Hoppe, 1904). The deviation in thinking and in publicly repeated demands reflects an increase in psychopathy in women (Finke, 1981; Wanke, 1981) as a result of their misinterpretation of their feminine role in modern Western society.

The statement about an increase in psychopathy in women, which is said to show up in an increasing amount of alcohol addiction in women, has a clear parallel to psychiatric arguments around the turn of the century about the causes of drinking and drunkenness in the working class. Psychiatrists as well as others in power suppose that women lack the moral strength to stand the test of public life. Since the effort needed for careers and for their work as housewives is too much for them, they easily indulge in immoral behavior. One such behavior is excessive alcohol consumption. Since it has always been claimed that women are not able to take as much alcohol as men (cf. Grotjahn, 1898; Hoppe, 1904, Wanke, 1970, 1981), they run a much higher risk of becoming alcoholics once they start to drink. Whatever motives drive them to drinking, their greater sensibility to alcohol makes them more vulnerable to its effects. Thus, either their hereditary psychopathy shows up in their drinking styles, or alcohol brings about psychopathy in them.

To prevent women from acting out their inner psychopathy or becoming psychopaths themselves, it is recommended to them to rethink out the issue of equality between the sexes and the proper role of women in our society. It is recommended to each woman that she be a humble and loyal wife and caring mother in the first place (cf. Rollmann, 1975; Schneider, 1981) and that she give up her professional career when she gives birth to her first child so that she can spend her time in childrearing and in making a perfect and beloved home for all family members. In times of economic crisis, as is the case today, the ideology of the feminine role (cf. Parsons, 1951; Parsons et al., 1955) is always "polished up" by those who gain from the inequality of the sexes.

The rhetoric regarding increasing rates of alcoholism in women in general, and in career women in particular follows once more the pattern of a debate between those who are in power and who are willing to defend their position by all means, and those who call for equal rights, here the realization of constitutional rights. By all appearances, women might lose the fight, as can be seen with regard to plans to force out of the labor force one of the partners in double-career families (e.g., plans of the state government of Lower Saxony). Such plans and political maneuvres will hit women much harder than men because of the fairly broad silent agreement on traditional role patterns for women and men in Western societies.

To enforce the double standard of judgment on the drinking habits of men and women, research on the fetal alcohol syndrome has been intensified in the last 10 years (cf. Bierich, 1978; Leiber, 1976; Majewski, 1980; Majewski et al., 1976;

Manzke et al., 1979, Scheppe, 1977; Seidenberg and Majewski, 1978). Since the beginning of the discussion on the detrimental effects of alcohol on offspring in the last century, it has been suspected that the drinking of the mother during pregnancy might significantly contribute to malformations of the fetus and the newborn (cf. Hoppe, 1904). The issue was brought up again in the late 1960s and stimulated further research efforts in the '70s. Taking everything together, there are reliable indications showing that some women who drink rather large amounts of alcohol, either constantly or periodically, during pregnancy give birth to malformed babies. Still, it is unclear in what way alcohol hinders the formation of organs and the development of the brain, and in which phase of the development of the fetus its toxic effects are most dangerous to it. With regard to the multitude of problems which are still open to question in the development of the fetal alcohol syndrome—for example, the father's contribution via drinking and drug taking to the malformation of the fetus (cf. *Time Magazine*, 1979); critical quantities and critical frequencies of alcohol intake by the mother; interactions of drugs and smoking, pill popping and drinking, and their effects on the fetus; psychological and socioeconomic problems of women in pregnancy and drinking—one would expect the researchers to draw only cautious conclusions from their findings. As always in the debate on alcohol, the arguments are not restricted to what is already scientifically proven; instead they are mixed up with irrational value judgments. Thus, the fetal alcohol syndrome is ascribed to the mother's drinking. Only women are held guilty for delivering malformed and malfunctioning babies. Consequently, preventive programs which are discussed in some papers (see Majewski, 1980; Manzke et al., 1979; Seidenberg and Majewski, 1978) addresss themselves to women only. It is recommended to help alcoholic mothers to get an abortion on eugenic grounds and to sterilize them if at all possible. Obviously, plans as old as the discussion on drinking and drunkenness are revived and presented by medical men as innocent preventive programs for the sake of alcoholic women—and for the race in particular.

Ideas about how to handle problems arising out of the relatively high alcohol consumption in our society have, after all, not changed much during the last 100 years. However, there is a change in the objects to whom they are addressed. In the last century, it was men of the working class who were said to be unable to control their drinking and, therefore, had to be put under control and sterilized. Today, it is women of all levels of social stratification who are said to misunderstand the constitutional guarantee of equal rights and, therefore, to misunderstand their feminine role, which, besides others, shows up in their drinking habits. Thus, an increasing number of women seem to be unable to control their drinking . These women, at least, have to be prevented from propagating—on eugenic grounds.

REFERENCES

ABEL, W. *Stufen der Ernährung*. Göttingen: Vandenhoeck & Ruprecht, 1981.

Aktionsprogramm zur Eindämmung und Verhütung des Alkoholmisbrauchs. Bundesministerium für Jugend, Familie und Gesundheit (ed.). Köln: Bundeszentrale für gesundheitliche Aufklärung, 1981.

ANTON, G.K. *Geschichte der preussischen Fabrikgesetzgebung*. Berlin: Rütten & Loening, 1953.

ARBEITSKREIS ALKOHOL. *Alkoholkonsum und Alkoholmissbrauch in der Bundesrepublik Deutschland und West-Berlin*. Bonn: Seidl, 1978.

ARNTZ, H. *Weinbrenner*. Stuttgart: Seewald, 1975.

ARRIVE, R. *Influence de l'alcoolisme sur la dépopulation*. Thèse, Paris, 1899.

BAER, A. *Der Alkoholismus, seine Verbreitung und seine Wirkung auf den individuellen und socialen Organismus*. Berlin: Hirschwald, 1878.

BAER, A., and LAQUER, B. *Die Trunksucht und ihre Abwehr*. Berlin: Urban & Schwarzenberg, 1907.

BASSERMAN-JORDAN, F. Von. *Geschichte des Weinbaus*. Frankfurt/Main: Keller, 1923.

BAUER, M. *Der deutsche Durst*. Leipzig: Seemann, 1903.

BIERGANS, R. *Bierbrauerei*. Stuttgart: Handwörterbuch der Staatswissenschaften, 1959.

BIERICH, J.R. Uber das embryo-fetale Alkoholsyndrom. In Deutsche Hauptstelle gegen die Suchtgefahren (ed.), *Familie und Suchterkrankung*. Hamm: Hoheneck, 1978, pp. 101-103.

BINDING, K., and HOCHE, A. *Die Freigabe der Vernichtung lebensunwerten Lebens, ihr Mass und ihre Form*. Leipzig: Thieme, 1920.

BIRNBAUM, K. *Über psychopathische Persönlichkeiten*. Wiesbaden: Bergmann, 1909.

BISMARCK, O. Von. *Die gesammelten Werke*. Bismarck an Scharlach, 7. 4. 1834. Berlin: O. Stollberg, 1924-1935, Vol. 14, p. 4.

BLOCHER, H. *Die Alkoholfrage in ihrem Verhältnis zur Arbeiterfrage*. Basel: Schriftstelle des Alkoholgegnerbundes, 1895.

BÖTTCHER, J.H. *Der Branntwein, ein sicherer Zerstörer des Wohlstandes, der Gesundheit, des häuslichen Glücks und der Zufriedenheit*. Hildesheim: Gerstenberg, 1839.

BRIEFS, G. *Das Spirituskartell*. Karlsruhe: Braun, 1912.

BRÜHL-CRAMER, C. Von. *Über die Trunksucht und eine rationelle Heilmethode: Geschrieben zur Beherzigung für jedermann*. Berlin: Nicolai, 1819.

BUNGE, G. Von. *Die zunehmende Unfähigkeit der Frauen, ihre Kinder zu stillen*. München: Reinhardt, 1909.

CHOROVER, S.L. *From Genesis to Genocid*. Cambridge: MIT Press, 1979.

CHRISTOFFEL, K. *Durch die Zeiten Strömt der Wein*. Hamburg: De Gruyter, 1957.

CLUSS, A. *Die Alkoholfrage*. Berlin: Parey, 1906.

DELBRÜCK, M. *Hygiene des Alkoholismus*. Jena: Fischer, 1901.

DEMME, R. *Über den Einfluss des Alkohols auf den Organismus des Kindes*. Stuttgart: Enke, 1891.

DER SPIEGEL. *Kauf-, Konsum- und Kommunikationsverhalten der Bundesbevölkerung*. Hamburg: Der Spiegel, 1973.

DER SPIEGEL. *Prozente*. Hamburg: Der Spiegel, 1977.

DER SPIEGEL. *Prozente (2)*. Hamburg: Der Spiegel, 1981.

ERHARDT, H. *Euthanasie und Vernichtung "lebensunwerten" Lebens*. Stuttgart: Enke, 1965.

ENGELS, F. Die Lage der arbeitenden Klasse in England, 1845. In *Karl Marx, Friedrich Engels, Werke*, vol. 2. Berlin: Dietz.

ENGELSING, R. *Zur Sozialgeschichte deutscher Mittel- und Unterschichten.* Göttingen: Vandenhoeck & Ruprecht, 1973.

FINKE, R. Alkoholismus bei Frauen–Statistische Ergebnisse aus stationären und ambulanten Institutionen. In Deutsche Haupstelle gegen die Suchtgefahren (ed.), *Frau und Sucht.* Hamm: Hoheneck, 1981, pp. 50-61.

Frau und Sucht. Deutsche Hauptstelle gegen die Suchtgefahren (ed.). Hamm: Hoheneck, 1981.

FRIESE, G., and LEMME, H. *Die deutsche Erbpflege.* Leipzig: Thieme, 1937.

FRÖHLICH, R. *Alkoholfrage und Arbeiterklasse.* Berlin: Verlag Expedition der Buchhandlung Vorwärts, 1904.

GÖHRE, P. *Drei Monate Fabrikarbeiter und Handwerksbursche.* Leipzig: Grunow, 1891.

GROTJAHN, A. *Der Alkoholismus nach Wesen, Wirkung und Verbreitung.* Leipzig: Wigand, 1898.

GROTJAHN, A. *Alkohol und Gesundheit.* Berlin: Verlag der Central-Kommission der Krankenhassen Berlins und der Vororte, 1906.

GROTJAHN, A. *Soziale Pathologie.* Berlin: Springer, 1923.

GÜTT, A., RÜDIN, E., and RUTTKE, F. *Gesetz zur Verhütung erbkranken Nachwuchses vom 14. Juli 1933.* München: Lehmann, 1934.

HAUFFEN, A. Die Trinkliteratur in Deutschland bis zum Ausgang des 16. Jahrhunderts. In *Vierteljahresschrift für Literaturgeschichte II*, 1889, pp. 489-516.

HERKNER, H. *Alkoholismus und Arbeiterfrage.* Hildesheim: Deutscher Verein gegen den Missbrauch geistiger Getränke, 1896.

HERKNER, H. *Die Arbeiterfrage*, 2 vols. Berlin: De Gruyter, 1921.

HERMBSTÄDT, F. Bermerkungen über die Versteuerung der Branntweinbrennereien durch den Blasenzins, und die Grundsätze, auf welche diese Versteuerung gestützt ist. In J. F. Dron (ed.), *Anleitung zur Kenntnis und Beurtheilung der wichtigsten Operationen in der Bierbrauerei und Branntweinbrennerei. Auf Befehl der höheren Verwaltungsbehörden ausgearbeitet.* Berlin, 1811, pp. 51-66.

HOFFMANN, W.G. *Das Wachstum der Deutschen Wirtschaft seit der Mitte des 19. Jahrhunderts.* Berlin: Springer, 1965.

HOPPE, H. *Die Tatsachen über den Alkohol.* Berlin: Calvary, 1904.

HUSS, M. *Chronische Alkoholkrankheit oder Alkoholismus chronicus.* Deutsch von G. v. d. Busch, 2 vols. Stockholm and Leipzig: Fritze, 1852.

KAUTSKY, K. Der Alkoholismus und seine Bekämpfung. *Die Neue Zeit* 9: 106-107, 1891.

KNOBLAUCH, H. *Die Organisation der deutschen Brauindustrie.* Greifswald: Adler, 1920.

KOCH, J.L.A. *Die psychopathischen Minderwertigkeiten.* Ravensberg: Maier, 1891.

KÖRNER, H.J.A. *Lebenskämpfe in der Alten und Neuen Welt. Eine Selbstbiographie*, 2 vols. Leipzig: Keil, 1865.

KRAEPELIN, E. *Psychiatrie*, 2 vols. Leipzig: Barth, 1915.

LAQUER, B. Einfluss der sozialen Lage auf den Alkoholismus. In M. Mosse, and G. Tugendreich (eds.), *Krankheit und soziale Lage.* München: Lehmann, 1913, pp. 473-495.

LEGRAIN, M. *Dégénérescence social et alcoolisme.* Paris, 1895.

LEIBER, B. Embryopathisches Alkoholismus-Syndrom in tausenden Fällen übersehen! *Medizin* 4: 1365-1371, 1976.

LEIXNER, O. Von. *Soziale Briefe aus Berlin.* Berlin: Pfeilstücker, 1891.

LENZ, F. Die Stellung des Nationalsozialismus zur Rassenhygiene. *Archiv f. Rassen- und Gesellschaftsbiologie* 25: 300-306, 1931.

LÖHR, H. *Über die Sellung und Bedeutung der Heilkunde im nationalsozialistischen Staat.* Berlin: Die Medizinische Welt, 1935.

MAJEWSKI, F. Alkohol als teratogene Noxe. In W. Keup (ed.), *Folgen der Sucht.* Stuttgart: Thieme, 1980, pp. 159-167.
MAJEWSKI, F., BIERICH, J.R., LÖSER, H., MICHAELIS, R., LEIBER, B., and BETTECKEN, F. Zur Klinik und Pathogenese der Alkoholembryopathie. *Münch. Med. Wschr.* 118: 1635-1642, 1976.
MANZKE, H., and SPRETER VON KREUDENSTEIN, P. Embryofetales Alkoholsyndrom. *Suchtgefahren* 25: 157-166, 1979.
MARTIUS, W. *Handbuch der deutschen Trink- und Trunksuchtsfragen.* Gotha: Perthes, 1891.
MOEBIUS, P.J. *Über Entartung.* Wiesbaden: Bergmann, 1900.
MOREL, B. *Traité des dégénérescences physiques, intellectuelles et morales de l'espèce humaine.* Paris: Baillière, 1857.
OBERDIECK, R. Beitrag zur Kenntnis des Alkoholismus und seiner rationellen Behandlung. *Arch. Psychiat. Nervenk.* 29: 579-632, 1897.
PAN, L. *Alcohol in Colonial Africa.* Helsinki: Finnish Foundation for Alcohol Studies, Vol. 22, 1975.
PARSONS, T., BALES, R.F., OLDS, J., ZELDITCH, M., and SLATER, P.E. *Family, Socialization, and Interaction Process.* New York: Free Press, 1955.
PARSONS, T. *The Social System.* New York: Free Press, 1951.
PLOETZ, A. *Grundlinien der Rassenhygiene.* Berlin, 1885.
PROGNOS. *Die Entwicklung des Alkoholkonsums in der Bundesrepublik Deutschland.* Basel: Prognos, 1979.
PUHLE, H.-J. *Agrarische Interessenpolitik und preussischer Konservatismus.* Hannover: Verlag für Literatur und Zeitgeschehen, 1966.
PUHLE, H.-J. *Politische Agrarbewegungen in kapitalistischen Industriegesellschaften.* Göttingen: Vandenhoeck & Ruprecht, 1975.
REHBEIN, F. *Das Leben eines Landarbeiters.* Jena: Diederichs, 1911.
REULECKE, J., and WEBER, W. (eds.). *Fabrik, Familie, Feierabend.* Wuppertal: Hammer, 1978.
RITTER, G.A., and KOCKA, J. (eds.). *Deutsche Sozialgeschichte.* München: Beck, 1974.
ROLLMANN, D. Für Mütter sollte der Beruf an zweiter Stelle stehen. *Die Zeit,* 7. 2. 1975.
RÜDIN, E. Aufgaben und Ziele der Deutschen Gesellschaft für Rassenhygiene. *Archiv f. Rassen- und Gesellschaftsbiologie* 28: 228-236, 1934.
SCHALLMAYER, W. *Vererbung und Auslese im Lebenslauf der Völker.* Jena, 1903.
SCHEPPE, K.J. Alkohol-Embryopathie. *Pädiat. Prax.* 18: 207-218, 1977.
SCHIVELBUSCH, W. *Das Paradies, der Geschmack und die Vernunft.* München: Hanser, 1980.
SCHNEIDER, K. *Klinische Psychopathologie.* Stuttgart: Thieme, 1967.
SCHNEIDER, W. Selbstverwirklichung–Nichts weiter als ein Wahn. *Frankfurter Allgemeine Zeitung,* 7. 11. 1981.
SEIDENBERG, J., and MAJEWSKI, F. Zur Häufigkeit der Alkoholembryopathie in den verschiedenen Phasen der mütterlichen Alkoholkrankheit. *Suchtgefahren* 24: 63-75, 1978.
STARKE, J. *Die Berechtigung des Alkoholgenusses.* Stuttgart: Hoffmann, 1906.
STEHR, A. *Alkoholgenuss und wirtschaftliche Arbeit.* Jena: Fischer, 1904.
STRUVE, E. *Bier, Bierbrauerei, und Bierbesteuerung.* Jena: Handwörterbuch der Staatswissenschaften, 1899.
TEUTEBERG, H.J., and WIEGELMANN, G. *Der Wandel der Nahrungsgewohnheiten unter dem Einfluss der Industrialisierung.* Göttingen: Vanderhoeck & Ruprecht, 1972.
Time Magazine. Fatherly risk. July 2, 1979, p. 36.

TIMM, U. *Deutsche Kolonien.* Autoren-Edition, 1982.

VOGT, I. Alkoholkonsum, Industrialisierung und Klassenkonflikte. In G. Völger (ed.), *Rausch und Realität.* Köln: Rautenstrauch-Joest-Museum, 1981.

VOGT, I. Einige Fragen zum Alkoholkonsum der Arbeiter. *Geschichte und Gesellschaft* 8: 134-140, 1982.

VOIGT, K. *Italienische Berichte aus dem spätmittelalterlichen Deutschland.* Stuttgart: Klett, 1973.

WANKE, K. Alkoholismus bei Frauen–Analyse klinischer Erfahrungen. In Deutsche Hauptstelle gegen die Suchtgefahren (ed.), *Alkoholismus bei Frauen.* Hamm: Hoheneck, 1970, pp. 68-80.

WANKE, K. Unterschiedliches Suchtverhalten bei Frau und Mann. In Deutsche Hauptstelle gegen die Suchtgefahren (ed.), *Frau und Sucht.* Hamm: Hoheneck, 1981, pp. 11-27.

WASSERMANN, L. *Die deutsche Spiritusindustrie.* Leipzig: Duncker & Humblot, 1909.

WEHLER, U. Der Aufstieg des Organisierten Kapitalismus und Interventionsstaates in Deutschland. In H. Winkler (ed.), *Organisierter Kapitalismus.* Göttingen: Vandenhoeck & Ruprecht, 1974 (a), pp. 36-51.

WEHLER, U. Sozialdarwinismus im expandierenden Industriestaat. In I. Geiss and B.J. Wendt (eds.), *Deutschland in der Weltpolitik des 19. und 20. Jahrhunderts.* Düsseldorf: Bertelsmann, 1974 (b), pp. 133-142.

WEINDLING, P. Theories of the cell state in imperial Germany. In C. Webster (ed.), *Biology, Medicine and Society.* Cambridge: Cambridge University Press, 1981, pp. 99-156.

WLASSAK, R.P. *Grundriss der Alkoholfrage.* Leipzig: Hirzel, 1929.

WIESER, S. Über das Trinkverhalten der allgemeinen Bevölkerung und Stereotype des Abstinenten und des Trinkers. *Fortschr. Neurol. Psychiat.* 36: 485-509, 1968.

WIESER, S. *Das Trinkverhalten der Deutschen.* Herford: Nicolai, 1973.

WURZBACHER, G. Suchtenwicklung und Rolle der Frau aus sozialwissenschaftlicher Sicht. In Deutsche Haupstelle gegen die Suchtgefahren (ed.), *Frau und Sucht.* Hamm: Hoheneck, 1981, pp. 28-40.

ZIEGLER, H.E. *Die Vererbungslehre in der Biologie und in der Soziologie.* Jena: Fischer, 1918.

The International Journal of the Addictions, 19(5), 571-575, 1984

Research Note

Student Substance Use: Stability and Change across College Years

Kenneth E. Friend,* PhD

Clarkson University
Potsdam, New York 13676

Parviz A. Koushki,† PhD

University of Riyadh
Riyadh, Saudi Arabia

Abstract

Entering freshmen, second-semester freshmen, and sophomores through seniors were surveyed regarding their recent alcohol and drug use. Among entering freshmen, 81% drank and 34% used drugs. Compared to groups that had been at college longer, entering freshmen were a significant 16% lower for alcohol and 12% lower for drugs than the other groups, but all other groups showed no significant differences regardless of year in school. When analyzed separately by sex, all results were identical to this overall pattern except that drug use among women did not appear to increase substantially from entering students to later years. These results indicate a relatively rapid influence of the college environment which then leads to stability of substance use behavior.

*To whom reprint requests should be sent.
†Former affiliation: Civil and Environmental Engineering Department, Clarkson College of Technology, Potsdam, New York.

 0020-773X/84/1905-0571$3.50/0

INTRODUCTION

In recent years, there have been a number of surveys of high school and college students providing useful information on patterns of alcohol, marijuana, and other drug use (e.g., Johnston, Bachman, and O'Malley, 1977; USDHEW, 1980; Vener, Krupa, and Climo, 1982). Aside from caffeine, the most popular social drugs are alcohol and marijuana, and there is reason to be concerned about their health and societal costs (Vener et al., 1982).

Surveys such as those cited here have generally shown that three-quarters or more of U.S. high school/college students use alcohol, and that one-third to one-half of the same people use drugs (usually marijuana). There appear to be no systematically large differences between high school and college students in different studies, and Vener et al. (1982) have reviewed evidence indicating the time stability of use levels in the sense of recent history and in terms of the age range of these young people. We note that these surveys have often sampled a set of age/school grade levels (e.g., college freshmen through seniors) which might have some year-by-year differences, and that one large recent study (Vener et al., 1982) was conducted in the spring time after all had been in college at least a semester. These are not problems per se for the studies, but without specific year-by-year analyses and comparison of entering students versus those at school for some time, it is difficult to detect specific change/stability in one social setting.

Since college is a whole new socialization experience for most people, we wished to determine the degree to which alcohol and drug use levels changed when freshmen came to college and the degree of change after the freshman year. We obtained a cross-sectional survey of college freshmen through seniors in the spring semester and of freshmen in the beginning of their first semester.

METHODS

All subjects were students at four local colleges in a rural, far upstate New York area. One group (beginning freshmen) was solicited during the first 1½ months of school from required social science courses (autumn 1980). These volunteer subjects were paid a small amount to come to a group questionnaire completion session where they were instructed not to put their names on the questionnaire and were assured of complete anonymity of response. This group had 286 subjects (106 females). The other groups in this study consisted of 459 students (233 females) from all 4 years of college who were interviewed and asked to fill in the questionnaire (spring 1980). Of these 459, somewhat more than half were freshman and sophomores (62%) since one of the colleges was a 2-year school. Again, anonymity of response was guaranteed to these respondents. The data to be analyzed here are self-reports of alcohol use or abstinence

Table 1

College Student Substance Use by Group

Group	Sample	Percent alcohol use	Percent drug use
1. Entering freshmen	286	81.5	34.3
2. 2nd-semester freshmen	140	97.9	49.3
3. Sophomores	146	95.2	43.8
4. Juniors	90	97.8	43.3
5. Seniors	83	98.8	49.4
6. Pooled data for groups 2-5		97.1	46.4

in the last 30 days and of drug use in the same period. Virtually all drug use was marijuana. Only 2% reported using some other drug but not marijuana.

RESULTS

Looking at alcohol first, we find virtually no differences in Table 1 among the four groups of second-semester freshmen and later classes (all $\chi^2 < 1$). In contrast, the lower alcohol use rate for entering freshmen was significantly different from each of the other four groups at $p < .001$ using χ^2 tests. It appears that nearly 16% of entering freshmen are influenced by the college environment to begin alcohol use, but the use rate is stable after that.

To see whether the same pattern of results was found for females and for males, Table 2 shows the results for entering freshmen males and females, and for the pooled data from the four groups of later college students (see Note 1). The female-to-male alcohol use rates do not differ for entering freshmen or for later students (both $\chi^2 < 1$). However, there are very significant differences ($p < .001$) for both males and females between entering freshmen and other students, showing that the overall difference in alcohol use rates is due to essentially identical differences for males and females.

Table 2

Substance Use Analyzed by Sex, Comparing Entering Freshmen to Other College Students

Group	Percent alcohol use	Percent drug use
Entering freshmen males	80.0	35.0
Other college males	96.5	53.1
Entering freshmen females	84.0	33.0
Other college females	97.9	39.9

The drug use figures in Table 1 show a similar pattern to that seen for alcohol. The four groups of second-semester freshmen and later classes have no differences from each other that even approach significance. When pooling the data from these four groups, the entering freshmen rate is clearly different at $p < .01$. These data appear to indicate a 12% increase in the drug use rate during the freshman year, but the drug use rate remains stable thereafter during the college years.

These drug use figures were also analyzed by sex, as shown in Table 2. Here, there appears to be a statistical interaction between sex and time status in college in that entering freshmen males and females do not differ ($\chi^2 < 1$), whereas later college males and females do ($\chi^2 = 7.50, p < .01$). Further, the analyses of each sex showed a significant difference for the males ($\chi^2 = 12.53$, $p < .001$), while the 6.9% difference for females was not statistically significant ($\chi^2 = 1.20$). These results were confirmed by applying another method of analysis to the data, analysis of variance (Note 2), which showed a main effect of sex on drug use (higher among males), a main effect of time status in college on drug use (lower for entering freshmen than others), and a statistical interaction showing a greater time effect for males. In sum, the general pattern found for alcohol is found here (differences between two points in the freshman year but not between later years), but the differences in the general pattern are particularly strong for males and do not achieve statistical significance for females in this sample. This lack of statistical significance for females, however, does not negate a general conclusion of "stability of substance use across the college years except during the freshman year."

CONCLUSIONS

If we take the entering freshmen data as indicating substance use established during high school, these results indicate two things. First, as others have found (e.g., Johnston et al., 1977), alcohol and drug use is relatively prevalent among high school students (apparently 81% and 34%, respectively, in the sample). If much of college student substance use is rooted in behavior begun during earlier years, it may be resistant to change.

Second, however, there is a detectable change in substance use as people move to the college environment, the only insignificant finding in these data being for female drug use. However, these significant changes seem to occur all within the freshman year since the use rates in later years were stable. There is no evidence of a continuing slow influence of the college environment. Therefore, those wishing to alter the effect of college on substance use should develop programs which pay special attention to the freshman year.

Generally, studies looking for increases or decreases in substance use in new environments should be designed with the possibility in mind that these changes may occur quickly and then be followed by new equilibrium. Also, studies analyzing college students should note the special differences that may exist for first-semester freshmen, and not simply pool their data with other groups.

ACKNOWLEDGMENT

This study was funded in part by National Cancer Institute grant CA29321, for which the first author is principal investigator.

NOTES

1. These data were pooled for purposes of performing statistical tests since the sample size in each college year would be too small to give sufficient statistical power for separate sex analyses. The trends for each sex, however, show stability in alcohol and drug use among the four college years, consistent with the overall data shown in Table 1.
2. Strictly speaking, analysis of vairance is inappropriate for a dichotomous dependent variable. However, as Cohen and Cohen (1975, p. 230) indicate, the robustness of this analytic model usually precludes problems with this violation of its assumptions.

REFERENCES

COHEN, J., and COHEN, P. *Applied Multiple Regression/Correlation Analysis for the Behavioral Sciences*. Hillsdale, NJ: Erlbaum, 1975.

JOHNSTON, L.D., BACHMAN, J.G., and O'MALLEY, P.M. *Drug Use among American High School Students 1975-1977.* Washington, D.C.: U.S. Department of Health, Education, and Welfare (National Institute on Drug Abuse), 1977.

U.S. DEPARTMENT OF HEALTH, EDUCATION, AND WELFARE. *Marijuana and Health* (Eighth Annual Report to the U.S. Congress, National Institute on Drug Abuse). Washington, DC: USDHEW, 1977.

VENER, A.M., KRUPA, L.R., and CLIMO, J.J. Drugs (prescription, over-the-counter, social) and the young adult: Use and attitudes. *Int. J. Addict.* 17: 399-415, 1982.

The International Journal of the Addictions, 19(5), 577–583, 1984

Research Note

Drinking Patterns among Student Nurses

Mary R. Haack,* RN, MS

University of Illinois at the Medical Center
Chicago, Illinois 60612

Thomas C. Harford, PhD

National Institute on Alcohol Abuse and Alcoholism
Rockville, Maryland 20857

Abstract

The present study examined the use of alcohol among student nurses in a senior class of a college of nursing. A majority of the students indicated a stable pattern of alcohol use, and 13% reported alcohol-related problems either at school or at work.

Current literature reveals an increased interest in the problem of the impaired nurse (American Nurses Association, 1982; Jaffe, 1981; Wright, 1982). The psychologically demanding nature of the clinical environment and the technical tasks carried out by nurses contribute to the stress associated with this profession. Several studies have been devoted to the negative consequences of stress experienced by nurses; that is, alcoholism, drug addiction, depression, and burnout (Isler, 1978; Kramer, 1974; Levenstein, 1980; Levine, Preston, and Lipscomb, 1975; Maslach, 1976). While there are no reliable data on the incidence and prevalence of alcohol abuse within the nursing profession at the present time, Bissell and Jones (1981) estimate that there are some 75,000 alcoholic nurses in the United States.

*To whom requests for reprints should be addressed at the University of Illinois, College of Nursing, 845 Damen Avenue, Chicago, Illinois 60612.

 0020-773X/84/1905-0577$3.50/0

In view of the high estimates of alcohol abuse among nurses in the United States, studies of the drinking practices of student nurses are particularly appropriate for understanding the development of alcoholism. With the exception of a few studies (Engs, 1981; Horii, Toni, and Haga, 1976), there is little in the U.S. literature on the drinking patterns of student nurses. Engs (1981) examined the patterns of drug use among medical, nursing, and pharmacy students in Australia and noted that alcohol was the most commonly used drug. Sixty-five percent of the student nurses used alcohol on a monthly basis.

Within the United States the proportion of college women who drank at least occasionally increased from 61% in the 1949-1952 period (Straus and Bacon, 1953) to 73% in the early 1970s (Hanson, 1974). Engs (1977) has noted that there has been a steady increase in the percentages of female collegians who drink; in a survey of 13 U.S. colleges, Engs found the 75% of the women reported drinking at least once a year. Wechsler and McFadden (1979), in a survey of New England colleges, reported that less that 5% of these students were abstainers and that a majority drank on a weekly basis or more often (70% among men and 50% among women).

The purpose of the present study was to examine the use of alcohol among student nurses in the United States and to compare these drinking patterns with surveys of other collegiate samples.

METHOD

The subjects in this study were senior students enrolled full time in the undergraduate program of a college of nursing. The majority of the students were between 21 and 23 years of age (73%). A brief questionnaire on the use of alcohol was administered to the students in classroom settings in the fall of 1981. Of the total population of senior students ($N = 110$), 103 participated in the study. The items included in the questionnaire are presented in the Appendix.

As part of another study (Haack, 1982), these students also completed the Staff Burnout Scale for Helath Professionals (Jones, 1980). Twenty items from this scale measure burnout, and 10 items form a lie scale. Information from this scale was used to corroborate the information obtained from the drinking questionnaire. One item from this scale ("After work I often feel like relaxing with a drink of alcohol") correlated positively and significantly ($p < .01$) with each of the drinking items in the present questionnaire. The item intercorrelations are presented in Table 1.

Approximately 5% of the sample had lie scores which suggested an attempt at dishonesty in responding (Jones, 1980). A high score indicates denial of feelings everyone has had at one time or another. The lie score correlated negatively and significantly ($p < .01$) with the number of drinking days ($r = -.26$)

Table 1

Item Intercorrelations of Drinking Measures[a]

	Age	Lie	Relax	Heavy	Bar	Freq.	Beer	Wine	Liquor	Total	Regular
1. Age	1.00										
2. Lie	.04	1.00									
3. Relax	.10	–.30*	1.00								
4. Heavy	–.21**	–.17	.58*	1.00							
5. Bar	–.33*	–.05	.32*	.63*	1.00						
6. Frequency	–.01	–.26*	.51*	.56*	.46*	1.00					
7. Beer	–.08	–.27*	.36*	.60*	.43*	.58*	1.00				
8. Wine	.06	–.05	.33*	.39*	.38*	.65*	.25*	1.00			
9. Liquor	–.18**	–.04	.17	.30*	.23*	.35*	–.04	.15	1.00		
10. Total	–.14	–.23*	.46*	.71*	.55*	.81*	.84*	.64*	.36*	1.00	
11. Regular	.12	–.11	.42*	.43*	.44*	.43*	.35*	.33*	.16	.44*	1.00
12. Problem	.05	–.17	.16	.17	.18	.19**	.23**	.04	.08	.21**	.22**

[a]Item descriptions: (1) age in years; (2) lie scale from SBS-HP (Jones, 1980); (3) "relax after work with drink" from SBS-HP (Jones, 1980) (1 = disagree to 7 = agree); (4) frequency of 6 or more drinks per occasion in past month; (5) frequency of going to bars; (6) number of days drinking in past week; (7) number of beers consumed in past week; (8) number of wine drinks in past week; (9) number of liquor drinks in past week; (10) total number of drinks in past week; (11) regular drinking (1 = no; 2 = yes); (12) problem at school or work (1 = no; 2 = yes).

*$p < .01$.

**$p < .05$.

and with the total number of drinks consumed ($r = -.23$). Students who tended to fake good responses tended to underreport drinking experience.

RESULTS

Drinking Frequency

Three percent of the students indicated that they were abstainers, and 11% reported that they were infrequent drinkers (not in the past month). Nineteen percent reported drinking in the past month but not in the past week, and 67% reported drinking in the past week. Beer and wine were preferred beverages. Among drinkers, 22% drank beer only, 23% drank wine only, 10% drank liquor only, and 45% drank combinations of beverages.

While the proportion of abstainers is comparable to that of New England college women (Wechsler and McFadden, 1979), the present sample had a higher proportion of weekly drinkers. Forty-seven percent of the New England women at the senior grade level reported drinking less than weekly, compared to 33% in the present sample. The student nurse sample also had a higher proportion of students who drank 4 or more days in the past week (13%) than did the New England sample (22%). When compared to nursing students in Australia (Engs, 1981), the present sample had a higher proportion of monthly users (86% vs 65%).

Students were asked to indicate the age at onset of regular drinking, defined as having two or more drinks per week. Approximately 45% of the students indicated that they had not adopted a pattern of regular drinking. Among the regular drinkers, 18% indicated that they adopted a pattern of regular drinking before age 18, and 37% reported a pattern of regular drinking at age 18 or older.

Another indicator of the establishment of a regular pattern of alcohol use is the frequency of going to public settings licensed for the sale of alcohol (bars, cocktail lounges, etc.). Thirty percent indicated that they never went to bars, 22% reported going once in the past month, 32% reported two to three times in the past month, and 16% reported once or twice a week.

Drinking Amounts

The average number of drinks per occasion (total weekly drinks by number of drinking days) was distributed as follows: none, 33%; one drink, 10%; two drinks, 19%; three drinks, 19%; four drinks, 7%; five drinks, 6%; six or more drinks, 6%;

A measure more typical of heavier drinking is provided by the item which indicated the frequency of having six or more drinks per occasion in the past month. Approximately 53% of the students reported no occasions of this type, 21% reported one occasion in the past month, 12% reported two to three occasions, and 14% reported four or more occasions.

Comparisons with other surveys are difficult due to variations in the measures of heavier drinking. Wechsler and McFadden (1979) defined "heavy" drinkers as having consumed more than six cans of beer, five glasses of wine, or five drinks containing distilled spirits per occasion. Frequent-heavy drinkers consumed this amount at least once a week. Approximately 10% of the senior college women fell in this drinking category. Engs (1977) defined "heavy" drinking as having five or more drinks per occasion more than once a week, and "moderate-heavy" drinking as three to four drinks per occasion at least once a week. Among the women in that survey, approximately 18% were moderate-heavy drinkers and 4% were heavy drinkers.

Slightly higher proportions of the student nurse sample may be defined as heavier drinkers when compared to the New England college sample of senior women. Approximately 12% of the student nurses reported an average consumption of five or more drinks in the past week, and 14% reported four or more occasions of heavier drinking in the past month. Slightly higher proportions of the student nurses may also be defined as moderate-heavy drinkers according the Engs (1977). Approximately 26% of the student nurses reported an average consumption of three or four drinks in the past week.

The student nurses were asked to indicate if alcohol ever interfered with their school work or work on a job. Approximately 10% reported that alcohol interfered with school work and 4% with their job. Only one student reported problems both at school and at work. The combined proportion of students with either problem was 13%.

CONCLUSIONS

This study has shown that the student nurses in this sample have adopted a pattern of alcohol consumption that is comparable to that of other female collegians. While the frequency of drinking and the proportion of heavier drinkers were somewhat higher when compared to other studies, the drinking measures were based on recent (last 7 days) experience and not on average consumption patterns.

The development of prevention programs for young health professionals is clearly needed. The results of the present study indicate that a significant proportion of student nurses may be at risk with respect to alcohol-related consequences. Young health professionals, like student nurses, represent important target populations for study. The issue of the impaired nurse is serious because it is related not only to the professional life of the individual nurse but also to the ethical and humanistic care of patients.

At the present time, most undergraduate programs offer 2 to 4 clock hours on the subject of addictions. Some schools provide no information on this topic. The lack of education on addiction inhibits a student nurse or nurse who has a drinking problem from recognizing it or knowing what to do about it. The inability of the nursing profession to effectively identify and provide treatment for impaired colleagues is a serious loss to the field. The work of Bissell and Jones (1981) indicates that many of the addicted nurses graduated in the top third of their classes and were highly respected for their excellent work before the work was affected by an alcohol or drug problem. Future studies need to examine the social support networks of family and peers, and their influence on the development of alcohol abuse.

APPENDIX: QUESTIONNAIRE ITEMS

1. Have you ever had a drink of an alcoholic beverage, including beer, wine, and liquor? (Yes or no.)
2. How old were you when you first started drinking on a regular basis; that is, began having two or more drinks a week? (Age in years or does not drink two or more a week.)
3. Have you had any alcoholic beverage, including beer, wine, or liquor, during the last 30 days? (Yes or no.)
4. How often have you had 6 or more drinks on one occasion during the last 30 days? (Never, once, 2 or 3 times, 4 or 5 times, 6 or 7 times, 8 or 9 times, 10 or more times.)
5. How often in the last 30 days did you go to bars, taverns, or cocktail lounges (do not include restaurants)? (Never, once this month, 2-3 times during the month, once or twice a week, several times a week, almost every day.)
6. During the last 7 days, ending with yesterday, on how many days did you drink alcoholic beverages? (Number of days.)
7. During the last 7 days, how many cans or bottles of beer did you have? (Number of drinks.)
8. During the last 7 days, how many glasses of wine did you have? (Number of drinks.)
9. During the last 7 days, how many drinks did you have containing liquor, such as whiskey, vodka, gin, brandy, etc.? (Number of drinks.)
10. A. Has drinking ever interfered with your school work? (Yes or no.)
    B. Has drinking ever interfered with your work on a job? (Yes or no.)

REFERENCES

AMERICAN NURSES ASSOCIATION, *Handbook for Delegates for Use at ANA Convention,* Washington, DC, June 1982, p. 34.

BISSELL, L., and JONES, R.W. The alcoholic nurse. *Nursing Outlook* February 1981, pp. 96-101.

ENGS, R.C. Drinking patterns and drinking problems of college students. *J. Stud. Alcohol* 38: 2144-2156, 1977.

ENGS, R.C. *The drug taking patterns of medical, nursing and pharmacy students in Brisbane, Australia.* Paper presented at the National Nurses Society on Alcoholism Forum of the National Council on Alcoholism, New Orleans, LA, April 9, 1981.

HAACK, M.R. *Student nurse alcohol consumption and burnout.* Paper presented at the 28th International Institute on the Prevention and Treatment of Alcoholism, Munich, West Germany, July 5-9, 1982.

HANSON, D.J. Drinking attitudes and behaviors among college students. *J. Alcohol Drug Educ.* 19: 6-14, 1974.

HORII, T., TANI, N., and HAGA, H. Survey of concern for drinking and alcoholism. II. Students of school for nurse. *Japanese J. Stud. Alcohol* 11: 25-30, 1976.

ISLER, C. The alcoholic nurse: What they try to deny. *RN* 41(7): 48-55, 1978.

JAFFE, S. Help for the helper: First hand views on recovery. *Am. J. Nursing* 82(April): 578-579, 1981.

JONES, J.W. *The Staff Burnout Scale for Health Professionals.* Park Ridge, IL: London House Press, 1980.

KRAMER, N. *Reality Shock.* St. Louis: Mosby, 1974.

LEVENSTEIN, A. Alcohol and tension. *Supervisor Nurse* 11(3): 46-47, 1980.

LEVINE, D., PRESTON, P., and LIPSCOMB, S. Historical approach to understanding drug abuse among nurses. *Am. J. Psychiatry* 131(9): 1036-1037, 1975.

MASLACH, C. Burned-out. *Hum. Behav.* September, 1976, pp. 16-22.

STRAUS, R., and BACON, S.D. *Drinking in College.* New Haven: Yale University Press, 1953.

WECHSLER, H., and MC FADDEN, M. Drinking among college students in New England: Extent, social correlates and consequences of alcohol use. *J. Stud. Alcohol* 40: 969-996, 1979.

WRIGHT, W. Nurses' drug problems are cloaked in denial. *The Journal* February 1982, p. 16.

The International Journal of the Addictions, 19(5), 585-590, 1984

Note

Prediction of Readmission in a Cohort of Alcoholics: A 2-Year Follow-Up

Richard A. Holland,* MA

Richard C. Evenson, PhD

Department of Psychiatry
University of Missouri School of Medicine at the Missouri Institute of Psychiatry
St. Louis, Missouri 63139

Abstract

A cohort of 1,192 first admissions to metropolitan public alcohol treatment programs was examined after 2 years. With the sample subdivided by number of readmissions, discriminant analysis based on demographic data, social history, and current drinking behavior provided only modest prediction of group membership (κ = .46), but may be sufficient to provide an alerting function for recidivism.

INTRODUCTION

A persistent problem in the treatment of alcoholism is the effect of a core group of chronic alcoholics who continue to reappear and eventually comprise the majority of all admissions. In the literature dealing with the follow-up of alcoholics after discharge, readmission rates often approach 60%. Rosenblatt, Gross, Malenowski, Broman, and Lewis (1971) found that 46% of 805 males studied had one or more earlier admissions. Vallance (1965), in a 2-year follow-up of 68 male alcoholics, found that half were readmitted. Earlier work here (Holland, Evenson, and Izadi, 1979) found that 62% of 409 alcoholics in treatment had a history of prior admissions.

*To whom correspondence should be addressed at the Missouri Institute of Psychiatry, 5400 Arsenal Street, St. Louis, Missouri 63139.

 0020-773X/84/1905-0585$3.50/0

Obviously, such recidivists do not respond well to the usual treatment offered. If this hard-core group of treatment-resistant alcoholic clients could be identified in advance, special attention could be provided and eventually, special programs developed.

The purpose of the present study was to determine whether the likelihood of an alcoholic patient being readmitted at a later time could be predicted by some combination of demographic and clinical variables.

METHOD

The sample selected was all first admissions to alcohol treatment wards at two large metropolitan public mental health facilities in St. Louis during the period 1973-1974. These programs were the only alcohol treatment programs provided by the Missouri Division of Mental Health in the greater St. Louis area. Data recorded for each patient were retrieved from the automated information system maintained by the Missouri Department of Mental Health (Hedlund, Sletten, Evenson, Altman, and Cho, 1977). Briefly, the system connects the major public mental health installations in the state to a central computer. An automated case registry is maintained, and various clinical instruments are keypunched and stored. Of particular interest were data collected with the Alcohol History Form (AHF), a self-report instrument developed to assess alcohol debilitation and drinking history. Earlier work has outlined the development (Evenson, Altman, Cho, and Montgomery, 1973) and reliability (Holland, Datta, Izadi, and Evenson, 1979) of the instrument, as well as the Missouri Alcohol Severity Scale (Evenson, Holland, and Cho, 1979), a measure scored from the Alcohol History Form. The Alcohol History Form includes an overall measure of severity of alcoholism, as well as items covering drinking history and background, drinking patterns and symptoms of alcoholism, interpersonal relationships, legal problems, and contact with helping agencies. Complete face-sheet data were also available, including demographic and socioeconomic variables. A total of 155 variables were included in the initial data pool.

During the 2-year period, 1,192 patients were admitted, discharged, and followed via the computerized data base for an additional 2 years through 1976. The number of readmissions to the facilities were noted: no readmissions (N = 782), one readmission (N = 227), and more than one readmission (N = 183). The sample was 88% male, 63% White, and 38% unemployed at admission. The age range was 3% age 18-29, 17% age 30-39, 30% age 40-49, 37% age 50-64, and 13% age 65 and over. Mean education was 10.1 years. Marital status included 26% married and 46% divorced.

Using demographic variables from the admission face sheet and the clinical/historical items from the Alcohol History Form, an analysis of variance was used to select the 80 items with the highest univariate F value across the readmission group classifications. These 80 items were then used in a stepwise discriminant analysis (Dixon, 1972) to determine the combination of variables best able to predict group membership (readmissions). The statistical program also allowed the random division of the sample into two halves; the discriminate function was developed on one half and cross-validated on the other.

Since the three-group classification for admissions is somewhat arbitrary, a similar analysis was done for two other classifications: (1) no readmissions versus any readmissions; and (2) no readmissions, 1 readmission, 2-3 readmissions, and 4 or more readmissions.

RESULTS AND DISCUSSION

The alternate categories of readmission frequency discussed in the preceding section resulted in less accurate prediction, and the results presented here are based on "no readmissions versus one readmission versus more than one readmission."

Maximum prediction occurred at the fifth step of the statistical program, and the five variables comprising the discriminant function are shown in Table 1, along with the item means for each readmission group. It should be noted that the results discussed here were cross-validated, as discussed earlier.

The multivariate prediction for each group can be compared with the actual group readmission rate in Table 2. The data in Table 2 represent the cross-validation sample ($N = 582$). The overall classification accuracy in 72%. However, the value of kappa (Cohen, 1960), which corrects for chance agreement, is only .46, indicating a modest level of prediction. As can be seen in Table 2, the discriminant function was able to correctly predict 87% of the "no readmission" group, 67% of the "one readmission" group, and 21% of the "more than one readmission" group. This level of agreement may, in fact, be enough to serve as an "alerting" index for clients who may need special attention.

Table 3 shows the largest correlations ($> .25$) with other items for the five predictor items used in the discriminant function. The correlates help clarify the nature of the successful predictor items. Item 4 seems clearly related to severity. Item 2 may be related to the fact that facility B serves a more impoverished area and does not receive detoxification patients directly from the police, as does facility A.

Table 4 shows recidivism rates broken down by type of admission: detoxification only and alcohol treatment center patients. It can be seen that detoxification patients have relatively greater multiple readmissions (18% compared to 10%). Presumably, this is reflected in the predictor item "admission to facility B."

We also calculated the mean years of problem drinking by number of readmissions. Those with no readmissions reported an average of 9.2 years (SD

Table 1

Predictor Items and Group Membership Mean Values

Step no.	Item	Number of readmissions[a] None		1		> 1	
1	Referral source other than self or friend	.21	(.41)	.90	(.30)	.93	(.26)
2	Admission to facility B	.25	(.43)	.20	(.40)	.12	(.33)
3	Spouse going to leave because of drinking	.26	(.44)	.34	(.48)	.30	(.46)
4	Drinking first a problem at age 20-29	.07	(.26)	.18	(.38)	.18	(.39)
5	No arrests or charges because of drinking	.09	(.28)	.21	(.41)	.25	(.44)

[a]Standard deviations in parentheses.

12.2) of problem drinking. Those with one readmission reported an average of 13.0 (SD 12.8) years of problem drinking. Those with more than one readmission reported an average of 14.2 (SD 14.1) years of problem drinking.

Since the discriminate analysis does best in predicting those who do not return, with decreasing accuracy for the recidivist groups, it seems likely that the predictor variables used do not include those most closely related to recidivism. This is consistent with earlier work be Adamson, Fostakowsky, and Chebib (1974), who found poor prediction of drinking outcome using life history and drinking behavior variables. They report motivational and attitudinal variables as best discriminators of abstinent versus nonabstinent groups. However, their study employed a very small sample (N = 38) and was not cross-validated.

Table 2

Predicted and Actual Readmission of Alcoholics[a]

		Predicted None	1	> 1	
Actual	None	324	44	3	371
	1	21	75	16	112
	> 1	11	67	21	99
		356	186	40	582[b]

[a]% correct = 72%; κ = .46.
[b]Replication half-sample.

Table 3

Correlates of Predictor Variables (r ⩾ .25)

1. Referral source other than self or friend
   a. Occupation: sales (.31)
   b. Military service (–.31)

2. Admission to facility B
   a. Referral source: relative or friend (–.89)
   b. Military service (–.52)
   c. Occupation: sales (.50)
   d. 3 days since last drink (.32)
   e. Cause of drinking: myself (.30)
   f. Severe hangovers (.28)
   g. Headaches (.27)
   h. Usually drink in bars or restaurants (.26)
   i. Not eating regularly (.25)
   j. No help from doctor, priest, minister, spouse (.25)
   k. Blackouts (.25)

3. Spouse leaving because of drinking
   a. Live with spouse and kids (.32)
   b. 24 hours since last drink (.29)
   c. Unemployed (.26)

4. Drinking first a problem at age 20-29
   a. No help from doctor, priest, minister, spouse (.37)
   b. Severe hangovers (.34)
   c. Headaches (.33)
   d. Shakes (.31)
   e. Not eating regularly (.25)
   f. No visits to hospital or clinic (.25)

5. No arrests or charges because of drinking
   a. No visits to hospital or clinic (.29)
   b. Fights when drinking (.28)

Table 4

Initial Admission Status by Number of Readmissions (N = 1,192)

	Number of readmissions					
	0		1		> 1	
Detoxification	525	(63%)	161	(19%)	146	(18%)
Alcohol treatment	257	(71%)	66	(18%)	37	(10%)

Siegel and Alexander (1982) found recidivism to be related to history of prior admissions, length of index admission, and receipt of aftercare services, for a sample of 252 patients. They found a 45% readmission rate for their sample, compared to the 34% found in the present study. It should be noted that our study includes first admissions only.

It seems likely that readmission to alcohol inpatient treatment is a process rather than a discrete event. That is, there is a complex interaction over time between levels of support available or utilized, including inpatient services, outpatient services, family or support networks, and precipitants such as physical/emotional well-being, economic conditions, and forces of social control.

In general, our results seem to indicate that in predicting readmission to alcohol treatment, social history and drinking patterns may not play the most dominant role, although they may be useful in alerting staff to likely recidivists.

REFERENCES

ADAMSON, J.D., FOSTAKOWSKY, R.T., AND CHEBIB, F.S. Measures assoicated with outcome on one year follow-up of male alcoholics. *Br. J. Psychiatry* 69: 325-337, 1974.

COHEN, J. A coefficient of agreement for nominal scales. *Educ. Psychol. Measurement* 20(1): 37-47, 1960.

DIXON, W.J. (ed.). *BMD: Biomedical Computer Programs.* Berkeley: University of California Press, 1972.

EVENSON, R.C., ALTMAN, H., CHO, D.W., and MONTEGOMERY, J. Development of an alcoholism severity scale via an iterative computer program for item analysis. *Q. J. Stud. Alcohol* 34(4): 1336-1341, 1973.

EVENSON, R.C., HOLLAND, R.A., and CHO, D.W. A scale for measuring the severity of alcoholism and evaluating its treatment. *J. Stud. Alcohol* 40(11): 1077-1081, 1979.

HEDLUND, J.L., SLETTEN, I.W., EVENSON, R.C., ALTMAN, H., and CHO, D.W. Automated psychiatric information systems: A critical review of Missouri's Standard System of Psychiatry (SSOP). *J. Oper. Psychiatry* 8(1): 5-26, 1977.

HOLLAND, R., DATTA, K., IZADI, B., and EVENSON, R.C. Reliability of an alcohol self-report instrument. *J. Stud. Alcohol* 40(1): 142-144, 1979.

HOLLAND, R.A., EVENSON, R.C., and IZADI, B. Characteristics of detoxification patients referrred to alcoholism treatment programs. *J. Stud. Alcohol* 40(9): 914-917, 1979.

ROSENBLATT, S.M., GROSS, M.M., MALENOWSKI, M.S., BROMAN, M., and LEWIS, E. Marital status and multiple psychiatric admissions for alcoholism: A cross validation. *Q. J. Stud. Alcohol* 32: 1092-1096, 1971.

SIEGEL, C., and ALEXANDER, M.J. Factors relating to recidivism among alcoholics. In *Proceedings of the Seventh Annual Multi-state Information System National Users Group Conference.* Orangeburg, NY: Information Sciences Division, Rockland Research Institute, 1982, pp. 229-236.

VALLENCE, M. Alcoholism: A two year follow-up study of patients admitted to the psychiatric department of a general hospital. *Br. J. Psychiatry* 111: 348-356, 1965.

The International Journal of the Addictions, 19(5), 591–593, 1984

Note

A Task Approach to Drug Use Intervention

Stanley Einstein,* PhD

Middle Eastern Summer Institute on Drug Use

Abstract

A schema is presented to help intervention agents and agencies plan and carry out programs which focus upon a number of tasks which need to be adequately fulfilled by the individuals and/or systems in order to facilitate healthy growth, maturation, and functioning.

A pragmatic way of viewing and planning drug use intervention is from the perspective of *tasks.* Mental health specialists, as well as educators, have in a variety of ways suggested that a certain number of tasks have to be adequately fulfilled by the individual in order for healthy growth and maturation to occur. These tasks include:

1. The establishment of emotional and psychological independence from parents and other adults as well as from peers.
2. The achievement of self-definition; a stable self-concept/self-identity.
3. The development of self-motivation and self-determination.
4. The establishment of an appropriate set of values to be used as a guide for behavior and of a self-control system used to implement the ethical/value system(s) which has been selected/developed.
5. The development of empathy as well as involvement in reciprocal interpersonal relationships.
6. The establishment and acceptance of an appropriate sexual identity and the development of meaningful and satisfying sexual relationships.

*Address correspondence to the author at 113/41 East Talpiot, Jerusalem, Israel.

 0020-773X/84/1905-0591$3.50/0

Table 1

A Schematic Framework for Developing a Task Approach to Drug Use Intervention

	Key task concepts									
Selected intervention factors	Independence	Identity	Self-determination	Values	Reciprocity	Capacities	Skills	Appropriate behavior	Trust	Other (specify)
Criteria										
Process										
Techniques										
Intervention agents										
Roles										
Policies										
Needed support system										
Site of intervention										
Temporal sequences										
Ongoing evaluation process										
Outcome: Success Failure										
Budget: Source(s) Amount										
Feedback system(s) Micro Macro										

7. The development of new and necessary intellectual capacities and skills.
8. The ability to function satisfactorily with others and to behave appropriately in relating to one's peers as well as other generations.
9. The acquisition of training or engagement in a training program that will develop the skills for achieving economic independence.
10. The development and acquisition of an open-ended range of coping skills, strategies, and styles in order to effectively function and adapt within a relatively unlimited number of types of intra- and interpersonal worlds with their associated lack of predictability, control, and various levels of ambiguity.
11. The development of trust in oneself and in others.

Table 1 is designed to help the reader determine what role(s) s/he may play in the achievement of these tasks. Each task should be well defined in terms of criteria. The process, available and theoretical, for achieving the specific task should be clearly spelled out. This includes selection of the most effective techniques and understanding of the time it will take to achieve the specific task, the most appropriate site for effective intervention, and who the most likely intervention agent(s) can be and should be. Within this approach the reader will surely find a role for him/herself as well.

One can, by expanding or somewhat changing the focus of the key concepts, also use them as goals for group or national growth and maturation. Obviously the notion that the tasks which are listed are the key ones for achieving health for individual and/or group/national functioning is an assumption. The reader who chooses to disagree with the importance of these tasks or who adds other ones will have to develop and be sure of the validity of his/her own assumptions.

The International Journal of the Addictions, 19(5), 595–599, 1984

Note

A Functional Approach to Drug Use Intervention

Stanley Einstein,* PhD

Middle Eastern Summer Institute on Drug Use

Abstract

A schema is presented designed to help intervention agents and agencies plan and carry out programs which relate to a variety of human functions which historically have been associated with a broad range of chemical substances: drugs, medicines, social substances, sacramental substances, etc.

A most reasonable way of approaching drug use intervention is by focusing upon the *function(s)* of drug use. Such a view helps us to put aside our feelings and thoughts about specific types of substances and particular types of people as well as the manner in which the "drug" was used.

In simple terms, this approach starts with the assumption (and/or is based upon the analysis of available data) that drug use has been able to, and continues to meet adaptational needs of individuals, groups, cultures, and societies (Table 1). We, as potential intervention agents, have the option of reviewing the *meaning(s)* and *importance* of each of these functions for ourselves as well as for others. We also have the option, as well as the responsibility, to consider what nonchemical, nondrug, nonsubstance alternatives exist to meet a particular function. This is not to suggest that there is anything inherently wrong with or bad about the current "chemical" solution. Indeed it may be the best, most efficient, safest, quickest, etc., manner of achieving a function which we agree is important to us or which someone else has decided is important for us—as well as for them.

*Address correspondence to the author at 113/41 East Talpiot, Jerusalem, Israel.

 0020-773X/84/1905-0595$3.50/0

Table 1

Categorizing Chemical Substances by Functions

Functions	Examples
Aesthetic	Achieving aesthetic experiences (American Indians [peyote] : strengthen dancing, playing music, learning, painting, and bead design; jazz musicians [marijuana] : achieving special effects in music; Huxley [mescaline] : to see beauty not available to ordinary man).
Aphrodesiac	Directing, increasing, and reinforcing sensual feelings and love making. This is basically a placebo effect. Beauty drugs (cosmetics) are given a love- and affection-winning role.
Cultural	Developing and maintaining drug use and abstinent cultural/subcultural activities, rituals, and life-styles.
Recreational	Facilitating recreational (leisure-type) activities, roles, and rituals.
Religious	Part of sacramental rituals and symbolism; developing a oneness with God/Supreme Force.
Psychological support	To provide support during severe stress situations which the individual (personality/biochemical structure) experiences temporarily or permanently (chemotherapy: tranquilizers, energizers, antidepressants, mood stabilizers, psychedelics, "death therapy").
Ego disruption	"Getting out of the rut"; sensation seeking (alcohol, hallucinogens, heroin).
Therapeutic	Primary, secondary, and tertiary prevention (medical and dental treatment; self-treatment).
Institutional	Meeting institutional needs/values (medicating patients at night in hospitals; medicating hyperactive schoolchildren).
Political	Developing, maintaining, and preventing the achievement of political needs and aspirations ("treating" dissidents in the USSR with psychotropics; reintroduction of opium into China by the British and then by the Japanese; Prohibition in the USA; politicizing drug use intervention). Maintaining a political status quo.
Ideological	Developing, maintaining, and reinforcing an ideological position/thesis ("Religion is the opium of the people" [Marx] ; "Alcohol is the devil's brew" [Temperance Movement] ; "Turn on, tune in, drop out" [Timothy Leary]).
Economic control	To maintain economic life-styles of nations, governments, companies, etc. (Peru [cocaine chewers] ; tobacco and alcoholic beverage industries, pharmaceutical industry [amphetamines]).

(continued)

Table 1 (continued)

Functions	Examples
Social control	Manipulation of psychological states through drugs for the control and direction of the individual (or group) whose personality and/or behavior is being affected (control of acting-out patients or of prisoners; prevention of acting up by "dissatisfied" populations).
Population control	Preventing, maintaining, or increasing the population to meet individual and/or systemic needs and goals.
War and other conflict functions	Biochemical warfare, poison gas, poison-tipped arrows; "drugging" soldiers before and during battles; disabling hostage holders.
Research	Researching behavior (LSD and psychosis).
Chemical catalysts/ facilitators	Preventing, facilitating, increasing, and minimizing the action of various chemical substances (enzyme actions).
Other	(Specify.)

What a functional approach can do for us, if we permit ourselves to become engaged by it, is to question the life-styles, patterns of adaptation, and coping skills of individuals and small and large groups/systems. It should permit us to analyze such modern truisms as *progress through chemistry,* for the individual, the primary group, and the nation. A functional approach would not question the chemical formula but certainly would question the formulation of progress. Table 2 appears to be a complicated table. It isn't. It lists a variety of functions which drugs, medicines, social substances, and other chemicals have been given through man's historical development. A number of selected factors have been listed to help the reader determine for him/herself, or with the help of others, the actual and potential meaning(s) and implications of the specific function which is being met by chemical means. When any given row is completed, or when the reader completes the entire table s/he should have a much better understanding about how various human functions have been met or can be met, and what our roles might be in such efforts.

At the very least such an approach should help us to integrate the fact that drug use is not simply the end result of certain types of people, using certain types of substances in certain ways and for certain reasons—all of which should be handled by someone else.

Table 2

Schematic Framework for Planning a Functional Use Model for Drug Use Intervention

Types of functions met by drugs	Program initiator (why/who)	Type of program (what)	Program focus (who/what)	Techniques (screening)	Goals	Policies, decisions	Staff (who)	Roles	Site (where)	Temporal factors (when/how long)	Needed coopera-tion (others)	Ongoing evalua-tion (what/when)	Criteria (success/failure)
Aesthetic													
Aphrodesiac													
Cultural													
Recreational													
Religious													
Psychological support													
Ego disruption													
Therapeutic													
Institutional													

Political													
Ideological													
Economic control													
Social control													
War and other conflict functions													
Population control													
Research													
Chemical catalysts/ facilitators													
Other (specify)													

INFORMATION FOR AUTHORS SUBMITTING MANUSCRIPTS

Send a clear double-spaced typewritten original and one duplicate to Ms. Nancy Reid-Rappolt, Editorial Assistant, *International Journal of the Addictions,* c/o Winch, Smith, Ostermann and Mates, MD's, 4141 Geary, Suite 326, San Francisco, California 94118. Also send one duplicate to the Chief Editor, Dr. Stanley Einstein, Building 113/41, East Talpiot, Jerusalem, Israel. DOUBLE-SPACE the entire manuscript; do not use single spacing anywhere, including references.

Include authors' academic degrees and present affiliation. If applicable, cite auspices under which work being reported was done. Specify address to which requests for reprints should be sent.

Begin your TITLE with a word useful in indexing. A 75- to 100-word ABSTRACT should be provided, which precedes each article. A summary is then not necessary. Major and minor headings may be used in the text; indicate major headings by typing in capitals.

Use METRIC UNITS of measure. If measurements were made in English units, give metric equivalents.

Cite all TABLES and FIGURES in the text. Tables should have titles, and figures should have brief legends. In tables, give each column a heading. Indicate units of measure in parentheses in the heading for each column. Do not use vertical rules. Do not use horizontal rules other than those in the heading and at the bottom. Submit PHOTOGRAPHS as glossy prints, untrimmed and unmounted; identify each with pencil lightly on the back and indicate top.

ARTWORK will not be returned unless specifically requested, and will be disposed of three months after publication.

REFERENCES in the text should be enclosed in parentheses and include the author's surname and the date of the item cited. Keep footnotes to a minimum. Footnotes should be collected at the end of the manuscript in their numerical order of appearance.

The BIBLIOGRAPHY (double-spaced) should be given at the end of the article in alphabetical order. Journal references should include authors, title, name of journal abbreviated according to *Chemical Abstracts List of Periodicals*, inclusive page numbers, and date. Book references should include authors, title, place of publication, publisher, and date.

AUTHOR RESPONSIBILITY: It is the sole responsibility of the author(s) to obtain written permission from the author(s), publisher(s), etc. for figures, tables, or any other information excerpted from previously published works which are used in the manuscript(s) considered for publication. It is understood that the manuscript(s) considered for publication in the *International Journal of the Addictions* have not been previously published nor are they under simultaneous publication consideration elsewhere.

Statements and opinions expressed in the articles and communications herein are those of the author(s) and do not necessarily express those of the Editor or publisher.

THE INTERNATIONAL JOURNAL OF THE ADDICTIONS

Volume 19 Number 5 1984

CONTENTS

Outcome Evaluations in Substance Abuse: A Comparison of Alcoholism, Drug Abuse, and Other Mental Health Interventions: M. S. Goldstein, M. Surber, and D. M. Wilner 479

Predictors of Adolescents' Intentions to Smoke: Age, Sex, Race, and Regional Differences: C. C. Presson, L. Chassin, S. J. Sherman, R. Olshavsky, M. Bensenberg, and E. Corty 503

Professional Psychotherapy and Its Relationship to Compliance in Treatment: C. J. Rogalski 521

Alcohol Use by Juvenile Offenders: B. Segal, S. S. Hobfoll, and F. Cromer 541

Defining Alcohol Problems as a Repressive Mechanism: Its Formative Phase in Imperial Germany and Its Strength Today: I. Vogt 551

Research Notes

Student Substance Use: Stability and Change across College Years: K. E. Friend and P. A. Koushki 571

Drinking Patterns among Student Nurses: M. R. Haack and T. C. Harford 577

Notes

Prediction of Readmission in a Cohort of Alcoholics: A 2-Year Follow-Up: R. A. Holland and R. C. Evenson 585

A Task Approach to Drug Use Intervention: S. Einstein 591

A Functional Approach to Drug Use Intervention: S. Einstein 595

MARCEL DEKKER, INC., New York and Basel

CODEN: INJABN 19(6) i-ii, 601-708 (1984)
ISSN: 0020-773X

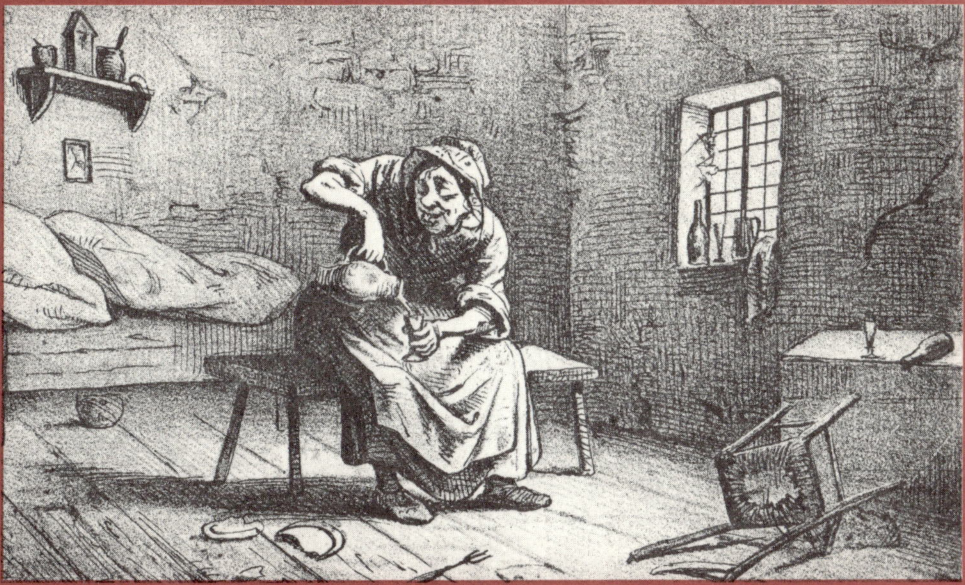

THE INTERNATIONAL JOURNAL OF THE Addictions

Volume 19 Number 6 1984

THE INTERNATIONAL JOURNAL OF THE ADDICTIONS

September 1984

Aims and Scope. This journal is a comprehensive medium for worldwide communication among both concerned laymen and professionals in research, training, and treatment in the field of addiction and substance misuse.

Indexing and Abstracting Services. Articles published in *The International Journal of the Addictions* are selectively indexed or abstracted in:

• Adolescent Mental Health Abstracts • ASCA • Bibliographic Index of Health Education Periodicals (BIHEP) • BioSciences Information Service of Biological Abstracts (BIOSIS) • Classified Abstract Archive of the Alcohol Literature • Current Contents/Clinical Practice • Excerpta Medica • Index Medicus • International Pharmaceutical Abstracts • ISI/BIOMED • Journal of Abstracts of the All-Union Institute of Scientific and Technical Information of the USSR • Psychological Abstracts • Science Citation Index • Selected List of Tables of Contents of Psychiatric Periodicals • Social Sciences Citation Index • State Central Scientific Medical Library/International Book Exchange—USSR

Articles published in *The International Journal of the Addictions* are listed in Selected List of Tables of Contents of Psychiatric Periodicals.

Manuscript Preparation and Submission. See end of issue.

Subscription Information. *The International Journal of the Addictions* (ISSN: 0020-773X) is published eight times annually in February, April, May, July, August, September, November, and December by Marcel Dekker, Inc., 270 Madison Avenue, New York, New York 10016. The subscription rate for Volume 19 (1984), containing eight numbers, is $225.00 per volume (prepaid). The special discounted rate for individual professionals and students is $112.50 per volume. To secure this special rate, your order must be prepaid by personal check. Add $20.00 for surface postage outside the United States. For airmail to Europe, add $32.48; to Asia, add $40.48.

Mailing Address. *Please mail payment with order to:* Marcel Dekker Journals, P. O. Box 11305, Church Street Station, New York, New York 10249.

Contributions to this journal are published free of charge. Second-class postage paid at New York, New York and additional mailing offices. POSTMASTER: Send address changes to *The International Journal of the Addictions*, P. O. Box 5005, Cimarron Road, Monticello, New York 12701.

Library of Congress Catalog Card Number 66-9896

Cover illustration courtesy of the Picture Collection, The Branch Libraries, New York Public Library.

THE INTERNATIONAL JOURNAL OF THE Addictions

The International Journal of the Addictions, 19(6), 601–611, 1984

Women and Alcohol Abuse—Factors Involved in Successful Interventions

Sue Dobbs Robinson, BA

The Ohio State University
Columbus, Ohio 43210

Abstract

This paper examines factors involved in successful interventions that led 18 alcoholic women to seek treatment. Literature was lacking concerning intervention with women, though there was one general source on intervention. A hypothesis on the benefit of families was contradicted. In the research, families were usually nonexistent or a barrier to recovery. Findings indicated that successful interventions ranged from a choice of treatment versus jail to seeking help due to internal feelings.

LITERATURE REVIEW

Literature was found stressing a nonjudgmental yet confrontive approach to intervention. It did not, however, cite information specifically about women and intervention (Johnson, 1973). Alcoholism is more often linked to psychological stress and a specific precipitating circumstance in women than in men, indicating a possibility that social and environmental factors can more readily be used with women to reverse their drinking patterns (Beckman, 1975). Women at one center who got divorces recovered more successfully than those who returned to their marriages (Hornik, 1977). Additionally, in cases in which alcoholic women are married, husbands often reduce the chances that their wives will obtain treatment because men deny a wife's alcoholism more often than women deny a husband's problem, and men cover up more for their wives (Badiet, 1975). Similarly, the parents of single alcoholic women often take over

 0020-773X/84/1906-0601$3.50/0

their responsibilities for them (Hornik, 1977), likewise reducing the chances for successful treatment. However, being in a program with only women has helped many change the low image of themselves and other women that they previously held (Sandmaier, 1977).

Many alcoholic women go to physicians with symptoms other than, but resulting from, their alcoholism and end up with a prescription for tranquilizers and an ultimate cross-addiction (Fraser, 1975). Women alcoholics are also admitted more often to hospitals as psychiatric patients, and for longer times, than male alcoholics (Beckman, 1975). Emergency wards are a possible source of referrring patients to treatment for their alcoholism in instances where these women arrive injured and drunk.

The Women's Alcoholism Program of CASPAR (Cambridge and Somerville for Alcoholism Rehabilitation) has had an active outreach program. They found that many organizations had regarded alcohol as a moral problem that they should not treat, and that alcohol problems were often not recognized. Since this outreach program began, numbers of women seeking treatment have increased substantially, with a large number of women being referred by the community agencies that had received training from the Women's Alcoholism Program (Sandmaier, 1977).

METHODOLOGY

This analysis is primarily qualitative. No statistical analysis was done in this research. In the summer of 1980 interviews were conducted with 18 recovering alcoholic women who were contacted through Operation Safety Valve, Lesbian Peer Support, Alcoholics Anonymous members, and friends known to the author to have personal experience with alcoholism. The majority of interviews were arranged by telephone; a minority were arranged face-to-face. All were conducted in as private a setting as possible, usually in the subjects' homes or places of business.

In order to ensure anonymity, the interview guides were numbered. Entree was obtained in advance of the interviews through a combination of a personal introduction by the interviewer, an explanation of the research, and a positive reference of the interviewer's character by a third party. Also available was a letter of introduction from Sue Blanshan, PhD, the advisor in this research.

The interviewer's attitude and nonverbal communication were nonjudgmental, and mention of the interviewer's personal experience with alcoholism was made in some instances. Interviews were designed with the intention of encouraging subjects to self-report on their drinking history and the people and/or events that led them to get help for their drinking problems. The interview form was quite open ended. Interviews generally lasted about 1 hour, so subjects were given ample time to respond.

ANALYSIS OF DATA: FINDINGS AND PROBLEMS

Families

Though three of the subjects were married at the time of the interview, these women were sought out by the interviewer for this reason. It was very difficult to find women who were married at the time they entered treatment and were still married at the time of the interview.

Children and surrogate children seemed to have little influence on many of the women, being unable to influence them to accept treatment, though subjects often reported that their children now help keep them sober. In two instances, however, women entered treatment primarily due to their feelings that they were not caring for their children properly. One of these subjects felt humiliated into treatment when her teenage son referred to her as an alcoholic. Another was embarrassed when her son reported that he had been asked in school what he had eaten for breakfast and his response had been "Three Oreo cookies and a dill pickle."

Additionally, the emancipated adult daughter of one subject confronted the subject and her husband directly, telling them, "If you don't get the booze out of the house, you will never see me again." When the subject's spouse denied having a problem, the daughter replied, "*Both* of you," and stood ready to back up her threat.

Helping Professions

A total of five women reported having spent time in psychiatric units. Four received no help for their alcoholism in these units. One of these women reported being taken to psychiatric wards on three occasions drunk on a stretcher: her alcoholism was never mentioned.

Five women reported seeing counselors who either were unaware of their alcoholism or did not know how to deal with it. Six reported seeing doctors who did not help. These findings confirm previous research indicating that alcoholic women often have a great deal of contact with professional people who have an opportunity to intervene in the interest of guiding them to treatment (Fraser, 1975; Beckman, 1975), but do not do so.

Medical Factors

Doctors and counselors have great opportunities for intervention but often do not utilize them. Fifteen of the subjects had experiences with professionals who either did not recognize the problem or had no idea how to deal with it. Some were even told not to quit drinking!

Some reported receiving prescriptions from doctors and psychiatrists. One, who was polyaddicted, reported that she had periods during which she was so high on the pills her psychiatrist had prescribed that she had no need to drink!

Tables 1-4 give specifics on much of the information gained in this study. Support for versus barriers to seeking and continuing treatment are covered in Table 1. Table 2 covers responses to drinking/alcoholism, including a listing by subject of personal responses and behavior. Background characteristics of subjects are covered in Table 3, including number of types of previous treatments and length of sobriety. Table 4 covers drinking history and other problem drinkers in the family.

Table 1

Support/Barriers for Seeking and Continuing Treatment

Type	No. of subjects
Support	
Self	
Desire for sobriety	18
Concern about children	4
Working in alcoholism field	5
Familial	
Daughter (age 12)	1
Adult daughter/direct intervention	1
Parents (living away)	1
Sister	1
Spouse	1
Other individuals	
Boyfriend	1
Close friend	4
Institutional	
Threat of prosecution	1
Threat of jail	1
Mental hospitalization	2
Employer held job	1
Group membership[a]	
Alcoholics Anonymous	17
Operation Safety Valve	6
Lesbian Peer Support	2
Barriers	
Personal	
Pride	1
Educational fulfillment	1
Anonymity desired	1
Low self-esteem	1
Ignorance	2

(continued)

Table 1 (continued)

Type	No. of subjects
Familial	
Spouse "best drinking buddy"	2
Addicted child	1
Threat of divorce	1
Affluence–parents supporting subject	2
Addicted nuclear family	1
Spouse hiding bottles	1
Institutional	
Fear of prosecution	1
Hospital misdiagnosis	2
Recorded own consumption for school project/not confronted	1
Nurse couldn't get information through profession	1
Open work schedule	1
AA didn't return call	1
Unhelpful doctors	6
Financial	
None	11
Spouse refused to pay medical expenses	2
Other	
Ob-Gyn and physician/husband whitewash of alcohol-induced miscarriage	1
Blackout-induced "streaking"[b]; nonconfrontive neighbors	1
No barriers	1

[a]Operation Safety Valve is a women's program designed to supplement AA membership; Lesbian Peer Support refers to a substance abuse division of LPS.
[b]"Streaking" is used in this context to indicate going around the neighborhood naked.

Table 2

Responses to Drinking/Alcoholism

Others' responses	
Type	No. of subjects
Familial	
Anger, disgust	4
Helplessness	1
Double standard	1
Unaware	1
Talk/nag/show concern	10
Denial	3
Confrontation	1
No response	1

(continued)

Table 2 (continued)

Others' responses	
Type	No. of subjects
Friends, etc.	
Helplessness	1
Unaware	1
Talk/nag/show concern	11
Took to counselor	1
No response	1
Employers	
No employer	2
Helped get nursing license back	1
Threat of law	1
Potential firing (learned indirectly)	1
Suspended or fired/not confronted	2
Felt blacklisted/no employment, no explanation	1
Intervention/job held for *S*	1
No response	10
As employer, *S* fired employee who "got too nosy"	1

Professionals' responses	
Type	No. of professionals
No treatment sought	1
No help/nursing license revoked	1
AA/treatment suggested	6
Social worker "gave push"	1
No help given	28

Personal responses/behavior (by subject)	
Subject no.	Responses
1	Several detox centers
	Loss of jobs
	Stealing drugs on job
2	Drank heavily in high school
	Virtually stopped eating
	DTs
	2 mental hospitalizations
3	Withdrawing, obsessions, wanting to die
	Was given Mellaril/quit using it
	Signed self into state hospital
4	DWIs[a]
	Forgery arrest
	Got into fights

(continued)

Table 2 (continued)

Personal responses/behavior (by subject)	
Subject no.	Responses
5	2 mental hospitalizations Overdoses/always let someone know
6	Not liking self when she drank Feeling of better off dead than alive
7	5 psychiatrists 2 mental hospitals Coming out of blackouts in midsentence
8	Loose sexual behavior Letting children down
9	Concerned about losing job Called AA Felt "corners were wearing away"
10	Anorexia Hospitalizations, psychiatrists Fired/became unemployable "Streaking" in blackouts
11	Unemployable "Gamut of psych. units"
12	Went into DTs from valium Sought help
13	Lots of trouble with school & law Suicide attempt Saw counselor
14	Depression Suicide attempts Sought help till she found right place
15	Polyaddicted/getting pills from doctor 8 psychiatrists in 10 years
16	Feeling of throwing life away Despondency
17	Several decisions to quit Functioning "on automatic" Sought AA
18	Physically ill Agreed to AA, went 1 year Return to drinking, then AA

[a]DWI is used here to indicate an arrest for driving while intoxicated.

Table 3

Background Characteristics of Subjects

Characteristic	No. of subjects	Characteristic	No. of subjects
Marital status		Educational status	
Married	3	Less than H.S. graduate[a]	3
Separated	1	H.S. grad., no college[a]	5
Divorced	8	Some college[a]	2
Never married	3	4 year degree	2
Widowed	2	Nurse's training (RN)	3
Previous long-term "live-in"	1	Master's degree or higher	3
		Vocational status:	
Age		Business owner	1
19-25	3	Professional-level employment	11
26-35	4	Unemployed	4
36-45	8	Underemployed	1
46-55	3	Secretary	1
Over 55	0	Varied employment	1
Ethnicity: Unknown (16 subjects White, 2 Black)	18	Medical: Unknown	18
		Length of sobriety	
		Under 6 mo	4
		6 mo to 1 yr	2
Religion (past and present)		1-2 yr	2
Catholic	6	2-4 yr	4
Apostolic	1	4-7 yr	3
Nazarene	1	7-10 yr	2
Unitarian	1	10-15 yr	0
None	4	16 yr	1
Jewish	0	Over 16 yr	0

Previous treatment

Type	No./length of treatment episodes	No. of subjects
Inpatient	11	1
	1	2
Outpatient	1	1
AA	10 yr	1
	1 yr	1
Detox center	3	1
	1	1
Mental hospitalization	3	1
	2	2
	1	2
Psychiatrists	5	1
	1	4
Medical hospitalization	1	2
No previous treatment		7
Results: Return to drinking in all cases		

[a]In these 3 categories, there are 5 *S*s whose exact educational status is unclear.

Table 4

Drinking History

Type	No. of subjects
Origins of Drinking	
Crisis related	
Separation and divorce	2
Husband had affair/girlfriend pregnant	1
Drugs prescribed for paternal death	1
Response to being repeatedly raped by brother	1
Non-crisis related	
During childhood	1
Other related	
Peer pressure	5
Occupational availability (waitress)	1
Unknown	3
Age initial use	
Unknown (early)	1
12-15	5
16-19	8[a]
20-29	2
30-39	1
40-49	1
Age problem drinking began	
Unknown	1
12-15	4
16-19	7
20-29	3
30-39	2
40-49	1
% life problem drinking	
Under 10	2
11-20	3
21-30	4
31-40	6
41-50	2
51-55	1
Over 55	0
Other problem drinkers in family	
Spouses	1
Siblings	3
Parent(s)	6
Extended family	7
Only after subject was adult	4
None	2

[a]Four of these subjects were 18.

IMPLICATIONS AND CONCLUSIONS

The Johnson Model of Intervention (Johnson, 1973) has been very successful but has only limited application. It requires a minimum of three people to tell the alcoholic a series of incidents that resulted from drinking, show concern, and press for treatment. Many people do not have that many knowledgeable and concerned people in their lives. More research is needed concerning one-to-one intervention methods, especially in the area of leading women to treatment.

In this study it was found that a one-to-one confrontation can have an effect, though the alcoholic will not necesarily listen to everything she hears. A cumulative effect often occurs so that at some point the alcoholic hears one comment too many or has one experience too many, and can no longer ignore her problem. In dealing with an alcoholic friend, colleague, or client, it is crucial not to be afraid to directly state the concern, not to be afraid to "call a spade a spade." A nonjudgmental attitude is not always necessary, either, as witnessed by the woman whose son humiliated her.

The women in this study were either getting into trouble with the law, contacting professionals, or were surrounded by people who know that there was a problem but either did not know what the problem was or were unable or unwilling to intervene. Family members were often ignorant of what to do; some saw alcoholism as a moral problem.

Professionals in medicine and the mental health fields have an obligation to learn about alcoholism, how to detect it and how to guide alcoholic women into treatment. Apparently their training often leaves them unprepared for this. They are often in the position to diagnose alcoholism in a person who presents with a different complaint, such as family problems or physical ailments. Since some people were directed to help by professionals in these fields, many other professionals could help their clients in this same way.

Employers and law officials also overlook opportunities to intervene to guide these women to treatment. Extensive outreach programs are needed in all these areas.

Child care was not a problem for most of the women, leading to a possible conclusion that women with child care problems probably do not receive help.

Due to instances in which a woman is married and living with a husband who controls the money, programs are needed that take the woman's word as to her financial need, rather than basing it on family income. The way many financial aid programs are set up, a woman married to a controlling husband with a high income cannot get the help she needs without his consent. Family income is not always an adequate indicator of a woman's financial need.

Specialized programs for women were clearly beneficial to a substantial percentage of the women interviewed. Others felt no such need or rejected the idea completely. The benefit of these programs is clear, however, for those women who feel the need. Though Alcoholics Anonymous appears to be a good program for most female alcoholics (it was rejected completely by only one of the subjects), several chose to supplement it with another program for women.

Since alcoholism is a major problem for women, community outreach and education programs are needed to make nonalcoholics as well as alcoholics aware of the symptoms of alcoholism. Professionals in the medical and mental health fields need to be educated concerning the symptoms to look for in their alcoholic patients and the best approaches for successful intervention and treatment.

REFERENCES

BADIET, P. Women and legal drugs: A review. In A. McLennan (ed.) and L. Pinder (comp.), *Women: Their Use of Alcohol and Other Legal Drugs.* A Provincial Consultation. Toronto: Addiction Research Foundation, 1976.

BECKMAN, L. *J. Stud. Alcohol* 36: 799, 802, 1975.

FRASER, W. The alcoholic woman: Attitudes and perspectives. In A. McLennan (ed.) and L. Pinder (comp.), *Women: Their Use of Alcohol and Other Legal Drugs.* A Provincial Consultation. Toronto: Addiction Research Foundation, 1976.

HORNIK, E. *The Drinking Woman.* Association Press, 1977.

JOHNSON, V. *I'll Quit Tomorrow.* New York: Harper and Row, 1973.

SANDMAIER, M. Women helping women: Opening the door to treatment. *Alcohol Health Res. World* 2(3): 23, 1977.

The International Journal of the Addictions, 19(6), 613–631, 1984

The Abstinence Phobias: Links between Substance Abuse and Anxiety

Sharon Martinelli Hall,* PhD

Langley Porter Institute
University of California
San Francisco, California 94143

Abstract

This paper presents a new model to explain the observed relationship between anxiety and substance abuse. Specifically, the concept of "abstinence phobias," common across psychoactive substances, is developed. The evidence needed to support this concept is outlined, and relevant data from studies of opiate, alcohol, and tobacco dependences are reviewed. Parallel data obtained from the treatment of obesity are discussed. It is concluded that the abstinence phobia merits further study; clinical implications are also considered.

This paper suggests a hypothesis about the often observed relationship between abuse of psychoactive drugs and anxiety, a relationship which has puzzled investigators across the field of substance abuse, including those studying alcoholism (e.g., Conger, 1956), narcotic addiction (e.g., Wikler, 1965), and nicotine dependence (e.g., Ikard, Green, and Horn, 1969). Generally, hypotheses about anxiety and substance abuse fall into one of two classes: (1) those which suggest that substance abusers are characterologically more anxious than normals (e.g., Martin, Haertzen, and Hewett, 1978) and (2) tension-reduction hypotheses, which propose that the substances involved are simply the preferred means of anxiety reduction for substance abusers, who need not necessarily be higher in "trait anxiety" than nonabusers (e.g., Conger, 1956).

*Address requests for reprints to the author at Behavioral Treatment Research, 1454 Fifth Avenue, University of California, San Francisco, California 94143.

 0020-773X/84/1906-0613$3.50/0

It is not the intent of this paper to evaluate the research relevant to either of these two lines of thought. Suffice it to say that these are chaotic areas, reflecting definitional and measurement problems, and, to quote Marlatt's (1976) evaluation of data relevant to the tension-reduction hypothesis, "Almost any finding can be found" (p. 274).

In addition, however, some of the confusion surrounding the relationship between anxiety and substance abuse may emanate from the continued focus on anxiety as an etiological factor in substance abuse, rather than as a result of it. This paper discusses one mechanism by which drug abuse may, in fact, produce anxiety (see Note 1).

THE ABSTINENCE PHOBIA

Once a person has become psychologically or physiologically dependent upon a substance, and consciously recognizes this dependency, anticipation of termination of drug use, or even reduction in dose, can produce anxiety, via at least two mechanisms. First, relatively mild symptoms of drug withdrawal can elicit fear. Fear may become conditioned because such symptoms have previously been followed by very aversive events (e.g., severe withdrawal symptoms), or the drug user believes they will be. Such beliefs may come about because the drug user is exposed to misinformation about withdrawal. Such misinformation can be transmitted verbally (i.e., via street lore) or more indirectly (i.e., via film portrayals of detoxifying addicts). Second, the anticipation of being "drug free" can produce fear because drug-free status demands behavior avoided by drug use and/or by membership in the culture that surrounds its use. This is especially the case with heroin, where the street culture rewards behaviors other than those adaptive in the larger society. Thus, this component of the phobia can be linked with perceived discomfort about specific interpersonal skills needed for important life events; that is, those needed to keep a job, to raise children, or to form interpersonal relations that do not revolve around drugs. A closely related mechanism is the loss of facilitation of difficult, frequently encountered situations provided by drug use. These components of the phobia parallel Bandura's (1977) descriptions of phobias as perceptions of low self-competency in an important area. Factors related to the genesis of the two possible components of the abstinence phobia are shown in Fig. 1.

For any one substance, either or both kinds of fears may be found and may interact with dose changes. Detoxification from methadone maintenance provides a clear example. The first process is straightforward: As methadone dose decreases, mild withdrawal symptoms are experienced and the detoxifying methadone maintenance client may experience conditioned fear reactions to these. In the second process, psychological and pharmacological factors can interact. The detoxifying client inevitably attempts to move to a different set of

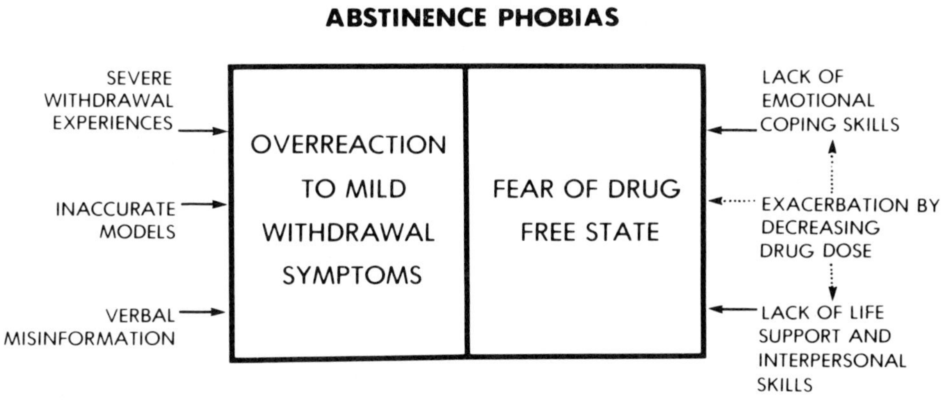

Fig. 1. Genesis of abstinence phobias.

acquaintances, work and leisure activities, and cultural standards. In making this move, he/she encounters situations which were previously avoided (e.g., conflicts with employers) or never experienced (e.g., applying for a loan), and/or for which adequate skills cannot be performed without anxiety. The anxiety-provoking nature of these experiences is enhanced by increases in emotional sensitivity due to decreasing drug levels. Thus, while the first component of the abstinence phobia simply reflects an overreaction to withdrawal symptoms, the second reflects a fear reaction to stressful situations, which may be intensified by dosage decreases.

The abstinence phobia manifests itself in symptoms analogous to those found in other phobias, including high levels of anxiety about the phobic object, a tendency to avoid the phobic object—unless other factors such as social pressure or one's own values operate against avoidance—and a preoccupation with the phobic object when avoidance is not possible or otherwise feasible.

Abstinence phobias probably fall on a continuum of fear specificity (similar to that proposed by Beck and Rush, 1976) from an extreme consisting of a specific fear that the client can clearly state when questioned ("I am afraid of messing up again") to more diffuse anxiety reactions, where the client has difficulty in verbalizing the cues that result in anxiety. The latter is especially true in the case of withdrawal symptom anxiety, where the stimuli are frequently internal and poorly labeled, and the person may be less able to clearly articulate the relationship between cognitions of danger and experienced anxiety.

EVIDENCE

The usefulness of the concept of the abstinence phobia rests on a matrix of indirect evidence. Such evidence can take one of several forms: (1) At least a "clinically interesting" minority of detoxifying individuals should report feeling anxious. (2) If they are able to verbally tie this anxiety to various factors related to withdrawal symptoms, to specific situations related to being drug-free or to historical factors which would logically lead to phobia development, the evidence for the concept is stronger. (3) Reports of anxiety in double-blind studies where expectations about dose and dose level are separately manipulated provide evidence for an abstinence phobia conceptualization, if anxiety is shown to be more closely related to the former than the latter. Double-blind studies are important because increases in anxiety during withdrawal can reflect pharmacological processes; most commonly used psychoactive drugs, with the exception of some psychedelics and amphetamines, have been shown to decrease anxiety pharmacologically, and drug withdrawal results in a temporary increase of the suppressed characteristics. (4) Addicted individuals should show avoidance behavior, that is, inability to reach zero dose, especially in more or less "free" situations such as outpatient settings. Although one might argue that relapse alone is evidence for the concept (i.e., constitutes an escape response), the argument is tautological, and the high relapse rates seen across the addictions probably reflect many complex factors. (5) Another line of evidence is identification of a syndrome which meets the criteria for phobic or anxiety response, such as the criteria provided by DSM-III for diagnosis for phobic disorders. (6) Evidence that anxiety behaves differently than physical symptoms, or is not closely related to physical symptoms, provides indirect evidence of a psychological as opposed to the physical etiology, although psychological mechanisms other than abstinence phobias must be considered. Such evidence includes differing courses of anxiety during and following detoxification than for physical symptoms. Clustering of anxiety-related variables apart from physical variables in statistical analyses using multivariate techniques and fluctuations in anxiety independent of dose are examples. (7) Evidence of skill deficits and discomfort about them are consonant with the predictions of the model, as are relationships between skill deficits and detoxification failure. (8) Finally, evidence that the abused drug acts to ameliorate skill deficits also supports the concept.

Each of the major addictions—to opiates, alcohol, and tobacco—is examined for evidence related to these points. Parallels in overeating are also considered.

OPIATES

The most compelling data in support of the abstinence phobia model are those from detoxifying methadone maintenance clients.

Clinical reports of increased anxiety have been present in almost every report of the detoxification process published since the inception of methadone maintenance in 1968 (Cushman and Dole, 1973; Goldstein, 1972; Kleber, 1977;

Kremen and Bayer, 1973; Lowinson, Berle, and Langrod, 1976; Muskelly, 1972; Riordan and Rapkin, 1972). In addition to direct reports of experienced anxiety, problems which may represent the effects of anxiety have been reported consistently. These include loss of appetite (Kremen and Bayer, 1973; Muskelly, 1972), impotence (Muskelly, 1972; Riordan and Rapkin, 1972), and insomnia and nausea (Cushman and Dole, 1973; Kremen and Bayer, 1973; Muskelly, 1972; Resnick, Kestenbaum, Gaztanaga, Volanka, and Freedman, 1974; Riordan and Rapkin, 1972).

While clinical reports do demonstrate the prevalence of anxiety, they do not separate pharmacological effects from psychological ones. At least one study, however, convincingly demonstrates the role of the latter in detoxification-induced discomfort, including anxiety. Senay, Dorus, Goldberg, and Thornton (1977), over a 30-week period, compared volunteer detoxifying methadone maintenance clients who were randomly assigned to either no maintenance, blind maintenance, blind rapid withdrawal (10% dose reduction per week), or blind gradual withdrawal (3% dose reduction per week). Blind gradual withdrawal and blind maintenance did not differ on a number of "withdrawal symptoms" reported, including anxiety, narcotics cravings reported, and average rate of heroin use. Pharmacologically, then, slow withdrawal need not produce increased anxiety, and at least some of the anxiety noted in clinical reports is thus probably due to psychological factors.

Another line of evidence is that related to avoidance. In methadone maintenance, it was the well-documented inability of clients to reach zero dose that first gave rise to the notion that abstinence fears may complicate treatment (Hall, 1979; Jackman, 1973; Milby, Garrett, and Meredith, 1980; Milby, Rice, and Garrett, 1979). Zero dose is generally reached by a minority (25-40%) of those detoxifying (Berger and Schweger, 1973; Brown, Bernardi, Greenberg, and MacArthur, 1957; Chappel, Skolnick, and Senay, 1973; Isiadinso, 1977; Kleber, 1977; Kremen and Bayer, 1973; Lowinson et al., 1976; Rabin and Stimmel, 1974; Resnick et al., 1974; Riordan and Rapkin, 1972; Stimmel, Rabin, and Engel, 1973).

The prevalence of specific detoxification-related fears has been studied by Milby and his co-workers (Milby, Garrett, and Meredith, 1980; Milby, Rice, and Garrett, 1979), who reported observations of an "iatrogenic detox phobia" among methadone maintenance clients. They defined the phobia as appearing in patients who: (1) have been treated for a time in methadone maintenance; (2) report unrealistic fears of the detoxification process; (3) have a history of brief abstinence or aborted detox attempts. After studying samples of detoxifying methadone clients drawn from a single clinic, these investigators concluded that the phobia could be reliably detected—with agreement ranging from 67% to 97%, depending on the method used—and that it was present in 26-27% of the sample. Milby et al.'s criteria were fairly exclusive, since ability to verbalize fears was necessary and clients who were not detoxifying were not assessed. Actual prevalence may have been somewhat higher, since severely phobic clients would probably be prevented from entering into detoxification status by anxiety.

Reports from treatment modalities for opiate detoxification other than methadone maintenance are relatively rare. However, the few data available from outpatient heroin detoxification indicate that anxiety increases during detoxification from heroin, and this increase appears to be related to factors other than decreasing dose. Dorus, Senay, and Showalter (1979) collected ratings of a variety of symptoms, including anxiety, during a double-blind comparison of 90-day methadone-assisted detoxification from heroin (84 days of gradually decreasing methadone dose, 6 placebo days) and standard 21-day detoxification (21 days of gradually decreasing methadone dose, 69 placebo days). Percent of subjects reporting anxiety and related symptoms (tenseness or nervousness) was 31.8 and 38.1, respectively, at week 3. At week 6, 43.8% of both conditions reported anxiety. Comparability of reported anxiety levels is especially interesting, since, at both assessment points, the 21-day group was receiving placebo, while the 90-day condition was receiving methadone.

Again, in detoxification from heroin, failure to reach zero dose is the rule rather than the exception; percentages completing detoxification range from 69 to 0 but generally are less than 40% (Hall, Bass, Hargreaves, and Loeb, 1979; Hargreaves, Lowe, Gaynor, and Fulwiler, 1977; Sheffet, Quinones, Lavennar, Doyle, and Prager, 1977; Wilson, Elms, and Thompson, 1975).

Most writers have assumed that heroin addicts are markedly deficient in social and interpersonal skills; however, studies reporting evaluations of skill levels have not been directly reported. Platt and L'Abate (1976) reviewed data relevant to psychopathology and family history of heroin addicts, both of which very likely influence social skill levels. From the data they present, it is reasonable to conclude that addicts come from families where development of adequate social skills is not likely, and that this lack is reflected in poor social relationships and in forms of psychopathology, such as diagnoses of "inadequate personality," where skill lacks are a primary factor. Further, comparisons of addict samples with normative populations indicate that they are deficient in interpersonal problem-solving skills (Platt, Scura, and Hannon, 1973).

Few investigators have studied the effects of opiates on social behavior. However, at least one study indicated immediate increases in social interaction following morphine injections, followed by a decline during chronic self-administration (Babor, Meyer, Mirin, McNamee, and Davies, 1976).

In summary, with respect to narcotic treatment clients, it is clear that anxiety is a consistently reported symptom during detoxification; it appears to be less related to dose than to expectations and psychological factors, and it may be implicated in relapse. Further, preliminary studies indicate that abstinence phobia may be a reliably diagnosable entity among methadone maintenance patients. Although no investigators have studied skill levels directly, inferences from family and other studies suggest that interpersonal skill levels are low. The development of abstinence anxiety is not surprising. Mild withdrawal symptoms can come to elicit anxiety by virtue of previous pairing with severe, uncontrolled symptoms, especially during incarceration. Even if the opiate user has never experienced severe symptoms, the mythology surrounding opiate use is sufficiently severe to provide a very potent expectation, as are the reports of friends about their detoxification experiences.

Many heroin addicts who participate in the "street" life have ample opportunity to develop a complex set of behaviors which are not adaptive in the larger society (Preble and Casey, 1969). Disruptive and relatively poor family histories provide little skill learning to offset the learning with more widely adequate skills. During detoxification, awareness of skill lacks it probably heightened, and any facilitation resulting from the drug itself is removed. Further, since most narcotic addicts experience multiple detoxification attempts, failure experiences due to these skill lacks may well be common.

SMOKING CESSATION

Evidence of an abstinence phobia is not as strong in other areas as it is in narcotic treatment clients. This is due less to negative findings than to lack of relevant data. However, increases in anxiety following smoking cessation are well documented; there is some evidence for anxiety as independent from dose and for avoidance of zero dose being related to anxiety. Wynder, Kauffman, and Lesser (1967) interviewed 224 ex-smokers within 5 years of termination of smoking. Although a sizable proportion (24%) reported experiencing no symptoms at all, 53% reported increased nervousness and irritability during and immediately following cessation. Myrsten, Elgerot, and Edgren (1977) followed habitual smokers for 15 days, during which one 5-day nonsmoking period was interspersed between two 5-day smoking periods. Increases in anxiety and tension were reported by 4 of 14 subjects during the nonsmoking period. Henderson, Bachman, Barstow, Hall, and Jones (1979) documented significant increases in anxiety, depression, and anger from pre- to posttreatment for chronic, heavy smokers, and Schacter (1977) has described quite vividly the anxiety and emotional upheaval experienced during nicotine withdrawal.

Parallel increases in anxiety are found in laboratory studies. Shiffman and Jarvik (1976) measured four withdrawal-related factors as a function of usual dose (light vs heavy smokers) following smoking cessation: stimulation, craving, "physical symptoms" (e.g., faster heart rate), and psychological symptoms (e.g., anxiety, restlessness, and discontentment). The shape of the function for physical symptoms differed slightly from those for craving and psychological symptoms. Stimulation (alertness) did not resemble any of the other functions. It did differentiate light and heavy smokers, while the other factors did not. The similarity between psychological factors and craving provides some support for involvement of psychological factors in the abstinence anxiety, especially if craving is viewed as expectancy of pleasant effects, as Marlatt (1978) has argued. Further, the lack of a dose-response relationship suggests that psychological etiologies should be considered.

Further evidence for a lack of relationship between anxiety and dose is found in the work of Ague (1973), who asked smokers to rate their moods prior to, following, and 1 hour after smoking cigarettes of one of four nicotine levels ranging from no nicotine to high nicotine. Smoking tended to decrease anxiety and aggression, but anxiety reduction as a function of dose did not occur. Since oral manipulative activities alone reduce anxiety (Freeman, 1948, cited by Gilbert, 1979), Ague's work suggests that factors other than a pharmacological effect of nicotine dose may be operative in anxiety during withdrawal.

Although studies on emotional reactions following smoking cessation are few, a great deal of outcome research exists on smoking treatment, and a great deal of evidence is available with respect to difficulties in reaching zero dose and concerning relapse. It should be noted that it is a misconception that "smoking cessation (but not maintenance) is easy." While rapid smoking in the laboratories of some investigators, working with well-motivated subjects, has produced high, almost complete quit rates (Hall, Sachs, and Hall, 1979; Schmahl, Lichtenstein, and Harris, 1972), smoking cessation is not easy. Most approaches appear to produce cessation rates considerably lower.

The research on personal and historical characteristics related to cigarette smoking does not allow a strong argument for the deficit in interpersonal and other skills among cigarette smoking treatment clients. Smokers are a much less well defined group than are heroin addicts or alcoholics. Most studies report comparison of current nonsmokers with a general category of "current smokers" or with smokers broken down into two categories (light vs heavy); criteria for individuals falling into each category vary markedly from study to study. Further, while narcotic addicts and alcoholic populations are generally defined by inclusion in treatment programs, subjects in studies of the personal and social characteristics of smokers have generally been college students not seeking treatment, who admitted they smoked on a questionnaire or in an interview. Such studies are not relevant to the present discussion, since one would expect abstinence fears to occur primarily among heavy, chronic users of a substance who have had repeated failures at detoxification and unpleasant postdetoxification experiences.

When more comparable populations are examined, some data relevant to social skill deficits emerge: Dudley, Aicken, and Martin (1977) divided chest clinic patients into those who (1) never had smoked, (2) those who had smoked but quit due to symptoms, (3) those who quit for other reasons, and (4) those who continued to smoke despite pressure exerted by the clinic. Ability to quit was related to "psychosocial assets," as measured by the Berle Index (Berle, Pinsky, Wolff, and Wolff, 1952) as well as to ability to express depression.

Similarly, Jacobs (1972) found a constricted, socially isolated style to be the second greatest amount of variance in predicting treatment failure in his sample of male, heavy smokers (over a pack a day for 20 years or more). (The factor accounting for the largest proportion of variance was a defiant, danger-seeking, impulsive trait constellation associated with manifest distress.)

Since nicotine administration has been known to suppress fear and anger responses to conditioned stimuli in both humans and animals (Hutchinson and Emley, 1973), the possibility that nicotine facilitates and improves the quality of social interactions for heavy, chronic smokers can be considered a viable one.

Logically, it would seem that abstinence anxiety, concerning both withdrawal symptoms and skill deficits, could develop in smokers, although it may well be less frequent and less intense than is the case with narcotic addicts. In contrast with the rich street lore about methadone and heroin withdrawal, until recently some governmental agencies have denied that a nicotine withdrawal syndrome exists (e.g., USPHS, 1964). To be sure, nicotine withdrawal has not been reported to reach the severity of opiate withdrawal. However, considering the many "last time I quit" stories of smoking treatment clients, it does seem plausible to suggest that sufficient informal negative modeling exists and perpetuates fears in some clients. With respect to skill-related factors, until recently nicotine was not a socially disapproved drug, so smokers did not create a separate culture where specific behaviors were learned and others more appropriate to general society were forgotten or never acquired. However, some segment of the chronic, heavy smoking population is isolated, withdrawn, and lacking in social skills and assets. Since abstinence from nicotine also has been shown to result in increases in anger, irritability, and concentration difficulties (Larson and Silvette, 1971), the presence of such symptoms may have predisposed already unskilled individuals to increased levels of social and interpersonal conflicts, thus providing the basis for an anticipatory anxiety reaction to termination of cigarette smoking.

ALCOHOL

Reports from existing alcohol detoxification studies consistently document a high level of anxiety during detoxification (Björkvist, 1975; Feuerlein, 1974; Hague, Wilson, Dudley, and Cannon, 1976; Hershon, 1977; Nathan, Titler, Lowenstein, Solomon, and Rossi, 1970). Approximately 25-33% of detoxifying alcoholics report anxiety (Feuerlein, 1974; Hershon, 1977).

Statistics relating to attempts to reach zero dose are not meaningful in alcohol detoxification, especially when considered in comparison with methadone, heroin, and nicotine. Unlike treatment for the latter three substances, in current practice, detoxification from alcohol always takes place in an inpatient setting. Thus, leaving treatment involves more and different barriers. Also, the alcoholic has his or her last drink prior to entering the hospital; this differs from the opiates and nicotine, where the dosage is under the client's control and usually gradually reduced.

Data pertaining to the role of withdrawal anxiety in alcoholism are less extensive than for nicotine and certainly for opiates. There is some evidence that alcoholics become more, rather than less, anxious, as they ingest alcohol (Nathan et al., 1970). While this might reflect a fear of ultimate withdrawal and its pains, other interpretations seem possible. What is clear, however, are the marked deficits in interpersonal skills and the anxiety related to those deficits experienced by alcoholics.

Not only are alcoholics probably lacking in important social skills, but discomfort about performance of these skills and the situations in which they are needed frequently lead to relapse. O'Leary, O'Leary, and Donovan (1976) reviewed the data related to social skill acquisition and psychosocial development in male alcoholics and prealcoholics. They concluded that prealcoholic teenagers were less socially skilled than their peers, had fewer appropriate models, and viewed the world in a simplistic, hypermasculine fashion. Due to a tendency to choose other heavy drinkers as friends, these boys continued to have a relatively restricted range of models, and to continue to fall behind others of their own age in social development. Alcoholics themselves become characterized by immature and restricted social responses, which may or may not be enhanced by drinking.

Not only are skill deficits present, but alcoholics feel considerable discomfort about situations requiring social skills, especially assertive skills in negative situations, and this discomfort can increase drinking. Miller, Hersen, Eisler, and Hilsman (1974) found that when alcoholics and nonalcoholics were exposed to situations requiring assertive responses, and then were told that their responses were below standard, both groups experienced anxiety, but only the alcoholic group showed an increase in drinking over a nonstressful condition.

Other studies indicate that discomfort about skill deficits, if not the deficits themselves, may be primary. Hamilton and Maisto (1979) found no significant overall differences in assertiveness in alcoholics and nonalcoholics, but a consistently greater perceived discomfort about assertiveness-requiring situations, especially negative ones, for alcoholics. These results support Martorano's (1974) conclusion that failure of assertiveness training with alcoholics reflects a failure to reduce discomfort about skills, rather than skill deficits per se.

Several studies have reported increases in social behavior following administration of ethanol (Griffiths, Bigelow, and Liebson, 1974, 1975; McNamee, Mello, and Mendelson, 1968; Nathan et al., 1970). For example, Griffiths et al. (1974) found that in alcoholic subjects, social behavior increasesd on days drinking was permitted, as compared to days when alcohol was not available. When alcoholics could chose between socialization and the opportunity to earn money, alcohol shifted behavior toward the social option (Griffiths et al., 1975).

Along these same lines, Stitzer, Griffiths, Bigelow, and Leibson (1980) found that both alcohol and secobarbitol (pharmacologically similar drugs with substantial abuse potential) increased amount of talking in a dyadic situation, but chlorpromazine (low abuse potential) did not.

SOME PARALLELS TO OBESITY

Some investigators consider obesity an addictive behavior because it is assumed to reflect misuse of food. This is not the place to argue the merit of this categorization or of the actual relationship of food intake to obesity.

What is relevant to the major hypothesis of this paper is the possibility that an anxiety response which parallels the skill deficit anxiety component of the abstinence phobia exists in some obese people. It should be noted that the parallel to the withdrawal component of the abstinence phobia—for example, anxiety produced by hunger pangs—does not seem likely to be a potential barrier to weight loss. Analytic writers suggest that the internal sensations resulting from the physiological changes of hunger are anxiety producing for obese individuals (Kaplan and Kaplan, 1957). This anxiety is assumed to be the result of early childhood experiences (e.g., hunger followed by extreme deprivation due to inadequate parenting, etc.). While it is perfectly logical that such conditioning might occur under adverse conditions, and that the physiological sensations of hunger might be anxiety provoking, it would seem likely that this response would eventually extinguish, since many obese individuals go on repeated diets in their adult lives and no unusually aversive experiences follow the hunger responses.

Evidence about anxiety during dieting is somewhat conflicting but generally appears to support the notion that anxiety does increase. In reviewing the relevant literature, Stunkard and Rush (1974) noted that approximately 50% of obese individuals dieting under medical supervision on an outpatient basis experience some sort of emotional symptoms, with 21% (Stunkard, 1957) to 41% (Silverstone and Lascelles, 1966) reporting increased anxiety during dieting. Stunkard considered these proportions underestimates, reasoning that the substantial proportion of dropouts from obesity programs is "mute testimony" that psychological difficulties are occurring.

While it is difficult to see how this anxiety during dieting could arise from experienced hunger, what is more likely is the possibility that weight changes, especially large ones, are anxiety provoking for many of these individuals, because they demand skills never learned, or forgotten. The author's own clinical experience indicates that desensitization about social situations related to weight loss (e.g., sexual advances) is occasionally necessary before treatment can proceed (Hall, 1979). Haber (1978) offered more objective data about such "new state" anxieties in her interview series of 12 patients, all of whom had lost

100 pounds or more. She reported considerable ambivalence about weight loss, with feelings of excitement and rebirth, conflicting with anxiety about the new possibilities represented by being thin. As Haber notes, increased anxiety may reflect both new rules and new relationships. Patients must rework relationships that remain stable and/or expose themselves to new relationships they are not used to dealing with. Thus, it is possible that at least some obese individuals harbor feelings similar to those experienced by substance abusers. One might argue that they would be more common in childhood-onset obese individuals who may well never have developed the skills to maintain adult social relationships, especially sexual ones.

TREATMENT IMPLICATIONS

Diagnosis

A question of importance to both researchers and clinicians is the diagnosis of abstinence phobias in substance abuse patients. The diagnostic criteria developed by Milby et al. (1980) for methadone maintenance patients represent the most extensive effort in this direction and promise to have both research and clinical applicability. However, diagnosis of abstinence phobias may be simpler among methadone maintenance patients than in patients attempting to detoxify directly from heroin, or for smokers or alcoholics. The reason for this is primarily logistical. Participation in methadone maintenance provides an opportunity to observe previous failures in detoxification and instances of inability to detoxify from methadone despite a considerable length of time spent in treatment and attainment of satisfactory psychosocial rehabilitation.

Absence of opportunity to observe such phenomena among heroin addicts in other treatment modalities and among users of other substances implies that more indirect diagnostic tools must be used in these instances. Questionnaires asking directly about such fears can be developed and may be of value, especially in relatively verbal and insightful patients (Note 2). Historical variables (e.g., previous aborted detoxification attempts) can be tapped by such questionnaires or by interview techniques, and tentative diagnostic criteria can be worked out on the basis of clusters emerging from such data.

Treatment Planning and Staff Training

The abstinence phobia concept has two clear implications for treatment planning. These are: (1) staff must be prepared to provide patients accurate information about what to expect during and after the detoxification process, and (2) anxiety reduction treatment and or skill enhancement procedures should be available when needed. In the absence of trained personnel or sufficient staff time, referrals to knowledgeable practitioners should be available.

An issue that complicates the provision of information about detoxification is that, in many instances, such information is not available in forms or sources easily accessible to treatment staff. Staff information sources about the detoxification process may differ little from those of patients; both may well be derived from inaccurate models presented in the media and from misinformation passed from patient to patient to staff. Important goals for staff training, then, are to provide accurate information about the detoxification process, to direct them to appropriate resources, and to encourage staff to communicate this information to patients. It may be important to use paraprofessional staff who are ex-users to communicate such information, since they may well have the greatest credibility among patients.

Countering inaccurate beliefs with accurate information may do much to decrease fears of the withdrawal process and to decrease overreactions to mild symptoms in many patients (Note 3). However, psychotherapeutic interventions may be required for others, those for whom overreactions to withdrawal symptoms are not modifiable by provision of information or those for whom fear of the drug-free state reflects real skill lacks. Several case studies already exist in the literature which describe therapeutic interventions for abstinence-related fears in methadone maintenance patients; techniques reported to be useful include systematic desensitization (Panyard and Wolf, 1974), implosive therapy (Hirt and Greenfield, 1979), and meditative techniques (Shapiro and Zifferblatt, 1976). Such techniques would seem easily adaptable for users of other substances.

Other treatment techniques which have been widely used in substance abuse settings would seem to have potential value, especially in relation to enhancement of emotional and interpersonal coping skills. These include anger management training (e.g., Novaco, 1977) and skills in handling anxiety-producing situations related to relapse (Chaney, O'Leary, and Marlatt, 1978), as well as general assertiveness and social skills training (e.g., Wolpe, 1969).

In many instances, effective modalities for anxiety reduction may well differ somewhat from those used in traditional settings. The substance abuse patient sees reduction of drug use as a goal. The connection between anxiety and reduction of drug use will have to be clearly and convincingly presented to the clients; treatments themselves may have to be modified so that they fit into multifocal programs aimed at reduction of substance abuse. It is most likely that treatment techniques will have to be brief and carefully targeted at the anxieties of concern.

Staff training issues with respect to such interventions vary depending on the category of staff considered; professional staff with training in psychotherapeutic interventions may be well advised to familiarize themselves with such techniques, while other staff members may best serve as initial diagnosticians and referral sources.

Success, Failure, and Their Clinical Implications

Continued incomplete attempts to terminate drug use and accompanying anxiety perpetuate a vicious circle of perceived low self-efficacy and increased anxiety. Careful consideration of possible abstinence phobias may provide a means of breaking into this vicious circle. Continued failure to acknowledge the existence of these phobias and to deal with them effectively will only accelerate this unfortunate circle.

CONCLUSIONS

This paper has discussed a model of psychogenic anxiety in detoxification from opiates, nicotine, and alcohol, and has considered the evidence relevant to it. A great deal of the evidence is, as yet, tentative. However, it would seem that a reasonable conclusion is that abstinence anxiety may play a role in preventing substance abusers from reaching zero dose. The evidence is strongest in the case of opiate addiction, but there are grounds for a potential role for such anxiety in detoxification from alcohol and nicotine, and a roughly parallel process may be operative in impeding weight loss.

This model suggests several areas worthy of further study. (1) Determinations should be made of the extent to which abstinence phobias exist, and the extent to which they reflect withdrawal versus skill deficit anxiety in different substance groups; (2) the extent to which such anxiety interfers with detoxification, and is implicated in relapse, should be determined; (3) given that substance abuse treatment clients are found to suffer from abstinence phobia, and that such phobias are found to be related to relapse, etiological studies that relate such anxiety to specific personality, familial, and social characteristics should be conducted.

Clinically, not only is determination of prevalence of interest; also of importance is the development of anxiety-reduction methods specific to abstinence anxieties.

One specific implication of this formulation is that anxiety reduction will frequently be a goal of treatment in the course of, or prior to, treatment of substance abuse. However, effective modalities of anxiety reduction may well differ from those used for traditional phobias. The substance abuse client sees reduction of drug use as a goal. The connection between anxiety and reduction of drug use will have to be clearly and convincingly presented to the client. Also, the treatments themselves must be designed so that they fit into multifocal programs aimed at reduction of substance abuse. It is most likely that they will have to be brief and carefully targeted at the anxieties of concern.

ACKNOWLEDGMENTS

The author wishes to thank Dr. William Hargreaves for his comments on initial drafts of this paper; and Drs. Ricardo Muñoz, John Bachman, and Barbara Havassy, and Ms. Jean Tschaan for their comments and suggestions on the final draft. This work was supported by USPHS Research Grant 1-RO1-DA01910 and by ADAMHA Research Scientist Development Award 1 KO2 DA00065.

NOTES

1. In this paper, *anxiety* refers primarily to either subjective reports of discomfort, apprehension, or tension; or avoidance or escape behavior in response to objectively innocuous stimuli. The action of the abstinence phobia should also be reflected in physiological measures. However, interactions between drug effects and changes in psychophysiological measures are sufficiently complex that it would seem that physiological measures are less than optimal.
2. Pilot versions of abstinence phobia questionnaires for cigarette smokers and methadone maintenance clients are available from the author.
3. The therapeutic effects of such information on phobias in general have been documented, particularly by Wolpe (1958).

REFERENCES

AGUE, C. Nicotine and smoking: Effects upon subjective changes in mood. *Psychopharmalogicia* 30: 323-328, 1973.

BABOR, T.F., MEYER, R.E., MIRIN, S.M., MC NAMEE, H.B., and DAVIES, M. Behavioral and social effects of heroin administration and withdrawal. *Arch. Gen. Psychiatry* 33: 363-367, 1976.

BANDURA, A. Self-efficacy: Towards a unifying theory of behavioral change. *Psychol. Rev.* 84: 191-215, 1977.

BECK, A.T., and RUSH, A.J. A cognitive model of anxiety formation and anxiety resolution. In I.G. Sarason and C.D. Speilberger (eds.), *Stress and Anxiety* (Vol. 2). Washington, DC: Hemisphere, 1976.

BERGER, H., and SCHWEGER, M.J. Voluntary detoxification of patients on methadone maintenance. *Int. J. Addict.* 6: 1045-1047, 1973.

BERLE, B.B., PINSKY, R.H., WOLFF, S., and WOLFF, H.G. The Berle Index: A clinical guide to prognosis in stress diseases. *J. Am. Med. Assoc.* 149: 1624-1628, 1952.

BJÖRKGVIST, S.E. Clonidine in alcohol withdrawal. *Acta Psychiatr. Scand.* 52: 256-263, 1975.

BROWN, E.M., BERNARDI, M., GREENBERG, M., and MAC ARTHUR, M. Studies of methadone terminations. *Br. J. Addict.* 70: 83-88, 1957.

CHANEY, E.F., O'LEARY, M.R., and MARLATT, G.A. Skill training with alcoholics. *J. Consult. Clin. Psychol.* 46: 839-843, 1978.

CHAPPEL, J.N., SKOLNICK, V.B., and SENAY, E.C. Techniques of withdrawal from methadone and their outcome over six months to two years. *Proc. Natl. Conf. Methadone Treatment* 5: 482-489, 1973.

CONGER, J.J. Alcoholism: Theory, problems and challenge. II. Reinforcement theory and dynamics of alcoholism. *Q. J. Stud. Alcohol* 17: 296-305, 1956.

CUSHMAN, P., and DOLE, V.P. Detoxification of rehabilitated methadone maintained patients. *J. Am. Med. Assoc.* 226: 747-752, 1973.

DORUS, W., SENAY, E.C., and SHOWALTER, C. *A double blind comparison of 21 day detoxification and 90 day gradual withdrawal by recently addicted patients.* Unpublished manuscript, 1979.

DUDLEY, D.L., AICKEN, M., and MARTIN, C.J. *J. Psychosomat. Res.* 21:367-375, 1977.

FEUERLEIN, W. The acute alcohol withdrawal syndrome: Findings and problems. *Br. J. Addict.* 69: 141-148, 1974.

FREEMAN, G.L. *The Energetics of Human Behavior.* Ithaca, NY: Cornell University Press, 1948.

GILBERT, D.G. Paradoxical tranquility and emotion reducing effects of nicotine. *Psychol. Bull.* 86: 643-661, 1979.

GOLDSTEIN, A. Heroin addiction and the role of methadone in its treatment. *Arch. Gen. Psychiatry* 29: 291-297, 1972.

GRIFFITHS, R.R., BIGELOW, G., and LIEBSON, I. Assessment of effects of ethanol self-administration of social interactions in alcoholics. *Psychopharmacologia* 38: 105-110, 1974.

GRIFFITHS, R.R., BIGELOW, G., and LIEBSON, I. Effect of ethanol self-administration on choice behavior: Money vs. socializing. *Pharmacol. Biochem. Behav.* 3: 443-445, 1975.

HABER, S. *Fear of thinness: An alternative approach to the treatment of obesity.* Paper presented at the American Psychological Association Meetings, Toronto, 1978.

HAGUE, W.H., WILSON, L.G., DUDLEY, D.L., and CANNON, D.S. Post detoxification drug treatment of anxiety and depression in alcohol addicts. *J. Nerv. Ment. Dis.* 162: 354-359, 1976.

HALL, S.M. The abstinence phobia. In N. Krasnegor (ed.), *Behavioral Approaches to Analysis and Treatment of Substance Abuse.* Washington, DC: Department of Health, Education, and Welfare, 1979.

HALL, S.M., BASS, A., HARGREAVES, W.A., and LOEB, P.C. Contingencies and information feedback in outpatient heroin detoxification. *Behav. Ther.* 10: 443-451, 1979.

HALL, S.M., and HALL, R.G. Outcome and methodological considerations in the behavioral treatment of obesity. *Behav. Ther.* 5: 352-364, 1974.

HALL, R.G., SACHS, D.P.L., and HALL, S.M. Medical safety of rapid smoking. *Behav. Ther.* 10: 249-259, 1979.

HAMILTON, F., and MAISTO, S.A. Assertive behavior and perceived discomfort of alcoholics in assertion required situations. *J. Consult. Clin. Psychol.* 47: 196-197, 1979.

HARGREAVES, W.A., LOWE, S.L., GAYNOR, J.L., and FULWILER, R.W. *Outpatient methadone detoxification in San Francisco: Its impact on treatment services for heroin addicts.* Unpublished manuscript, University of California, San Francisco, 1977.

HENDERSON, J.B., BACHMAN, J.B., BARSTOW, R., HALL, S.M., and JONES, R.T. *Effects of smoking cessation on the chronically ill.* Paper presented at meeting of the Association for the Advancement of Behavior Therapy, San Francisco, 1979.

HERSHON, H.I. Alcohol withdrawal symptoms and drinking behavior. *Q. J. Stud. Alcohol* 28: 953-971, 1977.

HIRT, M., and GREENFIELD, A. Implosive therapy treatment of heroin addicts during methadone detoxification. *J. Consult. Clin. Psychol.* 47: 982-983, 1979.

HUTCHINSON, R.R., and EMLEY, G.S. Effects of nicotine on avoidance conditioned stimuli and aggression response measures in animals and man. In W.L. Dunn (ed.), *Smoking Behavior: Motives and Incentives.* New York: Wiley, 1973.

IKARD, F.F., GREEN, D.E., and HORN, D. A scale to differentiate between types of smoking as related to management of affect. *Int. J. Addict.* 4: 646, 1969.

ISIADINSO, O.O. Success rates of detoxification from methadone maintenance on an ambulatory care unit. *J. Natl. Med. Assoc.* 36: 175-176, 1977.

JACKMAN, J.M. A hypothesis concerning the difficulty of withdrawal from maintenance on methadone. *Proc. Natl. Conf. Methadone Treatment* 1: 86-90, 1973.

JACOBS, M.A. The addictive personality: Prediction of success in a smoking withdrawal program. *Psychosomat. Med.* 34: 30-38, 1972.

KAPLAN, H.I., and KAPLAN, H.S. The psychosomatic concept of obesity. *J. Nerv. Ment. Dis.* 125: 181-201, 1957.

KLEBER, H.D. Detoxification from methadone maintenance: The state of the art. *Int. J. Addict.* 12: 820-870, 1977.

KREMEN, E., and BAYER, R. New choices for methadone maintenance patients: Planned, voluntary, long-term detoxification. *Proc. Natl. Conf. Methadone Treatment* 1: 667-674, 1973.

LARSON, P.S., and SILVETTE, H. *Tobacco: Experimental and Clinical Studies.* (Suppl. II). Baltimore: Williams and Wilkins, 1971.

LOWINSON, J., BERLE, B., and LANGROD, J. Detoxification of long-term methadone patients: Problems and prospects. *Int. J. Addict.* 11: 1009-1018, 1976.

MARLATT, G.A. Alcohol, stress and cognitive control. In I.G. Sarason and C.D. Spielberger (eds.), *Stress and Anxiety* (Vol. 3). Washington, DC: Hemisphere, 1976.

MARLATT, G.A. Craving for alcohol, loss of control, and relapse: A cognitive behavioral analysis. In P.E. Nathan, G.A. Marlatt, and T. Loberg (eds.), *Alcoholism: New Directions in Behavior Research and Treatment.* New York: Plenum Press, 1978.

MARTIN, W.R., HAERTZEN, C.A., and HEWETT, B.B. Psychopathology of narcotics addicts, alcoholics and drug abusers. In M.A. Lipton, A. DiMascio, and K.F. Killam (eds.), *Psychopharmacology: A Generation of Progress.* New York: Raven Press, 1978.

MARTORANO, R.D. Mood and social perception in four alcoholics: Effects of drinking and assertion training. *Q. J. Stud. Alcohol* 35: 445-457, 1974.

MC NAMEE, H.B., MELLO, N.K., and MENDELSON, J.H. Experimental analysis of drinking patterns on alcoholics: Concurrent psychiatry. *Psychiatry* 124: 81-87, 1968.

MILBY, J.B., GARRETT, C., and MEREDITH, R. Iatrogenic phobic disorders in methadone maintenance treated patients. *Int. J. Addict.* 15(5): 737-747, 1980.

MILBY, J.B., RICE, J.R., and GARRETT, C. *Iatrogenic phobic disorders in methadone maintenance treated patients.* Paper presented at the American Psychological Association, 1979.

MILLER, P.M., HERSEN, M., EISLER, R.M., and HILSMAN, G. Effects of social stress on drinking of alcoholics and social drinkers. *Behav. Res. Ther.* 12: 67-72, 1974.

MUSKELLY, T.E. Motivations and their relationship to methadone maintenance withdrawal problems. *Proc. Natl. Conf. Methadone Treatment* [No vol. no.]: 79-81, 1972.

MYRSTEN, A., ELGEROT, A.L., and EDGREN, B. Effects of abstinence from tobacco smoking on physiological and psychological adrenal levels in habitual smokers. *Psychosomat. Med.* 39: 25-38, 1977.

NATHAN, P.E., TITLER, N.A., LOWENSTEIN, L.M., SOLOMON, P., and ROSSI, A.M. Behavioral analysis of chronic alcoholism: Interaction of alcohol and human contact. *Arch. Gen. Psychiatry* 22: 419-430, 1970.

NOVACO, R. A stress inoculation procedure for the training of anger management in law enforcement officers. *Am. J. Comm. Psychol.* 5: 327-346, 1977.

O'LEARY, D.E., O'LEARY, M.R., and DONOVAN, D.M. Social skill acquisition and psychosocial development of alcoholics. *Addict. Behav.* 1: 111-128, 1976.

PANYARD, C., and WOLF, K. The use of systematic desensitization in an outpatient drug treatment center. *Psychotherapy: Theory Res. Practice* 11: 329-330, 1974.

PLATT, J., and L'ABATE, C. *Personality and Psychopathology in Heroin Addicts*. New York: Wiley, 1976.

PLATT, J., SCURA, W.C., and HANNON, J.R. Problem solving thinking of youthful incarcerated heroin addicts. *J. Comm. Psychol.* 1: 278-281, 1973.

PREBLE, E., and CASEY, J.J. Taking care of business–The heroin users' life in the streets. *Int. J. Addict.* 4: 1-24, 1969.

RABIN, J., and STIMMEL, B. A follow-up of patients discharged from methadone maintenance. In E. Senay, V. Shorty, and H. Alksne (eds.), *Developments in the Field of Drug Abuse*. Cambridge, MA: Schenkman, 1974.

RESNICK, R., KESTENBAUM, R., GAZTANAGA, P., VOLANKA, J., and FREEDMAN, A. Experimental techniques for rapid withdrawal from methadone maintenance: Results of pilot trials. In E. Senay and V. Shorty (eds.), *Developments in the Field of Drug Abuse*. Cambridge, MA: Schenkman, 1974.

RIORDAN, C.E., and RAPKIN, R. Detoxification as a final step in treating the successful long-term methadone patient. *Proc. Natl. Conf. Methadone Treatment* [No vol. no.]: 36-40, 1972.

SCHACTER, S. Nicotine regulation in heavy and light smokers. *J. Exp. Psychol.* 106: 5-12, 1977.

SCHMAHL, D.P., LICHTENSTEIN, E., and HARRIS, D.E. Successful treatment of habitual smokers with warm, smoky air and rapid smoking. *J. Consult. Clin. Psychol.* 38: 105-111, 1972.

SCHWARTZ, J.L. Smoking cures: Ways to kick an unhealthy habit. *NIDA Research Monograph Series: Research on Smoking Behavior*. Washington, DC: USPHS, 1977.

SENAY, E., DORUS, W., GOLDBERG, F., and THORNTON, W. Withdrawal from methadone maintenance: Rate of withdrawal and expectation. *Arch. Gen. Psychiatry* 34: 361-367, 1977.

SHAPIRO, D.H., and ZIFFERBLATT, S.M. An applied clinical combination of Zen meditation and behavioral self-management techniques, reducing methadone doses in drug addiction. *Behav. Ther.* 1: 694-695, 1976.

SHEFFET, A., QUINONES, M., LAVENNAR, M.A., DOYLE, K., and PRAGER, H. An evaluation of detoxification as an initial step in the treatment of heroin addiction. *Am. J. Psychiatry* 133: 337-340, 1970.

SHIFFMAN, S.M., and JARVIK, M.E. Smoking withdrawal symptoms in two weeks of abstinence. *Psychopharmacology* 50: 35-39, 1976.

SILVERSTONE, J.T., and LASCELLES, B.D. Dieting and depression: An assessment of affective disturbance occurring during the clinical trial of a new anoretic preparation. *Br. J. Psychiatry* 112: 513-519, 1966.

STIMMEL, B., RABIN, J., and ENGLE, C. The prognosis of patients detoxified from methadone maintenance: A follow-up study. *Proc. Natl. Conf. Methadone Treatment*, 1973.

STITZER, M.L., GRIFFITHS, R.R., BIGELOW, G.E., and LEIBSON, I. *Comparison of ethanol, secobarbitol, and chlorpromazine on human speaking in a dyadic social interactive situation.* Unpublished manuscript, 1980.

STUNKARD, A.J. The "dieting depression": Incidence and clinical characteristics of untoward responses to weight reduction regimens. *Am. J. Med.* 23: 77-86, 1957.

STUNKARD, A.J., and RUSH, J. Dieting and depression re-examined. A critical review of reports of interviewed responses during weight reduction for obesity. *Ann. Int. Med.* 81: 526-533, 1974.

UNITED STATES PUBLIC HEALTH SERVICE. *Smoking and Health: Report of the Surgeon General.* Washington, DC: USPHS, 1964.

WIKLER, A. Conditioning factors in opiate addiction and relapse. In D.M. Wilner and G.G. Kassenbaum (eds.), *Narcotics.* New York: McGraw-Hill, 1965.

WILSON, A., ELMS, T., and THOMPSON, G. Outpatient vs. hospital detoxification: An experimental comparison. *Int. J. Addict.* 10: 13-21, 1975.

WOLPE, J. *Psychotherapy by Reciprocal Inhibition.* Stanford, CN: Stanford University Press, 1958.

WOLPE, J. *The Practice of Behavior Therapy.* New York: Pergamon, 1969.

WYNDER, E.L., KAUFFMAN, P.L., and LESSER, R.L. A shortterm follow-up study on ex-cigarette smokers. *Am. Rev. Respir. Dis.* 96: 645-655, 1967.

The International Journal of the Addictions, 19(6), 633–652, 1984

"Turning on" Other Persons to Drugs

Harwin L. Voss, PhD

Richard R. Clayton, PhD

University of Kentucky
Lexington, Kentucky 40506

Abstract

Data obtained in a recent national survey are examined to test two hypotheses about drug transmission. The hypothesis that transmission of drug use to others is most likely to occur within a short period of time after initial use is supported. For each drug or drug class, at least one-half of the users who transmitted drug use to others did so within a span of 2 years after they began to use the drug. One-fourth of the marijuana users "turned on" others. Marijuana users are more likely to transmit their drug use than are users of other illicit drugs, but most drug users never "turn on" others. The hypothesis that drug transmission occurs only within a short period of time after onset of use is rejected. Among marijuana users who "turned on" others, 29% of them did so 5 or more years after they first used marijuana.

A key idea regarding the transmission of drug use is that neophytes are often introduced, or "turned on," to illicit drugs by friends or associates. Transmission in friendship networks has been demonstrated among opiate users (Ball and Chambers, 1970, p. 173; Brown, Greene, and Turner, 1976; O'Donnell, 1969, pp. 77-81; Pescor, 1943; Sacher et al., n.d.; Terry and Pellens, 1928, pp. 110-136). Similarly, the National Commission on Marihuana and Drug Abuse (1972, p. 278) reported that initial use of marijuana "ordinarily occurs in the course of normal social relationships." In the commission's national survey, 78.5% of the youth and 62.4% of the adults indicated that the first time they tried marijuana, the drug was given to them. These figures are underestimates because persons who did not respond to the relevant question (9.8% of the

 0020-773X/84/1906-0633$3.50/0

youth and 30.6% of the adults) were not excluded in the calculation of the percentages. Two-thirds of the adults and four-fifths of the youth were introduced to marijuana by friends, acquaintances, or family members (see Note 1). In a national study of drug use among young men, only 12% of the marijuana users said that they purchased the drug when they initially used it. Eighty-eight percent of the respondents who had used marijuana reported that it was given to them the first time they used it. For psychedelics, stimulants, sedatives, heroin, and cocaine, 60-70% of the users indicated that the drug was given to them the first time they used it (Note 2; O'Donnell et al., 1976, p. 62). Clearly, friends and acquaintances play an important role in users' initial experiences with illicit drugs.

DRUG TRANSMISSION IN THE HONEYMOON PERIOD

Another idea about the transmission of drug use is that new users introduce others to the drug only, or almost exclusively, within a short period of time—perhaps 1 or 2 years—after they begin to use it. Shepard and Voss (1978, p. 432) have tentatively accepted a variant of this hypothesis: "Although the evidence is limited, it has been suggested that persons who have used heroin for less than a year are the ones most likely to 'infect' others—their enthusiasm is contagious. Thus, heroin use spreads like an epidemic in which a 'carrier' infects persons in his or her friendship network."

There are several reasons why the idea of a restricted time span for drug transmisssion is plausible. For several different kinds of drugs, the initial period of use has been aptly described as a "honeymoon" (Lindesmith, 1968, p. 25). In this period, the users may enjoy the drug as much as they ever will but may encounter few, if any, ill effects. They are enthusiastic about the drug and may believe they are doing their friends a favor by acquainting them with the drug. With the passage of time, a user's interest in turning on others may diminish, and the opportunities to do so may also be restricted. After a few years of experience with a drug, users may, as a result of physical ill effects, legal difficulties, or other problems, adopt a different view of the drug. In that event, they might warn their friends not to use it. If they are deeply enmeshed in a drug subculture and spend most of their time with other users, there may be few nonusers among their friends and acquaintances whom they could turn on to the drug. Among any remaining nonusers, many of them would probably have had previous opportunities to try the drug. If they had not done so, they would not be promising candidates, even if an individual wanted to continue to turn on others.

A carefully phrased statement of the idea of a restricted time span in the transmission of drug use is provided by Hunt and Chambers (1976, p. 12), who conclude "that the interval between 'generations' of users was typically less than a year." They correctly qualify this conclusion, because "typically" means that approximately 80% of the new users appear in generations of about a year. They also note that there are some striking exceptions, particularly in areas that have a long history of heroin use. Further, Hunt and Chambers correctly observe that most heroin users do not initiate use in others. For example, of the 56 users in de Alarcon's (1969) sample, 20 of them transmitted heroin use to others. After they present some estimates based on mathematical models but no additional empirical data, Hunt and Chambers (1976, p. 25) present a questionable conclusion: "Each user is likely to transmit new use only during a brief initial period–typically during his first year of use." Although the word "typically" is a useful qualifier, inclusion of the word "only" could be misinterpreted, and this usage may be questioned (Note 3).

In this paper the studies that provide empirical support for the idea that transmission occurs within a restricted time span are reviewed and critiqued (see Table 1), and data obtained in a recent national survey are examimed to shed light on two hypotheses pertaining to drug transmission: (1) Drug transmission is *most likely* to occur within a short period of time after onset of drug use, and (2) drug transmission occurs *almost exclusively* within a short period of time after onset of use. Some descriptive information about the men who reported that they had turned on other persons to drugs is also provided.

RELEVANT EMPIRICAL STUDIES

While the suggestion that the transmission of drug use is an early and passing phase of drug use is highly plausible, the empirical data upon which it rests are rather limited. Hunt and Chambers (1976) based their assertions primarily on their secondary analysis of three studies of the spread of heroin microepidemics in: (1) Crawley, England (de Alarcon, 1969); (2) Chicago (Hughes, Crawford, Barker, Schumann, and Jaffe, 1971); and (3) Grosse Pointe, Michigan (Levengood, Lowinger, and Schoof, 1973). In each of these studies, the spread of heroin use was traced from one person to a number of others and from these "second-generation" users to still others. With a few exceptions, the year of first heroin use was established for each individual. This permitted measurement of the interval between initial use and initiation of someone else.

These three studies do not provide an adequate empirical basis for Hunt and Chambers's assertion that the process of transmission is essentially restricted to a brief, initial period following the onset of drug use. For one thing, none of these studies was designed to test the hypothesis that only new users transmit drug use to others. For example, the study in Grosse Pointe was based on a sample of 60 of an estimated 300 users in the population aged 15 to 19. The problem is not the size of the sample, but the sampling technique. The 60 youth were not a random sample of users, but were identified by means of

Table 1

Prior Studies of Transmission of Drug Use

Study	Technique used	Data collected	Results	Study limitations
Author: de Alarcon Years: 1962-1967 Drug: Heroin Location: Crawley, England Number: 58	Clinical records of the Crawley Psychiatric Service or direct questioning of subjects	Age at first use of heroin, identification of initiator, and subject's transmission of heroin to others	Heroin use spreads from individual to individual like a contagious disease; one man, initiated in another community, essentially initiated the epidemic in Crawley.	Subjects restricted to clinic patients in one "new town" in England; 53 of the 58 subjects were males; all subjects were 15 to 20 years of age; study covers a short time span, as most of the users began heroin use near the end of the study period.
Authors: Hughes et al. Years: 1967-1971 Drug: Heroin Location: Chicago, Illinois Number: 64	Personal interviews	Family background: neighborhood conditions; peer group dynamics; prior drug use; police contacts; initiator to heroin and	In microepidemics, group members are heavy poly-drug users prior to introduction of heroin; heroin is introduced to the group from multiple	Subjects recruited from patients in the Illinois Drug Abuse Program, and additional users identified by

		subject's transmission of heroin to peers	sources; individuals are initiated by friends, not heroin dealers; macroepidemics are aggregates of several independent microepidemics.	"snowball" sampling; small sample size; subjects all residents of Chicago.
Authors: Levengood, Lowinger, and Schooff Years: 1966-1971 Drug: Heroin Location: Grosse Pointe, Michigan Number: 60	Personal interviews	Drugs used and age at first use; identification of initiator to heroin and subject's transmission of heroin to peers; extent of heroin use and source of support	A wide range of drugs was used by the subjects; heroin use spread from individual to individual largely within existing peer groups; most of the 22 regular users initiated others to provide a source of income to purchase heroin; there were also 24 occasional users and 14 former users in the sample; all of the former users were regularly employed or attending school.	Subjects identified by other users or through "snowball" sampling; small sample restricted to young (15 to 24) Caucasians in one affluent suburb; 52 of 60 subjects were males; study covers a short time span as most users began heroin use near the end of the study period.

snowball sampling. With this technique, each user who was identified was asked to provide the name of the person who had initiated him and to identify any persons he had turned on. As Hunt and Chambers indicate, this uncovers interrelated users and excludes isolated users. Whatever bias this introduces is unknown. Because of similarities in research design, the other two studies almost necessarily involve similar sampling problems.

However, the most serious problem is that all three studies deal with relatively short time periods, and in two of them, most of the users did not begin to use heroin until the last year or two of the period studied. A person cannot be observed turning on someone else to heroin more than a year after the person's first use of heroin unless the observer waits for at least a year. Specifically, in the study in Crawley (1962-1967), in the years 1962, 1963, and 1964, one person began to use heroin each year, and two persons began to use it in 1965. Then, in 1966, 25 persons began to use heroin, as did another 26 persons in 1967, the year in which the study ended. de Alarcon wanted to determine how an epidemic begins and spreads, and for that purpose, the sample was quite adequate. Unfortunately, it is not adequate to estimate the interval between initial heroin use and its transmission to others. Thirteen of the 25 persons who began heroin use in 1966 initiated someone else. Because 1967 was the last year observed, their transmission of drug use could not have occurred more than a year after their initial use of heroin. Seven of the 26 persons who began to use heroin in 1967 introduced one or more persons to heroin and necessarily did so in the year they first used heroin.

Of the 58 persons in de Alarcon's sample, only five of them could have transmitted heroin use to another person more than a year after their initial use. It is instructive to examine these five persons whose initial use of heroin occurred prior to 1966. Four of them did not transmit their drug use to anyone. Introduced to heroin by a person who resided outside Crawley, the fifth person essentially initiated the entire epidemic. This man began his use of heroin in 1962. In 1966 he introduced four other persons in Crawley to heroin use, and two of these persons became the main line of transmission in the Crawley epidemic. As four of the five early users of heroin did not initiate anyone else, this was the only person with an interval of 4 years between use and transmission. It is essential to recognize that of the cases in which transmission occurred, it was the only one that could have involved a 4-year period of time.

In the study conducted in Grosse Pointe (1966-1971), the distribution by year is similar to the one in Crawley. For eight users, dates of initial use or transmission were not determined. Exclusive of these undated cases, the number of new users by year were: 1966, 1; 1967, 2; 1968, 1; 1969, 9; 1970, 22; and 1971, 5. With the exception of the four earliest users, there could not be instances of transmission after an interval longer than 2 years. As was the case in

Crawley, one individual, who began to use heroin in 1966, essentially initiated the entire epidemic.

The study conducted in Chicago provides a more adequate basis for the examination of transmission intervals than do the others because it covers a slightly larger number of years and the years of onset are spread over the years, rather than being concentrated in the last 2 years of the study. New users were distributed as follows: 1964 or earlier, 8; 1965, 8; 1966, 2; 1967, 9; 1968, 12; 1969, 10; 1970, 7; and 1971, 8. Of the persons who transmitted heroin use, most of them did so within an interval of 1 to 2 years, or less. This was also the case for the persons who used heroin sufficiently early to permit longer intervals to appear. The data show that if a user is going to transmit drug use, this is most likely to occur within a short span of time after initial use of the drug. However, the data also reveal that transmission is not confined to a brief time interval, as there were three intervals of 6 years and two intervals of 7 years.

THE DATA

To examine the transmission hypotheses on the basis of additional data, attention is shifted to a recent nationwide survey of drug use among 2,510 young men. The sample was drawn from Selective Service records to provide a probability sample of men who were born in the years 1944 through 1954 in the continental United States and who registered with Selective Service at the age of 18. The sample is representative of young men in the United States, exclusive of Alaska and Hawaii, who were 20 to 30 years of age in late 1974 and early 1975, when the interviews were conducted. Approximately 84% of the men in the target sample were interviewed; failure to locate individuals accounted for more than one-half of the missing cases. Less than 7% of the prospective respondents refused to be interviewed. A detailed description of the sampling procedures is available (O'Donnell et al., 1976, pp. 3-11).

Each respondent was asked if he had ever turned on anyone to any drug. If a positive response was elicited, he was asked which drug or drugs were involved. In addition, information about the first and last year in which he had turned on anyone was obtained. Information was recorded for as many as five drugs or drug classes. It should be specified what the questions do and do not reflect. Clearly, the questions elicit information about the drugs or drug classes a man has transmitted to other people, but information regarding the number of people he turned on was not obtained. Among the respondents who reported turning on someone to a drug, the number who named additional drugs declined as the question was repeated. Few respondents named four or five drugs. This suggests that little information was lost by gathering data about only five drugs.

To test the hypothesis that drug transmission is most likely to occur within a short period of time after onset of use, the interval between the first use of a drug and the first time a user turned on someone else was calculated. The results are presented in Table 2 for seven drugs, or drug classes. It should be noted that the category of marijuana includes both marijuana and hashish. The intervals shown in Table 2 were obtained by subtraction of the year in which the respondent first used the drug from the year in which he first turned on someone to it. There is, then, a certain imprecision in the intervals. An interval counted as 1 year could reflect a period of a few days or months, or it could reflect a period of slightly less than 2 years. It is presumed that such measurement errors are random and balance each other. In any case, they could not affect the argument to be presented on the basis of these data.

Just as some men who were not users of drugs sold drugs illegally, a few nonusers turned on others to drugs. The men who subsequently became users are shown in Table 2 as turning on others before use. Most of these men turned on some one in the year prior to their own use. Intervals could not be calculated for the men who failed to specify either the year in which they initially used the drug or the year in which they turned on others to it. In each column in Table 2, the largest number is found either in the same year or in the interval of 1 year. Most of the users who transmitted drug use to others did so within a time span of 2 years after they began to use the drug. For each drug or drug class, at least one-half of the transmissions are found within this limited period. Thus, the data from the national survey of drug use among young men provide strong support for the hypothesis that transmission of drug use to others is most likely to occur within a short period of time after initial use.

This is not, however, all that the data in Table 2 indicate. First, it is essential to recognize that, for each drug or drug class, most of the users never turned on anyone else. Of the seven drug classes, marijuana is the one most likely to be transmitted. Of the 1,382 men who reported some experience with marijuana, 26% said they had turned on others to this drug. The comparable percentages are lower for the other classes of drugs. In view of the fact that one-fourth of the marijuana users turned on others, it is apparent that drug transmission is not a rare occurrence. It is equally important to recognize that most users of illicit drugs do not transmit their drug use to others. Second, it should be noted that of the marijuana users who initiated others, approximately 30% of them did so after an interval of 3 years or more after their initial use. This was also the case for 20-25% of the transmissions of psychedelics, stimulants, and sedatives. These findings are contrary to the hypothesis that drug transmission occurs almost exclusively within a short period of time after onset of use. For heroin, the opiates, and cocaine, there are relatively few initial transmissions of drug use in intervals of 3 years or more. In the following section it is argued that the latter

Table 2

Interval between Initial Use of a Drug and First Turning On Others

Interval	Marijuana	Psychedelics	Stimulants	Sedatives	Heroin	Opiates	Cocaine
Before use	9	4	5	1	–	1	2
Same year	87	22	12	5	9	5	13
1 year later	91	30	16	3	6	7	9
2 years later	61	19	9	3	2	1	7
3 years later	44	9	16	3	2	–	–
4 years later	36	6	1	–	–	1	–
5 years later	9	6	1	1	–	–	1
6 years later	8	–	–	1	–	–	–
7 years later	6	–	–	–	–	–	–
8 years later	1	–	2	–	1	–	–
9 years later	1	–	–	–	–	–	–
10 years later	–	–	–	–	–	–	–
11 years later	1	–	–	–	–	–	–
12 years later	–	–	–	–	–	–	–
No use reported	2	3	2	1	1	1	1
Date(s) unknown	7	3	3	3	–	–	–
Totals	363	102	67	21	21	16	33
Percentage of users who ever turned on others	26	18	9	4	14	3[a]	9

[a]Quasi-medical users of opiates are excluded.

finding should not be construed as support for the hypothesis that drug transmission is confined to a brief time interval.

To test the hypothesis that drug transmission occurs almost exclusively within a short period of time after initial use, the interval between the first use of a drug and the last time the user turned on someone was calculated. The results are presented in Table 3. The intervals shown in Table 3 were derived by subtraction of the year in which the respondent first used the drug from the year in which he last turned on someone to it. Again, there is a certain degree of imprecision in the intervals because years, rather than precise dates, are used to derive them. In each column in Table 3, the largest numbers are found either in the same year or in the intervals of 1 year to 4 years. This suggests that the last transmission of drug use occurs within a few years of a person's initial use of the drug. This conclusion holds for all of the drugs or drug classes. On the other hand, with only three exceptions, in every column, at least one man is found in each of the time intervals of 1 year to 5 years.

The largest number of drug transmissions in Table 3 involve marijuana. If one excludes the two nonusers and the nine men who did not specify the year in which they last turned on someone to marijuana, then 103 instances of transmission, or 29% of the 352 dated transmissions, occurred 5 or more years after the respondent first used marijuana. There are even two respondents who turned on others to marijuana 12 years after their initial use of the drug. To understand what is involved in these two cases, it is essential to note that while a few of the interviews were conducted as late as May 1975, almost all of them were completed several months earlier. For practical purposes, 1974 may be treated as the last year in which the men could have turned on anyone to drugs. For the two men to have turned on someone to marijuana 12 years after their initial use means they would have to have begun marijuana use by 1962. Twenty-four respondents meet this requirement, but there were only four transmitters who had used the drug as early as 1962. Two is obviously a small number, but these two men constitute one-half of the transmitters who could have turned on others 12 years after they initially used marijuana. To reiterate, most users of illicit drugs, including marijuana, do not transmit their drug use—only 4 of the 24 men who used marijuana as early as 1962 turned on another person to marijuana. To produce an interval of 11 or more years, the transmitters would have had to use marijuana by 1963; there were only nine transmitters who had done so. Of these nine men, five turned on someone to marijuana 11 or more years after they began to use the drug.

Application of this logic led to the construction of Table 4, which shows the number of men who turned on others 5 or more years after they began to use marijuana. For convenience, the latest possible year in which the respondents could have used marijuana for the first time to produce a particular interval is listed. Both the number of users and the number of transmitters who

Table 3

Interval between Initial Use of a Drug and Last Turning On Others

Interval	Marijuana	Psychedelics	Stimulants	Sedatives	Heroin	Opiates	Cocaine
Before use	3	1	2	–	–	1	1
Same year	28	13	9	2	7	5	8
1 year later	51	22	10	4	4	4	8
2 years later	56	19	8	3	1	2	8
3 years later	55	17	10	3	4	1	–
4 years later	56	11	8	–	1	1	2
5 years later	32	9	4	2	1	–	3
6 years later	29	2	1	3	–	–	1
7 years later	22	1	2	–	–	–	–
8 years later	9	–	–	–	1	–	–
9 years later	5	–	1	–	1	1	–
10 years later	1	–	1	–	–	–	1
11 years later	3	–	–	–	–	–	–
12 years later	2	–	–	–	–	–	–
No use reported	2	3	2	1	1	1	1
Date(s) unknown	9	4	9	3	–	–	–
Totals	363	102	67	21	21	16	33

Table 4

Intervals between Initial Use of Marijuana and Last Turning On of Others to It

Interval	Number of transmissions (cumulative)	Latest possible year of onset	Men who used in or before that year (cumulative)		Transmitters as percentage of users and transmitters available	
			Users	Transmitters	Users	Transmitters
12 or more years	2	1962	24	4	8	50
11 or more years	5	1963	43	9	12	50
10 or more years	6	1964	72	15	8	40
9 or more years	11	1965	126	32	7	34
8 or more years	20	1966	208	59	10	34
7 or more years	42	1967	344	109	12	39
6 or more years	71	1968	541	174	13	41
5 or more years	103	1969	759	242	14	43

had used marjiuana in that year or earlier are shown; the transmitters are a subset of the users. While the transmitters are of primary interest, the number of users is shown as a reminder that most users do not transmit drug use to others. In the last column, the percentage of transmitters who turned on others in each time interval is shown in relation to the number of both users and transmitters available at that time. In other words, for the interval of 5 years or more, the number of transmitters who had used marijuana prior to 1969 serves as the denominator, and the numerators are, respectively, the number of users and of transmitters available. The figures in the first and third columns are cumulative; that is, a man who turned on someone 12 years after his initial use of marijuana is included in the other intervals. In these intervals, the percentage of users who turned on others ranges from 8 to 14, an indication that most users do not transmit drug use to others. On the other hand, of the 242 transmitters who had used marijuana prior to 1969, or 5 years before they were interviewed, 43% of them had turned on others to marijuana at least 5 years after their first use of marijuana. The lowest figure in the last column is 34%. The data pertaining to the men who transmitted marijuana use indicate, insofar as this drug is concerned, that turning on others is not confined to a brief honeymoon period.

Not shown are tables similar to Table 4 that were constructed for each of the other drugs. In each table, the pattern was similar. Most of the men who turned on someone did so in the same year as the one in which they first used the drug or within the next 4 years. Nevertheless, of the transmitters who used a drug sufficiently early to permit an interval of at least 2 years, sizable percentages of them turned on others at least 2 years after initial use of the drug—the percentages range from 33 for opiates to 72 for cocaine. The psychedelics are something of an exception in that, of the transmitters who could have had a rather long interval between initial use and the last time they turned on someone, relatively few did so. Only 1 of 14 men who could have had an interval of 7 years did so, and the same was true of only 3 of 25 transmitters who could have had an interval of 6 years.

Some relatively small numbers deserve mention. For the stimulants, two transmitters had intervals of 9 or 10 years between initial use of these drugs and the last time they turned on someone to them. These two men are significant because they represent one-half of the transmitters who could have had such an interval. Similarly, for sedatives, the five transmitters with intervals of 5 or 6 years represent one-half of the transmitters who had used sedatives sufficiently early to permit such an interval. There were only three transmitters who could have turned on others to heroin as many as 8 or 9 years after they began to use the drug, and two of them did so. These figures are not presented to estimate the proportion of drug transmitters who turn on others many years after their initial use of a drug. Such estimates cannot be based on these small numbers. However, these figures are important to correct an impression one might gain from Table 2. Casual inspection of that table might suggest that it is rare to find a long interval between the onset of use and transmission, and that the few instances that occur are insignificant. The numbers are small, but this is the case because time constraints make it impossible for them to be much larger. An equally accurate way to describe the lower portion of Table 2 would be to assert that, given the low proportion of drug users who transmit drug use to others, these figures are almost as large as they could be, in view of the age composition of the sample and the age of onset for the various drugs.

CHARACTERISTICS OF TRANSMITTERS

Of the 2,510 men in the sample, 520 of them turned on others to one or more drugs. Thus, approximately one-fifth of the men directly transmitted drug use to others. In Table 5, differences in the percentage of respondents who turned on others to drugs are shown for a number of demographic variables, and the transmitters are compared with the men who did not transmit drug use in terms of reported criminal activity and use of illicit drugs. In the first panel in Table 5, the men are classified into four age groups, and it is apparent that transmission occurred more frequently among the younger men. In terms of race, there is little difference between Whites and Blacks, but fewer of the men categorized as "other" reported that they had turned on others to drugs. There is a linear relationship between the extent of drug transmission and the prestige of the respondents' fathers' occupations: except for one slight reversal, this is also the case for the size of the city in which the respondents lived to the age of 18. As city size increases, the proportion of men who report turning on others increases. Similarly, more of the men whose fathers had the most prestigious occupations had turned on others than was the case for men whose fathers had less prestigious occupations. In contrast, the level of education achieved by the respondent is not strongly related to drug transmission. The men who had completed some college were more likely to report that they had turned on others, but it is instructive to note that there is only one percentage point difference between the high school dropouts and the men who had graduated from college. Current marital status is also related to transmission. The married men were least likely to report drug transmission, while more than one-third of the men who were cohabiting had turned on others (see Clayton and Voss, 1977). Church attendance is also related to drug transmission, as twice as many men who never attended church had turned on others than was the case for those who attended church each week. More of the men who were unemployed or were students reported turning on others than did the men who were employed. However, there is little difference in the extent of drug transmission according to the prestige of the respondent's occupation (see Voss, 1981).

Table 5

Demographic Characteristics, Criminal Activities, and Illicit Drug Use of Respondents Who Turned On Others to Drugs

	Number	Percentage who turned on others
Birth year: Age in 1974		
1944-1946: 28 to 30 years old	541	11
1947-1949: 25 to 27 years old	692	18
1950-1952: 22 to 24 years old	740	26
1953-1954: 20 to 21 years old	537	26
Race		
White	2,103	21
Black	303	20
Other	104	12
Father's occupational prestige		
No information	93	23
1 (low)	635	16
2	594	18
3	600	22
4 (high)	588	26
Size of place of residence to age 18		
1 million or more	187	26
100,000 to 999,999	610	23
25,000 to 99,999	466	20
2,500 to 24,999	730	21
Less than 2,500	456	16
Outside United States	46	6
Missing information	15	15
Respondent's education		
Less than high school	394	18
High school graduate	933	20
Some college	713	26
College graduate	470	19
Marital status		
Married	1,309	16
Cohabiting	120	37
Other	1,081	25
Church attendance		
Weekly	430	13
Monthly	471	16
Less than monthly	798	22
Never	811	26
Respondent's occupational prestige		
Unemployed	213	28
Student	172	24
1 (low)	558	20
2	528	22
3	502	20
4 (high)	537	18

(continued)

Table 5 (continued)

	Number	Percentage who turned on others
Nontraffic arrest		
Yes	786	35
No	1,724	14
Crime conviction		
Yes	303	38
No	2,207	18
Criminal activities		
None reported	446	3
One or two reported	1,164	15
Three or more reported	900	37
Illicit drug use[a]		
None used	1,988	12
One used	209	38
Two or more used	313	62
Sold drugs		
Yes	495	58
No	2,015	12
Reported addiction		
Yes	589	35
No	1,921	16

[a]In this measure, use of marijuana is excluded. Also excluded is experimental use (less than 10 times) of other illicit drugs. The drugs included in this measure are psychedelics, stimulants, sedatives, heroin, other opiates, and cocaine.

The respondents were asked if they had ever been arrested for a nontraffic offense or convicted of a crime and whether they had committed any of 10 specific criminal acts, regardless of whether they had been apprehended. The men who responded positively to these inquiries were more likely to report that they had turned on others than the men who denied arrest, conviction, or involvement in the 10 criminal acts. It is noteworthy that 62% of the men who reported use of two or more illicit drugs, other than marijuana, had turned on others to drugs. Similarly, 58% of the men who had sold drugs had turned on others. Finally, a higher percentage of the men who reported addiction to one or more drugs had turned on others than had the respondents who stated that they were never addicted.

BEHAVIORAL CORRELATES

The associations between drug transmission and 11 kinds of behavior (some of which may be considered unconventional) are shown in Table 6. Two of the items—registering to vote and political campaigning—clearly reflect conventional

Table 6

Behavioral Correlates of Drug Transmission

	Total		Percentage who turned on others	
	N	%	Yes	No
Have you ever:				
a. Lived in a commune?	129	5	43	20
b. Attended an outdoor rock concert or festival?	1,173	47	32	10
c. Meditated, or explored an Eastern religion or philosophy?	396	16	38	18
d. Joined a street gang?	273	11	36	19
e. Registered to vote?	1,795	72	20	22
f. Followed a vegetarian, macrobiotic, or organic diet?	200	8	47	18
g. Campaigned or worked for a political candidate, issue, or cause?	553	22	25	20
h. Taken part in a political demonstration?	368	15	36	18
i. Studied astrology, ESP, or the occult?	406	16	34	18
j. Bummed around the United States or elsewhere?	399	16	41	17
k. Thought pretty seriously about committing suicide?	211	8	38	19

activities. The respondents have not been mere passive observers of the political scene: 72% have registered to vote, 22% have participated in some kind of political campaign, and 15% have taken part in a political demonstration.

Almost one-half of the respondents have attended an outdoor rock concert or festival. Approximately one of every six respondents has meditated, or explored an Eastern religion or philosophy; studied astrology, ESP, or the occult; and "bummed around" the United States or elsewhere. On the other hand, relatively few of the men have ever belonged to a street gang, followed a macrobiotic diet or organic diet, contemplated suicide, or lived in a commune.

There is a consistent relationship between participation in these kinds of activities and transmission of drug use to others. With the exception of registering to vote, the percentage of men who report each of the other kinds of behavior is always higher for those who have transmitted drug use than for those who have not.

DISCUSSION

To test two closely related hypotheses regarding drug transmission, data obtained in response to a question about "turning on" others are utilized. To turn on another person means that an individual supplies someone with a drug on the first occasion the person uses it. To turn on others is certainly an important part of the transmission of drug use, but transmission also includes the diffusion of attitudes and values that support use of illicit drugs, and it is not necessarily restricted to provision of a drug to a neophyte. In this sense, transmission includes a case in which a person hears about a drug from friends or acquaintances, becomes curious about it, and takes some of a sibling's or friend's supply in order to try it.

In this paper, the term "transmission" is used descriptively and not in the medical sense of contagion. In view of the fact that most drug users do not report transmission to others, a contagion model seems to be inappropriate. The availability of a person who has used a drug and is willing to introduce a neophyte to the drug is only one factor in the spread of drug use. Information regarding the nature of the relationship between the transmitter and the neophyte is not available, and the relative importance of drug transmitters in the spread of drug use cannot be compared with other influences, such as the neophyte's curiosity about the drug and social pressure from peers to experiment with the drug.

The data regarding turning on others were obtained from one partner in a dyadic relationship. The respondents who indicated that they had turned on others—for example, to marijuana—presumably had specific other persons in mind. It is not known whether these persons, had they been identified and contacted, would have stated that they had been turned on by the respondent. The question, as phrased, elicits the respondent's perception. It is possible that some individuals believe that they were turned on to a drug by a man who, if asked, would deny that he had ever turned on anyone to that drug. In short, to state that one has turned on someone to a drug is to report a perception or an interpretation, and the same thing is true of a denial. In neither case would the perception or interpretation of the other person necessarily be identical. It would be useful to know what leads individuals to perceive that they have turned on another person. It might be helpful to obtain detailed descriptions of situations in which one or more persons first use a drug, and to identify those persons, if any, who consider that they turned on the neophytes.

The available data pertain to the number of drugs to which the respondents turned on others, and the data do not reflect the number of persons whom they initiated to illicit drugs. It is, of course, possible that new users turn on a large number of persons in the year following onset of drug use and relatively few persons in later years, even though some cases may occur. However, this is an empirical question, and the requisite data are not available. In the realm of speculation, one could translate the folk adage that misery loves company into the proposition that active recruitment of new users would occur a number of years after a person began to use a drug.

In any event, the data obtained in a national survey of drug use among young men provided strong support for the hypothesis that transmission of drug use to others is most likely to occur within a period of a year or two after initial use. Marijuana users are more likely to transmit their drug use than users of six other classes of drugs. In view of the fact that one-fourth of the marijuana users turned on others, it is apparent that drug transmission is not a rare event, but it is equally important to recognize that most users of illicit drugs do not transmit their use to others. The hypothesis that drug transmission occurs almost exclusively within a short period of time after onset of user was rejected. Among the marijuana users who turned on others, 29% of them did so 5 or more years after they first used marijuana. Similarly, sizable percentages of the transmitters of other illicit drugs turned on others at least 2 years after initial use of the drug.

NOTES

1. These figures would have been higher if those who provided no answer had been excluded, as 9.8% of the youth and 27.0% of the adults did not specify who introduced them to marijuana.
2. The comparable figure for the opiates was 48%, but this figure is deflated because quasi-medical use of opiates was not excluded. Quasi-medical use of opiates, or use "on one's own" but essentially for medical purposes, was extensive in this sample–37% of the men who used opiates fell in this category (O'Donnell et al., 1976, p. 29). Some 16% of the users of opiates obtained them initially by means of a prescription.
3. We are indebted to the late John A. O'Donnell for stimulating our interest in the issues as well as for a number of the ideas expressed in this paper. See O'Donnell's (1977) critique of the estimation procedures employed by Hunt to assess heroin epidemics.

REFERENCES

BALL, J.C., and CHAMBERS, C.D. *The Epidemiology of Opiate Addiction in the United States.* Springfield, IL: C.C. Thomas, 1970.

BROWN, B.S., GREENE, M.H., and TURNER, N.J. The spread of addiction–The role of the "Average Addict." *Am. J. Drug Alcohol Abuse* 3: 521-528, 1976.

CLAYTON, R.R., and VOSS, H.L. Shacking up: Cohabitation in the 1970s. *J. Marriage Family* 39: 273-283, 1977.

DE ALARCON, R. The spread of heroin in a community. *Bull. Narcotics* 21: 17-21, 1969.

HUGHES, P.H., CRAWFORD, G.A., BARKER, N.W., SCHUMANN, S., and JAFFE, J.H. The social structure of a heroin copping community. *Am. J. Psychiatry* 128: 43-50, 1971.

HUNT, L.G., and CHAMBERS, C.D. *The Heroin Epidemics: A Study of Heroin Use in the United States, 1965-75.* New York: Spectrum Publications, 1976.

LEVENGOOD, R., LOWINGER, P., and SCHOOF, K. Heroin addiction in the suburbs–An epidemiological study. *Am. J. Public Health* 63: 209-213, 1973.

LINDESMITH, A.R. *Addiction and Opiates.* Chicago: Aldine, 1968.

NATIONAL COMMISSION ON MARIHUANA AND DRUG ABUSE *Marihuana: A Signal of Misunderstanding.* New York: New American Library, 1972.

O'DONNELL, J.A. *Narcotic Addicts in Kentucky.* Washington, DC: U.S. Government Printing Office, 1969.

O'DONNELL, J.A. Comments on Hunt's estimation procedures. In J.D. Rittenhouse (ed.), *The Epidemiology of Heroin and Other Narcotics.* Rockville, MD: National Institute on Drug Abuse, 1977, pp. 59-62.

O'DONNELL, J.A., VOSS, H.L., CLAYTON, R.R., SLATIN, G.T., and ROOM, R.G.W. *Young Men and Drugs: A Nationwide Survey.* Rockville, MD: National Institute on Drug Abuse, 1976.

PESCOR, M.J. A statistical analysis of the clinical records of hospitalized narcotic addicts. *Public Health Rep.* Suppl. No. 143, 1943.

SACHER, C.G., BROWN, B.S., GREENE, M.H., and DU PONT, R.L. *Initiation into heroin use.* Unpublished paper, n.d.

SHEPARD, J.M., and VOSS, H.L. *Social Problems.* New York: Macmillan, 1978.

TERRY, C.E., and PELLENS, M. *The Opium Problem.* New York: Bureau of Social Hygiene, 1928.

VOSS, H.L. Drugs, crime and occupation prestige. *J. Psychoactive Drugs* 13: 267-275, 1981.

The International Journal of the Addictions, 19(6), 653-664, 1984

Alcohol Use among Graduate Business Administration Students

Mary L. Waring, PhD

Gilda Petraglia, PhD

Graduate School of Social Services

Lynn Cohen, PhD

Graduate School of Business Administration

Everett Busby, MSW

Graduate School of Social Services

Fordham University at Lincoln Center
New York, New York 10023

Abstract

This study of fully employed master's students in a graduate school of business administration found no significant differences in the drinking levels of men and women. The majority are heavy drinkers. There is a tendency for female and Jewish students to prefer wine. Despite the role that beverage alcohol plays in the corporate world, few students were interested in alcohol education.

Although drinking by undergraduate students has long been a focus of study, beginning in 1953 with Straus and Bacon and continuing to the present with Wechsler and Roman (1981), very few studies have been carried out on undergraduate or graduate students in the professions. Among recent studies on alcohol and drug use by college students, one authored by Segal, Huba, and Singer (1980) did not describe the sample's demographic characteristics. Other researchers such as Arafat (1979) reported only on males within their sample. Dodge, in 1979, did specify the major course of study of his all-male Catholic college sample in a study of college drug use. Yet, presently there are almost no

0020-773X/84/1906-0653$3.50/0

published studies of drinking patterns among master's students in business administration. Among the professions, generally, only a few studies have been reported. These include: Bissell, Lambrecht, and Von Wiegand (1973), who reported on alcoholic hospital employees; and Bissell and Jones (1976), and Glatt (1977), who studied alcoholic physicians. Isler (1978) has studied the alcoholic nurse, and Bissell, Fewell, and Jones (1980) have surveyed alcoholic social workers who acknowledged membership in Alcoholics Anonymous.

Since graduate business administration students either occupy or are preparing for middle management and top management positions in the corporate sector, it would seem important to know something about their drinking patterns and their attitude toward alcohol education. In a 1979 survey the Opinion Research Corporation discovered that 18% of management executives expressed concern about their use of alcohol (Kiechel, 1982). Charles Shirley (1982) studied 25 executives who were members of Alcoholics Anonymous and found that on the average they had waited 7 years to seek help. Despite the advancing stages of their alcoholism, they were steadily promoted, in part due to their geniality and their being enjoyable drinking companions. Nevertheless, the loss of functioning by alcoholic executives is a real problem (*Canadian Business,* 1981). Problems with alcohol misusers are not confined to male executives. A Rand Corporation study in 1977 showed that a married working woman between the ages of 21 and 34 is twice as likely to have a drinking problem as is her counterpart who does not work. That more working women who abuse alcohol remain unidentified is thought by some to relate to the scarcity of female supervisors in the work force, since supervisors appear to be reluctant to confront employees of the opposite sex (Daniloff, 1981). There is evidence that the corporate sector is beginning to recognize alcohol abuse as a problem. Today there are at least 4,600 Occupational Alcoholism Programs (OAPs) operative in industry and business. Of these, 4,300 have been developed since 1971 (Rich, 1980) in companies such as Eastman Kodak, Minnesota Mining Manufacturing, ITT, General Motors, J. C. Penney, Morgan Guaranty, and Equitable Life. In addition, Employee Assistance Programs (EAPs) have also proliferated (Hellan, 1980). EAPs counsel employees at every job position level about any type of personal problem. However, problems related to alcohol abuse account for most of their referrrals.

Given that alcohol misuse has consequences for effective decision making, time lost due to illness, and accidents, it would seem that knowledge about the drinking patterns and attitudes toward alcohol education among those being educated in business administration is important. It is the purpose of this study to explore these isssues.

METHOD

In the fall of 1981 a questionnaire survey was carried out on students enrolled in the school of business administration of an independent university on its New York City campus. The students were employed full time in the business sector and attended school at night. All were graduate students who were working toward their master's degree over the 3-year period. Most held administrative positions and wanted to upgrade their skills.

The survey was conducted in several courses required of graduate business school majors. The survey questionnaire, comprised of 15 multiple choice items, was designed for easy, rapid completion (see the Appendix). The questionnaire asked for demographic information and emphasized items on the nature of alcohol use such as type of beverage used, frequency, quantity, and circumstances of drinking. There also was a query about previous and/or desired education about corporate drinking.

On a pretest, 10 randomly selected students, not used in the final sample, read and completed the questionnaire, criticizing it for clarity. Throughout, confidentiality was assured in that no names were requested. Students were asked to specify their sex. In gaining their cooperation it was explained that participation in the survey was voluntary. They could leave blank any questions that they did not choose to answer. One hundred forty-seven students handed in completed questionnaires, for a response rate of 78%. It is possible that students who did not participate introduced some bias. However, the 78% response rate is acceptable and may indicate the high topical interest of the survey. Since the students were in required courses, they were a representative sample of the school's student body, which later data analysis did confirm. Although there is no direct objective validation of the questionnaire instrument, there is inferential evidence which suggests that the self-reports of these students provided valid data. One is the full response to all the items on the questionnaire. Another is that the questionnaire deals with a legal substance, alcohol.

As a part of the data analysis, a measure of the level of drinking needed to be developed that would permit categorizing the alcohol user as a light, modeate, or heavy drinker. Vogel-Sprott (1974) points out that a Pearson product-moment correlation between an individual's dose and frequency scores yields a value of −.005, indicating a need for both measures in defining drinking practices. Thus, if heavy drinking was defined only on the basis of quantity, persons so classifed could be entirely different from those considered to be heavy drinkers solely on the basis of a frequency criterion. Therefore, from the data on frequency of alcohol use and the quantity drunk at one sitting, a measure of drinking level was developed.

In this study, light drinking was defined as using alcohol on special occasions or holidays only, and up to four times weekly at a rate of one or two drinks. Moderate drinking was alcohol use from once weekly to daily at the rate of three drinks. Heavy drinking was alcohol use from once weekly to daily at the rate of four or more drinks.

FINDINGS

Sample Characteristics

As shown in Table 1, it was found that of the 147 respondents, 145 used beverage alcohol. Thus, 2 (1.4%) were abstainers. Of the users, 65 (44.8%) were males and 80 (55.1%) were females. Among all users, on ethnicity, 137 (94.4%) were Caucasian, 2 (1.3%) were Hispanic, 4 (2.7%) were Black, and 2 (1.3%) were Asian. Regarding religion, 78 (53.8%) identified themselves as Catholic, 29 (20%) as Jewish, 20 (13.7%) as Protestant, and 18 (12.4%) as having no religion. In terms of age, the range was from 21 years to 49 years. Within this range, those aged 20 through 31 were then categorized as younger students and those aged 32 through 49 as maturer students. One hundred thirteen (77.9%) were in the younger category, while 32 (22.0%) were maturer.

Within the school, graduate students concentrate in finance, marketing, or a combination of management with accounting or finance. In this sample there was no datum for 1 (.7%) student, while 65 (45.5%) were majoring in finance, 51 (35.1%) were in marketing, and 27 (18.6%) were in management/accounting

Table 1

Personal Characteristics of Alcohol Users (N = 145)

	Males		Females		Total	
	N	%	*N*	%	*N*	%
Age range						
Younger (20-31)	40	45.4	48	54.5	88	100
Maturer (32-49)	25	43.8	32	56.1	57	100
Older (50+)	–	–	–	–	–	–
Ethnicity/race						
Hispanic	2	100.0	–	–	2	100
Black	2	50.0	2	50.0	4	100
White	61	44.5	76	55.4	137	100
Asian	1	50.0	1	50.0	2	100
Religion						
Protestant	9	45.0	11	55.0	20	100
Jewish	14	48.2	15	51.7	29	100
Catholic	33	42.3	45	57.7	78	100
None	9	50.0	9	50.0	18	100
Business school major						
Finance	30	61.0	36	38.0	66	100
Marketing	22	43.1	29	56.9	51	100
Marketing/accounting/financing	13	48.1	14	51.9	27	100
No data	–	–	1	100.0	1	100

or finance. On all of the preceding characteristics the respondents were representative of the entire population of this urban school of graduate business administration.

Alcohol Use

Frequency, Location, and Circumstances of Drinking

Only two (1.3%) students were nonusers. Among the 145 (98.7%) users, there were some differences in the frequency with which they drank, as shown in Table 2. For the 80 women, 20 (25%) reported drinking once or twice weekly, while 12 (15%) drank less than weekly. However, of the 65 men, 15 (23.0%) drank as infrequently as once or twice weekly, with 7 (10.8%) drinking less than weekly. Most of the women (40; 50%) and men (33; 50.7%) drank three or four times weekly. Few, only 10 (15.8%) of the men and 8 (10.0%) of the women, drank daily. It appears, then, there are very slight differences between the males and females who drink, with slightly fewer women drinking daily. Both the males and females appear to drink at very similar levels of increased frequency.

More women (54; 67.5%) than men (30; 46.2%) drank in restaurants. Slightly more men (18; 27.6%) than women (16; 20%) drank at home. Close to one-quarter of the males but only an eighth of the females used bars at their main drinking location.

Table 2

Frequency, Location, and Circumstances of Drinking, by Sex (N = 145)

	Males (*N* = 65)		Females (*N* =80)	
	N	%	*N*	%
Frequency				
Less than weekly	7	10.8	12	15.0
Once or twice weekly	15	23.0	20	25.0
Three of four times weekly	33	50.7	40	50.0
Daily	10	15.3	8	10.0
Circumstances				
With friends	35	53.8	44	55.0
With relatives	8	12.3	20	25.0
Alone	22	33.8	16	20.0
Location				
Bars	17	26.2	10	12.5
Restaurants	30	46.2	54	67.5
At home	18	27.6	16	20.0

Asked with whom they drank and whether they drank alone, a majority, about 55% of both the males and females, reported that they drank with friends. However, twice as many women than men drank with relatives. About one-third of the men and one-fifth of the women reported drinking alone. None of these differences was statistically significant.

Level of Alcohol Consumption

Earlier a typology for classifying drinking behavior was presented. It utilizes the dimensions of quantity and frequency to specify students as light, moderate, or heavy drinkers. Table 3 shows this information in relation to demographic characteristics. For men and women it was found that most were heavy drinkers. Very few, under 10%, were moderate drinkers. However, slightly more women (15%; 12) than men (7.7%; 5) were light drinkers, while the opposite was true for heavy drinkers. Over three-quarters (77.5%; 62) of the women drank heavily, while nine-tenths of the men (90.7%; 59) were heavy drinkers. These differences clearly are not significant. This is in contrast to earlier studies of adult drinking patterns (Cahalan, Cisin, and Crossley, 1969), which found men to be significantly heavier drinkers than women.

Table 3

Age, Sex, Ethnicity, Religion, and Level of Beverage Alcohol Use

	Level of use (N = 145)					
	Light (N = 17)		Moderate (N = 7)		Heavy (N = 121)	
	N	%	N	%	N	%
Age						
Younger	14	12.1	4	3.5	98	84.4
Maturer	3	10.3	3	10.3	23	79.3
Sex						
Male	5	7.7	1	1.5	59	90.7
Female	12	15.0	6	7.5	62	77.5
Ethnicity/race						
Hispanic	–	–	–	–	2	100.0
Black	2	50.0	–	–	2	50.0
White	15	10.9	7	5.1	115	83.9
Asian	–	–	–	–	2	100.0
Religion						
Protestant	2	10.0	3	15.0	15	75.0
Jewish	11	33.3	4	12.1	18	54.5
Catholic	2	2.7	–	–	74	97.3
None	2	12.5	–	–	14	87.5

By age, 84.4% (98) of the younger students were heavy drinkers, while 79.3% (23) of the maturer students drank heavily. Few of either the younger students (3.5%; 4) or the maturer students (10.3%; 3) drank moderately. Nearly equal proportions, about 10% of younger and maturer students, were light drinkers. On the whole, then, age was not a significant factor in this sample with regard to level of drinking.

On ethnicity/race, among the 4 Blacks, half used alcohol lightly and half used heavily. For the Whites, 10.9% (15) were light users, 5.1% (7) were moderate users, and 83.9% (115) were heavy users. Both Hispanics drank heavily.

The religious affiliation of the sample and levels of drinking showed the following. Nearly equal percentages, about 12%, of the Protestants and the nonreligious were found to be light drinkers. More of the Jews, one-third; but very few Catholics, 2.7%, were light drinkers. The largest concentration of heavy drinkers (97.3%; 74) was found among the Catholics, followed by those who professed having no religion. However, none of these differences on religion and drinking reached statistical significance.

Beverage Preferences

As shown in Table 4, among the women there was a preference for a particular beverage. Over half (47; 58.7%) preferred wine, with exactly a quarter reporting using several types of alcohol. Very few women preferred liquor (10; 12.5%) or beer (3; 3.7%). In contrast, the men had no one beverage of choice. Nearly equal numbers preferred beer (25; 38.5%) or all forms of alcoholic beverages (20; 30.8%). This is in contrast to findings on New England college men, for whom beer was clearly the beverage of choice (Wechsler and McFadden, 1979). Ethnicity/race was confounded by sex in this sample. Thus, Whites had a slight preference either for wine (39.4%) or for all forms of beverage alcohol (28.5%).

The younger students (48; 42.5%) chose wine. However, the maturer students showed a slight preference for all forms of liquor at the rate of 31.2% (10). Religion did not affect beverage choice. Among Catholics, only small numbers preferred beer (15; 19.7%) or liquor (8; 10.5%), with more using all forms (25; 32.9%) and the largest number (28; 36.8%) selecting wine. Among the Jews and those who reported no religion, there was no significant difference on choice of beverage. Eighteen (54.5%) of the Jews and 7 (43.7%) of the nonreligious used wine. Similarly, about a third of the Catholics and the nonreligious used a combination of beverage alcohol. Among the Protestants, 7 (35%) chose beer, followed by wine and all forms of alcohol (4, or 20% for each). On the whole, then, there appears to be no one beverage of choice for these graduate students, although there is a tendency for women and for Jewish students to prefer wine.

Table 4

Type of Alcohol Preferred, by Personal Characteristics (N = 145)

	Beer		Wine		Distilled spirits		All forms	
Characteristic	*N*	%	*N*	%	*N*	%	*N*	%
Sex								
Male	25	38.5	8	12.3	12	18.4	20	30.8
Female	3	3.7	47	58.7	10	12.5	20	25.0
Age								
Maturer	9	28.1	7	21.9	6	18.7	10	31.2
Younger	18	15.9	48	42.5	16	14.1	31	27.4
Ethnicity								
Hispanic	2	100.0	–	–	–	–	–	–
Black	1	25.0	1	25.0	1	25.0	1	25.0
White	23	16.8	54	39.4	21	15.3	39	28.5
Asian	–	–	–	–	–	–	2	100.0
Religion								
Protestant	7	35.0	4	20.0	5	25.0	4	20.0
Jewish	3	9.1	18	54.5	5	15.1	7	21.2
Catholic	15	19.7	28	36.8	8	10.5	25	32.9
None	2	12.5	7	43.7	2	12.5	5	31.2

Alcoholism Education

Students were asked whether they had had any courses in alcoholism. Further, they were asked whether they would like a course in corporate alcoholism. These result are show in Table 5.

Among the total sample of 147, 11 did not respond to these questions. For the remaining 136, it was found that 24 (17.6%) students had had previous alcoholism course work. Of these, 14 (10.3%) wanted further course work on

Table 5

Experience or Courses in Alcoholism, by Wants Alcohol Course in Corporate Life (N = 136)

	Wants course			
	Yes		No	
Course work	*N*	%	*N*	%
Had	14	10.3	10	7.3
Never had	18	16.0	94	69.1

alcoholics. Among the 112 students with no education in the field of alcoholism, only 18 (16%) expressed a wish for it. Thus, even though nearly all of these students used beverage alcohol and even though the consequences of its misuse pose a large problem for business and the corporate world, these students did not view it as a subject of interest.

DISCUSSION

This study of graduate-level business administration students was undertaken to address the dearth of research on the drinking patterns of those who are preparing for and practicing in the professions. This survey, using brief, self-administered questionnaires, attained a response rate of 78%. Because its sample was drawn from an independent, urban university in the Northeast, its findings may be generalizable only to similar populations.

With these cautions in mind, several conclusions can be drawn. An overwhelming majority of the respondents (98.6%) used beverage alcohol. This is an even greater percentage of users than that reported by Wechsler and McFadden (1979) in their study of drinking among nearby New England college students. In this study both males and females (median age 27) drank at similar levels of frequency, usually three or four times weekly. Considering that business luncheons accompanied by martinis are thought to be a part of corporate life (Nulty, 1976), it was surprising to find that fewer men than women reported drinking in restaurants. It might be that these men were beginning to consider their health and their weight within the context of their careers, while these women were taking on the behaviors that have been seen to characterize the male corporate executive conditioned to alcohol with the business lunch (*Economist,* 1980). In this study a large majority of both the women and men were found to be heavy drinkers, even though slightly fewer women drank heavily while slightly more women drank lightly. These decreasing differences in drinking patterns between males and females can be attributed in this study to the fact that women were drinking oftener rather than that they were drinking more at each sitting.

Further research needs to be undertaken on the drinking habits of female executives in order to discover whether their rates of alcohol abuse are approaching those of their male counterparts. At the same time, more research needs to be undertaken on the drinking patterns and abuse of alcohol within the corporate sector. The extent to which practicing members of given professions perceive that there are particular expectations with regard to drinking also needs to be researched. It is conceivable that such expectations override cultural factors such as age, race/ethnicity, and sex.

Although it appears that American preferences for beverage alcohol are changing, with an upsurge in the use of wine and vodka (Nulty, 1976), in this study, only women, those over age 32, and Jewish students clearly preferred wine, while men and those under age 31 used beer or all forms of beverage alcohol.

Despite the important role that alcohol use and abuse is now known to play in the corporate world, fewer than 20% of these students had this type of education or wanted it. This would appear to represent an important blind spot in the education of actual and would-be corporate managers and executives. It is these people who not only make critical business decisions, but also hold ultimate responsibility for the work performance of countless employees. Further, if education in alcoholism does in fact affect drinking patterns (Waring, 1978), then schools that offer such training may have the potential for assisting in the prevention and reduction of alcohol abuse.

APPENDIX: DRINKING PATTERN SURVEY

Sex: _ _
M F

1. Use beverage alcohol (beer, wine, liquor)
   a. I do
   b. I do not
2. I usually drink:
   a. Daily
   b. Once or twice weekly
   c. 3 or 4 times weekly
   d. Only on holidays
   e. Only on special occasions
   f. Other (specify)
3. When I drink, I most frequently use:
   a. Beer
   b. Wine
   c. Liquor
   d. A combination
4. I usually drink:
   a. Before noon
   b. With noon meal
   c. In the afternoon (1-5 p.m.)
   d. Before the evening meal
   e. With the evening meal
   f. After the evening meal
5. I usually drink:
   a. With friends
   b. With relatives
   c. Alone
   d. Combination of a,b,c

6. I usually have the following number of drinks at one sitting:
   a. 1
   b. 2
   c. 3
   d. 4
   e. 5
   f. More

7. I usually drink:
   a. At home
   b. In bars
   c. In restaurants

8. Most of my classes are on:
   a. Mondays
   b. Tuesdays
   c. Wednesdays
   d. Thursdays
   e. Fridays
   f. Saturdays

9. I am an MBA candidate:
   a. 1st year
   b. 2nd year
   c. 3rd year

10. My concentration is:
   a. Finance
   b. Marketing
   c. Management
   d. Accounting
   e. Quantitative methods
   f. Other (specify)

11. I consider myself to be:
   a. Black
   b. Hispanic
   c. Caucasian
   d. Asian
   e. Other (specify)

12. With regard to religion, I am:
   a. Catholic
   b. Jewish
   c. Moslem
   d. Protestant
   e. Other (specify)
   f. None

13. My age is:
   a. 20-25
   b. 26-31
   c. 32-37
   d. 38-43
   e. 44-49
   f. 50-55
   g. 56-61
   h. 62 or over

14. Regarding alcoholism education:

I have had some course work	YES	NO
I have had no course work	YES	NO
I would like a course on alcoholism in corporate life	YES	NO

15. I am presently employed in the area of:

a. Finance	d. Management (general)
b. Marketing	e. Accounting
c. Quantitative	f. Other (specify)

We very much appreciate your help in completing our questionnaire. Many thanks.

REFERENCES

ARAFAT, I. Drinking behavior in high school, college and adult groups. *Free Inquiry Creative Soc.* 7(1): 87-91, 96, May 1979.

BISSELL, L., FEWELL, C., and JONES, R. The alcoholic social worker: A survey. *Soc. Work Health Care* 5: 421-432, 1980.

BISSELL, L., and JONES, R. The alcoholic physician: A survey *Am. '. Psychiatry* 133: 1142-1146, 1976.

BISSELL, L., LAMBRECHT, K., and VON WIEGAND, R. The alcoholic hospital employee. *Nurs. Outlook* 21: 708-711, 1973.

CAHALAN, D., CISIN, I.H., and CROSSLEY, H.M. *American Drinking Practices: A National Study of Drinking Behavior and Attitudes* (Rutgers Center of Alcohol Studies, Monogr. No. 6.). New Brunswick, NJ: The Center, 1969.

Canadian Business. How to help your executive on the road–and the wagon. 54: 150-151, March 1981.

DANILOFF, R. Managing alcoholism in the work place. *Working Woman* July 1981, p. 78.

DODGE, D. The variation of Midwest Catholic University's drug use pattern from other Catholic university findings. *Int. J. Addict.* 14(6): 867-875, 1979.

Economist. Ex drinkers' one-martini lunch. 275: 18, April 12, 1980.

GLATT, M.M. Characteristics and prognosis of alcoholic doctors. *Br. Med. J.* 1: 507, February 19, 1977.

HELLAN, R. Employee Assistance Programs. *Manage. World* 9: 18-20, October 1980.

ISLER, C. The alcoholic nurse: What we try to deny. *RN* July 1978, pp. 48-55.

KIECHEL, W. III. Looking out for the executive alcoholic. *Fortune* January 11, 1982, pp. 117-120.

NULTY, P. Changing habits of American drinkers. *Fortune* October 1976, pp. 156-166.

RICH, P. Dealing with alcoholism in U.S. industry. *U.S.A. Today* July 1980, pp. 26-29.

SEGAL, B., HUBA, G., and SINGER, J. Reasons for drug and alcohol use of college students. *Int. J. Addict.* 15(4): 489-498, 1980.

SHIRLEY, C. Topex Study: "Hitting bottom in high places." *Labor Manage. Alcoholism J.* (11)4: 130-135, 1982.

STRAUSS, R., and BACON, S.D. *Drinking in College.* New Haven: Yale University Press, 1953.

VOGEL-SPROTT, M. Defining "light" and heavy drinking–research implications and hypotheses. *Q. J. Stud. Alcohol* 35: 1388-1392, 1974.

WARING, M. The effects of alcohol education on the drinking patterns of undergraduate students in the human services. *Int. J. Addict.* 13(5): 849-854, 1978.

WECHSLER, H., and ROMAN, M. Extensive users of alcohol among college students. *J. Stud. Alcohol* 42: 149-156, 1981.

WECHSLER, H., and MC FADDEN, M. Drinking among college students in New England: Extent, social correlates and consequence of alcohol use. *J. Stud. Alcohol* 40: 969-996, 1979.

The International Journal of the Addictions, 19(6), 665-674, 1984

Can Personality Tests Predict Treatment Dropouts?

Robert J. Craig,* PhD

West Side VA Medical Center

School of Public Health
University of Illinois at Chicago

Chicago, Illinois

Abstract

Patients who completed a detoxification/rehabilitation drug abuse program were compared with program dropouts on a new personality instrument, the Millon Clinical Multiaxial Inventory. No differences were found between groups on any of the 20 comparison variables, replicating previous results with the MMPI. Data are presented showing that discriminant function predictors lose their potency within 3 years and maybe sooner. It is concluded that clinical judgments must form the basis of predicting dropouts until it can be demonstrated that personality tests can make reliable predictions on treatment dropouts.

In a heterogeneous population, the presence of substance abuse problems and a diagnosis associated with sociopathic character traits have been associated with premature termination from a variety of mental health treatment components (Baekeland and Lundwall, 1975). This knowledge is not particularly helpful in substance abuse programs where the population tends to be homogeneous with respect to substance use disorders and where most of the patients tend to have character disorders. Thus, substance abuse programs have to rely on more sensitive predictors.

*Address reprint requests to the author: Chief, Drug Abuse Program (123), West Side VA Medical Center, 820 S. Damen Avenue, Chicago, Illinois 60612.

0020-773X/84/1906-0665$3.50/0

Table 1

Overview of Studies Using Personality Tests to Predict Treatment Dropouts among Drug Abusers

Author (year)	Setting	Subjects	Test	Predictor	Results
Craig (in press)	Inpatient detox/rehab ward	200 opiate addicts	MMPI	*D* ↑ in dropouts	Few MMPI diff. predictors did not hold after 3 years.
De Leon et al. (1973)	TC	208 addicts	MMPI *SC* I-E Scale Beck, Dep. Inv. MAACL Anx., Dep., and Hos. Scales	*SC* ↑; *BDI* ↑; Anx. and Dep. ↑	Dropouts had more psychopathology on all measures.
Foureman et al. (1981)	TC	200 heroin addicts	MMPI	*F, Hs, D, Hy, Pa, Pt, Sc* ↑	Less psychopathology assoc. with Rx retention; MMPI could not predict precise range of retention.
Jarvis et al. (1975)	Air Force residential program	170 drug abusers, mostly heroin	MMPI	*F* ↑; *Pd* ↑	Psychopathic traits characterize dropouts.

Keegan and Lachar (1979)	Inpatient polydrug abusers	174	MMPI	*F, Pd, Pa, Sc, Ma* ↑	Greater psychopathology assoc. with dropouts.
Lin (1975)	Hosp. ward	190 addicts and alcoholics	MMPI	*F* and *Pd* ↑ (trend only)	Dropouts tend to be higher in psychopathology and sociopathic traits.
McFarlain et al. (1977)	Multimodal program	52 heroin addicts	MAACL Anx., Dep., and Hos. Scales	Multiple	Trend toward more psychopathology in dropouts.
Pittel (1972)	MMT	66 addicts	MMPI	*Pa, Pt, Sc* ↑	Relative absence of psychopathology in more successful patients.
Ward and Hemsley (1981)	Inpatient unit	38 polydrug abusers	EPI	*P* ↑; *E* ↑	High "psychoticism" and extroversion related to Rx completion.
Zuckerman et al. (1975)	3 TCs	59 M, soft drugs 59 M, hard drugs 28 F, polydrugs	MMPI	*F, Pa, Pt* ↑	Quitters show more psychopathology at time of admission.

In attempting to search for predictors of treatment attrition in drug abuse programs, investigators have studied demographic variables and biographic correlates of dropping out of treatment. A review of some of the prototypal studies has revealed that: (1) Results of the various predictors failed to generalize from one study to the next; (2) results from any particular study are often not cross-validated with independent samples within the same treatment program; and (3) predictors of stay/leave tend to be different, depending on the type of program studied (detoxification, drug-free, methadone maintenance, or therapeutic community) (Craig, in press).

In has been argued elsewhere that the measurement of the drug-abusing personality should be systematically related to other variables of interest (Craig et al., 1982). Treatment dropout is one such variable that has program management and clinical consequences. If we could determine reliable predictors of program completion, then we could allocate resources and efforts to those patients who would be most likely to benefit from treatment. Predicting treatment completion is clinically important because studies show that patients who complete a detox program are three times as likely to be drug-free 1 year later as people who drop out (Baekeland and Lundwall, 1975).

Several studies have used personality tests to "predict" treatment dropouts, and these are summarized in Table 1. From these 10 studies, the following conclusions are made:

1. Most studies report a significant trend toward significance for dropouts to score at higher levels of psychopathology on most of the psychological tests, with the *F* Scale of the MMPI often showing higher elevations in the dropouts.
2. Nine of the 10 studies did not report a cross-validation sample. The one study that replicated the discriminant function with independent samples at 3-year intervals, using MMPI predictor variables, found a reduction of about 50% in predictive accuracy after 3 years. The discriminant function that provided 75% accuracy in prediction in the cross-validation also resulted in a 50% reduction in predictive accuracy when applied to the original sample of 3 years earlier. These results imply that valid predictors at one moment in time either may not generalize to independent samples or may not be valid in later years (Craig, in press).

In reviewing the dropout process clinically, it appears that personality traits and characteristics—especially impulsivity, low frustration tolerance, lack of planning ahead, disengagement from secondary process thinking, and generalized ego controls—would seem to mediate between environmental/interactional precipitants and the decision to drop out of treatment. Thus, basic personality style might be able to predict treatment dropouts over and above more global conclusions, such as "psychopathology."

The Millon Clinical Multiaxial Inventory (MCMI) (Millon, 1977) is a 175-item self-report inventory that results in the determination of eight basic personality styles, three pathological personality syndromes, and nine transient clinical states. It was believed that MCMI scale scores, tapping personality styles and clinical states, might likely differentiate patients who drop out of treatment from those who remain in treatment. Information with regard to instrument reliability and validity is extensively presented in the test manual (Millon, 1977).

METHOD

Subjects

Subjects consisted of 100 opiate addicts (heroin, methadone, Talwin), who were treated in an inpatient detox and rehabilitation treatment unit in 1982. All *S*s were male, average age was 33, 31% were married, 15% worked full time, average education level was 11 years, 33% were first admissions, 90% had criminal histories, and they averaged 8 years of chemical abuse. Ethnicity was 90% Black, 7% White, and 3% Latino. All *S*s were of lower SES.

Expected length of stay (LOS) was 2 weeks for employed patients and 3 weeks for unemployed patients, with maximum LOS of 30 days. Average LOS was 17.5 days. Patients who do not complete the expected LOS for their respective category (employed-unemployed) in this program are given a discharge against medical advice (AMA).

The program admits about 350 drug-dependent veterans yearly. Patients are detoxed concurrent to rehab. The rehabilitation phase consists of group therapy three times a week; individual counseling two times per week; daily health educational groups with modules in physical health, vocational development, and psychology of the drug abuser; milieu therapy; and attendance in Narcotics Anonymous.

Procedure

All *S*s were individually administered the MCMI on a random basis as part of a larger research project. All protocols were computer scored, and only valid profiles were used in subsequent analyses.

RESULTS: BASE RATE SCORES

The MCMI uses the concept of "base rate scores," which are transformed scores "determined by known personality and syndrome prevalence data and by using cutting lines designed to maximize current diagnostic classification" (Millon, 1977). A base rate (BR) score of 60 represents the raw score mean of all patients who participated in the test construction studies. According to Millon, the greater the BR score on the MCMI, the greater the probability that the patient has the characteristics measured by the scale.

From the 100 MCMI addict profiles, 71 patients completed the program and 29 were given AMA discharges. Analysis indicated no significant differences between dropouts and completers on any demographic variable reported in the preceding section. A univariate ANOVA was conducted, controlling for the effects of age and using the BR scale scores of the 20 MCMI scales, for both the completers and dropouts. The results of this analysis appear in Table 2.

The analysis revealed no significant difference on any MCMI scale between the two groups. This replicates an earlier work in this area with equivalent samples demonstrating no statistical differences between completers and dropouts on the MMPI (Craig, in press).

In order to conduct a more refined prediction, a stepwise discriminant function analysis (DFA) was conducted to differentiate between groups. This resulted in an eight-variable function (age, dependent, histrionic, passive-aggressive,

Table 2

MCMI Scale Scores for Program Completers and Dropouts

Scale	Completers	Dropouts	*F*	Sign
Schizoid	50.21	54.86	< 1.00	NS
Avoidant	51.94	53.83	< 1.00	NS
Dependent	53.76	61.38	1.72	NS
Histrionic	67.11	60.62	2.48	NS
Narcissistic	71.25	65.83	1.56	NS
Antisocial	69.80	63.21	2.23	NS
Compulsive	46.32	47.93	< 1.00	NS
Passive-aggressive	64.32	64.08	< 1.00	NS
Schizotypal	48.13	50.90	< 1.00	NS
Borderline	61.24	59.00	< 1.00	NS
Paranoia	67.86	63.65	1.40	NS
Anxiety	73.92	69.38	< 1.00	NS
Somatoform	59.31	60.45	< 1.00	NS
Hypomania	58.86	52.96	< 1.00	NS
Dysthymia	65.22	67.03	< 1.00	NS
Alcohol	87.98	82.27	2.88	NS
Drug abuse	86.86	81.03	2.58	NS
Psychotic thinking	56.98	56.83	< 1.00	NS
Psychotic depression	53.77	54.38	< 1.00	NS
Psychotic delusion	59.76	57.72	< 1.00	NS

borderline, anxiety, somatoform, and dysthymia), which produced an overall 76% classification accuracy. This is quite similar to the level of prediction using DFA in similar reports. Unfortunately, many researchers may not have presented all of the relevant data that can be obtained from DFA. Table 3 presents DFA results from a previous MMPI study and the DFA results on the MCMI in the present study.

Note that the MMPI does a better job in predicting people who stay than it does in predicting people who will leave. MMPI predictions for those that will leave are essentially no better than chance and in one case grossly misclassified the leave group in a cross-validation sample 3 years later. In the present study, the MCMI did a reasonable job in predicting both stay and leave groups, but the sample size was too small for purposes of cross-validation.

Table 3

Predicting Program Status with MMPI and MCMI Using Discriminant Function Analysis

Study 1 MMPI

Predictive accuracy 87% (N = 100)

	Predicted		
	1978	Stay	Leave
Actual	Stay	94%	6%
	Leave	40%	60%

→

Predictive accuracy 44% (N = 100)

	Predicted		
	1981	Stay	Leave
Actual	Stay	93%	7%
	Leave	87%	13%

Study 2 MMPI

Predictive accuracy 75% (N = 100)

	Predicted		
	1981	Stay	Leave
Actual	Stay	87%	13%
	Leave	57%	43%

→

Predictive accuracy 38% (N = 100)

	Predicted		
	1978	Stay	Leave
Actual	Stay	66%	34%
	Leave	50%	50%

Study 3 MCMI

Predictive accuracy 88% (N = 100)

	Predicted		
	1982	Stay	Leave
Actual	Stay	90%	10%
	Leave	13%	87%

DISCUSSION

Personality tests have shown an initial promise of providing predictors of relevant treatment outcome indices, such as completing or dropping out of a program. However, many of these predictors are not useful for individual decision making. Furthermore, although several previous research studies have found elevations on the MMPI *F* Scale to be associated with subsequent premature termination from drug abuse treatment programs (particularly from therapeutic communities), our own research had previously found that neither the *F* Scale nor 28 other MMPI variables differentiated a group of dropouts from a group of program completers (Craig, in press). The results of the current study, using the MCMI, are identical. None of the 20 MCMI scales differentiated dropouts from completers.

Using a more sophisticated statistic, such as discriminant function analysis, dramatically improves the predictive accuracy of personality tests, but these conclusions may be "false positives." DFA is designed to come up with accurate predictions. The key question is whether any of these individual equations cross-validate to independent samples–and, if so, over what period of time do they remain accurate predictors? We have presented evidence that 3 years later, the predictive accuracy of personality tests, based on a discriminant function, is reduced by about 50%.

We are inclined to believe that personality tests may not be useful in predicting dropouts from drug abuse programs because a decision to drop out may be more environmental or interactional than one that is based on a personality predisposition. Our previous work in this area found that simply knowing how often the primary therapist was present or absent, or knowing how often any of the clinical staff were present or absent, accurately predicted dropouts about 75% of the time (Craig, Rogalski, and Veltri, 1982). This result was cross-validated and substantiated, implying an interactional dynamic with treatment dropout. Other research found that environmental factors tended to influence Black addicts to remain in treatment, while for White addicts, intrapsychic factors had greater influence in staying or leaving. This might suggest that personality tests may be more useful in predicting dropout for White addicts, whereas environmental factors may be more predictive of Black addicts dropping out of treatment.

IMPLICATIONS

Personality tests have not proven reliably useful in identifying predictors of treatment dropouts in drug abuse treatment programs. Our own studies have found no differences between program completers and program dropouts using MMPI and the MCMI. We did find differences between groups when we studied environmental and interactional variables. Therefore, at this point, it would seem that clinicians should look for more environmental/interactional predictors and make their decisions accordingly.

Prospective studies are needed in this area. So far, all studies are retrospective. They have applied their statistics after the fact. An important test of any prediction is whether it can tell clinicians in advance who is at risk for premature dropout. No study has done this to date.

The dropout needs more definition in the research literature. Patients who come into a program with no intention of completing it are probably examples of poor screening and selection criteria. They also are in a different psychological plane than the person who gets a phone call from home and then says he has to "take care of business." Yet both are listed as a "dropout." This implies that, until empirical research provides us with useful answers, programs will need to adjust selection criteria based on clinical judgments. Programs may wish to provide some alternative programming for patients viewed as high risks for dropout. This might include such ideas as placing high-risk patients in an outpatient setting for a period of time to test motivation for treatment and establishing an admissions process over several successive days—again as tests for motivation; or programs may attempt a role induction technique to teach clients to be "good patients" (Zweben and Lis, 1981).

ACKNOWLEDGMENTS

Appreciation is extended to George Meschel, PhD, and Armie Johnson for assistance with computer processing of the MCMI protocols, and to Barbara Kendra for secretarial services.

REFERENCES

BAEKELAND, F., and LUNDWALL, L. Dropping out of treatment: A critical review. *Psychol. Bull.* 82: 738-783, 1975.

CRAIG, R. Personality dimensions related to premature termination from an inpatient drug abuse treatment program. *J. Clin. Psychol.*. in press.

CRAIG, R., ROGALSKI, C., and VELTRI, D. Predicting treatment dropouts from a drug abuse rehabilitation program. *Int. J. Addict.* 17: 641-653, 1982.

DE LEON, G., SKODOL, A., and ROSENTHAL, M. Phoenix House: Changes in psychopathological signs of resident drug addicts. *Arch. Gen. Psychiatry* 28: 131-135, 1973.

FOUREMAN, W., PARKS, R., and GARDIN, T. The MMPI as a predictor of retention in a therapeutic community for heroin addicts. *Int. J. Addict.* 16: 893-903, 1981.

JARVIS, L., SIMNEGAR, R., and TRAWEEK, A. An MMPI comparison of U.S.A.F. groups identified as drug users. *Psychol. Rep.* 37: 1339-1345, 1975.

KEEGAN, J., and LACHAR, D. The MMPI as a predictor of early termination from polydrug abuse treatment. *J. Pers. Assess.* 43: 379-384, 1979.

LIN, T. Use of demographic variables, WRAT, and MMPI scores to predict addicts' types of discharges from a community-like hospital setting. *J. Clin. Psychol.* 31: 148-151, 1975.

MC FARLAIN, F., COHEN, G., YODER, J., and GUIDRY, L. Psychological tests and demographic variables associated with retention of narcotic addicts in treatment. *Int. J. Addict.* 12: 399-410, 1977.

MILLON, T. *Millon Clinical Multiaxial Inventory.* Minneapolis: National Computer Systems, 1977.

PITTEL, S. Three studies of the MMPI as a predictive instrument in methadone maintenance. In *Proceedings of the Fourth National Conference on Methadone Treatment,* 1972, pp. 443-446.

WARD, E., and HEMSLEY, D. Social and psychological factors associated with length of stay on an inpatient dependence treatment unit. *Int. J. Addict.* 16: 1281-1288, 1981.

ZUCKERMAN, M., SOLA, S., MASTERS, J., and ANGELONE, J. MMPI patterns in drug abusers before and after treatment in therapeutic communities. *J. Consult. Clin. Psychol.* 43: 286-296, 1975.

ZWEBEN, A., and LIS, S. The efficacy of role induction in preventing early dropout from treatment of drug dependency. *Am. J. Drug Alcohol Abuse* 8: 171-183, 1981.

The International Journal of the Addictions, 19(6), 675–688, 1984

Symbolic Interaction Theory: A Perspective on Drug Abuse and Its Treatment*

Robert J. Battjes, DSW

National Institute on Drug Abuse
Rockville, Maryland 20857

Abstract

Symbolic interaction theory is employed to explain the etiology of drug abuse and addiction. Selected interactionist concepts, which are especially pertinent to an understanding of drug abuse, are considered in relation to current drug abuse theory and the literature on the characteristics of drug abusers. The implications of this theoretical perspective for treatment are considered.

Review of existing drug abuse treatment programs and efforts at theory development suggest that symbolic interactionism is a theoretical perspective which can be employed to explain the etiology of drug abuse and addiction. As such, this theory can provide a useful framework to guide treatment and treatment research. Symbolic interaction theory and selected interactionist concepts, which are especially pertinent to the etiology of drug abuse, are detailed in this paper. Then the fit between symbolic interactionism and current drug abuse theory is discussed. The importance of the interactionist perspective in understanding the etiology of drug abuse is demonstrated through a review of the literature on characteristics of drug abusers. Finally, implications for treatment are considered.

*The interpretations and conclusions presented in this review do not necessarily represent the position of NIDA or the Department of Health and Human Services.

0020-773X/84/1906-0675$3.50/0

SYMBOLIC INTERACTIONISM

Symbolic interaction theory provides a framework for understanding individual behavior of drug abusers in terms of social interaction. According to this perspective, it is symbols–language, gestures, and expressions–which make human interaction possible. The use of common symbols enables people to develop a common orientation and thus understand and reinforce each other (Shibutani, 1961).

Through social interaction, symbols develop common meaning. Blumer (1969) noted that the "meaning of a thing for a person grows out of the ways in which other persons act toward the person with regard to the thing. Their actions operate to define the thing for the person" (p. 4). Meltzer (1978) stated: "By learning the symbols of his group, [a person] comes to internalize their definitions of events or things, including their definition of his own conduct" (p. 18). Symbols are not static, but they are continuously confirmed or revised in interaction.

The major focus of symbolic interaction theory is the process by which the individual's behavior is shaped through social interaction. In social interaction individuals are able to take the perspective of others in assessing their own behavior. Assuming the perspective of others enables individuals to assess the outcomes of alternate behaviors and to select an appropriate course of action. The responses of others serve to guide behavior. Initially, children are able to consider the perspectives of a few people, but as they mature they are able to integrate multiple perspectives and expectations. As multiple perspectives become integrated, they no longer are associated with specific individuals, and they become generalized. These generalized perspectives, which George Herbert Mead (see Blumer, 1969) referred to as the "generalized other," are internalized as the individual's self. Thus, an individual develops a concept of him/herself which Mead referred to as the "self," by internalizing the perceptions of others. The "self" includes the individual's attitudes, values, and norms. It serves to shape not only the individual's responses to his or her social world, but also the perception of the social world and feelings about it (Blumer, 1969; Jones and Day, 1977; Turner, 1978).

While symbolic interaction theory emphasizes the existence of common symbols and the importance of social interaction in shaping individual behavior, the uniqueness of individuals is also recognized by this theory. Shibutani (1961) emphasized that each individual has a unique background of experiences and a unique combination of significant others, and that there are constitutional differences among people. Blumer (1969) emphasized that each person's "environment" is determined by the meaning that the elements have for the person. Thus, two individuals living in the same space may live in different "environments." In order to understand a person, it is necessary to understand the environment as he or she perceives it.

Socialization

The concept of socialization has been developed to explain more fully the process by which the perspectives of others are internalized by the individual. Brim (1966) defined socialization as the process by which individuals acquire the culture of their group—the habits, beliefs, attitudes, and motives which are necessary to perform the roles expected by society. Clausen (1968) defined socialization as social learning in which mutual expectations are built up, become normative between the participants, and become internalized standards of the individual. It is a continuing process which results in the transmission of shared norms and standards. Goode (1966) emphasized that "the significance of socialization is thus not only that the individual acquires a commitment to the norms of society ... but that he accepts the rightness of applying a particular norm or norms to a specific situation" (p. 313).

Brim (1966) further explained the socialization process:

> The basic premise is that most of what is learned from socialization in childhood, and indeed throughout life, is a series of complex interpersonal relationships. . . . The result is the emergence of a series of "self-other" systems, in which the child is oriented toward the role prescriptions and evaluations of significant others in his environment. (p. 8)

Individuals learn what behavior is appropriate through interaction in social groups which shape behavior by rewarding that which is considered appropriate and punishing that which is considered inappropriate. Reward and punishment primarily take the form of granting or withholding esteem. An individual's satisfaction and sense of well-being are dependent on the esteem of others, and thus they are powerful motivators. Individuals learn to anticipate the responses of others to their behavior, and eventually they incorporate the assessments of others as the basis for their own self-assessment.

In any social situation individuals are influenced by the expectations of those present, the expectations of other significant people who are not present, and the internalized expectations of the generalized other which have been incorporated into the self-concept. Since internalized expectations, which Brim (1966) referred to as the "true self," are more significant to the individual than the expectations of persons in current interaction, the individual will tend to ignore current expectations which conflict with the "true self." Thus, the primacy of the internalized expectations provides a degree of stability and predictability to individual behavior.

Socialization is not a one-time process which occurs in childhood, but a continuing process which occurs throughout life. Early socialization is especially important in that the attitudes, values, and norms formed at that time are relatively stable and influence subsequent perceptions. However, these attitudes, values, and norms are subject to modification through subsequent experiences. While adult socialization does not generally alter the individual's basic identity, significant shifts in identity are not uncommon (Brim, 1966, 1968; Goode, 1966; Inkeles, 1968).

Reference Group

In explaining behavior, the concept of reference group is closely related to Mead's concept of the "generalized other" (Kuhn, 1978). Shibutani (1978) has provided a broad definition of the reference group and a statement of its impact on the individual. A reference group is:

> that group whose perspective constitutes the frame of reference of the actor. . . . Through direct or vicarious participation in a group one comes to perceive the world from its standpoint. Yet this group need not be one in which he aspires for acceptance. . . . a reference group becomes any collectivity, real or imagined, envied or despised, whose perspective is assumed by the actor. (p. 109)

The reference group influences not only the individual's perceptions, but also his or her thinking, judgments, and behavior. Because individuals seek to maintain self-esteem and seek confirmation of their worth from the reference group, the opinions of the reference group can supersede societal customs and laws in influencing individual behavior (Shibutani, 1961, 1978).

While the family is generally the primary reference group during childhood, the peer group emerges as an important reference group for the individual during adolescence. Faced with the transition from childhood to adulthood, with related anxieties and insecurities, adolescents turn to their peers for support and understanding. The peer group provides a system in which they can feel accepted and competent, and conformity to the group is highly prized. Thus, the adolescent peer group is especially powerful in influencing the behavior of its members (Ausubel, 1954; Clausen, 1968; Lippitt, 1968; Sherif and Sherif, 1964).

The influence of the peer group occurs within the context of prior socialization. In other words, the peer group's influence tends to be limited by the standards which the individual has previously internalized. Thus, the peer group is influential primarily with regard to behaviors which have not been addressed in prior socialization and with individuals whose prior socialization has been generally inadequate. The strength of the peer group's influence on the individual is also determined by a number of contemporaneous factors including the intensity of peer group involvement versus other involvements (Clausen, 1968), the degree of disruption of other ties such as family and school (Sherif and

Sherif, 1964), and the extent to which parents are uncertain about appropriate norms (Douvan and Adelson, 1966). Studies of college students have shown that homogeneous peer groups (Newcomb, 1966) and peer groups which are similar demographically to the individual (Pace and Baird, 1966) have more influence than heterogeneous and dissimilar peer groups.

Deviance

Several conceptions of deviance, which overlap somewhat with each other, stem from the interactionist theoretical perspective. One conception considers deviance as a failure of socialization. According to this perspective, inconsistent modeling by parents, inconsistency in the application of sanctions to disapproved behavior, and the diffusion of responsibility for socialization among various social institutions result in the individual's failure to incorporate social norms (Inkeles, 1968).

A second conception stems from Park's (1928) concept of "marginal man," an individual who attempts to adapt to two diverse cultural groups, resulting in inner turmoil and intense self-consciousness. Shibutani (1961) has emphasized that some individuals:

> find themselves in marginal status, a position that incorporates within it the contradictions of the structure of the community. . . . marginal men find it difficult to maintain an adequate level of self-esteem. In moves to maintain their acceptability, some of them search for special tasks which enable them to exploit their anomalous situations, some withdraw into a special group of marginal people, and some even withdraw into psychosis or destroy themselves. (p. 593)

A third conception is referred to as "labeling." According to this conception, an individual who commits a deviant act is labeled a deviant. His or her past behavior is reinterpreted by others in light of this deviant act. There are two possible effects of labeling. In labeling individuals, others convey an expectation of deviant behavior and push them into further deviant acts. Labeled individuals may also be shunned by conventional groups because of the deviant label and thus be deprived of socialization opportunities (Becker, 1963; Jones and Day, 1977).

The final conception focuses on deviance as a subcultural phenomenon. According to this conception, the individual is socialized into a deviant life-style by participation in or identification with a deviant social group. The primary proponent of this perspective was Edwin Sutherland. According to Sutherland's theory of differential association, criminal behavior is learned though a process of interaction with criminals in intimate, interpersonal groups. A person learns attitudes, motives, and rationalizations as well as techniques through this process.

Within American society there are mixed attitudes toward legal codes. People become delinquent when they have been exposed to an excess of attitudes which favor violation of the law over attitudes unfavorable to such violation (Sutherland and Cressey, 1970).

Similarly, Cloward and Ohlin (1966) emphasized that a new member of a delinquent subculture adopts the subculture's perceptions of the world. Appropriate values and beliefs are learned and serve to validate and rationalize participation in the prescribed activities of the group.

Becker (1963) noted the multiplicity of social groups, each with its own rules. An individual may violate the rules of one group when abiding by the rules of another. Some groups enforce their rules on other groups, such as the rules of adults that are imposed on youth and the rules of the middle class that are imposed on the lower class. Like Sutherland, and Cloward and Ohlin, Becker has emphasized that the individual learns to participate in a deviant subculture, acquiring deviant motives and interests. While some delinquents may have been socialized initially into a deviant group, most have been socialized into conventional as well as unconventional groups. Thus, they must learn rationalizations to neutralize conventional norms.

Life circumstances may cause a person to be exposed to a deviant group. Becker has stressed the importance of labeling in pushing a person into a deviant group; since the person labeled deviant is an outcast in conventional groups, he or she is likely to turn to a deviant group for acceptance.

A REVIEW OF DRUG ABUSE THEORY

A review of current theoretical perspectives on the etiology of drug abuse demonstrates the extent to which symbolic interaction theory has influenced the drug abuse field.

Becker (1963, 1980) emphasized the importance of social interaction for initiation into the use of marijuana and other drugs. Initiation to use is a learning process. The marijuana smoker must learn how to smoke to produce the real effect, how to recognize the effect and relate it to the drug, and how to consider the effect as pleasurable. Regarding other drugs, Becker pointed out that drugs have many effects, some of which may go unnoticed or not be attributed to the drug. Some effects which may initially be unpleasurable or frightening are redefined as not being so bad after all. An individual becomes a confirmed user only through participation in a subculture with other users so that the necessary redefinitions can occur.

Johnson (1980) also emphasized the importance of subcultures (reference groups) in drug abuse etiology. The peer or youth culture governs behavior patterns and friendship groups. Veiled competition within an unconventional subculture leads to experimentation with new behaviors (such as drug abuse) which may subsequently be defined as normal. Johnson identified four different drug subcultures: alcohol, marijuana, mixed drugs, and heroin.

Lukoff (1980) focused on the role of socialization in the etiology of drug abuse. Various agencies, including the family and the peer group, contribute to the socialization process. Lukoff raised two theoretical issues related to adolescent drug use. The first focuses on the declining legitimacy of parental authority, and the second focuses on the development of the peer culture with alternate values and goals.

Two of the three models of, or pathways to drug use identified by Gorsuch (1980) reflect the influence of symbolic interaction theory. According to the prodrug socialization model, the individual is socialized by family or peers to use drugs or into a set of personality traits (e.g., individualism and experimentation) conducive to drug use. According to the nonsocialized drug user model, the individual has been inadequately socialized regarding drug use issues. Whether or not he or she becomes an abuser depends upon such situational factors as peer pressure and availability.

Jessor and Jessor's (1980) problem behavior theory addresses the etiology of drug abuse and other deviant behaviors. Behavior is viewed as the result of the personality system (goals, values, beliefs, attitudes) and the perceived environment (primarily parent and peer influence). The Jessors stress that youth who are more oriented toward their peers than their families are more prone to problem behavior including drug abuse.

Kandel (1976, 1980) noted that peer behavior is the most important predictor of adolescent marijuana use. It does predict other drug use as well, but it is not as powerful a predictor. In predicting whether an adolescent will progress from marijuana to the use of other drugs, the quality of the relationship with the parents and level of personal and school performance become significant predictors.

Steffenhagen's (1980) self-esteem theory, derived from Adlerian psychology, stresses that both overprotective and neglected life-styles hinder early socialization and the development of self-esteem. Deviance is learned and its form is determined by the nature and frequency of deviant associations. Peer pressure is especially powerful in shaping behavior in adolescence because of the adolescent's strong need for acceptance.

Other theorists have incorporated aspects of symbolic interaction theory within broader theoretical perspectives. Smart (1980) emphasized the quest for group belonging as a motivating factor in heroin addiction. Huba et al. (1980) emphasized the importance of interpersonal forces, such as family, friends, cultural models, and behavioral reinforcers. Ausubel (1980) emphasized the importance of attitudinal tolerance within the individual's subcultural, racial, ethnic, and social-class milieu.

CHARACTERISTICS OF DRUG ABUSERS

A review of the drug abuse literature concerning characteristics of drug abusers demonstrates the usefulness of the interactionist framework for understanding drug abuse.

Considerable attention is focused on familial factors which affect the family's ability to socialize the individual and serve as a positive reference group. The relationship between drug abuse and broken homes or loss of a parent has frequently been reported regarding heroin addiction (Baer and Corrado, 1974; Braucht et al., 1973; Chambers and Moffett, 1970; Chambers et al., 1968; Chein et al., 1964; Craig and Brown, 1975; Helzer et al., 1976). This relationship has also been reported as a factor in amphetamine abuse (Brooks et al., 1976). Disturbance in the relationship between the parents of addicts was reported by Chein et al. (1964).

The parents of narcotic addicts have been reported as overprotective and overindulgent (Alexander and Dibb, 1975; Braucht et al., 1973; Ellinwood et al., 1966), and also as authoritarian (Ellinwood et al., 1966). For narcotic addicts and drug abusers, the family is portrayed as less cohesive and less close than families of nonabusers; parents are portrayed as providing less love, trust, and support; and parents are viewed with less esteem (Baer and Corrado, 1974; Braucht et al., 1973; Chein et al., 1964; Ellinwood et al., 1966; Jessor, 1976; Kandel, 1976; Lindblad, 1977; Spevack and Pihl, 1976). Braucht et al. (1973) and Lindblad (1977) pointed out that parents of narcotic addicts establish inadequate controls or limits on behavior. Similarly Jessor (1976) and Lukoff (1980) indicated that parents of drug abusers provide fewer behavioral controls than parents of nonusers. Cultural disparity between narcotic addicts and their parents (Vaillant, 1966) is another familial factor which impacts on the family's ability to socialize the individual.

The importance of peers and peer reference groups has also received considerable attention in the literature. Drug users have been found to have more drug-using friends than nonusers (Jessor, 1976; Spevack and Pihl, 1976). Kandel (1976) found that the best predictor of marijuana use is use by one's best friend. She also found that adolescents coordinate their choice of friends and their drug-using behavior. If these are incongruent, the adolescent will either break off the friendship or modify the drug use behavior (Kandel, 1976). Chambers et al. (1968) noted that Black heroin users typically initiate use in the company of a peer who is a user.

The drug subculture in heroin addiction has been found to provide a set of norms and values, and a source of respect and admiration (Stephens and Levine, 1971). Feldman (1973) found that heroin addicts chose drug use within the context of neighborhood life as a means to sustain and enhance their reputations. Richards (1977) noted that, among users of both marijuana and opiates, cults and cliques are likely to form and provide reinforcement for drug use behavior. In his study of lower-class addicts in Chicago, Finestone (1957) found the addicts detached from conventional society and aligned to a reference group which provided success-goals and social admiration which were beyond reach in the conventional society. Blumer (1967), in analyzing drug abusers, differentiated two basic types ("rowdy dudes" and "cool style"). He found that each type had its own peer group supporting it. Glaser et al. (1971) compared heroin addicts and their nonaddict siblings and found that the clearest difference was in the early reference groups. Addicts were involved in the illegitimate street culture at an early age, whereas their nonaddict siblings rejected the illegitimate world and sought legitimate employment.

Segal (1976) reported on a study of college students which demonstrated that student drug users have allied themselves with a counterculture which eschews achievement and conformity. Spevack and Pihl (1976) found that drug-using high school students are more likely than nonusing students to engage in recreational activities which are esteemed by the youth culture but not adults.

A number of personality characteristics of drug abusers have been identified which may serve to increase the influence of deviant peer groups. Drug abusers have been found to be more rebellious, less self-reliant, and less self-confident. They feel less accepted by others (Smith and Fogg, 1976) and more alienated (Block, 1976; Jessor, 1976), and are more likely to be experiencing an identity crisis (Mellinger et al., 1976). Disturbances in peer relationships have also been identified (Brooks et al., 1976; Lindblad, 1977) which may increase the pressure to conform to the peer group. While it has not been determined whether these personality traits precede or result from membership in a drug subculture, once established, they can be expected to affect the ongoing influence of the peer group.

As indicated in the preceding review, drug-abusing behavior results from the complex interaction of a variety of interpersonal and intrapersonal factors. There is no single circumstance or characteristic which is necessary or sufficient to the development of drug use. An individual has multiple reference groups, one or more of which may exert a prodrug influence while another(s) may exert an antidrug influence. Thus, some individuals exposed to a prodrug peer group are insulated from drug use because of the greater influence of an antidrug reference group, such as the family. Also, personality variables may predispose some individuals to peer group influence, while making other individuals relatively invulnerable to such influence.

IMPLICATIONS FOR TREATMENT

The literature reviewed suggests that drug abuse is a subcultural phenomenon. The individual drug abuser has internalized deviant attitudes, values, beliefs, and norms through identification with a prodrug reference group. The group also provides rationalizations which justify drug use behavior.

Drug abuse treatment and rehabilitation, viewed from the symbolic interactionist perspective, is a process of resocialization. It requires the modification of attitudes, values, beliefs, norms, and behavior. Treatment also requires modification of the individual's self-concept. Such changes can be difficult to achieve. The level of difficulty will, of course, vary depending on the level of commitment to a deviant subculture and the availability of positive reference groups.

Symbolic interaction theory suggests that the client's cultural framework and reference groups should be seen as a major focus in drug abuse treatment. Beginning with the intake process, treatment staff should clarify the client's existing values, beliefs, and norms, identifying those factors which support drug use and also those factors which support abstinence. It is also important that the client's system of rationalizations which justify continued drug use be explored fully. The client may have multiple reference groups which will impact on the resocialization process attempted through treatment. One or more reference groups may support continued use, whereas other groups may oppose use or may simply not address it. The client's family and peer group are two reference groups which can be expected to have major impact on resocialization. Thus, in the formulation of treatment plans and throughout treatment, staff should carefully consider the past, current, and potential influence of family and peers.

The family's past and current roles in socialization should be considered carefully. With some clients, family relationships have been positive, prior socialization has been generally adequate, but parental expectations regarding drug abuse issues have not been clearly established. In such cases it may be desirable to involve the family in treatment to help the parents clarify their expectations and establish limits around the use of drug. For these families, treatment would focus initially on drug use and its impact on both the user and the family. While some families may be able to share their concerns about drug use and its impact with little difficulty, treatment staff will often need to help the family identify and express the various ways in which drug use negatively affects them. The family is then ready to consider the establishment and enforcement of limits. Here the counselor helps the family to identify existing limits and mechanisms for enforcing them, to identify gaps and inconsistencies in limits, to identify ineffective or inconsistent enforcement procedures, and to develop clear and consistent limits and plans for their enforcement. Occasional follow-up sessions may be needed to review and reinforce progress.

With other clients, close family relationships have become attenuated and parental influence has declined. In these cases family therapy may be needed, not primarily to establish limits but to strengthen the bond between the client and family, and thereby enhance parental influence. The role of treatment staff with these families is to help them explore the relationships among family members, to identify both the strengths and strains within the family system, to reinforce and build on the affection and support that has existed within the family, and to develop constructive ways of resolving conflicts. In those families where conflicts have revolved around the issue of behavioral expectations, a secondary focus on limit setting may be needed.

With a third group of clients, family relationships have been disturbed and prior socialization has been inconsistent. In these cases intensive family treatment may be needed to focus on disturbances in the family system as well as to assist the parents in clarifying and enforcing limits. (See Stanton et al. [1982] regarding systems-oriented family treatment.) In the case of this third group, the therapist will need to consider the potential of the family for change. Some family systems may be so disturbed that family treatment is not feasible.

Since drug abusers are particularly vulnerable to the influence of their peer groups, they need to extract themselves from the drug subculture and align themselves with groups which support abstinence. Throughout treatment, staff should be alert to the influence of peers and the desirability of modifying peer group memberships. They should encourage the client to evaluate his or her peer relationships, withdraw from negative relationships, and strengthen relationships with nonusing friends. Formation of new peer relationships with nonusers will be essential for many clients. Program staff should help the client develop specific strategies and plans for altering these relationships.

Considering the importance of the peer group in maintaining self-esteem, withdrawal from the drug subculture can be a difficult process. Program staff will need to provide considerable support and encouragement in this process, and they should be sensitive to the client's need to have his or her self-esteem bolstered. Staff should encourage the client to draw on other sources of support, such as family members and nonusing friends. Other clients in treatment who are also attempting to change and former clients who are drug-free can serve as additional sources of support. Consideration should be given to linking the client with other current or former clients who have similar interests in order to encourage the formation of supportive peer relationships.

Because it is difficult to alter reference groups, program staff will need to focus repeatedly on peer relationships, helping the client to develop and implement specific plans for establishing new friendships. Special consideration should be given to socially isolated clients who may need concrete assistance in developing interpersonal relationships.

REFERENCES

ALEXANDER, B.K., and DIBB, G.S. Opiate addicts and their parents. *Fam. Process* 14: 499-514, 1975.

AUSUBEL, D.P. An interactional approach to narcotic addiction. In D.J. Lettieri, M. Sayers, and H.W. Pearson (eds.), *Theories on Drug Abuse: Selected Contemporary Perspectives* (DHHS Publ. No. (ADM) 80-967). Washington, DC: U.S. Government Printing Office, 1980.

AUSUBEL, D.P. *Theory and Problems of Adolescent Development.* New York: Grune and Stratton, 1954.

BAER, D.J., and CORRADO, J.J. Heroin addict relationships with parents during childhood and early adolescent years. *J. Genet. Psychol.* 124: 99-103, 1974.

BECKER, H.S. *Outsiders: Studies in the Sociology of Deviance.* New York: Free Press, 1963.

BECKER, H.S. The social bases of drug-induced experiences. In D.J. Lettieri, M. Sayers, and H.W. Pearson (eds.), *Theories on Drug Abuse: Selected Contemporary Perspectives* (DHHS Publ. No. (ADM) 80-967). Washington, DC: U.S. Government Printing Office, 1980.

BLOCK, J.R. Behavioral and demographic correlates of drug use among students in grades 7-12. In D.J. Lettieri (ed.), *Predicting Adolescent Drug Abuse: A Review of Issues, Methods and Correlates* (DHHS Publ. No. (ADM) 77-299). Washington, DC: U.S. Government Printing Office, 1976.

BLUMER, H. *Symbolic Interactionism: Perspective and Method.* Englewood Cliffs, NJ: Prentice-Hall, 1969.

BLUMER, H. *The World of Youthful Drug Abuse.* Berkeley, CA: University of California, School of Criminology, 1967.

BRAUCHT, N.G., BRAKARSH, D. FOLLINGSTAD, D., and BERRY, K.L. Deviant drug use in adolescence: A review of psychosocial correlates. *Psychol. Bull.* 79: 92-106, 1973.

BRIM, O.G., JR. Adult socialization. In J.A. Clausen (ed.), *Socialization and Society.* Boston: Little, Brown, 1968.

BRIM, O.G., JR. Socialization through the life cycle. In O.G. Brim, Jr., and S. Wheeler (eds.), *Socialization after Childhood: Two Essays.* New York: Wiley, 1966.

BROOKS, R., SZANDOROWSKA, B., and WHITEHEAD, P.C. Psychosocial dysfunctions as precursors to amphetamine abuse among adolescents. *Addict Dis.* 2: 465-478, 1976.

CHAMBERS, C.D., and MOFFETT, A.D. Negro opiate addiciton. In J.C. Ball and C.C. Chambers (eds.), *The Epidemiology of Opiate Addiction in the United States.* Springfield, IL: C.C. Thomas, 1970.

CHAMBERS, C.D., MOFFETT, A.D., and JONES, J.P. Demographic factors associated with Negro opiate addiction in the United States. *Int. J. Addict.* 3: 329-343, 1968.

CHEIN, I., GERARD, D.L., LEE, R.S., and ROSENFELD, E. *The Road to H: Narcotics, Delinquency, and Social Policy.* New York: Basic Books, 1964.

CLAUSEN, J.A. (ed.), *Socialization and Society.* Boston: Little, Brown, 1968.

CLOWARD, R., and OHLIN, L.W. Norms of delinquent subcultures. In B.J. Biddle and E.J. Thomas (eds.), *Role Theory: Concepts and Research.* New York: Wiley, 1966.

CRAIG, S.R., and BROWN, B.S. Comparison of youthful heroin users and nonusers from one urban community. *Int. J. Addict.* 10: 53-64, 1975.

DOUVAN, E., and ADELSON, J. *The Adolescent Experience.* New York: Wiley, 1966.

ELLINWOOD, E.H., JR., SMITH, W.G., and VAILLANT, G.E. Narcotic addiction in males and females: A comparison. *Int. J. Addict.* 1: 33-45, 1966.

FELDMAN, H. American way of drugging. *Society* 10: 32-38, 1973.

FINESTONE, H. Cats, kicks, and color. *Soc. Probl.* 5: 3-13, 1957.

GLASER, D., LANDER, B., and ABBOTT, W. Opiate addicted and nonaddicted siblings in a slum area. *Soc. Probl.* 18: 510-521, 1971.

GOODE, W.J. Norm commitment and conformity to role-status obligations. In B.J. Biddle and E.J. Thomas (eds.), *Role Theory: Concepts and Research*. New York: Wiley, 1966.

GORSUCH, R.L. Interactive models of nonmedical drug use. In D.J. Lettieri, M. Sayers, and H.W. Pearson (eds.), *Theories on Drug Abuse: Selected Contemporary Perspectives* (DHHS Publ. No. (ADM) 80-967). Washington, DC: U.S. Government Printing Office, 1980.

HELZER, J.E., ROBINS, L.N., and DAVIS, D.H. Antecedents of narcotic use and addiction. *Drug Alcohol Depend.* 1: 183-190, 1976.

HUBA, G.J., WINGARD, J.A., and BENTLER, P.M. Framework for an interactive theory of drug use. In D.J. Lettieri, M. Sayers, and H.W. Pearson (eds.), *Theories on Drug Abuse: Selected Contemporary Perspectives* (DHHS Publ. No. (ADM) 80-967). Washington, DC: U.S. Government Printing Office, 1980.

INKELES, A. Society, social structure, and child socialization. In J.A. Clausen (ed.), *Socialization and Society*. Boston: Little, Brown, 1968.

JESSOR, R. Predicting time of onset of marijuana use: A developmental study of high school youth. In D.J. Lettieri (ed.), *Predicting Adolescent Drug Abuse: A Review of Issues, Methods and Correlates* (DHEW Publ. No. (ADM) 77-299). Washington, DC: U.S. Government Printing Office, 1976.

JESSOR, R., and JESSOR, S. A social-psychological framework for studying drug use. In D.J. Lettieri, M. Sayers, and H.W. Pearson (eds.), *Theories on Drug Abuse: Selected Contemporary Perspectives* (DHHS Publ. No. (ADM) 80-967). Washington, DC: U.S. Government Printing Office, 1980.

JOHNSON, B.D. Toward a theory of drug subcultures. In D.J. Lettieri, M. Sayers, and H.W. Pearson (eds.), *Theories on Drug Abuse: Selected Contemporary Perspectives* (DHHS Publ. No. (ADM) 80-967). Washington, DC: U.S. Government Printing Office, 1980.

JONES, R.A., and DAY, R.A. Social psychology as symbolic interaction. In C. Hendrick (ed.), *Perspectives on Social Psychology*. Hillsdale, NJ: Lawrence Erlbaum Associates, 1977.

KANDEL, D. Developmental stages in adolescent drug involvement. In D.J. Lettieri, M. Sayers, and H.W. Pearson (eds.), *Theories on Drug Abuse: Selected Contemporary Perspectives* (DHHS Publ. No. (ADM) 80-967). Washington, DC: U.S. Government Printing Office, 1980.

KANDEL, D. Some comments on the relationship of selected criteria variables to adolescent illicit drug use. In D.J. Lettieri (ed.), *Predicting Adolescent Drug Abuse: A Review of Issues, Methods and Correlates* (DHEW Publ. No. (ADM) 77-299). Washington, DC: U.S. Government Printing Office, 1976.

KUHN, M.H. Major trends in symbolic interaction theory in the past twenty-five years. In J.G. Manis and B.N. Meltzer (eds.), *Symbolic Interaction: A Reader in Social Psychology*, 3rd ed. Boston: Allyn and Bacon, 1978.

LINDBLAD, R. *Self Concept and Drug Addiction: A Controlled Study of White Middle Socioeconomic Status Addicts* (DHEW Publ. No. (ADM) 77-474). Washington, DC: U.S. Government Printing Office, 1977.

LIPPITT, R. Improving the socialization process. In J.A. Clausen (ed.), *Socialization and Society*. Boston: Little, Brown, 1968.

LUKOFF, I.F. Toward a sociology of drug use. In D.J. Lettieri, M. Sayers, and H.W. Pearson (eds.), *Theories on Drug Abuse: Selected Contemporary Perspectives* (DHHS Publ. No. (ADM) 80-967). Washington, DC: U.S. Government Printing Office, 1980.

MELLINGER, G.D., SOMERS, R.H., and MANHEIMER, D.I. Drug use research items pertaining to personality and interpersonal relations. In D.J. Lettieri (ed.), *Predicting Adolescent Drug Abuse: A Review of Issues, Methods and Corrleates* (DHEW Publ. No. (ADM) 77-299). Washington, DC: U.S. Government Printing Office, 1976.

MELTZER, B.N. Mead's social psychology. In J.G. Manis and B.N. Meltzer (eds.), *Symbolic Interaction: A Reader in Social Psychology,* 3rd ed. Boston: Allyn and Bacon, 1978.

NEWCOMB, T.M. The general nature of peer group influence. In T.M. Newcomb and E.K. Wilson (eds.), *Collge Peer Groups.* Chicago: Aldine, 1966.

PACE, R.C., and BAIRD, L. Attainment patterns in the environmental press of college subcultures. In T.M. Newcomb and E.K. Wilson (eds.), *Collge Peer Groups.* Chicago: Aldine, 1966.

PARK, R.E. Human migration and the marginal man. *Am. J. Sociol.* 33: 881-893, 1928.

RICHARDS, L.G. Role of society. In S.N. Pradham and S.N. Dutta (eds.), *Drug Abuse: Clinical and Basic Aspects.* St. Louis: C.V. Mosby, 1977.

SEGAL, B. Personality factors related to drug and alcohol use. In D.J. Lettieri (ed.), *Predicting Adolescent Drug Abuse: A Review of Issues, Methods and Correlates* (DHEW Publ. No. (ADM) 77-299). Washington, DC: U.S. Government Printing Office, 1976.

SHERIF, M., and SHERIF, C.W. *Reference Groups.* New York: Harper and Row, 1964.

SHIBUTANI, T. Reference groups as perspectives. In J.G. Manis and B.N. Meltzer (eds.), *Symbolic Interaction: A Reader in Social Psychology,* 3rd ed. Boston: Allyn and Bacon, 1978.

SHIBUTANI, T. *Society and Personality.* Englewood Cliffs, NJ: Prentice-Hall, 1961.

SMART, R.G. An availability-proneness theory of illicit drug abuse. In D.J. Lettieri, M. Sayers, and H.W.. Pearson (eds.), *Theories on Drug Abuse: Selected Contemporary Perspectives* (DHHS Publ. No. (ADM) 80-967). Washington, DC: U.S. Government Printing Office, 1980.

SMITH, G.M., and FOGG, C.P. Teenage drug use: A search for causes and consequences. In D.J. Lettieri (ed.), *Predicting Adolescent Drug Abuse: A Review of Issues, Methods and Correlates* (DHEW Publ. No. (ADM) 77-299). Washington, DC: U.S. Government Printing Office, 1976.

SPEVACK, M., and PIHL, R.O. Nonmedical drug use by high school students: A three-year survey study. *Int. J. Addict.* 11: 755-792, 1976.

STANTON, M.D., TODD, T.C., and ASSOCIATES. *The Family Therapy of Drug Abuse and Addiction.* New York: Guilford Press, 1982.

STEFFENHAGEN, R. A. Self-esteem theory of drug abuse. In D.J. Lettieri, M. Sayers, and H.W. Pearson (eds.), *Theories on Drug Abuse: Selected Contemporary Perspectives* (DHHS Publ. No. (ADM) 80-967). Washington, DC: U.S. Government Printing Office, 1980.

STEPHENS, R., and LEVINE, S. The "street addict role": Implications for treatment. *Psychiatry* 34: 351-357, 1971.

SUTHERLAND, E.H., and CRESSEY, D.R. *Criminology.* Philadelphia: J.B. Lippincott, 1970.

TURNER, J.H. *The Structure of Sociological Theory,* 2nd ed. Homewood, IL: Dorsey Press, 1978.

VAILLANT, G.E. A twelve-year follow-up of New York narcotics addicts. III. Some social and psychiatric characteristics. *Arch. Gen. Psychiatry* 15: 599-609, 1966.

The International Journal of the Addictions, 19(6), 689-696, 1984

Research Note

Individual Characteristics of Aggressive Beer and Distilled Beverage Drinkers

R. O. Pihl,* PhD

Mark Smith, BA

Brian Farrell, BA

Department of Psychology
McGill University
Montreal, Quebec, Canada

Abstract

Sixty male social drinkers completed the MMPI and a drinking history and attitude questionnaire. These individuals were then randomly divided into four groups, receiving either a distilled or brewed beverage, or two comparable placebos. Subjects in the alcohol groups became equally intoxicated (BAC = .71) and rated themselves as significantly more intoxicated than placebo subjects. All subjects then participated in a Buss aggression task. Aggression scales were related to the pretask personality, history, and attitude measures. Differences were found between factors descriptive of subjects who became aggressive after consuming or believing they had consumed a distilled versus a brewed beverage. In particular, a history of lack of positive alcohol effects and social maladjustment were typical of high-aggressive distilled alcohol and alcohol-placebo subjects, while the presence of family problems and anxiety typified high-aggressive beer and placebo-beer subjects.

The association between alcohol use and violence is both common and pervasive. Significant correlations between alcohol consumption and assaults Mayfield, 1976; Shupe, 1954), rape (Gebhard, Gagnon, Pomeroy, and

*To whom requests for reprints should be sent at the Department of Psychology, 1205 Dr. Penfield Avenue, Montreal, Quebec H3A 1B1, Canada.

 0020-773X/84/1906-0689$3.50/0

Christenson, 1965), murder (Virkkunen, 1974), and suicide (Haberman and Baden, 1974) have been reported. In a World Health Organization report (1979), alcohol consumption was implicated worldwide in from 24% to 72% of assaults, from 13% to 50% of rapes, and from 28% to 68% of homicides. The nature of the relationships between alcohol and aggression is presently unclear, and as indicated by the foregoing percentages and the fact that most people do not become violent when they drink, the problem is individual, affecting only a proportion of alcohol consumers. The present study was designed to assess the interaction of background drinking factors and personality variables as contributors to increased aggression when intoxicated.

Table 1

Demographic and Alcohol Characteristics of 60 Male Social Drinkers

	Mean	SD	Range	Minimum
Age	24.2	4.6	16.0	18.0
Education (yr)	13.1	2.2	11.0	7.0
SES[a]	167.5	134.4	441.0	3.0
Consumption[b]	8.5	6.5	23.0	1.0

	Categories	Absolute frequency	Percent frequency
Marital status	1. Married	15	25.0
	2. Separated	1	1.7
	3. Common-law	3	5.0
	4. Divorced	1	1.7
	5. Single	40	66.7
Alcohol preference	1. Beer	37	61.7
	2. Wine	6	10.0
	3. Distilled alcohols	15	25.0
	4. Other	2	3.3
Drinking habit	1. Nondrinker	2	3.3
	2. Light social	23	38.3
	3. Average social	29	48.3
	4. Heavy social	5	8.3
	5. Alcoholism problem	1	1.7

[a] Socioeconomic standing was assessed using the revised Blishen and McRoberts Index (1976).
[b] Average number of 1.5-oz drinks, or equivalent, consumed per week.

METHOD

The characteristics of the 60 volunteer male subjects are illustrated in Table 1. The study was conducted in two sessions. During the first session, subjects were asked to complete the MMPI and a drinking history and attitude questionnaire. In addition to the three validity scales and 10 clinical scales of the MMPI, the following research scales were included: resentment and aggression, MacAndrew Alcoholism Scale, family problems, control, lack of ego mastery, anxiety, depression, manifest hostility, social alienation, social introversion, social status, social responsibility, and social maladjustment. The questionnaire dealt with the amount of weekly alcohol consumption; self-description of degree of drinking habit; and effect of drinking, including changed sociability, relief from frustration, decrease in tension, reduction in anger, improved clarity in thinking, and increase in enjoyable activities.

At the second, or drinking session, the level of aggression for subjects when intoxicated or after consuming a placebo beverage was ascertained. This procedure and the results of that aspect of the study are presented in Pihl, Smith, and Farrell (1984). Briefly, aggression was measured using a modified version of the Buss aggression machine where the subject was led to believe he was participating in a reaction-time test while another "individual" (actually nonexistent) was being tested for pain perception. The subject could choose one of five buttons to press as a measure of his reaction time, and each clearly marked button resulted in a different intensity of shock to the other "individual." The intensity of shock chosen and the duration of time the button was held down were the measures of aggression. In addition, an overall aggression score for each subject was obtained by multiplying the shock intensity chosen on each trial by its corresponding duration and dividing by the total number of trials. Before the aggression task originated, subjects were randomly assigned to one of four conditions: (1) alcohol condition–subjects were administered 1.32 mL/kg body weight of 95% United States Pharmacopoeia (USP) alcohol in a 1:5 (alcohol: orange juice) solution; (2) alcohol-placebo condition–subjects were administered orange juice of equal proportions as in the alcohol condition, the alcohol part being replaced by juice and 2 cc of 95% USP alcohol layered on the drink's surface; (3) beer condition–subjects were administered 21.3 mL of Brador (6.2% alc/vol) per kilogram of body weight; (4) beer-placebo condition–subjects were administered 21.3 mL of a mixture of 3 parts Texas Pride to 1 part Panther per kilogram of body weight. After a 20-min period for consuming the beverages and a further 20-min waiting period, Breathalizer readings were taken and intoxication rating scales were completed. Subjects then participated in the aggression task. Subjects in the alcohol and beer conditions achieved almost identical BAC readings, approaching legal intoxication (mean = .71 both before and after the task). These subjects also rated themselves as significantly more intoxicated than placebo subjects.

RESULTS AND DISCUSSION

A factor analysis was performed on scores from the three validity scales, 10 clinical scales, and 13 research scales from the MMPI, as well as scores obtained from the questionnaire. The initial factor matrix indicated a high degree of intercorrelation between MMPI scale scores. A varimax rotation yielded 17 MMPI scales and three variables from the Background Information Questionnaire which demonstrated multiple loadings and were dropped from further factor analysis. The remaining variables were again factor analyzed. Five factors accounting for 75% of the variance resulted from this analysis. The rotated factor loadings are presented in Table 2.

Intercorrelations (Pearson product-moment correlations) between all aggression measures were computed for each group; this revealed that the aggression score was the measure of aggression which correlated the highest with

Table 2

Rotated Factor Loadings from Factor Analysis

	I	II	III	IV	V
Hostility factor					
K scale	-.723	-.387	.272	-.074	.068
Resentment and aggression vs lack of resentment and aggression	.821	.383	.013	.019	.092
Lack of ego mastery – defective inhibition	.855	.151	.082	.135	.042
Manifest hostility	.884	.225	-.131	-.004	.069
Social responsibility	-.810	-.242	-.081	-.018	-.033
Social maladjustment factor					
Social introversion (*Si*)	.177	.914	.097	-.088	-.159
Social introversion vs interpersonal poise and outgoingness	.094	.928	.029	.049	-.118
Social status	-.191	-.732	-.070	-.125	-.104
Social maladjustment	.068	.955	.024	-.029	-.139
Aggression factor					
Hypochondriasis (*Hs*)	-.173	.112	.812	.137	-.025
Hysteria (*Hy*)	-.127	.009	.888	-.066	.033
Psychopathic deviate (*Pd*)	.348	.067	.712	-.232	-.036
Effects pattern					
Alcohol makes me less tense	.002	.058	-.069	.818	.098
Alcohol makes me less angry	.047	-.029	-.025	.794	-.022
Alcohol compliments other enjoyable activities	.111	.039	.069	.850	.133
Drinking factor					
Quantity of alcohol consumption per week	.369	-.021	.121	.152	.770
Drinking habit	-.046	-.109	-.002	.349	.775
Socioeconomic standing	.227	.148	.128	.218	-.543

other measures (mean r = .62), and thus it was used as the dependent variable in the stepwise regression analysis. Independent variables included the five factor scores and the 17 MMPI scale scores which were not included in the factor analysis. Regression analyses were computed for each of the drug conditions separately as well as for all conditions combined. To control for the effects of experimental manipulations on the aggression scores, the analysis was conducted in accordance with the procedure outlined by Kerlinger and Pedhazur (1973). The results of the regression analysis are presented in Table 3. Controlling for sample differences, the coefficients in the regression analyses indicated positive loadings for the psychasthenic scale and the drinking factor; and negative loadings

Table 3

Results of Stepwise Regression Analysis on Aggression Scores for All Groups Controlling for Sample Differences and for Each Group Separately

	Standardized coefficient	F value	Significance
All groups (N = 60)			
Dummy one	0.169	2.29	< 0.05
Dummy two	0.393	12.58	< 0.01
Dummy three	0.104	0.88	> 0.10
Aggression factor	−0.518	16.33	< 0.01
Psychasthenia	0.660	15.76	< 0.01
Depression	−0.307	4.40	< 0.01
Effects	−0.188	3.03	< 0.01
Drinking factor	0.186	2.74	< 0.05
Beer (N = 16)			
Drinking habit factor	0.408	7.83	< 0.01
Psychasthenia (*Pt*)	0.725	18.03	< 0.01
Family problems	0.654	15.34	< 0.01
Social adjustment	−0.635	15.08	< 0.01
Alcohol (N = 16)			
Social maladjustment	0.907	12.52	< 0.01
Depression	−0.631	6.54	< 0.01
Effects factor	−0.342	3.62	< 0.05
Placebo-beer (N = 16)			
Psychasthenia	1.179	59.59	< 0.01
Family problems	0.929	47.60	< 0.01
Social alienation	−0.975	37.11	< 0.01
Control	−0.438	15.94	< 0.01
Masculinity-femininity	−0.252	5.97	< 0.01
Placebo-alcohol (N = 12)			
Effects factor	−0.684	12.34	< 0.01
Social maladjustment	0.551	7.04	< 0.01
Depression	−0.442	4.37	< 0.05

for the depression scale, the aggression factor, and the effects factor. Therefore, regardless of drug manipulation, those individuals who scored high on the aggression task tended to score high on the psychasthenic scale, reported heavier consumption of alcohol, tended to come from lower socioeconomic backgrounds, and reported that alcohol did not generally produce positive effects; but scored low on MMPI measures of aggression and depression.

In the beer condition, the coefficients indicated positive loadings for the drinking factor, the psychasthenic scale, and family problems; and a negative loading for the social maladjustment factor. In the alcohol condition, the social maladjustment factor loaded positively, and the MMPI depression scale and the effects factor loaded negatively. In the placebo-beer condition, the coefficients indicated positive loadings for the psychasthenic scale and family problems; and negative loadings for MMPI measures of social alienation, control, and masculinity-femininity. In the placebo-alcohol condition, the social maladjustment factor loaded positively, and the MMPI depression scale and the effects factor loaded negatively.

Notable in the regression analysis is the basic lack of differentiation between drug and placebo consumers, accompanied by varying profiles for aggressive alcohol-placebo and beer-placebo drinkers. These findings support the growing body of literature demonstrating the importance of psychological factors such as expectancy and attribution in alcohol-related aggression (Lang, Goeckner, Adesso, and Marlatt, 1975; Pihl, Zeichner, Niaura, Nagy, and Zacchia, 1981). Also, of particular interest in these results is the differential profile of aggressive alcohol consumers versus beer consumers. Studies (Boyatzis, 1974; Takala, Pihkanen, and Markkanen, 1957) have reported increased aggressiveness to alcohol relative to the response to beer. In the present study, aggressive beer and aggressive placebo-beer drinkers scored high on variables measuring anxiety and the pressure of family problems; the coefficients for these variables were not significant in the regression analysis for the alcohol group. Further, the low scores on the social maladjustment and introversion factors for aggressive subjects in both beer groups were in the opposite direction to the high social maladjustment and introversion scores seen in the aggressive alcohol subjects.

Interestingly, the absence of a history of positive associations with alcohol use, indicated in the regression analysis by the negative coefficient for the alcohol effects factor, was the most significant determinant for increased aggression in the placebo-alcohol group. In addition, this factor entered significantly into the regression, on the third step, in the alcohol group. In comparison, this factor had not entered into the regression by the ninth step for either the placebo-beer or the beer group. Why the lack of positive associations is predictive of increased aggression in subjects who consume alcohol or believe they consume alcohol, as opposed to beer, is presently unanswerable.

The results of the present study may point to a differential conditioning history, where for some individuals alcohol consumption is associated with negative sociological or psychological events, which increases the likelihood of aggression. To continue this speculation, beer consumption is more likely associated with positive events or situations and thus evokes a different set of behaviors. Conditioning models of drug abuse are well known (Wikler, 1973), but in the case of alcohol, these need to be explored further in terms of a specific drug-related response such as aggression. Attributional factors may also be involved, as anthropological evidence (MacAndrew and Edgerton, 1969) has shown how differential meaning and function are attributed to different beverages, which affects both group and individual behavior.

ACKNOWLEDGMENT

This study was supported by a grant from the Brewers Association of Canada. Data were collected in 1981.

REFERENCES

BLISHEN, B.R., and MC ROBERTS, H.A. A revised socioeconomic index for occupations in Canada. *Can. Rev. Sociol. Anthropol.* 13: 71-79, 1976.

BOYATZIS, R.E. The effect of alcohol consumption on the aggressive behavior of men. *Q. J. Stud. Alcohol* 35: 989-992, 1974.

GEBHARD, P.H., GAGNON, J.H., POMEROY, W.D., and CHRISTENSON, C.V. *Sex Offenders: An Analysis of Types.* New York: Harper and Row, 1965.

HABERMAN, P.Q., and BADEN, M.M. Alcoholism and violent death. *Q. J. Stud. Alcohol* 35: 221-231, 1974.

KERLINGER, F.N., and PEDHAZUR, E.J. *Multiple Regression in Behavioral Research.* New York: Holt, Rinehart, and Winston, 1973.

LANG, A.R., GOECKNER, D.J., ADESSO, V.J., and MARLATT, G.A. Effects of alcohol on aggression in male social drinkers. *J. Abnorm. Psychol.* 84: 508-518, 1975.

MAC ANDREW, C., and EDGERTON, R.B. *Drunken Comportment: A Social Explanation.* Chicago: Aldine, 1969.

MAYFIELD, D. Alcoholism, alcohol, intoxication and assaulting behavior. *Dis. Nerv. Syst.* 37: 288-291, 1976.

PIHL, R.O., SMITH, M., and FARRELL, B. Alcohol and aggression: A comparison of brewed and distilled beverages. *Addict. Behav.* In press, 1984.

PIHL, R.O., ZEICHNER, A., NIAURA, R., NAGY, K., and ZACCHIA, C. Attribution and alcohol mediated aggression. *J. Abnorm. Psychol.* 90: 468-475, 1981.

SHUPE, L.M. Alcohol and crime: A study of the urine alcohol concentration found in 882 persons arrested during or immediately after the commission of a felony. *J. Crim. Law, Criminol. Police Sci.* 44: 661-664, 1954.

TAKALA, M., PIHKANEN, T.A., and MARKKANEN, T. *The Effects of Distilled and Brewed Beverages: A Physiological, Neurological and Psychological Study.* Helsinki: Finnish Foundation for Alcohol Studies, 1957.

VIRKKUNEN, M. Alcohol as a factor precipitating aggression and conflict behavior leading to homicide. *Br. J. Addict.* 69: 149-154, 1974.

WIKLER, A. Dynamics of drug dependence: Implications of a conditioning theory for research and treatment. *Arch. Gen. Psychiatry* 28: 611-616, 1973.

WORLD HEALTH ORGANIZATION. *Health Statistics: Annual Report.* Geneva: World Health Organization, 1979.

The International Journal of the Addictions, 19(6), 697–700, 1984

Note

Considering Motivation and Ability for Drug Use Intervention: Some Implications

Stanley Einstein,* PhD

Jerusalem, Israel

Two factors or concepts which are often considered or alluded to in drug use intervention are *motivation* and *ability*. The assumption/presumption most often is that successfully engaging a drug user in treatment, developing the needed therapeutic alliance, and achieving a successful outcome demands a highly motivated patient. The same can be said about "populations at risk" and drug use prevention efforts. By *ability* we most often mean the basic skills, capabilities, etc., for effectively utilizing specific intervention techniques, engaging in necessary roles, etc. The capable, highly motivated drug user is a likely candidate for successful therapeutic intervention, and his "vulnerable" non-drug-using peer/relative, with the same characteristics, is most likely to be "saved" through prevention efforts from *chemical coping*.

Since motivation and ability are not unitary factors, but rather are conceptual gradients, their interface presents us with some serious challenges. Schema 1 visually presents one way of schematizing the outcome of such an interface. For those who believe that drug users are as treatable as any other type of population, *given the necessary planning, conditions, and resources,* the upper left-hand cell presents relatively minimal problems. The challenges/problems are with the other three cells. What are the options for planning and carrying out effective treatment/intervention in the following cases?

- Under conditions of *high ability* and *low states of motivation* to change
- Under conditions of *low ability* and *high states of motivation* to change
- Under conditions of *low ability* and *low states of motivation* to change

*Address correspondence to the author at 113/41 E. Talpiot, Jerusalem, Israel.

 0020-773X/84/1906-0697$3.50/0

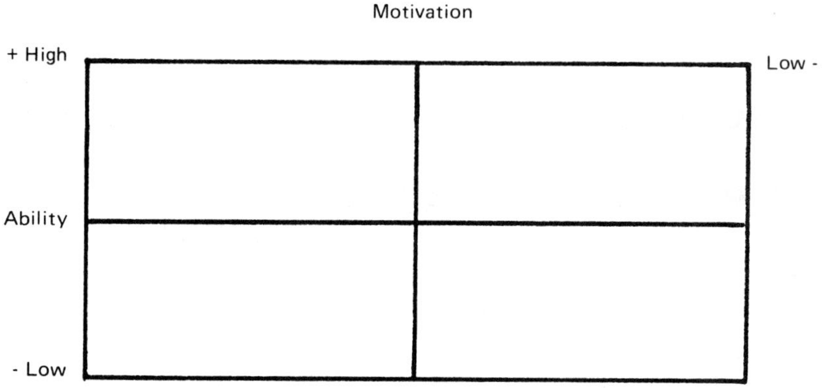

Schema 1. The interface between motivation and ability.

You the reader will no doubt find or create reasonable solutions for these varying conditions. Types of skill training, reassessment, and selection of goals suitable to specific motivation levels are examples of what can be done in order to reasonably utilize the available types and levels of abilities and motivation for intervention planning. The purpose of this note is not to report, to document, or to summarize proven recipes. The interested reader can find sufficient literature which suggests what *they* have done and/or *you* should do. This note is designed to remind the reader to be constantly aware, as s/he chooses strategies for drug user treatment planning, whether s/he is working within a static or dynamic context, with unitary concepts or with gradients, with controllable and/or measurable concepts.

In addition, this note is designed to raise the specter of associating concepts that traditionally are projected only onto the drug user/pre-drug user, with other participants in drug use intervention as well. Schema 2 is designed to stimulate the reader to consider what are the implications of the actual/potential interface of levels or types of motivation and ability for others who are or should be involved in the intervention process (planning, doing, outcome).

When one gets off the drug user's back and we begin to focus upon other actual or potential significant intervention partners, we may be faced with numerous uncomfortable considerations:

- Do we generally concern ourselves with assessing the levels of ability and motivation of individuals who are willing to treat drug users or prevent drug use?

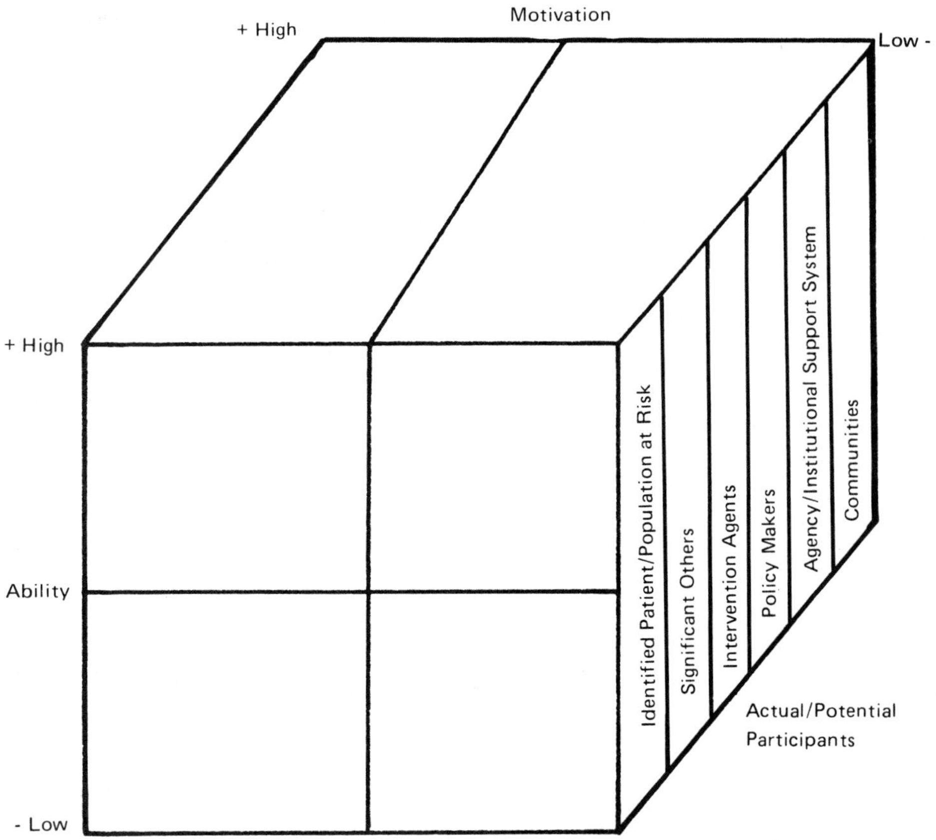

Schema 2. The interface between motivation and ability for all actual/potential intervention participants.

- What are some reasonable criteria for measuring levels and types of agency abilities and motivations, regarding the effective planning and carrying out of drug use intervention, and are they generally considered and used?
- What abilities and motivations (types and levels) do various types of communities need (and how can they be helped to achieve them?) in order to integrate/reintegrate stigmatized drug users, or not to isolate and reject the almost stigmatized pre-drug user?
- What are the necessary abilities and motivations (types, levels, and their interactions) needed by the general service/treatment agency support system to become actively and effectively involved in drug use intervention, in a given community, under conditions of the existence of specialized drug use/user programs or their absence?

You the reader can obviously raise an almost endless list of questions related to intervention planning, and the two factors/concepts which are being focused on, when you consider the possible combinations and permutations of:

Levels of Ability × Levels of Motivation × Types of Participants

And this is aside from simply looking at each of the participants, individually, in terms of high and low levels of ability and motivation. Intervention, as a planned and goal-oriented dynamic process, presumes various types and levels of interaction between the necessary participants within this process, with evaluatable as well as nonevaluatable outcomes.

Motivation and *ability* are but two examples of concepts, constructs, factors which do not seem to be adequately considered in drug use intervention planning and programs, or in evaluation efforts, notwithstanding the continued and continuous alluding to them. It would be most helpful if usable parameters could be suggested by readers, for research efforts within and between various cultures/environments, so that we could go beyond the semantics of these two terms.

The International Journal of the Addictions, 19(6), 701–707, 1984

Note

Outcome of Drug User Treatment: A Selection of Additional Needed Factors

Stanley Einstein,* PhD

Jerusalem, Israel

Documenting, understanding, and replicating the outcome of treating drug users/misusers continue to remain relatively rare phenomena. That is not to say that there isn't a steady flow of published reports and public presentations at numerous conferences (local, national, and international) which for semantic ease can be subsumed under the rubric of *drug addict/user treatment evaluation*. By and large these printed and verbal reports can be further subdivided into two major categories:

- A report about one program and/or type/family of techniques
- A comparison of types of programs/techniques

The interested reader will have no difficulties in collecting the growing literature made available to us by advocates as well as critics of specific programs, types of treatment programs, and types of treatment technologies. On the surface there is much material available. On closer viewing one can, and indeed should, ask whether we have the *necessary material* available to understand the outcome of the treatment of drug users/misusers. In a time of decreasing public resources, we owe it to ourselves to go beyond the simplistic comparisons between detoxification, outpatient (drug-free), outpatient (mixed modality), inpatient (mixed modality), methadone maintenance, therapeutic community, criminal justice programs, religious programs, etc.

The current literature inundates us with "facts" concerning dropping out of treatment, and its close relative, length of time remaining in treatment (and

*Address correspondence to the author at 113/41 E. Talpiot, Jerusalem, Israel.

 0020-773X/84/1906-0701$3.50/0

Table 1

Treatment Roles, Tasks, Styles, and Expectations: Selected Factors

Roles	Tasks	Styles	Expectations
Symmetrical–equal	Strive toward equality	Unqualified acceptance/rejection	Total cure
Asymmetrical–unequal	Rational/irrational inequality	Qualified acceptance/rejection	Partial cure
		Authoritarian/laissez-faire	Getting well
Partner–collaborator	Limit setting	Objective/disciplined subjectivity	Getting better
		Alternative expert	Relief
Advocate/negotiator/mediator	Reality testing	Problem oriented/technique	Compensation
Professional/aprofessional expert-	Reality creator	oriented	Symptom removal
"technician"	Promote–develop		Support
	Explore–discover	Seeks closure/tolerates ambiguity	Understanding
Problem solver/solution facilitator		Goal oriented	Change
	Compliance achievement		Life-style
Decision maker/facilitator	Carry out/stimulate	Accepting/questioning	Behavioral
Objective/subjective		Believer/doubter	Functional
Traditionalist/innovator	Open/close		Events
Nurturer	Carry out/develop	Directive/nondirective	Physical–material
Pace setter	Gratifier/nongratifier	Confront/avoid	Emotional
			Perceptual
Support giver	Continuity of treatment	Exaggerate/mirror/minimize	Spiritual
	Reinforce/inhibit	Interpretive/noninterpretive	Prevent
Helper		Tolerant–understanding	Eliminate
	Lead–maintain–follow	Flexible/inflexible	Minimize
Arbiter–conciliator		Disease oriented/person–system	Ameliorate
Educator–teacher	Consider–determine	oriented	Develop
Catalytic agent	Prevent–maintain–cure	Empathic/nonempathic	Control
	Ideology oriented/process		Inhibit
Mirror–resonating chamber	oriented	Formal/informal	Reinforce
	Initiate–react–respond	Genuine–authentic	Maintain
Healer	Trust	Judgmental/nonjudgmental	Stability–homeostasis
Change agent	Learn–know–evaluate	Respectful/disrespectful	Mobilize

Diagnostician	Accessible	Engaging	Goal oriented
	Isolate/integrate	Hopeful/pessimistic	Technique oriented
Control agent	Uncover/close	Patient/impatient	Process oriented
Model	Protect	Driving/relaxed	Outcome oriented
Consultant	Save	Energetic/placid	Person oriented
Communicator–transmitter	Develop therapeutic alliance	Personal/impersonal	System oriented
Credible	Facilitate opportunity for treatment	Sociable/nonsociable	Organ oriented
		Permissive/nonpermissive	Cell oriented
	Strategist	Warm/"neutral"/cold	Macro oriented
	Tactician	Active/passive	Micro oriented
		Physical/nonphysical	Theoretical–ideological
		Verbal/nonverbal	"Common sense"
		Expressive/nonexpressive	Realistic
		Casual/intensive	Unrealistic–magical
			Temporal aspects (past, present, immediate, future, atemporal)
		Distant/close	
		Individualist/loner/team member	Pain–discomfort
		Spontaneous/deliberate	Comfort
		Egalitarian	Manipulation
		Dogmatic	Respect
		Normalizing	Success
		Pragmatic	Failure
		Authoritarian	Side effects
		Reasoner–solver	Secondary gains
		Consult/evoke	Remission
		Contractual/mandated	Discover
		Decision maker/decision follower	Create
		Aggressive–assertive	Death
		Facilitate/manipulate	
		Adaptive/nonadaptive	
		Provoke/evoke	
		Seductive	
		Charismatic	
		Self-confident	
		Encouraging	

during what treatment phase); abstinence rates; rates of criminal involvement/activities; and conventional involvement/activities. What has been and remains difficult, if not impossible to understand from all of these reports, is What is the documented outcome related to—or even caused by? It is not as if the treatment outcome literature (general literature, and not drug user specific) has not indicated, suggested, hinted where we might look in order to find some reasonable answers. It surely has!

This brief note is designed to be a catalytic tool which hopefully will stimulate interested therapists and researchers in the substance use/misuse field to begin to look at the actual and potential effects of four factors which are integral to both the process and outcome of treatment. These four factors are:

- Roles
- Tasks
- Styles
- Expectations

Table 1 is designed as a semantic-conceptual tool and summary of what the broad treatment literature has often associated with these four factors. You the reader can easily add terms or delete terms.

During the treatment process there is an interface (actual and/or potential) between roles, tasks, styles, and expectations for all those who are involved (patient, significant others, therapist, policy makers, agency, community, etc.). This interface presumes that for any given *type of role,* there are suitable as well as unsuitable associated *tasks,* which can be carried out in a variety of *suitable/unsuitable* and *effective/ineffective styles* within a systemic milieu of *realistic/unrealistic expectations.* From this perspective alone the reader is asked to consider, as s/he peruses treatment evaluation reports, whether any information was presented about any of these four factors. Do we know, and/or adequately understand, the actual and potential roles, tasks, styles, and expectations which made up the treatment process?

Obviously these four factors, when related to the complexities of a structured change process (treatment), are not simply unitary concepts. They are interacting factors. Within such a context, irrespective of the technology being used and the ideological basis of the effort, we are obligated to consider, for each of the participants and for each of the four factors, those issues which relate to *responsibility, rights,* and *obligations,* and their implications. Schema 1 is designed to help the reader to consider the actual as well as the potential relationships and interfaces between these three selected parameters of treatment.

It may be useful for you the reader to schematically review the last few sentences. We started with whatever the "evaluation literature" continues to report about the treatment outcome of drug addicts/users, in terms of a

	Roles	Tasks	Styles	Expectations
Rights				
Responsibilities				
Obligations				

Schema 1. A visual schema for exploring and choosing elements basic to treatment planning.

traditional classification of types of programs. From the perspective of this brief note, such documentation is of little if any help to program planners, therapists, etc. The use of these traditional classifications—solely, without further delineation(s)—has advantages for two major groups primarily: the confirmed believers and professional/chronic critics. In order to better understand what has or hasn't happened during the treatment process, we have to know, among many other things, information about roles, styles, tasks, and expectations for all of the change process participants. Lastly, in order to more fully comprehend the parameters and effects of each of these four selected factors, singly and/or interacting with one another, we are obliged to collect pertinent data which validly document the parameters of responsibilities, rights, and obligations.

Why do we need such information? In order to understand, in a usable manner, the effective and ineffective role demands of various types of programs, public and private, which are designed/mandated/permitted to treat drug addicts/drug users.

Schema 2 is designed to help you the reader to begin to consider the drug user's actual and/or potential interfaces with selected treatment parameters and types of programs, using their traditional classifications. If we had the necessary reliable information which is associated with role-related treatment issues, we could then consider such significant treatment issues as: needed skills/abilities for all the participants; needed skill training; the options and processes for role induction; actual and potential "side effects" (planned/unplanned; known/unknown); relevancy (theoretical/empirical/"common sense"); and "costs."

If we choose to seriously investigate, document, and understand the effects and implications of *responsibility,* within a treatment context, we would have to consider such issues as: extent (quantitative and qualitative), needed skills/abilities, needed skill training, temporal aspects, "side effects," relevancy, and "costs."

When considering the factor of therapeutic style—a set of behaviors defining characterisitic change-oriented relationships—we would be obligated to fully

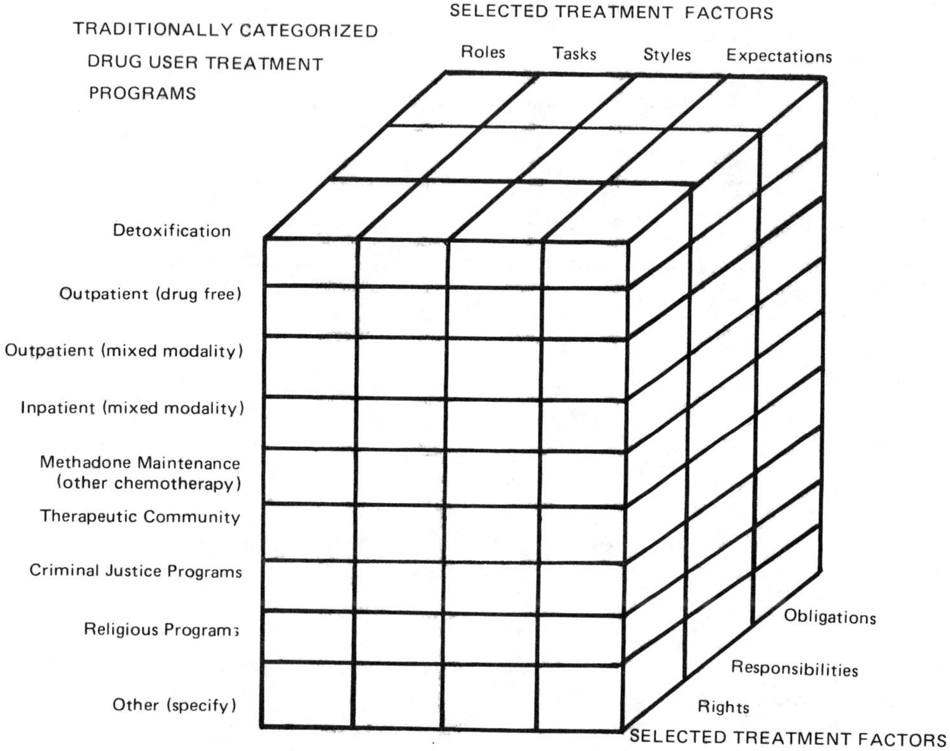

The reader is asked to fill out this schema for the following types of participants in the treatment-change process: patient(s) ——; significant other(s) ——; treatment agent(s) ——; policy maker(s) ——; treatment agency ——; treatment/service agency support system ——; community (s) ——.

Schema 2. The interface between selected treatment factors and traditionally categorized drug user treatment programs.

understand the as yet unresolved question in the treatment literature which pits the "good therapist" against the "relevant/adequate therapist" or "differential therapist." When one considers whether there are good therapists who can treat just about anyone, in their specific field, or whether there are therapists who are best with only certain types of conditions, patients, techniques, etc., the factor of therapeutic style is not a side issue.

Until we begin to collect all of the necessary information, we can (and probably will) continue to do that which we have done so well for so long. But we shouldn't fool ourselves, or others, by concluding that we are *evaluating* or that we are permitting objective researchers to evaluate what we are doing.

We can't fault ourselves, or be faulted, for inadequate planning. Planning, as distinct from reflexive reactions, presumes the existence and use of relevant basic data. Currently, notwithstanding the plethora of statistics, we don't have/collect the needed data which could help us with the treatment of drug addicts/users, the appropriate training of needed clinical staff and other change agents, the development of appropriate policies, the engagement of needed systems and communities, and the selection of relevant criteria for understanding and judging that which we have done as well as what we haven't done.

THE AMERICAN JOURNAL OF DRUG AND ALCOHOL ABUSE

Volume 10, Number 2, 1984

CONTENTS

A Longitudinal Study of Offspring Born to Methadone-Maintained Women. I. Design, Methodology, and Description of Women's Resources for Functioning 135
J. Marcus, S. L. Hans, C. B. Patterson, and A. J. Morris

A Longitudinal Study of Offspring Born to Methadone-Maintained Women. II. Dyadic Interaction and Infant Behavior at 4 Months 161
V. Bernstein, R. Jeruchimowicz Jeremy, S. L. Hans, and J. Marcus

A Longitudinal Study of Offspring Born to Methadone-Maintained Women. III. Effects of Multiple Risk Factors on Development at 4,8, and 12 Months 195
J. Marcus, S. L. Hans, and R. Jeruchimowicz Jeremy

The Index of Choice: Indications of Methadone Patients' Selection of Naltrexone Treatment 209
E. G. Singleton, M. F. Sherman, and G. E. Bigelow

Teacher Training in Affective Education for the Primary Prevention of Adolescent Drug Abuse 223
J. H. Malvin, J. M. Moskowitz, G. A. Schaeffer, and E. Schaps

Heroin Addicts and Nonaddicted Brothers 237
J. F. Maddux and D. P. Desmond

Strategies to Improve Compliance with Narcotic Antagonists 249
T. R. Kosten and H. D. Kleber

Therapeutic Communities: What Are the Retention Rates? 267
G. De Leon and S. Schwartz

Frequency of Heroin Use and Drug Users' Life-Style 285
E. W. Flaherty, L. Kotranski, and E. Fox

Books Received 315

MARCEL DEKKER, INC.

270 MADISON AVENUE, NEW YORK, N.Y. 10016

(212) 696-9000

U.S. Postal Service

STATEMENT OF OWNERSHIP, MANAGEMENT AND CIRCULATION

Required by 39 U.S.C. 3685)

1A. TITLE OF PUBLICATION: The International Journal of the Addictions	1B. PUBLICATION NO.: 0 0 2 0 7 7 3 X	2. DATE OF FILING: October	
3. FREQUENCY OF ISSUE: eight times per year	3A. NO. OF ISSUES PUBLISHED ANNUALLY: 8	3B. ANNUAL SUBSCRIPTION PRICE: $225.00	

4. COMPLETE MAILING ADDRESS OF KNOWN OFFICE OF PUBLICATION *(Street, City, County, State and ZIP+4 Code) (Not printers)*

270 Madison Ave. New York, NY 10016

5. COMPLETE MAILING ADDRESS OF THE HEADQUARTERS OF GENERAL BUSINESS OFFICES OF THE PUBLISHER *(Not printer)*

270 Madison Avenue New York, NY 10016

6. FULL NAMES AND COMPLETE MAILING ADDRESS OF PUBLISHER, EDITOR, AND MANAGING EDITOR *(This item MUST NOT be blank)*

PUBLISHER *(Name and Complete Mailing Address)*

Marcel Dekker, Inc. 270 Madison Ave. New York, NY 10016

EDITOR *(Name and Complete Mailing Address)*

Dr. Stanley Einstein 113/41 E Talpiot, Jerusalem, ISRAEL

MANAGING EDITOR *(Name and Complete Mailing Address)*

7. OWNER *(If owned by a corporation, its name and address must be stated and also immediately thereunder the names and addresses of stockholders owning or holding 1 percent or more of total amount of stock. If not owned by a corporation, the names and addresses of the individual owners must be given. If owned by a partnership or other unincorporated firm, its name and address, as well as that of each individual must be given. If the publication is published by a nonprofit organization, its name and address must be stated.) (Item must be completed.)*

FULL NAME	COMPLETE MAILING ADDRESS
Marcel Dekker	41 Londonderry Dr. Greenwich, Ct.
Maurits Dekker	14 Stepping Stone Ln. Greenwich, Ct.
Rozetta Dekker	14 Stepping Stone Ln. Greenwich, Ct.
	zip code 06830

8. KNOWN BONDHOLDERS, MORTGAGEES, AND OTHER SECURITY HOLDERS OWNING OR HOLDING 1 PERCENT OR MORE OF TOTAL AMOUNT OF BONDS, MORTGAGES OR OTHER SECURITIES *(If there are none, so state)*

FULL NAME	COMPLETE MAILING ADDRESS

9. FOR COMPLETION BY NONPROFIT ORGANIZATIONS AUTHORIZED TO MAIL AT SPECIAL RATES *(Section 423.12 DMM only)*
The purpose, function, and nonprofit status of this organization and the exempt status for Federal income tax purposes *(Check one)*

☐ (1) HAS NOT CHANGED DURING PRECEDING 12 MONTHS
☐ (2) HAS CHANGED DURING PRECEDING 12 MONTHS
(If changed, publisher must submit explanation of change with this statement.)

10. EXTENT AND NATURE OF CIRCULATION *(See instructions on reverse side)*	AVERAGE NO. COPIES EACH ISSUE DURING PRECEDING 12 MONTHS	ACTUAL NO. COPIES OF SINGLE ISSUE PUBLISHED NEAREST TO FILING DATE
A. TOTAL NO. COPIES *(Net Press Run)*	1170	1125
B. PAID AND/OR REQUESTED CIRCULATION 1. Sales through dealers and carriers, street vendors and counter sales	0	0
2. Mail Subscription *(Paid and/or requested)*	862	815
C. TOTAL PAID AND/OR REQUESTED CIRCULATION *(Sum of 10B1 and 10B2)*	862	815
D. FREE DISTRIBUTION BY MAIL, CARRIER OR OTHER MEANS SAMPLES, COMPLIMENTARY, AND OTHER FREE COPIES	70	64
E. TOTAL DISTRIBUTION *(Sum of C and D)*	932	879
F. COPIES NOT DISTRIBUTED 1. Office use, left over, unaccounted, spoiled after printing	238	246
2. Return from News Agents	0	0
G. TOTAL *(Sum of E, F1 and 2—should equal net press run shown in A)*	1170	1125

11. **I certify that the statements made by me above are correct and complete**

SIGNATURE AND TITLE OF EDITOR, PUBLISHER, BUSINESS MANAGER, OR OWNER

Iris Accordino

PS Form 3526, July 1984

(See instruction on reverse)

INFORMATION FOR AUTHORS SUBMITTING MANUSCRIPTS

Send a clear double-spaced typewritten original and one duplicate to Ms. Nancy Reid-Rappolt, Editorial Assistant, *International Journal of the Addictions,* c/o Winch, Smith, Ostermann and Mates, MD's, 4141 Geary, Suite 326, San Francisco, California 94118. Also send one duplicate to the Chief Editor, Dr. Stanley Einstein, Building 113/41, East Talpiot, Jerusalem, Israel. DOUBLE-SPACE the entire manuscript; do not use single spacing anywhere, including references.

Include authors' academic degrees and present affiliation. If applicable, cite auspices under which work being reported was done. Specify address to which requests for reprints should be sent.

Begin your TITLE with a word useful in indexing. A 75- to 100-word ABSTRACT should be provided, which precedes each article. A summary is then not necessary. Major and minor headings may be used in the text; indicate major headings by typing in capitals.

Use METRIC UNITS of measure. If measurements were made in English units, give metric equivalents.

Cite all TABLES and FIGURES in the text. Tables should have titles, and figures should have brief legends. In tables, give each column a heading. Indicate units of measure in parentheses in the heading for each column. Do not use vertical rules. Do not use horizontal rules other than those in the heading and at the bottom. Submit PHOTOGRAPHS as glossy prints, untrimmed and unmounted; identify each with pencil lightly on the back and indicate top.

ARTWORK will not be returned unless specifically requested, and will be disposed of three months after publication.

REFERENCES in the text should be enclosed in parentheses and include the author's surname and the date of the item cited. Keep footnotes to a minimum. Footnotes should be collected at the end of the manuscript in their numerical order of appearance.

The BIBLIOGRAPHY (double-spaced) should be given at the end of the article in alphabetical order. Journal references should include authors, title, name of journal abbreviated according to *Chemical Abstracts List of Periodicals*, inclusive page numbers, and date. Book references should include authors, title, place of publication, publisher, and date.

AUTHOR RESPONSIBILITY: It is the sole responsibility of the author(s) to obtain written permission from the author(s), publisher(s), etc. for figures, tables, or any other information excerpted from previously published works which are used in the manuscript(s) considered for publication. It is understood that the manuscript(s) considered for publication in the *International Journal of the Addictions* have not been previously published nor are they under simultaneous publication consideration elsewhere.

Statements and opinions expressed in the articles and communications herein are those of the author(s) and do not necessarily express those of the Editor or publisher.

THE INTERNATIONAL JOURNAL OF THE ADDICTIONS

Volume 19 Number 6 1984

CONTENTS

Women and Alcohol Abuse—Factors Involved in Successful Interventions: S. D. Robinson 601

The Abstinence Phobias: Links between Substance Abuse and Anxiety: S. M. Hall 613

"Turning on" Other Persons to Drugs: H. L. Voss and R. R. Clayton 633

Alcohol Use among Graduate Business Administration Students: M. L. Waring, G. Petraglia, L. Cohen, and E. Busby 653

Can Personality Tests Predict Treatment Dropouts?: R. J. Craig 665

Symbolic Interaction Theory: A Perspective on Drug Abuse and Its Treatment: R. J. Battjes 675

Research Note

Individual Characteristics of Aggressive Beer and Distilled Beverage Drinkers: R. O. Pihl, M. Smith, and B. Farrell 689

Notes

Considering Motivation and Ability for Drug Use Intervention: Some Implications: S. Einstein 697

Outcome of Drug User Treatment: A Selection of Additional Needed Factors: S. Einstein 701

MARCEL DEKKER, INC., New York and Basel

CODEN: INJABN 19(7) i-ii, 709-826 (1984)
ISSN: 0020-773X

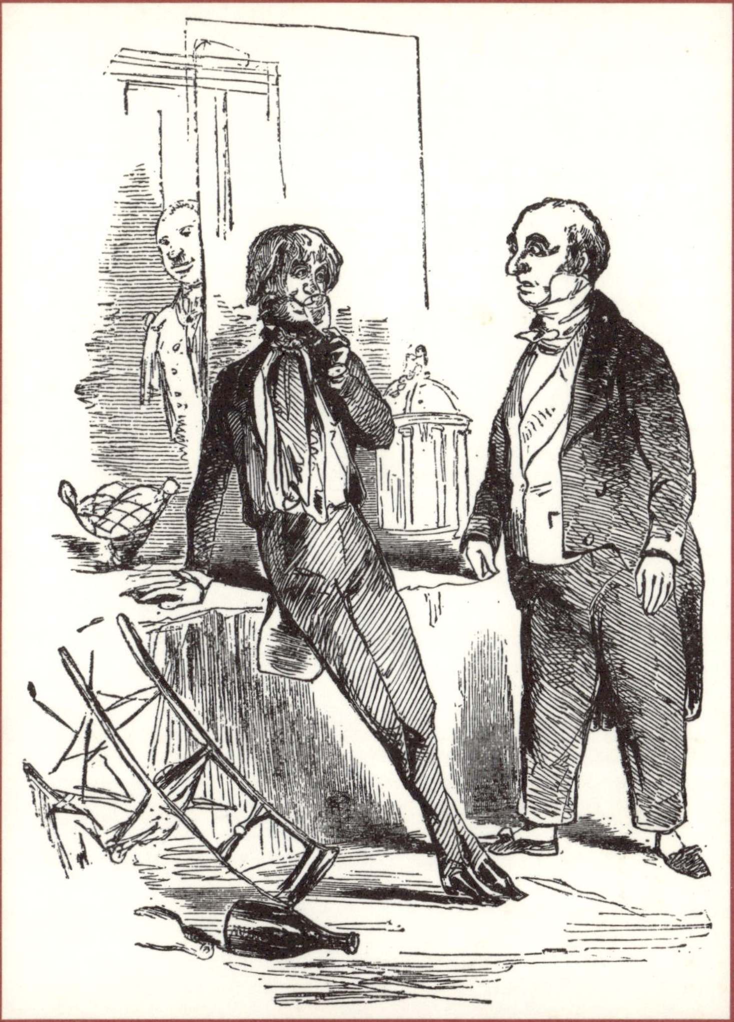

THE INTERNATIONAL JOURNAL OF THE Addictions

Volume 19 Number 7 1984

THE INTERNATIONAL JOURNAL
OF THE ADDICTIONS

November 1984

Aims and Scope. This journal is a comprehensive medium for worldwide communication among both concerned laymen and professionals in research, training, and treatment in the field of addiction and substance misuse.

Indexing and Abstracting Services. Articles published in *The International Journal of the Addictions* are selectively indexed or abstracted in:

• Abstracts Journal of the Institute of Scientific Information of the USSR Academy of Sciences • Adolescent Mental Health Abstracts • ASCA • Bibliographic Index of Health Education Periodicals (BIHEP) • BioSciences Information Service of Biological Abstracts (BIOSIS) • Classified Abstracts Archive of the Alcohol Literature • Current Awareness in Biological Sciences • Current Contents/Clinical Practice • Excerpta Medica • Index Medicus • International Pharmaceutical Abstracts • ISI/BIOMED • Psychological Abstracts • Science Citation Index • Selected List of Tables of Contents of Psychiatric Periodicals • Social Sciences Citation Index • State Central Scientific Medical Library/ International Book Exchange–USSR

Articles published in *The International Journal of the Addictions* are listed in Selected List of Tables of Contents of Psychiatric Periodicals.

Manuscript Preparation and Submission. See end of issue.

Subscription Information. *The International Journal of the Addictions* (ISSN: 0020-773X) is published eight times annually in February, April, May, July, August, September, November, and December by Marcel Dekker, Inc., 270 Madison Avenue, New York, New York 10016. The subscription rate for Volume 19 (1984), containing eight numbers, is $225.00 per volume (prepaid). The special discounted rate for individual professionals and students is $112.50 per volume. To secure this special rate, your order must be prepaid by personal check. Add $20.00 for surface postage outside the United States. For airmail to Europe, add $32.48; to Asia, add $40.48.

Mailing Address. *Please mail payment with order to:* Marcel Dekker Journals, P. O. Box 11305, Church Street Station, New York, New York 10249.

Contributions to this journal are published free of charge. Second-class postage paid at New York, New York and additional mailing offices. POSTMASTER: Send address changes to *The International Journal of the Addictions*, P. O. Box 5005, Cimarron Road, Monticello, New York 12701.

Library of Congress Catalog Card Number 66-9896

Cover illustration entitled: *The Mulligan and Mr. Perkins,* courtesy of the Picture Collection, The Branch Libraries, New York Public Library.

THE INTERNATIONAL JOURNAL OF THE Addictions

The International Journal of the Addictions, 19(7), 709–719, 1984

Adherence in a Behavioral Alcohol Treatment Program

Edward B. Fink,* MD

Section of Psychiatry and Human Behavior
Brown University, and
Day Hospital
Butler Hospital
Providence, Rhode Island 02906

Sandra Rudden, AB

Butler Hospital

Richard Longabaugh, EdD

Barbara McCrady, PhD

Robert Stout, PhD

Section of Psychiatry and Human Behavior
Brown University, and
Butler Hospital
Providence, Rhode Island 02906

Abstract

This report examines the correlates of early treatment termination by patients being treated for alcohol abuse or dependence. All of the study subjects were participants in a controlled experimental investigation of the differences in clinical outcome and treatment cost of extended inpatient and partial hospital treatment. A large number of

*To whom requests for reprints should be addressed: Chief, Day Hospital, Butler Hospital, 345 Blackstone Boulevard, Providence, Rhode Island 02906.

 0020-773X/84/1907-0709$3.50/0

clinical variables demonstrated no difference between groups, except for the greater likelihood of a DSM III Axis I diagnosis of alcohol abuse or dependence in the treatment completers. In contrast, three of four system variables differentiated completers from noncompleters. Patients treated by hospital-employed psychiatrists, in contrast to private psychiatrists, were more likely to complete the program; 4 sequential months in the middle phase of the study were associated with noncompletion of treatment; and patients who were detoxified on the preferentially designated unit were more likely to receive some specialized alcohol treatment. The authors interpret these data to indicate that treatment adherence is influenced by factors affecting the cohesiveness of the treatment delivery system. The failure of patient characteristic variables to predict treatment adherence may well be a result of their comparative insignificance in relation to system variables.

Nonadherence with recommended treatment is one of the most common problems in alcohol treatment delivery, with nonadherence rates of 52-75% in outpatient treatment and 14-39% in inpatient treatment (Baekelund and Lundwall, 1975). In spite of the research efforts of numerous investigators, the problems of nonadherence with recommended treatment is still poorly understood. In their comprehensive review, Baekelund and Lundwall (1975) summarized data which relate early dropout to: (1) younger age, earlier onset of alcoholism, and martial instability; (2) personality characteristics such as hostility, immaturity, decreased self-esteem, and social dependency; (3) more advanced stage of alcoholism, accompanied by passive-aggressive and psychopathic features, dependency on alcohol for relief from feelings of resentment, anxiety or depression, and difficulty forming close relationships; (4) lower socioeconomic status; (5) social isolation; (6) referral by other institutions, as opposed to self-referral; and (7) refusal to accept disulfiram treatment. They concluded, however, that alcohol abusers who prematurely terminate treatment are heterogeneous in their clinical characteristics and vary widely from one report to another. This conclusion has been reiterated more recently by others (Franklin, 1980; Smart and Gray, 1978).

The goal of this report is to examine correlates of treatment adherence in a behavioral alcohol treatment program. These include detailed parameters of patient characteristics and a separate set of treatment system variables. There is particular interest in the latter since they are not emphasized in previous papers.

METHOD

Subjects

All of the study subjects were participants in a controlled investigation of the differences in clinical outcome and treatment costs of extended inpatient and partial hospital treatment of alcohol abuse or dependence. Table 1 details the sociodemographic and clinical characteristics of the sample. All patients had been admitted to the inpatient service of a university-affiliated psychiatric hospital for detoxification or intensive hospital treatment. The average age of patients was 41 years. Two-thirds were males. Their drinking histories indicated

Table 1

Description of Study Sample

		%	Mean	SD
I.	Sociodemographic characteristics			
	Age (mean)	–	41.48	11.84
	Sex (% male)	68.2		
	Education ⩾ 12 yr	63.8		
	Ever married	81.2		
	Living with spouse	47.3		
	Living alone	24.1		
II.	Ethnic background			
	White	96.5		
	Black	3.0		
	Other	0.5		
III.	Vocational status			
	Full-time employment	63.1		
	Part-time employment	4.5		
	Housewife	11.1		
	No job	11.6		
	Retired, disabled, other	9.7		
IV.	Drinking measures			
	ETOH diagnosis	92.1		
	ETOH diagnosis or problem list	100.0		
	Prior ETOH-related hospitalizations	59.1		
	Prior Alcoholics Anonymous attendance	28.8		
	Prior use of other outpatient services	34.8		
	MAST		30.18	5.63
	Alcoholism Impairment Index		16.97	7.36
	Quantity-Frequency Index		8.11	7.58
	Days abstinent (past 180 days)		41.15	6.15
	Days with six drinks of more (past 180 days)		82.28	22.88
	Years drinking		16.53	11.87
	Global Assessment Scale		48.39	7.05

severe impairment. Average alcoholism screening score on the Michigan Alcoholism Screening Test (Selzer, 1971) was 30.18; and on the Quantity-Frequency Index (Cahalan et al., 1969) for the month prior to admission it was 8.11, or an average of over 16 standard drinks per day. Within the 6 months prior to treatment, their longest average period of abstinence was slightly more than a month. They reported an average of 16.53 years of prior drinking, and 59% reported one or more prior alcohol-related hospitalizations.

Despite their severe alcohol abuse, most patients were otherwise still fairly intact and functioning. Three-quarters had either a full-time job or were students or housewives. For 70% their primary income was earned. Sixty-four percent had completed high school. Eighty-one percent had been married at least once, and 47% were currently living with their spouses. Their residential status was stable as only 22% moved once or more in the 6 months prior to treatment.

Procedures

During a 14-month period, beginning February 1979, 260 patients admitted to the hospital met the screening criteria for the study. If they signed informed consent, comprehensive baseline data were collected (Longabaugh et al., 1983). These variables describe patient clinical characteristics in the five categories suggested by Pattison (1976), namely: Drinking Measures, Emotional Health, Interpersonal Health, Vocational Health, and Physical Health. Specific items are listed in Table 2.

All subjects received 1 week of detoxification and comprehensive medical and psychiatric assessment, and treatment on one of four inpatient units, after which those who had agreed to randomization were transferred to the specialized treatment program. Patients in both the partial hospital and extended inpatient experimental groups participated in the same alcohol treatment program, located in the partial hospital. Based upon a social learning model of alcohol abuse, treatment components included group sessions teaching behavioral analysis and behavior change skills and the application of these skills to the patients' individual life situations, goal-setting meetings, patient and family member education sessions, modeling of successful abstinence by volunteers who previously had serious drinking problems, and social skills training. Eighty percent of patients had family members or close friends involved in weekly multiple family group sessions and individual family sessions. Patients in the extended inpatient group returned to their 24-hour unit for nights and weekends.

The treatment staff consisted of two PhD-level psychologists, one psychiatrist, two registered nurses, two nursing assistants, and one master's-level social worker. All of these staff members were full time; five were females and three were males; the mean age was 29 years (range: 25-38 yr); three were married,

Table 2

Patient Characteristic Variables Used in Baseline Assessment

I.	Drinking measures[a]
	Alcohol Impairment Index (last 30 days) (Armor et al., 1976)
	Quantity-Frequency Alcohol Index (last 30 days) (Cahalan et al., 1969)
	Number of years drinking
	Frequency of days having 1-2 mixed drinks (last 30 days)
	Frequency of days having 3-6 mixed drinks (last 30 days)
	Frequency of days having more than 6 mixed drinks (last 30 days)
	Previous arrests (ever)
	Percentage of abstinent days
	Previous hospitalizations for alcohol problems (ever)
	Readmission frequency for alcohol problems (last year)
	Occurrence of alcohol-related offenses
	Occurrence of alcohol-related hospitalizations
	Previous noncompletion of treatment (last year)
	Primary diagnosis: alcohol related (index admission)
	Secondary diagnosis: alcohol related (index admission)
II.	Emotional health[a]
	Psychosocial Functioning Inventory (Feragne et al., 1983)
	Positive affect
	Negative affect
	Life satisfaction
	Subjective well-being
	Presence of recent stressful events
	Presence of a dysphoric mood
	Primary diagnosis: non-alcohol related (index admission)
	Secondary diagnosis: non-alcohol related (index admission)
	Global Assessment Scale (index admission) (Hargreaves and Fulwiler, 1977)
III.	Interpersonal health[a]
	Marital status (current)
	Education (yr)
	Living alone
	Psychosocial Functioning Inventory (Feragne et al., 1983)
	Spouse role
	Parent role
	Housemate/roommate role
	Subjective role performance
	Social role performance
	Social role satisfaction
	Summary role functioning
IV.	Vocational health
	Full- or part-time employment
	Current vocational status
	Number of days holding a job
	Job lost due to drinking
V.	Physical health
	Presence of medical problems/diagnosis
VI.	Other sociodemographic variables
	Age
	Sex

[a] Last 6 months unless otherwise indicated.

two were single, three were divorced. In addition, at any one time two or three recovered alcoholics worked as volunteers from 20 to 30 hours/week. They had a mean age of 58 years (range: 39-68 yr) and included five males and one female during the 14-month study period. All of the professional staff (PhD, MD, RN, and MSW) had considerable experience working with alcoholics prior to beginning the study (range: PhD, 5-7 yr; MSW, 1-2 yr). All staff members were screened prior to employment by the project chief (B.M.) to assure that their attitudes toward drinking and alcoholics were appropriate to their job descriptions and consistent with the project's treatment goal of abstinence.

At various phases of treatment, some subjects prematurely terminated their participation. They were categorized as treatment "completers" (completed detoxification and the behavioral treatment program) or "noncompleters." The length of stay for completion of the behavioral treatment program is determined for each patient by the treatment team after consideration of the patient's individual clinical characteristics and his/her family and vocational situations. The median stay for completers is 12 days, with a range of 6 to 21 days. The "noncompleters" included: (1) patients who met criteria for admission into the study but did not agree to randomization to the behavioral treatment program ($N = 62$), (2) patients who initially agreed to randomization but left treatment immediately after detoxification ($N = 24$), and (3) patients who attended the behavioral treatment program for less than 5 days ($N = 19$).

Measures

The 41 patient variables collected at baseline assessment are recorded in Table 2. In addition, four treatment system variables were measured. These included: (1) Admitting Psychiatrist and (2) Treating Psychiatrist: Patients are admitted to the hospital by either a full-time salaried hospital psychiatrist or a private attending psychiatrist. Each patient then is assigned in rotation to be treated by either a salaried hospital psychiatrist or a private attending psychiatrist. These two variables, Admitting Psychiatrist and Treating Psychiatrist, were assessed because of the strong administrative support that the hospital's medical director provided for this clinical research program. It was expected that the clinical practice of the hospital-employed psychiatrists, with regard to their recognition of alcohol disorders and their individual support of the behavioral treatment program, would be greater than that of the private psychiatric attendings. (3) Admission Date: The month of admission (viz.: early, middle, or late in the study period) was assessed. Since patient participation in a research study may be affected by staff effectiveness, and since the latter may change over time, patient acceptance of treatment may relate to the time in the course of study when he/she was admitted. (4) Treatment Unit Assignment: The possible detoxification setting for a given patient included one of four inpatient units. One unit had been designated at the beginning of the study to serve preferentially for the detoxification of most patients, with overflow patients assigned to one of the other three units. Staff on the designated unit, in contrast to staff on the other three units, maintained a systematic liaison with the specialized alcoholism treatment program staff and received more staff education regarding the treatment of alcohol abusers. Therefore, initial patient assignment to the specific detoxification unit was recorded in order to test its effect upon patient acceptance of the postdetoxification specialized behavioral treatment program.

RESULTS

Patient Variables

Of all the sociodemographic, clinical, and historical variables listed in Table 2, only diagnostic assignment separated completers from noncompleters. Chi square with Yates correction was used with all nominal measures; Student's *t* (two-tailed and pooled variance where appropriate) was used on all continuous variables. Table 3 reveals that completers ($N = 153$) were more likely to have a DSM-III Axis I diagnosis of alcohol abuse or dependence (American Psychiatric Association, 1980), in contrast to noncompleters ($N = 105$) ($\chi^2 = 19.08$, $df = 1$, $p < .001$). The latter more often had an Axis I primary or secondary diagnosis of affective disorder. None of the other 40 variables in Table 2 separated the completers from noncompleters.

System Variables

Three of the four system variables significantly differentiated completers from noncompleters.

Table 3

Alcohol Abuse or Dependence: DSM-III Axis I Diagnosis for Completers and Noncompleters (N = 258)

	Completers		Noncompleters	
	N	%	*N*	%
Alcohol diagnosis (Axis I)	134	66	68[a]	34
No alcohol diagnosis (Axis I)	19	34	37	66
Totals	153		105	

χ^2 (1 *df*) = 19.08, $p < .001$

[a]Missing data for two subjects.

Table 4

Treating Psychiatrist for Completers and Noncompleters (N = 258)

	Completers		Noncompleters	
	N	%	*N*	%
Salaried	93[a]	65	50	35
Private	60	52	55	48
Totals	153		105	

χ^2 (1 *df*) = 4.37, $p < .05$

[a]Missing data for two subjects.

Table 5

Admission Date for Completers and Noncompleters (N = 260)

	Completers		Noncompleters	
	N	%	*N*	%
Early	68	63	40	37
Middle	24	44	30	56
Late	63	64	35	36
Totals	155		105	

χ^2 (2 *df*) = 6.57, $p < .05$

Table 6

Mean Number of Days in Preferred Detoxification Unit and Receipt of Specialized Alcohol Treatment

	Treatment recipients (*N* = 172)	No treatment (*N* = 86)
Mean days on preferred unit	3.90	2.78

t (256 *df*) = 2.34, $p < .05$

1. Treating Psychiatrist (Table 4): Patients treated by salaried hospital psychiatrists, in contrast to private psychiatrists, were more likely to complete the program ($\chi^2 = 4.37, df = 1, p < .05$). There were no differences between the clinical practice of salaried psychiatrists and that of private psychiatrists regarding time spent with patients, frequency or length of team meetings, or billing procedures. As discussed later, however, we expect that there was a difference between these two groups of treating psychiatrists regarding their identification with the project's goals.
2. Admission Date (Table 5): Four sequential months in the middle phase of the study (viz.: June, July, August, and September) were associated with noncompletion of treatment ($\chi^2 = 6.57, df = 2, p < .05$).
3. Treatment Unit Assignment (Table 6): Patients who received some specialized alcohol treatment were more likely to have been detoxified on the preferentially designated unit ($t = 2.34, df = 256, p < .05$).

DISCUSSION AND SUMMARY

Treatment dropout or nonadherence represents a significant problem in health care delivery. As part of a larger study comparing the clinical and cost effectiveness of extended inpatient and partial hospital treatment of alcohol abuse or dependence, the current report focuses on the correlates of early termination of treatment. A large number of clinical variables demonstrated no difference between the groups, except for the greater likelihood of a primary or secondary DSM-III Axis I diagnosis of alcohol abuse or dependence in the treatment completers. These findings are consistent with Smart and Gray (1978), who failed to find significant relationships between early dropout and social stability, marital stability, resources, and social isolation using multivariate analysis.

In contrast, three out of four system variables revealed significant differences between treatment completers and noncompleters. The former were more likely to be treated by full-time hospital-employed psychiatrists, in contrast to private attending psychiatrists. They also were more likely to be detoxified on the specifically designated inpatient unit which maintained a stronger liaison with the alcoholism treatment program staff. Patients admitted during the middle months of the data collection period, which occurred during the summer, were more likely to be noncompleters.

Our interpretation as to why these three system variables should all be related to treatment adherence is that each is a measure of the cohesiveness in the hospital system. First, the hospital's medical director was strongly supportive of the research project. Salaried psychiatrists directly or indirectly reported to him. Therefore, they would be more influenced by his attitude than would treating psychiatrists who were in private practice. We believe that they conveyed this expectation that patients would participate in the research to the patients themselves.

Second, although patients treated on either the primary detoxification unit or one of the overflow units were randomly assigned to one of the two experimental groups, patients on the primary unit at any one time constituted a group of four to eight patients to be treated in the research program. The large majority of them wanted continued treatment, and it is likely that they supported one another's participation. Moreover, the nursing staff of the primary unit were more experienced in dealing with the alcohol abuser and the alcohol treatment program and therefore more likely to have the skills and attitudes which would foster patient participation in the research program. Group support, by both staff and patients, is a factor which we feel has significant impact upon research participation (Fink et al., 1977).

Finally, the period of highest rejection of the program coincided with the summer months when the greatest number of new staff were present in the hospital. New rotations among psychiatry residents and psychology interns began at this time. In addition, as a vacation period, more of the experienced nursing staff were more often away. This left the units staffed by a greater percentage of new staff who were not as well integrated into the system or not as reflective of the values of system members.

No doubt there could be other interpretations of these findings. What is most striking is that only 1 of 41 patient characteristic variables separated completers from noncompleters. Three out of four treatment system variables, on the other hand, all were consistent with each other and lend support to the hypothesis that treatment adherence was influenced by factors affecting the cohesiveness of the treatment delivery system.

Future research might explore system variables more objectively. For example, assessment of staff members of all disciplines regarding their attitudes toward each patient and the rationale for specific treatment goals could be included. We have suggested that differences between the private psychiatrists and salaried hospital psychiatrists regarding their attitude toward and commitment to the institutional project goals influenced our findings. Specific measures of these variables, however, were not included in this study. Likewise, we believe that differences in staff knowledge regarding alcoholism and inpatient management skills influenced treatment adherence, but these variables were not objectively assessed.

Of further interest is whether nonadherence at the time of the index hospitalization has any relationship to the use of outpatient aftercare or rehospitalization rates and other clinical outcome measures. Also, how would a patient's score on such measures be related to the system variables discussed here and to the knowledge, skills, and attitudes of the treating staff? Several of these questions regarding clinical outcome are being addressed in the analysis of the 24-month outcome data which is now in progress.

It appears to us that if system variables continue to be ignored by clinical investigators, we are likely to be further frustrated in our ability to understand why some patients complete treatment and others do not. The failure of patient characteristic variables to predict treatment adherence may well be a result of their comparative insignificance in relation to system variables.

REFERENCES

AMERICAN PSYCHIATRIC ASSOCIATION. *Diagnostic and Statstical Manual of Mental Disorders,* 3rd ed. Washington, DC: APA, 1980.

ARMOR, D.J., POLICH, J.M., and HAMBREL, H.B. *Alcoholism and Treatment.* Santa Monica, CA: The Rand Corporation, 1976.

BAEKELUND, F., and LUNDWALL, L. Dropping out of treatment: A critical review. *Psychol. Bull.* 82: 738, 783, 1975.

CAHALAN, D., CISIN, I., and CROSSLEY, H. *American Drinking Practices: A National Study of Drinking Behavior and Patterns.* New Brunswick, NJ: Rutgers Center for Alcohol Studies, 1969.

FERAGNE, M., LONGABAUGH, R., and STEVENSON, J. The Psychosocial Functioning Inventory. *Evaluation Health Professions* 6: 25-48, 1983.

FINK, E.B., CARPENTER, W.T., Jr., SACHS, M.H., and LANGSNER, C.A. Testability and group phenomenon in schizophrenia. *Comp. Psychiatry* 18: 23-29, 1977.

FRANKLIN, J.L. *Durability of treatment: A three stage cohort study of 260 alcoholic clients.* Paper presented at the Evaluation Research Society, Annual Meeting, Arlington, Virginia, November 1980.

HARGREAVES, W., and FULWILER, R. *A Global Assessment Scale for Substance Abusers.* San Francisco, CA: University of California at San Francisco, Langley Porter Neuropsychiatric Institute, 1977.

LONGABAUGH, R., MC CRADY, B., FINK, E., STOUT, R., MC CAULEY, T., and MC NEILL, D. Cost effectiveness of alcohol treatment in partial vs. inpatient settings: Six-month outcomes. *J. Stud. Alcohol* 44: 1049-1071, 1983.

PATTISON, E.M. A conceptual approach to alcoholism treatment goals. *Addict. Behav.* 1: 177-192, 1976.

SELZER, M.L. The Michigan Alcoholism Screening Test: The quest for a new diagnostic instrument. *Am. J. Psychiatry* 127: 1653-1658, 1971.

SMART, R.G., and GRAY, G. Multiple predictors of dropout from alcoholism treatment. *Arch. Gen. Psychiatry* 35: 363-367, 1978.

The International Journal of the Addictions, 19(7), 721–741, 1984

Alcohol Education Programs for University Students: A Review of Their Effectiveness

Michael S. Goodstadt, PhD

Anuppa Caleekal-John, MSc

Education Research Section
Addiction Research Foundation
Toronto, Ontario
Canada M5S 2S1

Abstract

A review of the experimental evidence concerning the effectiveness of 14 alcohol education programs for university students suggests that such programs, in spite of weaknesses in their experimental evaluation, offer the promise of significant impact on college students' reported alcohol-related behavior, as well as on their attitudes and knowledge. Programs are more likely to be effective if they include field (or laboratory) experience, as well as factual and experiential strategies, and if they occur over an extended period of time.

A very large number of education programs and activities have been undertaken on university campuses with the objective of preventing or ameliorating problems arising from alcohol abuse (Kraft, 1979). This has been especially true in the United States where, for example, the NIAAA "50+ Project" conducted an alcohol information program during 1974-1975 in 63 selected colleges across the United States, with participants from one university in each state, plus 12 private schools. Aims of the project were (1) to gather information regarding drinking practices and attitudes on campus; (2) to disseminate information

 0020-773X/84/1907-0721$3.50/0

about alcohol, alcohol use, and alcohol abuse; (3) to encourage universities to address the issue of alcohol use and abuse in the form of educational communication efforts. A follow-up conducted by Kraft (1977) found that the "50+ Project" stimulated alcohol abuse prevention programming in 81% of the participating universities. Activities involved at various campuses included information-sharing approaches, individual attitude/behavior change approaches, staff-training approaches, changing normative behaviors, institutional change approaches, and intervention approaches for problem drinkers. Follow-up activities and programs have been developed in many of the universities and colleges. These developments (American Alliance for Health, Physical Education, and Recreation, 1978) have included the following: (1) alcohol awareness activities, (2) alcohol education courses and workshops, (3) supervisory training functions, (4) counseling and referral, (5) program development and consultation, and (6) research and evaluation. Guidelines for the development of campus alcohol progams have been proposed (in addition to programs reviewed later in this section, see also Filstead et al., 1976; Mills et al., 1981; Snyder, 1980).

Donovan (1979, 1981) describes the development of a campus education/prevention/treatment forum at Brown University, Rhode Island (U.S.). The Brown Group on Alcohol consisted of faculty, students, and non-university members who had an interest in the formation of an alcohol interest group. Their activities ranged from information dissemination on a variety of topics related to the proper use of alcohol, to institutional policy making. Awareness campaigns were held by the group using films, posters, pamphlets, and speakers on alcoholism. Peer-counseling procedures were developed by the group, and a list of alternative forthcoming activities which were unassociated with alcohol was made available to students. Arrangements were made with the local Alcoholics Anonymous and Al-Anon organizations to organize a treatment group and the Brown Group of Alcoholics Anonymous.

The Rutgers University Committee on Use of Alcohol has also been engaged in activities similar to the Brown Group on Alcohol (Crossman, 1981). A recent report concerned with university policy change regarding alcohol use was submitted by the Rutgers Committee (1981); this recommended a student assistance program similar to employee assistance programs in industry, as well as institutional policy changes which would have a direct effect on changing the university environment to encourage appropriate use of alcohol on campus. Institutional policy recommendations included such items as steps to improve pub management by provision of recommended alternative nonalcoholic beverages and food, and the encouragement of self-regulation of "appropriate" rules regarding alcohol use for specific groups (residence halls, fraternities, sororities, clubs, and organizations).

A review of the literature has identified 14 studies (other then those involving programs for medical students—see later discussion) that have experimentally assessed the impact of a definable campus-based alcohol education program (see Tables 2-4 for summary of studies). The outcome of this research is synthesized in this paper; special attention is given to (1) study design characteristics and (2) experimental findings of the 14 studies.

EXPERIMENTAL EVALUATIONS OF CAMPUS-BASED ALCOHOL EDUCATION PROGRAMS

Theoretical Frameworks

In alcohol education, we are concerned with individual learning that brings about, or is required for, behavior whose ultimate effects will be a change in (1) personal development and (2) social relationships, and/or (3) eventual environmental modification. A family of models pervasive in such health education in general, and in alcohol education on campuses in particular, involve the expected relationships between changes in knowledge, attitudes, and behaviors.

In discussing knowledge-attitude-behavior models and their relationships to alcohol education, one can conceptualize them either as concerned with the *process* of alcohol education or as concerned with the *outcomes* of alcohol education (or concerned with both) (see Table 1). In either case, the three domains involved are the cognitive (e.g., knowledge), the affective (e.g., attitude), and the psychomotor (e.g., behavior). Change can occur either in or through any or all of these domains. Various submodels of the general knowledge-attitude-behavior change model include: (1) knowledge change leads to behavior change; (2) attitude change leads to behavior change; (3) knowledge change leads to attitude change, which, in turn, leads to behavioral change; and (4) behavioral change leads to attitudinal change, which, in turn, reinforces or produces further behavioral change.

The majority of the 14 campus-based alcohol programs reviewed here have espoused some version of the knowledge-attitude-behavior change model.

The problem for alcohol education in using these models lies in determining the relationships that exist between knowledge, attitude, and behavior change, and how these, in turn, are related to alcohol use (Gonzalez, 1978; Goodstadt, 1978).

Program Characteristics

As indicated in Table 2, the majority (12) of the 14 studies included some factual input in the form of lectures. The majority of studies (nine), in addition, have incorporated affective activities (e.g., values clarification) in some of the experimental groups (Dennison, 1977; Dennison and Prevet, 1980; Dennison et al., 1977; Engs, 1977; Gonzalez, 1980; Robinson, 1981; Rozelle, 1980; Rozelle and Gonzalez, 1979; Serdahely and Behunin, 1977). Field activities

Table 1

Scheme of Outcome and Process Variables in Alcohol Education Programming

	Outcome variables		
	Cognitive outcomes	Affective outcomes	Behavioral outcomes
Outcome criteria			
Increase in . . .	Correct information Awareness Understanding Acceptance, etc., re. alcohol, alcohol use, users, abusers, alcohol policies, etc.	Responsible attitudes Health-oriented values Aware of dissonance between values/attitudes and behaviors, etc., re. alcohol, alcohol use, users, abusers, policies, etc.	Responsible use Healthy alternatives Discussions re. alcohol Early identification Decision-making skills re. alcohol, alcohol use, users, abusers, policies, etc.
Decrease in . . .	Incorrect information Absence of information Etc.	Irresponsible attitudes Health-risky values Inaccurate stereotypes Etc.	Consumption (frequency/quantity) Irresponsible use Trend toward increased use Negative support behaviors Etc.

	Process variables[a]		
	Cognitive change	Affective change	Behavioral change
Process alternatives			
I	I_{cog} ⟶	⟶	⟶ O_{behav}
II.		I_{aff} ⟶	⟶ O_{behav}
III	I_{cog} ⟶	⟶ O_{aff} ⟶ I_{aff} ⟶	⟶ O_{behav}
IV		O_{aff} ⟵ ↓ I_{aff} ⟶	⟵ I_{behav} ⟶ O_{behav}

[a] I, input; O, outcome; cog, cognitive; aff, affective; behav, behavioral.

Table 2

College-Based Alcohol Education Program Evaluations: Program Characteristics

Study no.	Author(s)	Date of publication	Program description	Program intensity	Sample: Population	Sample: Sample size
1	Robinson	1981	Exp. 1: Lecture + explicit conclusions and recommendations Exp. 2: Lecture Exp. 3: Lecture + values clarification exercises Control: No treatment	2 h/wk for 2 wk = 4 h	Health class students	200
2	Rozelle and Gonzalez	1979	Exp. 1: Lecture + content-oriented discussion group Exp. 2: Lecture + experiential group Control: No treatment	2 h/wk for 10 wk = 20 h	Responsible Alternatives to Alcohol Abuse enrollees	41
3	Rozelle	1980	Exp. 1: Lecture + content-oriented discussion group Exp. 2: Lecture + experiential group Control: No treatment	2 h/wk for 10 wk = 20 h	Responsible Alternatives to Alcohol Abuse enrollees	144
4	Gonzalez	1980	Lecture, etc. + discussion and brainstorming	Single session of 4 h	Education Research program re. topics such as drinking and motivation; volunteers from university courses	126

(continued)

Table 2 (continued)

Study no.	Author(s)	Date of publication	Program description	Program intensity	Sample: Population	Sample: Sample size
5	Portnoy	1980	Lecture based on Health Belief Model and Communication Strategies	3 meetings in 1 wk; total 3 h, 20 min	Education students in Health Ed. course	276
6	Dennison et al.	1977	Exp. 1: Cognitive (lecture) + affective (e.g., values clarification) + field activities Exp. 2: (Control) cognitive + affective, no field activities	5 wk	Health Education course students	60
7	Dennison and Prevet	1980	Exp. 1: Cognitive (lecture) + affective (e.g., values clarification) + field activities Exp. 2: (Control) cognitive + affective no field activities	5 wk	Health Education course students	53
8	Sorgen	1979	Attended Alcoholism Rehabilitation Centre	10 days = 80 h	3rd-year student nurses (Canada)	63
9	Engs	1977	Film + values clarification exercises + discussion	Single session; 2-3 h	Education Research Program re. topics such as drinking and human sexuality; volunteers from university residence	83

10	Waring	1980	Cognitive + field trips	3 h/wk for 12 wk = 36 h	Alcoholism Seminar – human services students	103
11	Serdahely and Behunin	1977	Exp. 1: Lecture + discussion re. drugs Exp. 2: Lecture + values clarification + group discussions + peer-led classes re. drugs	Unknown	Drugs, Alcohol, and Tobacco course: 2 sections	143
12	Dennison	1977	Exp. 1: Cognitive (lecture) + affective (e.g., values clarification) + field activities Exp. 2: (Control) cognitive + affective, no field activities	12-15 h in classroom	Health Science course students	91
13	Serdahely	1980	Factual pharmacological approach to drug education	Unknown	Drugs, Alcohol and Tobacco course: 2 sections	41
14	Caleekal-John	1984	Interdisciplinary cognitive, including lectures, film, discussions, etc.	5 h/wk for 2 wk = 10 h	Physiology course	17

Table 3

College-Based Alcohol Education Program Evaluations: Experimental Design Characteristics

		Experimental design					Dependent variables		
Study no.	Author(s)	Experimental/control conditions	Randomization	Pretest	Posttest	Follow-up	Knowledge	Attitudes	Behavior
1	Robinson	3 Exp. conditions and 1 Control condition	None	√	√	3 mo	√	√	√
2	Rozelle and Gonzalez	2 Exp. conditions and 1 Control condition	Random assignment to 2 Exp. conditions; random selection of students from other course for Control condition	√	√	–	√	√	√
3	Rozelle	2 Exp. conditions and 1 Control condition	Random assignment to 2 Exp. conditions; random selection of students from other course for Control condition	√	√	3 mo	√	√	√
4	Gonzalez	1 Exp. and 1 Control condition	Random assignment to Exp. or Control	√	√	3 mo	√	√	√

5	Portnoy	Solomon 4-groups design (1 Exp.; 1 Control condition)	Random assignment to 4 groups (?)	√	√	6 wk	√	√	√
6	Dennison et al.	1 Exp.; 1 Control condition	Random assignment of 4 courses to Exp. or Control condition	√	√	1 mo	–	–	√
7	Dennison and Prevet	1 Exp.; 1 Control condition	Random assignment to Exp. or Control condition	√	√	1 mo	–	–	√
8	Sorgen	1 Exp.; 1 Control condition	None	√	√	–	√	√	–
9	Engs	1 Exp.; 1 Control condition	Assigned (randomly?) to Exp. or Control	√	√	3 mo	√	–	√
10	Waring	1 Exp.; 1 Control condition	None	√	√	–	√	√	√
11	Serdahely and Behunin	2 Exp. conditions	None	√	√	–	–	–	√
12	Dennison	1 Exp. and 1 Control condition (2 Exp. conditions)	Random assignment of 4 courses to Exp. or Control condition	√	√	–	–	–	√
13	Serdahely	1 Exp. condition	None	√	√	–	–	–	√
14	Caleekal-John	1 Exp. condition	None	√	√	1 mo	√	√	√

and experiences have been employed in eight studies (Dennison, 1977; Dennison and Prevet, 1980; Dennison et al., 1977; Gonzalez, 1980; Rozelle, 1980; Rozelle and Gonzalez, 1979; Sorgen, 1979; Waring, 1980). Three studies have compared alternative approaches to alcohol education; for example, an emphasis on experiential learning versus cognitively oriented small group discussions (Robinson, 1981; Rozelle, 1980; Rozelle and Gonzalez, 1979).

The majority of programs have extended over many weeks, with several hours of involvement per week. Two studies (Serdahely, 1980; Serdahely and Behunin, 1977) focused on drugs in general, rather than on alcohol exclusively.

Experimental Designs

The 14 studies were classified according to their experimental design into one of four groups (see Table 3):

Design A: More than one experimental condition and one control condition
Design B: One experimental and one control condition
Design C: Two experimental conditions and no control condition
Design D: No control condition; one experimental condition

Design D was considered to lack the minimum requirements for sound experimental design, since it included no control or comparison groups. Two studies compared two experimental approaches without a no-treatment control condition—allowing for a comparison between the relative effectiveness of the two approaches but unable to determine whether the experimental approaches were better than nothing. As can be seen from Table 3, half (i.e., seven) of the studies employed a single comparison between one experimental condition and one no-program comparison group. Finally, two studies compared two experimental approaches to each other and to a nontreatment control. It can also be seen from Table 3 that no study used random procedures to select the experimental groups—that is, all experimental groups were "availability" samples; only one study randomly selected a control group (from among possible control groups); eight studies (of the 11 studies employing control groups) randomly assigned groups (although frequently only two groups) to either experimental or control condition. These latter eight studies, therefore, come closest to including an acceptable experimental design.

Measures of Program Impact

Knowledge

Nine studies of the 14 studies reviewed attempted to bring about change in individuals' knowledge levels regarding the effects of alcohol on the body. One of the 14 studies attempted to bring about change in individuals' knowledge levels regarding alcoholism and alcoholics (Sorgen, 1979).

Attitudes

Seven studies focused on attitudinal change regarding responsible personal use of alcohol. One of the 14 studies attempted to bring about attitudinal change among the subjects regarding alcoholics and alcoholism (Sorgen, 1979).

Behavior

Of the 14 studies reviewed, 13 studies were specifically concerned with self-reported behavioral change regarding alcohol use. The studies employed indicators of the consequences of alcohol use occurring in various domains of student life (e.g., physical consequences, vomiting; educational consequences, missing classes due to hangover; legal consequences, DWI; and psychosocial consequences, disruptive behavior). Two of the 14 studies reviewed measured behavioral change regarding drug use among college students, including alcohol (Serdahely, 1980; Serdahely and Behunin, 1977). One of the 14 studies measured behavioral intention rather than behavioral change regarding alcohol use (Portnoy, 1980).

All studies employed at least preprogram and immediate postprogram measure of program impact; the majority of studies (i.e., eight) also employed longer-term postprogram follow-ups, ranging from approximately 1 month to 3 months (see Table 3).

Although the evidence concerning college-based alcohol education programs is not extensive, there are sufficient experimental studies to begin to assess the potential of such programs. It should be emphasized, however: (1) that none of the studies is without problems in research design and/or analysis and (2) that 6 of the 14 studies have emanated from two sources, namely the University of Florida Alcohol Abuse Prevention Program (Rozelle and Gonzalez) and the SUNY (Buffalo) Alcohol Instructional Model (Dennison et al.).

Impact of Experimental Programs

Knowledge, Attitudes, and Behavioral Change

Six studies attempted to achieve changes in each of the knowledge, attitude, and behavior domains, and also possessed both experimental and control groups. Four of these six studies were successful in achieving their three-part objective to at least some degree (Robinson 1981; Rozelle, 1980; Rozelle and Gonzalez, 1979; Waring, 1980). (See Table 4 for summary of findings.)

Table 4

College-Based Alcohol Education Program Evaluations: Program Impact

Study no.	Author(s)	Results: Knowledge	Results: Attitudes	Results: Behaviors
1	Robinson	Exp. 1: > Control at post (and follow-up?) Exp. 2: > Control at post Exp. 3: > Control at post	Some evidence that Explicit Instructions improved on some measures; that Implicit Instruction deteriorated on one measure	1. > Control at post 2. NS 3. NS No differences between Exp. conditions
2	Rozelle and Gonzalez	Exp. 1: Improved pre-post Exp. 2: No change pre-post Control: No change pre-post	1. No change 2. Improved pre-post 3. No change	1. No change 2. Improved pre-post 3. No change
3	Rozelle	Exp. 1: > Control at post and follow-up Exp. 2: > Control at post and follow-up	1. > Control at post and follow-up 2. > Control at post and follow-up	1. > Control only at follow-up 2. > Control only at follow-up
4	Gonzalez	> Control at post and follow-up	> Control at post and follow-up	No difference
5	Portnoy	> Control	No changes in HBM variables	Some suggestion that beer consumption declined in Exp. condition

6	Dennison et al.	Not asked	Not asked	No statistical tests applied: evidence suggests improvement in Exp. condition
7	Dennison and Prevet	Not asked	Not asked	No differences re. drinking severity and automobile-related disruptive drinking behavior; significant reduction in nonautomobile disruptive drinking behavior at post and follow-up
8	Sorgen	Exp. > Control	Significant differences between Exp. vs Control change scores on 4 of 10 measures	Not asked
9	Engs	Exp. > Control at post and follow-up	Not asked	No changes
10	Waring	Exp. > Control	Exp. > Control on some factors	Exp. improved more than Control re. heavy drinking
11	Serdahely and Behunin	Not asked	Not asked	No changes
12	Dennison	Not asked	Not asked	Fewer perceived intoxications among Exp. vs Control
13	Serdahely	Not asked	Not asked	No changes
14	Caleekal-John	Post > pre	Post > pre	Post > pre

Knowledge Change

All of the nine studies that attempted knowledge change were successful in achieving this objective.

Attitude Change

Seven of the eight studies that aimed at producing attitude change achieved their objective. Six of the seven attitudinally successful programs possessed experimental designs that included at least one control group. Only one program resulted in some evidence of negative attitudinal shifts in one condition (i.e., opposite to that intended) (Robinson, 1981).

Behavior Change

Nine of the 13 studies that included a focus on self-reported behavior change were at least partially successful in this regard. Eight of these nine studies possessed at least one control group. No program resulted in a negative behavioral change.

Three studies have compared the relative impact of alternative approaches to alcohol education. Robinson (1981) found evidence that a lecture which involved the explicit statement of conclusions and recommendations was more effective in producing change in all three domains than was a lecture that left the conclusions implicit (produced only positive knowledge, negative attitude, and no behavioral change). A lecture in conjunction with value clarification exercises produced only knowledge change.

Gonzalez (1982) summarizes a series of studies by Gonzalez and Rozelle. Among these, Rozelle (1980) found that in comparison to the control group, both experimental conditions (i.e., lecture + experiential, lecture + cognitive group) produced significantly higher levels of responsible attitudes and knowledge about alcohol. This difference was found immediately after the programs as well as 3 months later. There was also a "sleeper" effect such that 3 months later, but not immediately after the programs, fewer negative consequences of drinking were recorded by the experimental groups. No statistically significant differences were found, however, between the two experimental groups, although the experiential condition consistently produced more responsible attitudes and fewer negative consequences of drinking. Rozelle and Gonzalez (1979), in an earlier study, presented evidence that suggests that the lecture + experiential condition produced significant improvements in attitudes and negative consequences of drinking, while the lecture + cognitive condition resulted in improvements only in knowledge.

It is possible that a combination of program type (strategy) and program intensity has an effect on the achievement of behavior change (see, e.g., Schaps et al., 1981). Further analyses suggest the following conclusions: (1) The successful programs seem to be associated with providing field experience for students–three of these programs come from the same source (i.e., Dennison, 1977; Dennison et al., 1977; Dennison and Prevet, 1980). (2) The successful programs appear to be more intensive; that is, involve a greater number of hours spread over an extended period of time. (3) Successful programs do not appear to be more likely to possess inadequate experimental designs.

ALTERNATIVE APPROACHES TO COLLEGE ALCOHOL EDUCATION

Alternative Activities to Alcohol Use

The "alternatives" approach to alcohol and drug abuse is defined as including (Cohen, 1973):

> . . . those constructive and viable attitudes, values orientations, experiences, lifestyles, opportunities, activities, pursuits, and programs which can prevent significant drug abuse or diminish drug abuse by providing greater satisfaction than can drugs. (p. 1)

The "alternatives" approach attempts to take into consideration the type of gratification, needs, aspirations, and motives related to drug use. The motives related to alcohol use include: (1) physical relaxation; (2) enhancement of sexual experience; (3) psychological escape or release of emotional agony; (4) reduction of normal tension, anxiety, and conflict; (5) emotional relaxation; (6) mood alteration; (7) desire for privacy, (8) intensification of personal courage; (9) increase in self-esteem; (10) gain in peer recognition; (11) facilitation of social interaction; (12) reduction of boredom; (13) increase in enjoyment of artistic productions; and (14) desire for fun (Cohen, 1973). Cohen (1973) suggests each of these needs, motives, or aspirations could be fulfilled by an alternative non-drug approach.

Almost no experimental evidence exists concerning the value of the alternatives approach to drug education. A few recent studies have examined the potential value of transcendental meditation (TM) in this regard. Monahan (1977) tested the hypothesis that a transcendental meditation program may result in a decrease in overall patterns of legal and illegal psychoactive substance use in a population. Results showed that meditation decreased use of every substance whereas control subjects increased use of beer and wine and other substances. A significant relationship was found between regularity of meditation (twice a day) and the amount of decrease in use of nicotine, wine and beer, and marijuana. TM may be viewed as an alternative activity to alcohol use among college students. Lazar et al. (1977) examined the use of alcohol, tobacco, and marijuana among college students and adults before TM instruction and 4-12 weeks after the program. Results showed a significant decline for the use of all drugs and a high correlation between decreased anxiety and decreased drug use. Aron and Aron (1980) reviewed research associated with TM program participation and addictive behavior. Findings provided evidence supporting the positive effect of TM for substance abuse prevention and for treatment of drug abusers. Engs and Mulhall (1981) found no effect on drinking or smoking patterns as a result of either a 15-week active endurance program (i.e., jogging and physical conditioning exercises) or a passive participatory program (e.g., riflery, archery, and billards).

Drug Information Centers

Information in the literature regarding activities of and the need for college-based drug information centers is fragmentary. Schneiweiss (1980) describes the activities of the Northeastern University drug information center, which serves as a base for the provision of knowledge concerning drugs for faculty, students, and the community. It was found that, from September 1978 to February 1980, 55% of the requests for drug information came from the university faculty, indicating the need for the center to act as a support service for faculty.

Intervention (Counseling)

Mascalo (1979) suggests that positive and low-key programs are needed on university campuses to develop students' awareness of the risks and consequences of alcohol abuse. College counselors having the opportunity to identify problem drinkers, and basing their work upon their liaison with students and faculty-administration, are in an advantageous position to educate the university community about alcohol use and misuse. This can be done by: (1) training programs for volunteers and residence hall advisers; (2) workshops, minicourses, and in-service training for health, security, and housing staff; and (3) self-development counseling for students. Bellows (1978), who conducted a statewide training needs survey in Nebraska, points to the lack of systematic training in alcoholism counseling. Skuja et al. (1980) describes a community-university partnership model for training alcoholism counselors.

Inclusion in Medical Education

Alcohol education has, to a greater or lesser extent, formed a part of the curricula of faculties of medicine, nursing, social work, etc. Attempts have also been made to integrate it into other parts on the university curriculum. On other occasions, alcohol education courses or units have been established on a more independent basis.

Finn (1979) notes that both the single-discipline approach and the integration of alcohol education into a number of subject areas have advantages and drawbacks: The benefits of the single-discipline approach are primarily of an administrative and logistical nature, while those of the integrative approach are largely educational. Thierman et al. (1978) stress the importance of integrating alcohol education in university curricula since many students are likely to be future doctors, teachers, social workers, nurses, and other helpers who will encounter alcoholics and their families during the course of their careers. It is therefore argued that, if the needs of many of the future alcoholics are to be met, members of these professional groups should hold consistent and positive attitudes toward the alcoholic.

Pokorny et al. (1978) surveyed 105 U.S. medical and osteopathic schools and found that 49% had no alcohol or drug misuse instruction. A total of 672 substance misuse courses were reported by the remaining 51%. Only 17 schools had a continuing-education program in substance misuse. Alcohol and drug misuse education amounted to a mean of .6% of all required hours of instruction. Fisher et al. (1975) have shown that when medical students are exposed to alcohol and drug misuse education, their previously held negative attitudes toward alcohol and other drug users have been altered in a postive direction. Similar findings have been reported by Powell et al. (1974) and Distefano et al. (1975) for nursing and general hospital personnel, respectively. O'Neil et al. (1980) found that a course employing a programmed text on alcoholism resulted in significantly higher knowledge scores than did less extensive alcoholism exposure; no change in attitudes was detected. No effects were found to result from intensive alcoholism training programs for social caseworkers (Bailey, 1970) and paraprofessionals (Cooke et al., 1975).

Nocks (1980) suggests that universities offer alcohol education minicourses with a maximum length of 6 hours for medical students. The course should highlight various issues related to physicians' attitudes to alcohol abusers as a means of modifying the attitudes of the "would-be" physicians. Coggan et al. (1981) suggest a modular approach to alcohol education as the most appropriate means of integrating the unit into a family medicine clerkship. They also emphasize the need to integrate alcohol education in medical education since it is an excellent example of a chronic disease which has both biomedical and psychosocial components and which can affect the entire family unit.

SUMMARY AND IMPLICATIONS OF EXPERIMENTAL EVALUATIONS OF CAMPUS-BASED PROGRAMS

In contrast to alcohol and other drug education programs (see, e.g., Goodstadt, 1978, 1980; Schaps et al., 1981), campus-based alcohol education programs appear: (1) to be better designed, in employing at least one control group and some degree of random assignment; (2) to be more likely to be concerned with reported behavioral as well as attitudinal and knowledge change; (3) to be as (or more) intensive in their operation; and (4) to be more likely to be successful in achieving the desired behavioral, attitudinal, and knowledge changes. Reasons for all of these outcomes could be due to the programs' locus (i.e., campus base). It would not be surprising if campus staff were more likely to adhere to at least minimum program evaluation standards. Campus programs can also, if associated with ongoing curricula, extend over a greater period of time than is commonly possible in nonacademic (or even secondary school) settings. Finally, campus programs have a significant potential for impact since (1) they are less likely to encounter problems of comprehension than would be the case in general or noncampus populations, and (2) they are likely to be transmitting information with which students are already familiar and to be reinforcing attitudes and behaviors which existed in the recent past (i.e., in their graduating year of high school).

The evidence that exists suggests that programs that contain some amount of field (or laboratory) experience, along with factual information and effective experiential strategies, provide a powerful stimulus for change among university students. This effect appears to be more likely when programs are intense, involving a considerable amount of input over a large number of hours, spaced over an extended period of time. Almost no data exist concerning nonuniversity postsecondary college programs.

Published reports provide little insight into the factors associated with program inadequacies. This, of course, is characteristic of much sociobehavioral research, which favors the publication of successful (i.e., statistically significant) results and ignores the lessons to be learned from apparent failures. With few exceptions (e.g., Sheppard and Goodstadt, 1984), alcohol education research has ignored the richness of data at hand to program developers and evaluators regarding the barriers to program effectiveness. Program failure can occur at any point in the progression of program development and implementation, as a consequence of such factors as (1) inadequate conceptualization, (2) poor content or process development, (3) unsatisfactory implementation, and (4) inappropriate program evaluation. These failures can, themselves, be the result of a diversity of social and professional impediments.

A survey of university student-services administrators identified a variety of perceptions regarding program needs, including a denial of the existence of alcohol problems among students and, at the other extreme, problems of almost crisis proportions. The same survey suggested a wide range of barriers to program implementation and effectiveness, including: (1) limitations on financial and personnel resources, (2) student and staff attitudes and prejudices, (3) entrenchment of alcohol in general life-styles, (4) student union opposition (due to potential financial losses), and (5) lack of adequate information regarding the nature and extent of the problem (Caleekal-John and Goodstadt, 1983).

Further research is required to examine, more systematically and in more detail, the influence of: (1) alternative educational processes employed in programs; (2) alternative program characteristics such as "intensity" and duration; (3) training and background of instructors; and (4) sample characteristics, both demographic and alcohol related.

REFERENCES

AMERICAN ALLIANCE FOR HEALTH, PHYSICAL EDUCATION, AND RECREATION. *A Monograph on Alcohol Education and Alcohol Abuse Prevention Programs at Selected American Colleges.* Prepared for NIAAA. Washington DC: NIAAA, 1978.

ARON, A., and ARON, E. The Transcendental Meditation program's effect on addictive behavior. *Addict. Behav.* 5: 3-12, 1980.

BAILEY, M.B. Attitudes toward alcoholism before and after a training program for social caseworkers. *Q. J. Stud. Alcohol* 31: 669-683, 1970.

BELLOWS, D. *Evaluation of the Alcohol Training Program of the Psychology Department UNL.* Lincoln, NB: University of Nebraska Lincoln, Department of Psychology, 1978.

CALEEKAL-JOHN, A. An interdisciplinary cognitive approach to alcohol education in the university curriculum. *J. Alcohol Drug Educ.* In press, 1984.

CALEEKAL-JOHN, A., and GOODSTADT, M.S. *Perceived needs regarding alcohol problems and alcohol education programs on Ontario university campuses.* Substudy No. 1264, Addiction Research Foundation, Toronto, Canada, 1983.

COGGAN, P., DAVIS, A., and ROGERS, J. Teaching alcoholism to family medicine students. *J. Fam. Practice* 13: 1025-1028, 1981.

COHEN, A.Y. *Alternatives to Drug Abuse: Steps Toward Prevention* (NIDA). Washington DC: U.S. Government Printing Office, 1973.

COOKE, G., WEHMER, G., and GRUBER, J. Training paraprofessionals in the treatment of alcoholism. *Q. J. Stud. Alcohol* 10: 241-249, 1975.

CROSSMAN, L.H. Rutgers student alcohol project: Open systems perspective. *J. Alcohol Drug Educ.* 26(3): 23-29, 1981.

DENNISON, D. The effects of selected field experiences upon the drinking behavior of university students. *J. School Health* 47: 38-41, 1977.

DENNISON, D., and PREVET, T. Improving alcohol-related disruptive behaviors through health instruction. *J. School Health* 50: 206-208, 1980.

DENNISON, D., PREVET, T., and AFFLECK, M. Does alcohol instruction affect student drinking behavior? *Health Educ.* 8(6): 28-30, 1977.

DISTEFANO, D., CRAIG, S., HENDERSON, J., and PRYER, M. Effects of brief alcoholism training on general hospital personnel. *Psychol. Rep.* 37: 1321-1322, 1975.

DONOVAN, B.E. Brown Group on Alcohol: Development of an on-campus education/prevention/treatment forum. *J. Alcohol Drug Educ.* 24(3): 56-65, 1979.

DONOVAN, B.E. Establishing a university alcohol education/prevention program and some principles. *J. Alcohol Drug Educ.* 27(1): 62-77, 1981.

ENGS, R. Let's look before we leap: The cognitive and behavioral evaluation of a university alcohol education program. *J. Alcohol Drug Educ.* 22(2): 39-48, 1977.

ENGS, R.C., and MULHALL, P.F. Again–Let's look before we leap: The effects of physical activity on smoking and drinking patterns. *J. Alcohol Drug Educ.* 26(2): 65-74, 1981.

FILSTEAD, W.J., ROSSI, J.J., and GOBY, M.J. Alcoholism and alcohol problems on college campuses: Problems, priorities and recommendations. *J. Alcohol Drug Educ.* 21(2): 35-42, 1976.

FINN, P. Alcohol and education in the school curriculum: The single discipline vs. the interdisciplinary approach. *J. Alcohol Drug Educ.* 24(2): 41-57, 1979.

FISHER, T.C., MASON, R.L., KEELEY, K.A., and FISHER, J.V. Physicians and alcoholics: The effects of medical training on attitudes. *J. Stud. Alcohol* 36: 949-955, 1975.

GONZALEZ, G.M. What do you mean–prevention? *J. Alcohol Drug Educ.* 23(3): 14-23, 1978.

GONZALEZ, G.M. The effect of a model alcohol education module on college students' attitudes, knowledge and behavior related to alcohol use. *J. Alcohol Drug Educ.* 25(3): 1-2, 1980.

GONZALEZ, G.M. Alcohol education to prevent alcohol problems: A summary of some unique findings. *J. Alcohol Drug Educ.* 27(3): 2-12, 1982.

GOODSTADT, M.S. Alcohol and drug education: Models and outcomes. *Health Educ. Monogr.* 6: 263-279, 1978.

GOODSTADT, M.S. Drug education–A turn on or a turn off? *J. Drug Educ.* 10: 89-99, 1980.

KRAFT, D.P. Follow-up of a federal effort to encourage campus alcohol abuse prevention programs. *J. Am. College Health Assoc.* 26: 150-153, 1977.

KRAFT, D.P. Strategies for reducing drinking problems among youth: College programs. In H.T. Blane and M.E. Chafetz (eds.), *Youth, Alcohol and Social Policy.* New York: Plenum Press, 1979.

LAZAR, A., FARWELL, L., and FARROW, J.T. The effects of the Transcendental Meditation program on anxiety, drug abuse, cigarette smoking and alcohol consumption. In D.W. Orme-Johnson and J.T. Farrow (eds.), *Scientific Research on the Transcendental Meditation Program: Collected Papers,* Vol. 1. Livingston Manor, NY: MIU Press, 1977.

MASCALO, A. Role of the college counselor in alcohol abuse counseling and education. *J. Alcohol Drug Educ.* 24(3): 52-55, 1979.

MILLS, K.C., PFAFFENBERGER, B., and MC CARTY, D. Guidelines for alcohol abuse prevention on the college campus: Overcoming the barriers to program success. *J. Higher Educ.* 52: 399-414, 1981.

MONAHAN, R.J. Secondary prevention of drug dependence through the Transcendental Meditation program in Metropolitan Philadelphia. *Int. J. Addict.* 12: 729-754, 1977.

NOCKS, J.J. Instructing medical students on alcohol: What to teach with limited time. *J. Med. Educ.* 55: 858-864, 1980.

O'NEIL, P.D., SUTKER, P.B., KILPATRICK, D.G., and KEELER, M.H. Programmed self-instruction on alcoholism for medical students: A controlled evaluation. *J. Psychiatr. Educ.* 4: 201-212, 1980.

POKORNY, A., PUTMAN, P., and FRYER, J. Drug abuse and alcoholism teaching in U.S. medical and osteopathic schools. *J. Med. Educ.* 53: 816-824, 1978.

PORTNOY, B. Effects of a controlled usage alcohol education program based on the health belief model. *J. Drug Educ.* 10: 181-195, 1980.

POWELL, B., MUELLER, J., and SCHWERDTFEGER, T. Attitudes changes of general hospital personnel following an alcoholism training program. *Psychol. Rep.* 34: 461-462, 1974.

ROBINSON, J., III. A comparison of three alcohol instruction programs on the knowledge, attitudes and drinking behaviors of college students. *J. Drug Educ.* 11: 157-166, 1981.

ROZELLE, G.R. Experiential and cognitive small group approaches to alcohol education for college students. *J. Alcohol Drug Educ.* 26(1): 40-53, 1980.

ROZELLE, G.R., and GONZALEZ, G. A peer-facilitated course on alcohol abuse: An innovative approach to prevention on the college campus. *J. Alcohol Drug Educ.* 25(1): 20-30, 1979.

RUTGERS UNIVERSITY COMMITTEE ON THE USE OF ALCOHOL. *Report.* New Brunswick, NJ: State University of New Jersey, May 1981.

SCHAPS, E., DI BARTOLO, R., MOSKOWITZ, J., PALLEY, C.S., and CHURGIN, S. A review of 127 drug abuse prevention program evaluations. *J. Drug Issues* 11: 17-44, 1981.

SCHNEIWEISS, F. Activities of a college drug information center. *Drug Information* 14: 72-76, 1980.

SERDAHELY, W.J. A factual approach to drug education and its effects on drug consumption. *J. Alcohol Drug Educ.* 26(1): 63-68, 1980.

SERDAHELY, W.J., and BEHUNIN, O. Drug education: Reducing or increasing drug consumption? *J. Alcohol Drug Educ.* 23(1): 8-19, 1977.

SHEPPARD, M. A., and GOODSTADT, M.S. The dissemination and implementation of a school-based alcohol education program: Were we successful? In *Knowledge: Creation, Diffusion and Utilization*. In press, 1984.

SKUJA, A., FORD, W., SCOTT, S., and ELLIS, D. Action: A community/university partnership for training alcoholism counselors. *J. Alcohol Drug Educ.* 25(3): 41-47, 1980.

SNYDER, G.H. Developing alcohol courses in a two year college. *J. Alcohol Drug Educ.* 25(3): 13-19, 1980.

SORGEN, L.M. Student learning following an educational experience at an alcohol Rehabilitation Center in Saskatoon, Saskatchewan, Canada. *Int. J. Nursing Stud.* 16: 41-50, 1979.

THIERMAN, T., KERN, J.C., and PAUL, S.R. Promoting alcoholism education in the undergraduate and graduate curriculum. In A. Schechter, H. Alksne, and E. Kaufman (eds.), *Critical Concerns in the Field of Drug Abuse.* New York: Dekker, 1978. (Also, Alcoholism education in the undergraduate curriculum. *J. Drug Educ.* 6: 153-164, 1976.)

WARING, M.L. Impact of alcoholism training on college students preparing for human services careers. *Int. J. Rehab. Res.* 3: 395-396, 1980.

The International Journal of the Addictions, 19(7), 743–752, 1984

Family Mapping: Toward an Understanding of the Interactional Dynamic of the Alcoholic Marital Dyad

Kathryn M. Synol,* MA

Park Forest, Illinois 60466

Abstract

Family mapping is a structure which provides the therapist and the marital couple with information about family of origin issues which can then be used as a therapeutic point of reference.

That alcoholism is a family-based problem has been firmly established in the literature (Bowen, 1974; Jackson, 1958; Kelly, 1973; Steinglass, 1981), and that family therapy is the treatment of choice by many clinicians has been equally well noted (Keller, 1974; Stanton and Todd, 1982; Steinglass, 1981). The salient feature in these families is the existence of and the protection of the "alcoholic marriage." (For purposes herein the alcoholic marriage is defined as one in which the male is alcoholic and his spouse in nonalcoholic. The author does recognize that the alcoholic in such marriages can be either spouse and sometimes both spouses are alcoholic.)

Alcohol abuse and intoxication, when considered within the operational framework of such a marriage, manifests a dynamic logic of its own. Ewing and Fox (1968) concluded that the alcoholic marriage provides an arena in which the male alcoholic's dependency needs are satisfied by his wife's nurturing needs, which are in turn gratified by his dependency needs. It is in essence an implicit

*Address correspondence to the author at 245 Gentry Street, Park Forest, Illinois 60466.

 0020-773X/84/1907-0743$3.50/0

"dance" which carefully maintains its own rhythm (i.e., homeostasis) through the use of alcohol. Therapy then must be interactionally oriented rather than individually focused (Steinglass et al., 1971).

Yet to fully understand the interactional pattern of the alcoholic marriage, the clinician needs to return to the patterns of the parental relationships in the families of origin of each partner. Therein will be found the raison d'être of the present marital system.

Framo (1976) notes that the marital system is a reenactment of the needs and expectations formed in the original family system. Hence, the two systems are intricately intertwined. Since many alcoholics have at least one alcoholic parent, as do their nonalcoholic wives (Burk, 1972; Julius and Papp, 1981; Sloboda, 1974; Weiner et al., 1971), the mutual projection and transference of internal objects carried out in close relationships would result in seemingly "irrational" behavior and marital distress.

Family mapping is one technique which provides the clinician with abundant information about the family of origin of each partner in the marital dyad. This information is gathered in a nonthreatening structure and in a concise form.

It has also been this author's experience that family mapping:

1. Provides literal or concrete-thinking clients with a less abstract, more concretized method of looking at family patterns.
2. Decreases the amount of anxiety in the early stages of therapy as it is a highly structured technique.
3. Decreases anxiety regarding talking about the present marital system by focusing on the less threatening family of origin.
4. Provides both partners with new information about themselves and the other partner.
5. Helps clients to understand behavior which has been confusing to him/her.
6. Facilitates engaging the clients as the therapist and the clients participate in the mapping process together.
7. Provides the therapist with themes which will resurface at a future time (i.e., "grist for the mill").
8. Provides the groundwork for the clients to begin to view their relationship interactionally.
9. Provides the therapist with information about each partner's expectations of the marital relationship and what needs are being gratified by the homeostasis.

It should be noted that since family mapping can provide an overwhelming amount of what may prove to be anxiety-provoking material in a short space of time, caution needs to be exercised with clients who are borderline psychotic and/or who have a history of non-drug-induced psychosis. These individuals may lack the ego strength necessary to cope with the emotional intensity experienced as an awareness of family patterns and family influences develops.

Also, couples who present with the child as the identified patient are frequently resistant to focusing on their relationship and may reject the need for family mapping.

THE PROCEDURES

1. The therapist explains the purpose of the mapping to the couple.
   Example: In order that I might get to know each one of you better, I need to learn more about the families that each of you came from.
2. The therapist then explains that she/he will ask questions and the responses will be written on the blackboard.
   Note: This author prefers to record the information on a blackboard, allowing the client's task to remain focused on retrieving historical information and gaining awareness of some of the process and structure of the family of origin. Having the client record his/her own information may facilitate encoding the data, but it might also provide a task on which to defocus painful feelings.
3. The therapist determines which partner wants to map first.
4. The therapist explains the meaning of the symbols to be used.
5. The partner who is the observer is given paper and pen to copy the mapping as it is being done. (It is important to keep both partners involved.)
6. The following symbols are used:

○	Female	□	Male
∅	Deceased female	⧄	Deceased male

7. The following questions are asked and the responses are mapped on the blackboard:
   - What is your mother's name?
   - How old is she? (If deceased, how old was she when she died?)
   - What was her highest level of education?
   - What was her life occupation(s)?
   - Tell me five positive things about her.
   - Tell me five negative things about her.
     (Repeat this procedure for father.)
   - How long has the relationship between Mom and Dad lasted? (Or how long did it last?)
   - How would you describe it?
   - Who was born first?

- How long were your parents married before that birth?
- Who was born next?
- How many years between the children?
  (Do this until all siblings are included.)
- What are your brothers and sisters like?
- Who is closest to which parent?
- Who is your spouse like in your family?
- Who are you like?
- Who was the disciplinarian?
- What was the discipline like?
- What unspoken rules and myths existed in your family?
  (The therapist will have to help the couple get started with this in most cases.)

8. Note that throughout the mapping process, the therapist should be clarifying.
   Example:
   Client: My mother was kind and loving.
   Therapist: How did you come to know this; what kinds of things did she do or say that let you know that she was kind and loving?

Although these questions are designed to be the core of the family-mapping process, this is not to imply that the technique is a rigid structure. The number of additional probes possible is limited only by time, the client's ego strength, and the therapist's ability to be creative.

An understanding of how the client would have changed the family of origin, if she/he could have, could provide the therapist with valuable data about who the client is trying to save, trying to heal, trying to punish, trying to love, trying to gain love from, etc.

Although the family mapping is done only once, references to the uncovered dynamics are frequently made by the therapist during the therapeutic process.

It might prove useful to remap the family later in therapy to determine what changes in perception and integration have occurred for each of the partners. A remapping might also elicit new information which may then be more within the client's conscious awareness than earlier in therapy.

CASE EXAMPLE

The Dyad

April, age 26 years, and Scott, age 37 years, have entered treatment for Scott's alcoholism. He had completed an inpatient rehabilitation program and was attending Alcoholics Anonymous. There was, however, significant marital distress.

Scott has two children by a previous marriage who live out of state. They have three children from this marriage. April's teenage sister also lives with them. However, neither partner presents the children as problems.

April has a history of polydrug abuse and heroin addiction. She completed a drug rehabilitation program 6 years prior to entering treatment with Scott for his alcoholism. She remained drug-free during that period until Scott entered the hospital inpatient treatment unit. She then relapsed on heroin and used it periodically during the month that he was hospitalized.

They entered the first session enraged at one another. Scott had just learned of April's heroin relapse. April angrily announced that she wanted a divorce. She then stated that she did not know what she wanted and began to sob. She wept intermittently throughout the session.

Because of April's confusion and intrapsychic pain, the clinical decision was made to provide her with an individual therapist as well as to continue with the marital therapy.

The family mapping was not held until Sessions 3 and 4 to allow time for April to achieve some emotional release.

Figures 1 and 2 are diagrams of their family mapping, and the following sections provide an abbreviated review of some of the discoveries made by this couple about themselves and each other through the mapping process.

April

1. April was amazed at how little she knew about Scott.
2. April discovered that the only way to get taken care of (loved) in her family was to get sick. (Note on the diagram that once Mom got sick, Dad got close to her.) She was able to tie this into her present behavior and parenting practices.
3. April discovered that not telling Scott anything was identical to Mom not telling Dad anything for fear of an explosion.
4. April's family forces money on her and then demands repayment and intrudes into her life. They make her obligated to them so that she can never be free to them. (No one separates from this family.)
   Therapist: How old were you when you left home?
   April: It looks like I never did leave home, what with everybody pushing into my marriage and then demanding things, making me feel guilty.
5. April discovered that if she does not accept "financial help" from her father and sister, they will abandon her, ostracize her (see diagram for family rule No. 4). This happened to her sister, Marcia, who refused to be manipulated through money.
6. She discoverd that she is just like her father and that Scott is like her mother. She feels closest to Scott when he's sick and needy.

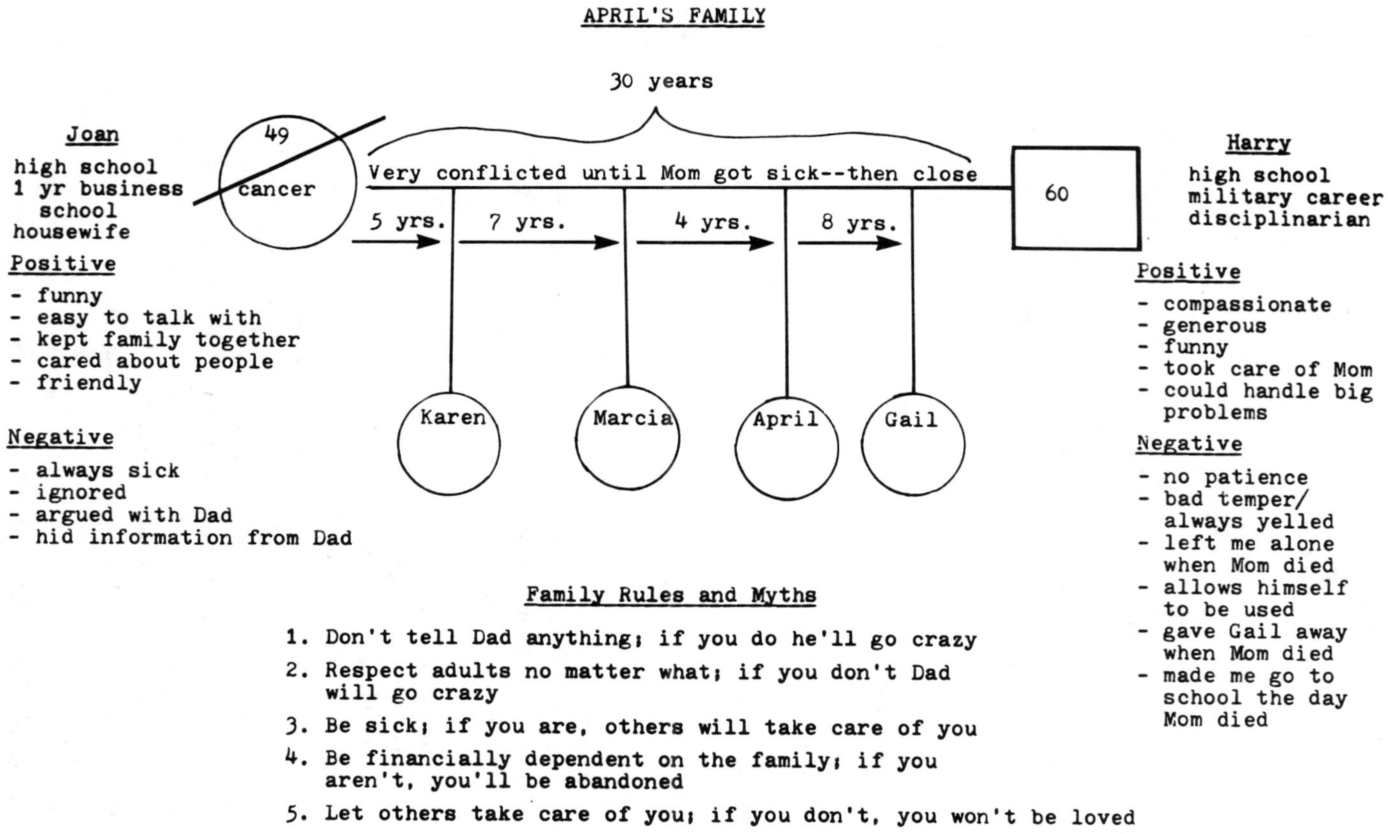

Fig. 1. April's family map.

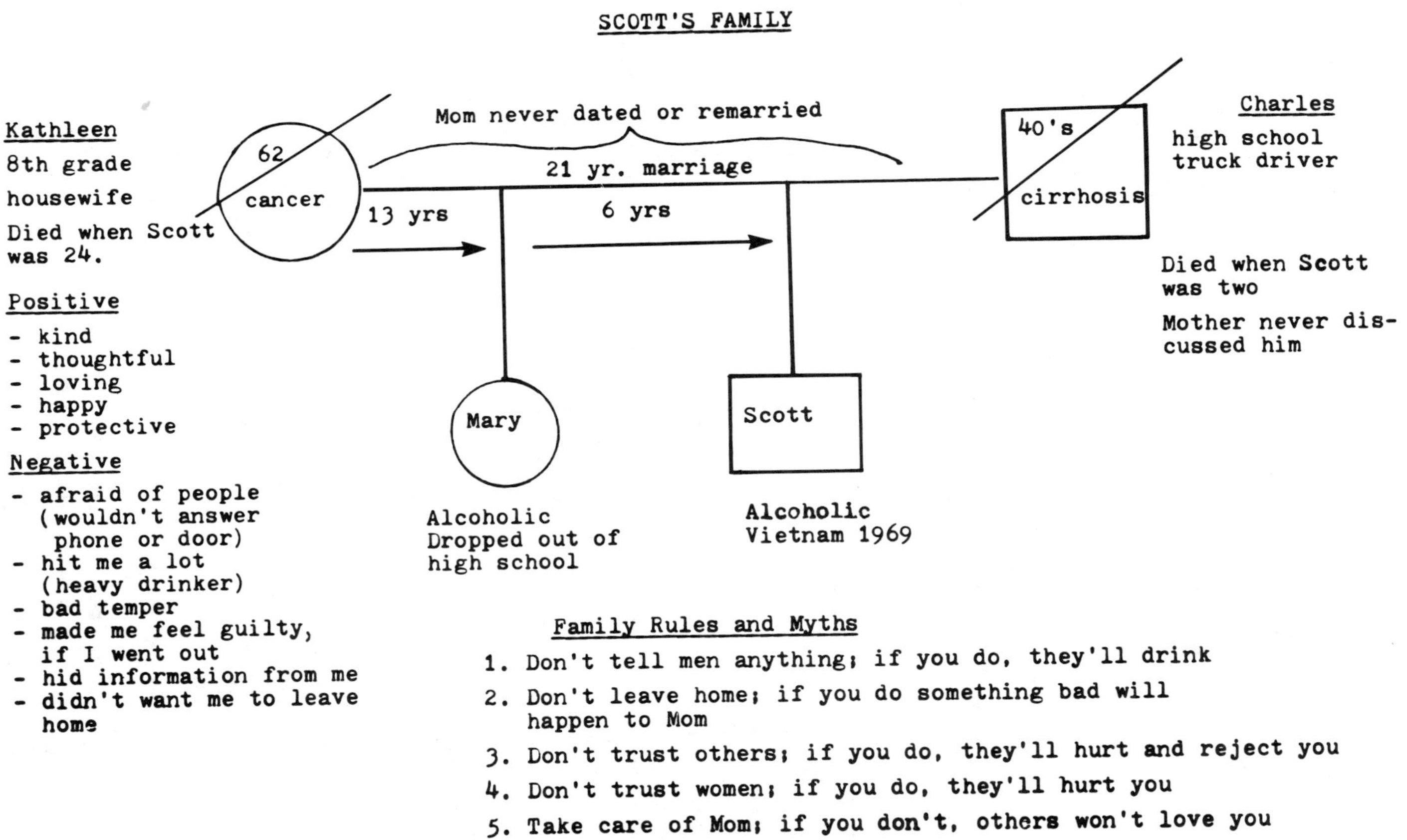

Fig. 2. Scott's family map.

Scott

1. Scott was amazed at how little he knew about April.
2. Scott believed that if he left April alone she would get sick. (Note: Mom had an asthma attack whenever he tried to go out with his friends, and she died when he went to Vietnam.) April fulfilled this prophecy by relapsing on drugs when Scott was hospitalized.
3. Scott discovered that April is like his mother. April hid information (because of her family of origin) and this enraged Scott, who would then drink to give expression to his anger. Scott's mother and sister always hid information from him.
4. Scott discovered that he has never left home. Someone has always taken care of him—Mom, the army, his first wife, a good friend, his second wife.

Outcome

At the time of this writing this couple is still in therapy. Both partners have been able to identify how they act out in the present marriage their roles and needs from their respective families of origin, and have realized that they have never completed adolescent separation (a theme which appears frequently in the family mappings completed by this author on clients presenting with alcoholism). They have had to resolve considerable anxiety about establishing closeness without one or both of them feeling the need to get sick in order to facilitate that happening.

April has been working on her violent temper, which surfaces when she feels "cheated." She has been able to connect this feeling with being ignored by Mom in favor of her oldest sister, Karen. Both she and Dad got attention from Mom through violent outbursts of temper.

Using Framo's criteria (1980) for marital improvement, the following progress, though tentative, has been noted:

1. More open communication
2. More genuine liking of each other
3. More empathic understanding of one another
4. An understanding of their irrational expectations based on family of origin issues

Major areas requiring significant improvement are:

1. The need to become more personally differentiated from each other
2. Adjustment to the reality of deidealized love.

It is very interesting that as this couple has made noticeable progress in their relationship, April's teenage sister, who lives with them, has become symptomatic. This has resulted in the whole family being included in family therapy.

CONCLUSION

Family mapping is not a panacea and does not bring about change in and of itself. It does, however, help the couple to gain insight into their own dynamic and to use that insight as a point of embarkation and as a point of reference throughout the therapeutic process.

This is particularly important in the alcoholic marriage and/or family because it is freqeuntly the case that the family believes that if the alcoholic would just stop drinking, everything in the family would normalize. When it does not, the family becomes confused and anxious; thus the stage is set for yet another relapse.

The success of family mapping is best assessed vis-à-vis the client's ability to identify family patterns and to understand that those patterns that were integral to the functioning of the family of origin are integral to the homeostasis of the family of procreation.

Some clients will be able to use the mapping as a point of reference with minimal assistance from the therapist throughout the therapy.

There are those clients who will reject the concept of the family of origin as the matrix of present-day actions and reactions. Some may eventually come to understand this concept later in therapy as the therapist uses it as a backdrop. If this understanding occurs, the clients will begin to make references to the family-mapping material independent of the therapist.

However, other clients will continue to reject the impact of the family of origin, despite all evidence to the contrary. The therapist then may need to use more concrete, problem-solving techniques or perhaps may need to clarify the client's therapeutic goals.

It is quintessential for any therapist who works with couples and/or families to have explored the multidimensional nature of his/her own family of origin. The dynamics of that family will affect the way in which the therapist interacts with the clients, just as it affects the therapist's intimate relationships.

Family mapping may evoke unresolved feelings in the therapist as she/he is reminded of the process and structure of her/his own family. Indeed, every family mapping will contain some element of the therapist's family of origin experience.

While doing a client's family mapping then, it is possible for the therapist to gain additional insight into some area of functioning of his/her own family which may not have been previously understood and/or integrated.

Such an understanding is essential for the identification of interfacement issues which may prevent therapeutic movement and which may even promote symptom maintenance.

REFERENCES

BOWEN, M. Alcoholism as viewed through family systems theory and family psychotherapy. *Ann. NY Acad. Sci.* 233: 115, 1974.

BURK, E. Some contemporary issues in child development and the children of alcoholic parents. In F.A. Seixas, G.S. Omenn, E.S. Burk, and S. Eggleston (eds.), *Nature and Nurture in Alcoholism.* New York: Annals of the New York Academy of Science, 1972.

EWING, J., and FOX, R. Family therapy in alcoholism. In J. Masserman (ed.), *Current Psychiatric Therapies,* Vol. 8. New York: Grune and Stratton, 1968.

FRAMO, J. Family of origin as a therapeutic resource for adults in marital and family therapy: You can and should go home again. *Family Process* 15:198-210, 1976.

FRAMO, J. Marriage and marital therapy: Issues and initial interview techniques. In M. Andolfi and I. Zwerling (eds.), *Dimensions of Family Therapy.* New York: Guilford Press, 1980.

JACKSON, J.K. Alcoholism and the family. *Ann. Am. Acad. Polit. Soc. Sci.* 315:90-98, 1958.

JULIUS, E., and PAPP, P. Family choreography: A multigenerational view of an alcoholic family system. In E. Kaufmann and P. Kaufmann (eds.), *Family Therapy of Drug and Alcohol Abuse.* New York: Gardner Press, 1981.

KELLER, M. (ed.). Trends in the treatment of alcoholism. In *Second Special Report to the Congress on Alcohol and Health.* Washington, DC: Department of Health, Education, and Welfare, 1974, pp. 145-167.

KELLY, D. Alcoholism and the family. *Maryland State Med. J. 22:* 25-30, 1973.

SLOBODA, S. The children of alcoholics: A neglected problem. *Hosp. Comm. Psychiatry* 25: 605-606, 1974.

STANTON, M., and TODD, T. *The Family Therapy of Drug Abuse and Addiction.* New York: Guilford Press, 1982.

STEINGLASS, P. Family therapy with alcoholics: A review. In E. Kaufmann and P. Kaufmann (eds.), *Family Therapy of Drug and Alcohol Abuse.* New York: Gardner Press, 1981.

STEINGLASS, P., WEINER, S., and MENDELSON, J. Interactional issues as determinants of alcoholism. *Am. J. Psychiatry* 128: 275-280, 1971.

WEINER, S., ET AL. Familial patterns in chronic alcoholism. *Am. J. Psychiatry* 127: 1646-1651, 1971.

The International Journal of the Addictions, 19(7), 753–765, 1984

Social Recovery and Therapeutic Mission

Larry W. Whorley, DSW

Fort Belvoir Counseling Center
The U.S. Army Engineer Center and Fort Belvoir
Virginia 22060

Abstract

Social recovery is defined as restoration to effective social functioning. The Social Recovery Inventory, an instrument derived from role and social exchange theories, is demonstrated as a method of measuring recovery vis-à-vis occupational, familial, and civic functioning. Conditions for social recovery are examined, with discussion of implications for treatment, in-service training, and administration.

Rehabilitation has been a major topic in the addiction literature. There has been much discussion of methods, techniques, strategies, and innovative approaches in the treatment of alcoholism and other drug addiction. However, this paper does not address rehabilitative means. Rather, attention is given to purposes, or ends.

This presentation proceeds from the assumption that the purpose, or mission, of addiction rehabilitation is enhancement of recovery. Recovery, then is the concern of this treatise. More specifically, reestablishment of interpersonal relations—that is, social recovery—is examined.

Social recovery has received some attention in the literature (Adams and McNear, 1977; Haasz et al., 1980; King et al., 1979; Miller et al., 1980; Moffett et al., 1974). In addition, a distinction between two related concepts, abstinence and recovery, has been discussed. Abstinence has been cited as an important prerequisite for recovery; yet abstinence and recovery are not synonymous (Haasz et al., 1980; King et al., 1979).

 0020-773X/84/1907-0753$3.50/0

Social recovery actually has been a somewhat confusing concept. Some writers have viewed it as general resocialization (Adams and McNear, 1977; Haasz et al., 1980), while others have defined it more strictly as informal social contacts (Moos et al., 1981). This paper approaches social recovery from an explicit theoretical perspective. An understanding of social recovery is devised through an integration of role and exchange theories.

In order to more clearly define social recovery, one may begin by viewing social recovery as reestablishment of social functioning. Most definitions of social functioning rely upon role theory. For example, the following definition is representative:

> Social functioning . . . designates those activities considered essential for performance of the several roles which each individual, by virtue of his membership in social groups, is called upon to carry out. (Typically the individual has roles in social groups related to such social institutions as the family, the church, the school, work, and leisure.) All role performance requires reciprocal activity, or social interaction, between individual and individual, individual and group, and individual and community. (Boehm, 1959, p. 46)

The preceding conceptualization provides some general framework, but it is difficult to operationalize the concept from this definition. Therefore, building upon this role theory foundation, this study conceptualizes and measures social functioning through a nexus of role and exchange theoretical concepts. Table 1 presents the key concepts used.

Table 1
Key Concepts

1. *Social Position:* A particular location within a social structure, such as husband, father, employee, supervisor, parent, teacher, etc.
2. *Social Role:* The behavioral expectations associated with a given social position
3. *Social Functioning:* Effective performance of role expectations associated with the various social positions in social living
4. *Social Recovery:* Restoration to effective social functioning as a result of rehabilitation
5. *Reward:* A positive reinforcer; a stimulus which increases behavior that immediately precedes it
6. *Cost:* Rewards forgone as a result of social interaction with a role partner
7. *Social Profit:* Rewards contributed by a role partner minus one's costs that are incurred as a result of interaction with a role partner
8. *Social Profitableness:* One's contribution to a role partner minus one's behavior which is costly to a role partner

SOCIAL FUNCTIONING

Following role theory, human interaction takes place through role performance, or enactment (Rose, 1962). People occupy various social positions (husband, father, employee, citizen, etc.) which carry a specific set of expectations for behavior in each position. This organized, learned, and expected behavior associated with a given position constitutes a role. Since positions/roles are reciprocal (husband-wife; parent-child; supervisor-worker), one interacts with many role partners.

Such reciprocal role enactment suggests an exchange process. Indeed, according to social exchange theorists, social behavior *is* exchange (Burgess and Bushell, 1969; Homans, 1961). Social exchange involves the giving, receiving, and withholding of such rewards as affection, respect, service (labor), information, goods, and money (Foa and Foa, 1974). The exchange perspective is a behavioral, quasi-economic approach in which social profit determines relationships.

Social profit is defined as "rewards minus costs." An individual's profit is determined by subtracting his costs (resulting from any destructive behavior of his role partner) from his rewards (contributed by the role partner) (Homans, 1961). A synthesis of role and exchange perspectives is possible: An individual who enacts the expected role behavior therefore contributes rewards to his role partner, while a violator of role expectations engenders costs for his role partner.

A related concept is that of social profitableness (Whorley, 1978). From the viewpoint of a role partner, an individual may perform or fail to fulfill role obligations. In behavioral-exchange terms, performance is profitable to others, while failure is unprofitable. An addict's social profitableness (to others) will be determined through balancing his contributions against any costs incurred by others. If contributions outweigh costs, the addict may be described as (generally) socially profitable; that is, such specific social functioning vis-à-vis the role situation would be adequate. Conversely, addicts whose costly behavior outweighs contributions are (generally) unprofitable to role partners. If unprofitableness becomes extreme, the addict may be ostracized, imprisoned, experience psychiatric hospitalization, or even be executed.

Therefore, performance of role expectations creates social profitableness. Social profitableness describes positive, effective social functioning, while social dysfunction would be indicated by a state of unprofitableness. A client's potential for changing a state of unprofitableness to effective social functioning will be determined by two propositions. These propositions maintain: (1) The greater the client's access to rewards (affection, respect, service, information, goods, and money), the greater potential for effective social functioning; and (2) the greater the client's tendency to withhold rewards from role partners, the lesser potential for social profitableness (effective social functioning).

Determination of social recovery is appropriate after a period of rehabilitation. In reality, the social profitableness/functioning of a treated addict would be examined. Social recovery would require positive social functioning (social profitableness) within any given role arena.

This paper presents a method for measurement of social recovery, derived from the foregoing conceptualization. An instrument, the Social Recovery Inventory, is presented and demonstrated. Also, conditions which affect inventory results are discussed.

SOCIAL RECOVERY INVENTORY

The Social Recovery Inventory explores three crucial arenas of social functioning. Social functioning is examined in regard to occupational, familial (family-related), and civic (citizenship) functioning of addicts in the community.

Since the previous discussion suggested that aspects of role performance be conceptualized as social profitableness, an attempt was made to formulate profitableness measures which together would depict total social functioning. Personnel at the U.S. Army Engineer Center and Fort Belvoir, Virginia, assisted in the development of indices for measurement of the three components of social functioning.

Each index includes contribution and cost scales; the cost scale score is subtracted from the contribution scale score to yield an index score of functioning. Each index score may vary from −21 to +21; positive index scores indicate profitableness, while negative index scores suggest overall unprofitableness. Note that social recovery requires positive index scores within the inventory.

The Occupational Performance Index (OPI) was constructed from consultation with a panel of 100 civilian employee supervisors. The supervisors suggested scale items and ranked items according to importance. The mean rank for each item was adopted as an item weight. Moreover, a previous version of this index applied to military personnel has been useful in determining occupational recovery from drug addiction (Whorley, 1981).

The army installation's child abuse-family violence team assisted in the development of both the Familial Performance Index (FPI) and the Civic Performance Index (CPI). This team of 20 human service professionals represented a broad range of disciplines, including medicine, nursing, social work, education, and legal representatives. The team was asked to suggest items for both contribution and cost scales. Following the same procedure taken in construction of the Occupational Performance Index, the mean rank for each of the two indices was designated the (item) weight value.

Figure 1 illustrates the Social Recovery Inventory format. The inventory should be completed after a reasonable period of rehabilitation. The following case demonstrates the potential of the inventory.

CASE STUDY

R.J. was a 34-year-old male who was married and the father of two children. He was employed by the U.S. government as a maintenance supervisor. After referral by his own supervisor, it was found that R.J. had been drinking heavily on a daily basis for at least 2 years. He also had admitted to improperly taking diazepam (Valium) in excess of prescription and while drinking. Subsequent medical evaluation indicated the presence of alcohol dependence (alcoholism; alcohol addiction) and Valium abuse.

In order to obtain baseline (pretreatment) measures of social functioning, the three indices constituting the Social Recovery Inventory were computed. R.J.'s supervisor reported the following information vis-à-vis the OPI: (Good Interpersonal Relations) - (Tardiness + Poor Attention + Job Inefficiency) = 4 - (4 + 4 + 4) = 4 - 12 = -8. The client's wife was consulted for FPI and CPI computations. She indicated the following FPI results: FPI = (Occasional Domestic Help) - (Failed Promises + Failed Self-Disclosure + Failed Listening + Failed Family Obligations) = 2 - (2 + 2 + 4 + 3) = 2 - 11 = -9. The Civic Performance Index (CPI) yielded: (Paid Taxes) - (Unpaid Creditors + Drunk Driving + Social Rudeness) = 3 - (3 + 6 + 4) = 3 - 13 = -10.

R.J. was admitted to detoxification, inpatient, and outpatient treatment for 6 months. R.J. abstained from alcohol and other drugs during this rehabilitation period. He also attended Alcoholics Anonymous meetings several times a week.

In order to determine the presence or absence of social recovery, the Social Recovery Inventory was calculated after the 6-month rehabilitation period. Applying the general formula Index = Contributions - Costs, the three indices of the inventory were computed.

R.J. showed dramatic improvement in both occupational and civic functioning. His OPI score, for example, improved from a pretreatment low of -8 to a postrehabilitation score of +12 (Good Attendance, Good Interpersonal Relations, and Good Productivity; no costly behaviors were reported by the supervisor). Civic adjustment exhibited a similar transformation. The client's wife reported that R.J. no longer behaved destructively in the community, while he now was reasonably courteous to non-family members, paid creditors, and observed laws, including safe driving practices. A resultant CPI was computed: CPI = (4 + 3 + 5) - 0 = +12. In both occupational and civic arenas, R.J. therefore may be described as "recovering."

However, in the area of family role functioning, the client did not obtain recovery. The client's wife reported that he continued to be uncommunicative (failing to listen and self-disclose) and reneged on promises to engage in family activities (dinner, picnics, etc). Yet, he reportedly fulfilled financial obligations and still occasionally helped in domestic tasks which were not his primary responsibility. A postrehabilitation FPI of -1 (as compared to an earlier FPI of

NAME: ____________
TEST
DATE: ____________

SOCIAL RECOVERY INVENTORY

CONSTRUCTIVE BEHAVIORS	SOCIAL FUNCTIONING		
	OCCUPATIONAL	FAMILIAL	CIVIC
	1. High Productivity(5) ____	1. Exhibits Physical and/or Verbal Affection (5) ____	1. Obeys Laws/Safe Driving Practices (5) ____
	2. Good Work Relations(4) ____	2. Fulfills Primary Obligations(4) ____	2. Courteous to Citizens(4) ____
	3. Versatile Skills(4) ____	3. Listens to Family(4) ____	3. Community Service(3) ____
	4. Good Attendance(3) ____	4. Discloses Feelings(4) ____	4. Pays Taxes(3) ____
	5. Special Achievements(3) ____	5. Spends Time with Family(2) ____	5. Pays Creditors(3) ____
	6. Impressive Unit Representative(2) ____	6. Assists Domestic Chores(2) ____	6. Political Participation (e.g., Voting)(3) ____
	(A) ____	(C) ____	(E) ____

DESTRUCTIVE BEHAVIORS	1. Absenteeism/Tardiness(4) ____ 2. Inattention to Duties(4) ____ 3. Low Productivity(4) ____ 4. High Accident Rate(3) ____ 5. Malingering(3) ____ 6. Poor Work Relations(3) ____ (B) ____	1. Physical Abuse(6) ____ 2. Verbally Degrades(4) ____ 3. Neglects Primary Obligations(4) ____ 4. Fails to Listen(3) ____ 5. Reneges on Promises(2) ____ 6. Fails to Self-Disclose(2) ____ (D) ____	1. Major Legal Violation (e.g., Felony)(6) ____ 2. Offensive Public Acts(4) ____ 3. Fails to Pay Creditors(3) ____ 4. Fails to Pay Taxes(3) ____ 5. Minor Legal Violation (Misdemeanor) (3) ____ 6. Reclusiveness(2) ____ (F) ____
INDICES	OCCUPATIONAL PERFORMANCE INDEX= A - B= ____ - ____ = ____	FAMILIAL PERFORMANCE INDEX= C - D= ____ - ____ = ____	CIVIC PERFORMANCE INDEX= E - F= ____ - ____ = ____
Circle the Appropriate Item(s) as Indicated by Positive Index Sign(s):	OCCUPATIONAL RECOVERY	FAMILIAL RECOVERY	CIVIC RECOVERY

Fig. 1. Social Recovery Inventory format.

−9) was computed. Although some improvement was detected, social recovery within this role arena di·' not occur.

Figure 2 summarizes the Social Recovery Inventory results as previously presented. Note that recovery requires a positive index sign.

DISCUSSION

The Social Recovery Inventory accounts for the complex nature of social functioning; all addicts exhibit *both* constructive and destructive behaviors in the course of interaction. It is the relative importance of behaviors and comparative balance between constructiveness and destructiveness which determines the labeling of an addict as generally "wholesome" or "spoiled."

This instrument also suggests a reward maximization-cost minimization strategy in practice. It is a familiar approach which directs the practitioner to help the addict to improve strengths while eliminating limitations. Directed attention to skills (contributions) also encourages a positive approach to practice as well.

An opportunity for program evaluation also exists, for comparison of index scores prior to and following intervention allows some conclusion on program effectiveness. Index scores may indicate a general category of adjustment (recovery; overall impairment) as well as degree of recovery, improvement without recovery, or deterioration. For example, the example of R.J. illustrates occupational and civic recovery and demonstrates familial progress (as indicated by FPI movement from −9 to −1).

The Social Recovery Inventory is but a preliminary development in the continuing clarification of social recovery. Although the instrument possesses several limitations (possible generalization restrictions and some insensitivity to multiple events), it offers a theoretically based operationalization of social recovery.

In moving from the definition of social recovery to the question of its causation, one may identify the conditions which determine it. Abstinence, as a prerequisite, has been reviewed. It is best understood as a necessary but not sufficient condition for social recovery; that is, the presence of abstinence does not ensure recovery, but its absence will prevent it. Then what other conditions exist?

A valuable resource in this inquiry may be found in the seminal work of Ripple (1955). Ripple hypothesized "that the client's use of casework service is determined by his motivation, his capacity, and the opportunities afforded him both by his environment and by the social agency from which he seeks help" (p. 173). Motivation here refers to client goals and pressure toward these goals (the client's interests, attractions, objectives, and desires). Capacity involves physical, intellectual, and emotional development (the client's abilities, skills, and strengths). Opportunity includes two categories of resources: service

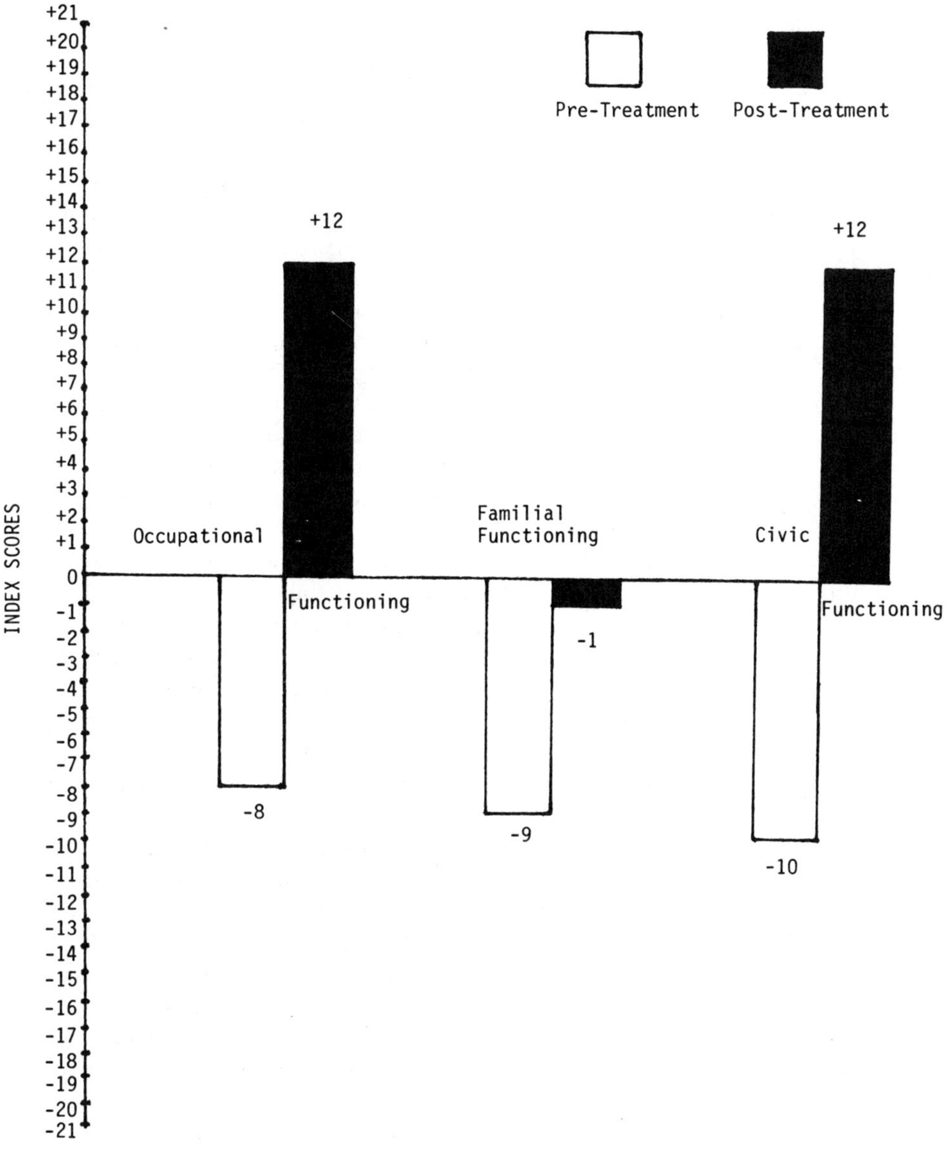

Fig. 2. Social Recovery Inventory results.

opportunity (level of staff competence, range of treatment methods, accessibility to clientele) and environmental opportunity (societal conditions which benefit or hinder clientele).

An analogy may be drawn to social recovery. In addition to abstinence, it is proposed that the addict's motivation, capacity, and opportunity are further determinants of social recovery. The presence of these four variables, then, provides a sufficient set of conditions for social recovery.

Discussion of the previous case study will illustrate this proposition. In particular, R.J.'s performance of familial roles (husband, father) seemed especially problematic, for the Social Recovery Inventory (i.e., the Familial Performance Index) indicated progress without recovery after treatment.

After some exploration with the addicted client, it was discovered that R.J. had lost interest in his desire for his wife. His motivation to fulfill the role of husband (and even father) therefore was affected adversely; R.J. often avoided coming home and participation in family activities because he feared that marital conflict would emerge. This also implied a limited emotional capacity to communicate and cope with interpersonal tension. His treatment plan therefore was amended to assist the wife and client to improve communication skills and learn to tolerate potential disagreement.

Another potential illustration might involve an addict who did not appear to recover occupationally. However, the reason might be unemployment or ethnic prejudice. Any deprivation of environmental opportunity may hinder social recovery even though enhanced motivation, capacity, and service opportunity exist with a drug-free, treated addict. Such circumstances as social problems (unemployment; racism, poverty) and irretrievable physical capacity (e.g., irreversible brain damage) lie beyond the addict's control.

In summary, treatment will involve an effort to enable the client to increase access to rewards while decreasing any tendency to withhold rewards from role partners. For example, helping the client to express such positive feelings as affection and approval will increase client contributions to role partners. Another therapeutic intervention, anger control therapy, relates to the other general objective, that of decreasing the client's reluctance to offer rewards to a role partner (e.g., a husband who pouts or who is violent due to inadequate impulse control). Given a particular pretreatment level of social functioning, what then realistically can be expected vis-à-vis social recovery? Theoretically, therapeutic impact will depend upon the client's access to rewards and the addicted client's willingness/reluctance to reward. Although access to rewards explicitly suggests opportunities (resources such as information, goods, and money), it also involves capacity in the sense that client capability to express affection and approval serves as a valuable reward for certain role partners. Finally, willingness/reluctance to reward role partners evokes the concept of motivation (the addicted client's interest or desire to reward).

Social recovery emerges as a complex and variable phenomenon. As may be inferred from the preceding examination, one man's (social) recovery may look quite different from another's. Each may be a recovering addict, but the two may differ in regard to involvement in social roles and performance within the same arena. One may be more family oriented, while the other may be deeply involved in civic activities (community service or politics). Thus, social recovery is a global concept which requires specification to have meaning.

In addition, practitioners would be well advised to identify carefully the addicted client's responsibility in rehabilitation. The discussion of irreparable physical capacity and diminished opportunity revealed the inability of addicted clientele to *totally* control *all* conditions for recovery. Therefore, it would be unwarranted to pronounce (to the addict): "You are responsible for your own recovery." Yet such a message has been promulgated, explicitly and implicitly, in the past.

Of course, the addict generally can control certain conditions. For example, the client can choose to accept agency services which seek to enhance motivation and capacity or work with the environment to increase opportunities. Also, the addict has control of the first drink or dosage. Even though prey to compulsion and irrational thinking, the addict can choose to use his own strengths or ask for help prior to beginning a cycle of uncontrolled, compulsive use stimulated by the first drink or drug dosage. Abstinence, then, can be considered "controllable." Indeed, abstinence (often referred to as "sobriety") can be considered the addict's responsibility ("You are responsible for your own sobriety"). In reflection of this viewpoint, a therapeutic approach has been developed to train addicts in relapse prevention (Marlatt and Gordon, 1980). The relapse prevention approach focuses upon helping the recovering addict to avoid taking that first dosage which begins the chain of uncontrolled, compulsive use.

The preceding examination of social recovery would suggest a need for staff to model and teach empathy as a social skill. If the client is to contribute to a role partner, he must be capable of recognizing the partner's expectations. Also, the recovering addict must ascertain those activities that are rewarding (or costly) to the role partner. With such awareness, the addicted client may be socially profitable.

Therefore, as a first step, in-service training can develop counselors as models through empathy training (Milnes and Bertcher, 1980). Second, staff education should include coaching clients in practicing social skills during clinical sessions. Such practice may involve a variety of modalities, including group interaction, role play (Corsini, 1966), or cognitive techniques (Frank, 1978).

A final implication stems from the importance of opportunity in social recovery. Since such "social" problems as poverty, racism, and massive unemployment restrict the client's social potential, they are clinical issues as well.

Treatment programs clearly would benefit from alleviation of these restrictions upon client opportunity. Therefore, staff participation in health and welfare councils or other community organizations involves administrative practicality as well as altruism.

SUMMARY

Therapeutic mission vis-à-vis social recovery has been defined from a perspective of role and exchange theories. Derived from this perspective, the Social Recovery Inventory has been demonstrated as an instrument for determination of rehabilitation progress.

The necessary conditions for social recovery have been reviewed, and implications for (addicted) client responsibility and adjustment have been discussed. Finally, clarification of role performance in arenas other than vocation, family life, and citizenship awaits further research.

REFERENCES

ADAMS, G.J., and MC NEAR, F.M. Transabling: An action therapy for resocialization. *Maryland State Med. J.* 26: 82, 1977.

BOEHM, W.W. *Objectives of the Social Work Curriculum of the Future,* Vol. 1 of the Curriculum Study. New York: Council on Social Work Education, 1959, p. 46.

BURGESS, R., and BUSHELL, D. *Behavioral Sociology.* New York: Columbia University Press, 1969, p. 274.

CORSINI, R. *Roleplaying in Psychotherapy.* Chicago: Aldine, 1966.

FOA, U.G., and FOA, E.B. *Societal Structures of the Mind.* Springfield, IL: C.C. Thomas, 1974, p. 80.

FRANK, S. Just imagine how I feel: How to improve empathy through training in imagination. In *The Power of Human Imagination.* New York: Plenum Press, 1978.

HAASZ, I. ET AL. Basic principles in resocializational: Rehabilitation of alcoholic patients. *Alcoholism: J. Alcoholism Related Addict.* 16: 62-65, 1980.

HOMANS, G. *Social Behavior: Its Elementary Forms.* New York: Harcourt, Brace, and World, 1961.

KING, B.L., ET AL. Alcoholics Anonymous, alcoholism counseling, and social work treatment. *Health Soc. Work* 4(4): 181-198, 1979.

MARLATT, G.A., and GORDON, J.R. Determinants of relapse: Implications for the maintenance of behavior change. In *Behavioral Medicine: Changing Health Lifestyles.* New York: Brunner/Mazel, 1980.

MILLER, M., ET AL. *Learning to Live Again: A Guide for Recovery from Alcoholism.* Hazel Crest, IL: Human Ecology Systems, 1980.

MILNES, J., and BERTCHER, H. *Communicating Empathy.* San Diego, CA: University Associates, 1980.

MOFFETT, A.D., ET AL. New Ways of reating addicts. *Soc. Work* 19: 389-396, 1974.

MOOS, R.H., ET AL. The process of recovery from alcoholism. *J. Stud. Alcohol* 42: 383-402, 1981.

RIPPLE, L. Motivation, capacity, and opportunity as related to use of casework service: Theoretical base and plan of study. *Soc. Serv. Rev.* 29: 172-193, 1955.

ROSE, A.M. *Human Behavior and Social Processes: An Interactionist Approach.* Boston: Houghton Mifflin, 1962.

WHORLEY, L.W. Social profitableness: Pathway to community acceptance of psychiatric patients. *Ment. Health Soc.* 5: 183-185, 1978.

WHORLEY, L.W. The Occupational Performance Index. *Labor-Management Alcoholism J.* 10: 204-208, 1981.

The International Journal of the Addictions, 19(7), 767–787, 1984

An Evaluation of the Alternatives Approach to Drug Abuse Prevention

Royer Cook,* PhD
Hazel Lawrence, MS
Carolyn Morse, MS
Janice Roehl, MS

Institute for Social Analysis
Reston, Virginia 22090

Abstract

An alternatives-oriented, school-based drug abuse prevention program, Positive Alternatives for Youth (PAY), was evaluated over a 2-year period. Using a random-assignment, pretest-posttest control group design, 135 PAY students and 106 control group students were assessed on several attitudinal and behavioral measures of drug use. During the first year significant differences were detected between PAY and control students. Fewer differences were found in the second year, although a special analysis showed evidence of impact on PAY students rated as more involved in program activities. Reasons for specific results are discussed and implications are drawn for the alternatives approach and the field of drug abuse prevention.

Since the mid-1960's approaches to prevent the abuse of drugs have taken many forms, from educational approaches to counseling-therapeutic approaches, and more recently, to efforts aimed at strengthening the individual's family and social environment. Among the more intriguing prevention efforts developed to

*To whom requests for reprints should be sent at the Institute for Social Analysis, 11739 Bowman Green Drive, Reston, Virginia 22090.

 0020-773X/84/1907-0767$3.50/0

date is the alternatives approach (Cohen, 1971; Cook and Morse, 1980; Dohner, 1972). Dohner expressed the essence of the alternatives concept when he stated that individuals use and abuse drugs because of the rewards and pleasures they provide, rewards and pleasures that are not available to them through nonchemical means, and that in order to prevent or reduce drug abuse, individuals must be provided with "positive alternatives" to drug abuse–ways of gaining the desired rewards and pleasures through healthy, nonchemical activities.

Briefly, the alternatives approach may be viewed as being based upon the following chain of events:

1. Drug abuse fulfills certain social, psychological, and physiological needs and wants; it can produce several positive states and reduce negative states.
2. A variety of nonchemical activities and experiences are also capable of fulfilling these needs and wants in a much healthier way.
3. By engaging in these nonchemical activities and experiences, an individual will fulfill the needs and wants, and will therefore not have to abuse drugs. Instead, he or she will proceed to a fuller, healthier adjustment and life-style.
4. Therefore, by making alternative activities available to youths in a community, there will be a decrease in the use and abuse of drugs.

A wide variety of activities and experiences from athletics to Zen have been suggested as alternatives, and many have found their way into prevention programs. The popularity (at least in concept, if not in practice) of the alternatives approach is probably attributable to its "positive" image, its theoretical attractiveness, and the disappointing performance of the other more traditional prevention approaches, such as drug education (Hanson, 1980). Yet there has been very little research–and virtually no rigorous evaluation research–on the efficacy of the alternatives approach.

The general purpose of this research was to conduct a field experiment to determine the impact of the alternatives approach on drug and alcohol use, and on several correlates of drug use.

BACKGROUND

When drug abuse first became a phenomenon of national concern in the mid-1960s, the initial predominant response aimed at its prevention was to embark on drug abuse education programs. The educational approach is essentially based on the rationale that a significant proportion of people–especially young people–use and abuse drugs because they are not sufficiently aware of the effects and damages of drug taking. Research has generally indicated that the impact of educational approaches on drug use and abuse is negligible or, at best, limited to certain subpopulations of youth (Braucht et al., 1973; Cook and

Morton, 1975; Goodstadt, 1974; Richards, 1971). Richards's early review of the state of the art of drug education was not encouraging, although she cautioned against the use of unrealistic criteria, such as attempting to detect immediate decreases in drug use. Braucht et al. (1973) cited the paucity of evidence in support of drug education while noting the dearth of methodological rigor among the evaluation studies. This investigator (Cook and Morton, 1975) found drug education in the Army to be largely ineffective in a combination of cross-sectional and pretest-posttest control group (nonrandom assignment) studies. Based upon this evidence and their review of the literature, Cook and Morton concluded that drug education was not an effective drug prevention technique. In his review of the prevention evaluation literature, Goodstadt (1974) concluded that there was an impressive lack of evidence indicating beneficial effects of drug education, but that the methodological flaws of the evaluations were so great that confident inferences of any sort were extremely difficult to make. Hanson's recent (1980) review of the efficacy of drug education was not encouraging.

Furthermore, when one analyzes the accumulated evidence on the etiology of drug abuse, there is little reason to believe that the use or abuse of drugs occurs out of ignorance or misperceptions of the effects and dangers of drug abuse. The key studies of Becker (1968), Jessor and Jessor (1977), Johnston et al. (1978), and Kandel (1978), and our work in the military (Cook, Hostetter, and Ramsay, 1975; Cook, Walizer, and Mace, 1976) have implicated a broad and complex range of personal and social conditions which contribute to drug abuse. A review of research on the social psychological factors which predispose individuals toward initial drug abuse has identified a wide range of conditions which might underlie drug abuse, including the family environment, peer associations, socialization to nontraditional norms, numerous personality characteristics, and availability of drugs (Gorsuch and Butler, 1976; Kandel, 1978). If any conclusion may be drawn regarding the accumulated evidence on the probable causes and correlates of drug abuse, it is that it has multiple causes, that for any given individual it may be rooted in any of a number of deficiencies in one's personality and environment.

In recent years, the character of drug abuse prevention has changed—or at least the cutting edge of prevention approaches—to include more affective, behavioral approaches. Instead of using simply an informational approach, innovative programs are attempting to strengthen the personal and social-environmental supports of youth. These approaches appear to be rooted more firmly in the social psychology of drug abuse and deviance. They recognize that the literature indicates that the common correlates (and perhaps causes) of drug abuse in youth are personal problems and social-environmental deficiencies. They are based on the logical rationale that an amelioration of these personal and social conditions will produce a diminution of drug abuse. These approaches are relatively new; there is not yet a substantial accumulation of published evaluation research in the literature. While some reports indicate that such approaches are promising, research to date has been flawed by many of the same deficiencies (lack of control, multiple measures, etc.) that have plagued the drug education evaluations (Schaps et al., 1980).

The alternatives approach is one of these recently developed approaches to drug abuse prevention.

THE ALTERNATIVES APPROACH

The basic notions underlying the alternatives approach were first mentioned in a series of articles appearing from 1968 through 1971 (Chanin, 1969; Cohen, 1971; DeRopp, 1968; Paine, 1971). However, it was probably Dohner (1972) who was mainly responsible for pulling together somewhat disparate ideas into a coherent statement of the alternatives concept. Dohner contended that individuals use and abuse drugs because of the rewards and pleasures they provide, rewards and pleasures that are not available to them through nonchemical means. In order to prevent or reduce drug abuse, individuals must be provided with "positive alternatives" to drug abuse—ways of gaining the desired rewards and pleasures through healthy, nonchemical activities.

The alternatives to drug abuse suggested by Dohner included personal awareness, interpersonal relations, self-reliance development, vocational skills, aesthetic experiences, intellectual experiences, social-political involvement, sexual expression, meditation, spiritual-mystical experiences, and creative experiences. As indicated by this list, a central conceptual problem with this approach is that almost any activity qualifies as an "alternative to drug abuse." According to Dohner, any of these activities may or may not supplant the need or desire to engage in drug abuse. These were Dohner's experienced-based speculations about the range of activities. Cohen (1973) later provided a list of 93 different alternative activites. And the publication *Alternative Pursuits for America's 3rd Century* presents the reader with an even more highly varied array of alternative concepts and activities (NIDA, 1974). Even if there are an infinite variety of activities which might possibly serve, in a particular instance, to supplant one's desire for drugs, surely there are some limited number that combine prevention efficacy with feasibility. Perhaps an even more important question is whether exposure to any (or any combination) of these experiences helps to prevent drug abuse.

METHOD

The object of the 2-year evaluation research project was the Positive Alternatives for Youth (PAY) program which presented alternatives classes in the public schools of Milwaukee, Wisconsin. The PAY program was evaluated in two cycles over a period of 2 years. In both cycles, the design used was a pretest-posttest control group design (Campbell and Stanley, 1966), a "true" experimental design in which students eligible for the program were randomly assigned to either the PAY alternative classes or to a no-treatment control group, and were assessed on the criteria of interest both before and at the end of the semester-long PAY classes. Analysis of variance and analysis of covariance were used to assess the significance of differences between the PAY students and the control students.

Program Description

The Positive Alternatives for Youth program is a series of alternatives classes presented to junior and senior high school students in the Milwaukee Public Schools. The classes meet two to three times a week during regular school hours and are conducted jointly by a Pay staff person and a teacher-trainee. The objectives of the Pay program were jointly developed by the research team and the PAY staff. They are listed here in order of importance as weighted by the PAY staff:

1. *To improve interpersonal skills:* Students in PAY classes will become more effective in establishing interpersonal relationships with peers and with adults. They will learn to communicate ideas and feelings more effectively, and to be more assertive in interactions with others.
2. *To improve self-esteem, feelings of power, and skills to make decisions about life and career:* Students in PAY classes will feel better about themselves and will feel that they have some control over their lives, rather than being at the mercy of forces over which they have no control. PAY students will also learn to make decisions about their life and will begin to perceive more career options available to them.
3. *To improve the number and variety of positive behaviors:* PAY students will more frequently engage in a larger variety of positive, healthful activities and will less frequently engage in deviant or delinquent acts. They will more frequently seek nonchemical means to alter mood and seek comfort.
4. *To prevent alcohol and drug abuse:* In comparison to control subjects, students in the PAY classes will engage in less alcohol and drug use. To the extent that drugs and alcohol are used, they will be used more responsibly by PAY students than by students in the control group.

The alternatives classes consisted of the following major units, presented over a semester:

- *Orientation:* Designed mainly to create a relaxed atmosphere and to begin building group cohesion.
- *Communications:* Awareness and practice of communicating feelings effectively, with a special emphasis on assertiveness.
- *Self-concept:* To help youths become more aware of their own qualities and to share perceptions about self and others.
- *Self-care:* Designed to help youths recognize and cope with states of depression and stress.
- *Activities:* Activities presented to the youths are of three types: (1) physical activities, (2) creative-expressive activities, and (3) consciousness alteration.

It should be noted that the prevention of drug and alcohol abuse was given a low priority as a program goal and was not a separate major unit in the curriculum (although the topic was addressed as part of other units, particularly the self-care unit).

The typical PAY class involved one or two experiential exercises, such as active-listening role plays and the "coat of arms" exercise (where each student draws a coat of arms that represents his/her own values and characteristics), interspersed with lecturettes and discussion. The atmosphere was loose and informal, with PAY staff and students on a first-name basis. The typical PAY class had 10-12 students, with 15 as an upper limit.

In the 1979-1980 school year, three high schools and one junior high school were involved in the PAY program. In the 1980-1981 school year, two junior high schools and one senior high school participated in the program (the other two senior high schools that participated during the previous year continued to operate the PAY program on their own). Thus, the emphasis shifted in the second year from the senior high school students to the younger junior high school students.

The PAY program staff consisted of a half-time program director, a full-time program coordinator, and a half-time alternative education specialist. The program coordinator and the alternative education specialist were responsible for the day-to-day implementation of the program, shaping the details of the curriculum and serving as cofacilitators of the PAY classes along with the teachers.

Design and Measures

The design used for the evaluation of the PAY program was a pretest-posttest control group design in which students were randomly assigned to either PAY classes or a control group. This "true" experimental design provides for a high degree of internal validity; that is, excellent protection from the threats (potential differences in history, maturation, selection, etc.) which prevent one from attributing observed differences between experimental and control subjects to the treatment in question. The design fares less well with regard to external validity.

The approach to the development and refinement of our instrument battery was characterized by several important considerations designed to ensure reliable and valid measurement. First, most of the instruments were previously developed instruments or modifications of such instruments. They included instruments that we had developed and used in previous research, as well as selected instruments from the literature that display evidence of reliability and validity. Second, before using them to collect data on the spring 1980 cohort, we administered several pretests to ensure clarity of items and comprehension by the respondent. Third, care was taken to ensure that the drug use data were valid. Students were assured that the data were confidential, that no one outside the research team would ever know what any person's response was. The first page of the instrument battery showed the name and code number; the second page, only the code number. As the battery was passed out to the subjects, they removed the first page and handed it in–further evidence that we were interested only in codes and not names.

The dependent variables and the set of instruments used to measure them were as follows:

1. *Drug and alcohol use:* Measured by the Drug Use Checklist.
2. *Activities participated in:* Measured by the Activities Checklist.
3. *Feelings and remedies:* Measured by a modified version of the Barnes and Olson Feelings and Remedies Scale, which assesses the degree to which the respondent uses chemical or nonchemical "remedies" in reaction to (or in search of) emotional states.
4. *Marijuana involvement:* Measured by the Marijuana Involvement Scale, adapted from the Jessor and Jessor instrument battery.
5. *Alcohol involvement:* Measured by the Alcohol Involvement Scale, also adapted from the Jessor and Jessor battery.
6. *Alternatives impact:* Measured by a specially developed scale designed to assess the broad but subtle impact of alternatives classes. This 73-item scale consists of the following subscales:
   a. *Social relations:* Assesses attitudes and perceptions of one's social skills.
   b. *Peer control:* Assesses attitudes toward resisting peer pressure.
   c. *Self-esteem:* A modification of Rosenberg's scale.
   d. *Future orientation:* Assesses the degree to which one is oriented toward the future.
   e. *Stress management:* Assesses how well one feels he or she has learned to cope with stress.

f. *Attitudes toward drugs:* A condensed version of a previously developed scale of attitudes toward drug use.
g. *Attitudes toward alcohol:* A specially developed scale of attitudes toward alcohol use.
h. *Responsible use:* Assesses the degree to which an individual accepts the notion of responsible use of drugs and alcohol.
i. *Activity attitudes:* Assesses attitudes toward activity, including the degree of acceptance of the alternatives concept.

Reliability and Validity of the Measures. The Drug Use Checklist was developed by Hurst, Cook, and Ramsay (1975) to assess the prevalence of drug use in the Army. In that research, the measure was shown to be reliable (test-retest reliability of .81) and valid (in comparison to urinalysis data) on a worldwide sample of 17,141 soldiers. The Activities Checklist consisted of a simple list of 15 different types of activities derived from Dohner's suggested alternatives; the respondent simply checked the frequency of involvement in the activity during the last 2 months from "not at all" to "daily." The Feelings and Remedies Scale was developed by Barnes and Olson (1977) and used in their alternatives research. The Marijuana Involvement Scale was developed and used in the Jessor and Jessor (1977) research. The authors reported a coefficient of reproducibility of .96, a coefficient of scalability of .86, and an alpha coefficient of .81. They also indicated that it "proved extremely useful as a criterion measure that goes beyond the simple distinction between users and non-users" (Jessor and Jessor, 1977). The Alcohol Involvement Scale was an adaptation of the Marijuana Involvement Scale, substituting alcohol and drinking in place of marijuana and "getting stoned." The Alternatives Impact Scale was specially developed for this research, although two subscales were modifications of previously developed scales. The Self-Esteem Subscale was a modified version of Rosenberg's (1965) scale, and the Attitudes Toward Drugs Scale was a condensed version of a scale developed by Cook and Theologus (1976). Alpha coefficients (estimates of internal consistency) computed on all the subscales were as follows: Social relations, .76; Peer control, .58; Self-esteem, .80; Future orientation, .45; Stress management, .65; Attitudes toward drugs, .82; Attitudes toward alcohol, .80; Responsible use, .57; and Activity attitudes, .75. Thus, about half of these subscales display very good reliability coefficients (.76 to .82), while the others are marginal (.45 to .65). Not surprisingly, the higher alpha coefficients are yielded by the longer subscales (8 to 12 items), and the lower ones by the very short subscales (3 to 4 items).

During the first year, the instrument battery did not contain the Marijuana Involvement or Alcohol Involvement Scales, and the Alternatives Impact Scale contained only 20 items (although the subscales of self-esteem and attitudes toward drugs and alcohol were included as separate scales in the first-year battery).

Including a background/demographics section, the entire battery required approximately 1 hour for completion.

Data Collection Procedures

Pretest and posttest outcome data were collected on PAY and control group students during the spring semesters of 1980 and 1981. Outcome data were not collected during the fall semesters mainly because they were, in effect, pilot semesters for the PAY program in both years, times when the program was being revised, new schools were added, teacher-facilitators were being trained, etc. In both years, all the PAY students and the control groups were volunteers, recruited on the basis of a "pitch" delivered to students in study halls at the beginning of the semester, designed both to inform them about the program's purposes and activities, and to motivate them to join PAY.

During the first year 154 students were pretested; 90 were PAY students and 64 were in the control group. Seventy-seven of the PAY students and 57 of the control group were posttested. During the second year 129 students were pretested; 70 were PAY students and 59 were in the control group. At the end of the semester 58 of the PAY students and 50 of the control group were posttested.

Subjects

The first-year experimental group consisted of 39 males and 38 females, and the control group contained 32 males and 25 females. There were 47 Whites, 29 Blacks, and 1 Oriental in the first-year experimental group; the control group contained 42 Whites, 14 Blacks, and 1 Oriental. The mean age of the experimental group was 15.6 years; for the control group, 15.0 years.

During the second year, the average age of experimental and control students was 13.9 years (14.0 for the experimental group and 13.9 for the control group). The experimental group consisted of 20 males and 38 females, of whom 28 were White, 29 Black, and 1 was Oriental. The control group contained 22 males and 28 females, of whom 33 were White, 14 were Black, 2 were Oriental, and 1 was American Indian. Thus, in the second year, the subject pool was younger (by 1.5 years) and contained more females.

Analysis. In the analysis of the first-year data, analysis of variance (ANOVA) of gain scores was the selected analytic technique. For the analysis of second-year data, analysis of covariance (ANCOVA) was employed, using the pretest score as the covariate.

RESULTS

Data were collected on the PAY program in each of 2 years. Because of changes in both the program and the instrument battery from the first year to the second, separate analyses were conducted on each year's data.

Year 1 Results

All the dependent measures were converted to gain scores (posttest minus pretest) and subjected to one-way analysis of variance, contrasting experimental (PAY) group scores with control group scores. Table 1 shows the variables for which significant differences were found; Table 2 shows the nonsignificant effects.

The Drug Use Checklist showed a significant difference between PAY and control students only on the substance of hard liquor, with PAY students showing a decrease and control students showing a slight increase in hard liquor use ($F = 6.72, p = .01$). There were no other differences across types of drugs on the Drug Use Checklist. On the Feelings and Remedies Scale, we found that alternatives students reduced their use of drugs and alcohol in response to negative emotional states, whereas control students increased drug and alcohol use in response to negative states ($F = 4.59$, $p = .03$). There were no differences in response to positive states; apparently recreational use of alcohol and drugs–to "feel good," to "have fun," etc.–is unaffected by the PAY classes. When we looked at specific clusters of negative emotions, we found that it was in response to anxiety in particular that the PAY students switched to more nonchemical

Table 1
Results of One-Way ANOVAs on Year 1 Data: Significant Effects

Variable	Experimental $\bar{X}$ (pre)	Experimental $\bar{X}$ (post)	Control $\bar{X}$ (pre)	Control $\bar{X}$ (post)	F	p
Hard liquor	1.53	1.40	1.49	1.55	6.72	.01
Drug/alcohol use in response to negative emotions	0.90	0.86	0.98	1.57	4.59	.03
Drug/alcohol use in response to anxiety	0.43	0.32	0.48	0.86	4.25	.04
Self-esteem (posttest)		30.80		28.87	4.77	.03
Alternatives impact (posttest)		64.11		59.99	11.58	.0009

Table 2
Results of One-Way ANOVAs on Year 1 Data: Nonsignificant Effects

Variable	F	p
Activity	0.045	0.8316
Drug use (overall)	0.673	0.4137
Tobacco	0.034	0.8537
Beer/wine	0.298	0.5865
Inhalant use	0.248	0.6194
Stimulant use	0.023	0.8794
Depressant use	1.327	0.2517
Marijuana use	0.011	0.9175
Hallucinogen use	0.045	0.8329
Opiate use	0.435	0.5107
Cocaine use	2.340	0.1289
PCP use	0.756	0.3864
Qualude use (no use)	0	0
Drug attitudes	0.232	0.6310
Feelings/remedies (drug and alcohol use in response to . . .):		
Positive emotions	0.178	0.6780
Hostility	1.784	0.1844
Depression	0.124	0.7251
Adventure seeking	0.949	0.3321
Camaraderie	1.340	0.1498
Pleasure seeking	0.521	0.4719
Pain	0.158	0.6915

remedies ($F = 4.25, p = .04$). Alternatives students displayed higher self-esteem scores than the control students ($F = 4.77, p = .03$). They also scored higher on the Alternatives Impact Scale ($F = 11.58, p = .0009$).

The one-way ANOVAS showed no significant differences between PAY students and controls on the Activities Checklist, Attitudes Toward Drugs Scale, or on any substance use indices (except for hard liquor).

Selected two-way ANOVAS showed effects of Sex (as well as Program) on self-esteem, with boys scoring significantly higher than girls ($F = 9.15, p = .003$). When we divided all students into High or Low Activity, based upon whether they scored above or below the median on the Activity Checklist, we found that the High-Activity group had a significantly higher score on the Alternatives Impact Scale ($F = 4.69, p = .03$).

In addition to these analyses, two types of dropout analyses were conducted: (1) PAY students were compared with PAY dropouts on dependent variable pretest scores, and (2) PAY dropouts were compared with control dropouts (those who did not appear for posttesting).

PAY dropouts differed from PAY students significantly on the variable of hard liquor use ($F = 6.84$, $df = 1, 71$, $p = .01$), with the dropouts ($N = 13$) using more hard liquor at pretest than those who stayed in PAY ($N = 78$). Similarly, the dropouts had significantly lower scores on two of the self-esteem subscales: "Being known" ($F = 4.07$, $df = 1, 72$, $p = .047$) and "Well-being" ($F = 6.03$, $df = 1, 72$, $p = .016$). They did not differ on other dependent variables. These results suggest that one reason the PAY classes had more success in decreasing hard liquor use and increasing self-esteem was that some of the more difficult youths left the program. Although this does not change the fact that those who stayed in PAY (the large majority) achieved positive changes on these indices in comparison to the control group, it dampens those findings somewhat. In addition, it should serve to alert PAY staff that some of the students who were most in need of the program were dropping out—not an uncommon problem with a variety of prevention and treatment programs.

The comparison of PAY dropouts with control dropouts also showed PAY dropouts to exceed control dropouts on the pretest index of hard liquor use. However, there were only seven control dropouts, most of whom were from the junior high school sample (all PAY dropouts were in the senior high school sample). Thus, the age differences in the two groups combined with the very low *N* rendered this particular dropout analysis somewhat meaningless.

Year 2 Results

Analyses of the second-year PAY DATA were of three major types: (1) one-way ANCOVAs on the dependent variables contrasting PAY and control students; (2) three-way ANCOVAs testing the main effects of the program (PAY vs control), race, and sex; and (3) one-way ANCOVAs contrasting high-involvement PAY students with low-involvement PAY students. In all analyses, pretest scores were used as the covariate. The last analysis was based upon a division of the PAY students on the basis of ratings by facilitators and observers.

One-way ANCOVAs comparing PAY students with control students revealed differences only on the Activity Checklist, with PAY students showing an increase in activity level above that of control students. ANCOVA contrasts of PAY and control students on all other dependent variables were nonsignificant. The three-way ANCOVAs testing the main effects of the program, race, and sex identified a few significant differences for both race and sex across several dependent variables, but very little in the way of significant interactions between program and sex or race. However, the program effect on drug attitudes approached significance ($p < .10$) when the sex and race variance was partitioned out, with PAY students showing a slightly less favorable attitude toward drugs, while control students exhibited a slight increase in positive attitudes toward drugs.

When these analyses were completed, it was evident that the impact of the PAY program in the second year was not overwhelming—at least as indicated by our battery of dependent measures. Still, there were the findings of the previous year: If the PAY program was not effective, why had several dependent variables shown significance in the first year? There were, of course, several possible explanations for some decrease in program impact from the first to the second year (e.g., change in target populations; see later discussion), yet none seemed quite strong enough to warrant a conclusion that the program had simply lost its effectiveness, particularly when both observers and facilitators were reporting perceived movement on the part of many of the PAY students. Perhaps the PAY program was having an impact on only those students who were involved in the program—those who paid attention to, and meaningfully participated in, the PAY exercises. To test this thesis, two sets of "involvement" indicators were developed for each student, based upon the ratings of students by facilitators and by observers. Mean ratings on the dimensions of participation, understanding, and attention were computed for each student and combined into a single index of involvement. Thus, each PAY student had two indices of involvement, one based upon the facilitators' ratings and the other based upon the observers' ratings. PAY students were then divided by the overall mean involvement score into a High-involvement group and a Low-involvement group. One-way ANCOVAs were then computed on the dependent variable set, using involvment as the main effect. This involvement index should not be construed as simply an estimate by the facilitators or observers of how great an impact the program was having on the students. It was an indicator of how engaged they were in the process; and although the index is correlated with impact, it was not derived by simply identifying the most promising students.

The analysis based upon facilitator-designated involvement produced several significant differences between the two groups, virtually all of them in the expected direction:

- *Future orientation:* High-involvement students showed a greater increase in orientation toward the future than Low-involvement students, as indicated by scores on the Future Orientation Subscale of the Alternatives Impact Scale ($F = 4.04, p = .05$).
- *Attitudes toward alcohol use:* High-involvement students showed less favorable attitudes toward alcohol use than Low-involvement students, as indicated by scores on the Alcohol Attitudes Subscale of the Alternatives Impact Scale ($F = 4.90, p = .03$).
- *Responsible use:* High-involvement students exhibited more change toward more responsible use of drugs and alcohol than Low-involvement students,

as indicated by scores on the Responsible Use Subscale of the Alternatives Impact Scale ($F = 3.91, p = .05$).

- *Attitudes toward activity:* High-involvement students exhibited more positive attitudes toward activity (liking to do physical and creative activities) than Low-involvement students, as shown by scores on the Activity Attitudes Subscale of the Alternatives Impact Scale ($F = 4.31$, $p = .04$).
- *Alcohol involvement:* High-involvement students increased their alcohol involvement less than did the Low-involvement students, as shown by scores on the Alcohol Involvement Scale, although the differences only approached significance ($F = 3.16, p = .08$).
- *Marijuana use:* High-involvement students decreased their use of marijuana while Low-involvement students increased their use of marijuana, as shown by scores on the marijuana item on the Drug Use Checklist, although the difference only approached significance ($F = 2.92, p = .09$).

The analysis of High/Low-involvement groups as identified by the *observers* revealed differences only on the Feelings and Remedies Scale. In contrast to the Low-involvement group, the High-involvement group reported an increase in both (1) their use of nondrug remedies in response to negative emotional states ($F = 2.83$, $p = .098$), and (2) their use of drug remedies when seeking positive emotional states ($F = 4.53, p = .04$).

As shown in Table 3, in nearly all of these cases (with the exception of the Responsible Use means) the control group pretest and posttest means paralleled the Low-involvement group means.

Although these results must be viewed with a great deal of caution, they provide some support for the position that the PAY program may have had considerable impact on those youth who were actively involved in the program; that is, those who actually "received" the treatment in the full sense.

Unlike the first year, analysis of dropouts was not conducted on the second-year data. Although the decrease in sample sizes from pretest to posttest was roughly the same in both years, the decreases in the second year were not, for the most part, due to students "dropping out"; that is, voluntarily leaving the PAY classes or being dismissed from the program, as was the case during the first year. Of the 12 PAY students who were not posttested, two students were not posttested because their assignment had not been random, but at the request of the school administration; six students attended the PAY classes, but were not posttested because they either did not bring their parental permission forms or were absent during the posttest data collection period; one student was transferred to another school; and three took the pretest but never attended the PAY classes. Only the last three could legitimately be called dropouts.

Table 3
Mean Scores on Dependent Measures for Three Groups of Students

	High-involvement	Low-involvement	Controls
Future			
Pre	3.705	3.281	3.723
Post	4.117	3.489	3.998
Alcohol attitude			
Pre	2.088	2.044	2.191
Post	2.029	2.254	2.316
Responsible Use[a]			
Pre	2.486	2.591	2.607
Post	2.315	2.626	2.442
Alcohol involvement			
Pre	1.657	1.409	1.578
Post	1.768	1.542	1.733
Activity subscale			
Pre	4.168	4.042	4.223
Post	4.277	4.010	4.195
Marijuana use			
Pre	1.212	1.083	1.170
Post	1.182	1.167	1.293

[a]On the Responsible Use Subscale, a lower score indicates more responsibility.

DISCUSSION

At the end of the first year of research on the PAY program, the following "implications" had been drawn (Cook and Morse, 1980):

> We judged these preliminary results to be encouraging; they demonstrated to us that classroom-based alternatives as presented in the PAY program hold promise for preventing certain types of drug and alcohol abuse, particularly in reaction to negative emotional states. However, these first year's results were also characterized by notable negative findings. The impact on overall drug and alcohol use was slight, at best, and there was no evidence of effects on general attitudes toward drug use....
>
> Our basic interpretation of these mixed results is that the PAY classes had some impact on alcohol use, on chemical reactions to negative states, and improved self-esteem and social skills because these were the areas where the PAY classes were concentrated.

In the second year, the "encouraging" results of the initial year seemed at first glance to have diminished considerably, although the special involvement analyses showed program effects across a broad array of dependent variables—for High-involvement students. Those students who actively participated in the alternatives program moved toward a more future-oriented attitude, viewed alcohol use more negatively and healthful activity more favorably, and exhibited a more responsible attitude toward the use of drugs and alcohol. There were also indications that their use of alcohol and marijuana decreased, although across both years, the detectable effects of the program on reported drug and alcohol use were slight. These small effects on use must, however, be viewed with the understanding that it is quite difficult for a *prevention* program to show impact on reported drug and alcohol use in such a short period of time (5 months), particularly when use rates are so low.

There were several possible reasons for differences in apparent impact between the two years. First, the curriculum was altered somewhat in the second year to include more activities. However, our close examination of the PAY program (through classroom observations as well as curriculum review) revealed that the program did not significantly bolster the activity component—certainly not activities of the strenuous, physical kind. The lack of physical activity was attributed to both the unavailability of gymnasium facilities and the ambivalent views of the PAY staff, who were not as enthusiastic about the physical components as the affective-verbal components. Second, although the program coordinator changed from the first to the second year, that change was probably not a key contributor to the variation in results; most of the classes were actually taught by the assistant and the teachers. The most probable explanation for the less strong effects in the second year is the age difference between the target populations. In the first year, the students were predominantly high school students, mostly juniors and seniors; in the second year they were mostly junior high school students. Perhaps the concepts and experiences of the PAY program are too complex for or seen as irrelevant by many adolescents 13 to 14 years of age; perhaps only the more advanced (socially and cognitively) adolescents are prepared to engage in, and learn from, such experiences—that is, those youths in the High-involvement group. Of course, such an interpretation is not consonant with the current prevailing view that prevention programs should begin at the elementary and junior high school levels. But this evidence indicates that programs which address the more complex concepts of self and interpersonal skills may not be as effective with the younger populations.

What then can be said at this point about the efficacy of the PAY program and, by implication, about school-based alternatives programs of this type?

At a general level, it would be misleading to characterize the impact of the PAY program as simply "mixed" or "diminished"; there was also evidence that the PAY program can have some impact on the ways in which youths view themselves and their use of drugs and alcohol. When the program is directed toward high school age youth (as it was the first year), they are more likely to seek out nonchemical means of coping with negative emotional states, use less hard liquor, and feel improved self-esteem. There are also indications (the evidence is less definite on this score) that youths who become involved in the program show movement away from the use of alcohol and marijuana, display less favorable attitudes toward alcohol use and more favorable attitudes toward participating in activities, and show an increased orientation toward the future. They also exhibit tendencies toward more responsible use of drugs and alcohol.

These are tantalizing findings: Youth moving away from the use of chemicals toward activity and responsibility, gaining increasing respect for the broader hazards of drug and alcohol use to a healthful, satisfying life. But why does the evidence for impact flicker so—why are program effects so uneven?

We suspect that the central reason for the muted impact (beyond the age effects) lies in the program's thrust toward rather sweeping fundamental change and away from a focus on the issue of drug and alcohol use. During the past decade, many programs which focused on the prevention of drug and alcohol abuse (in both purpose and content) drew further away from the explicit mention of drugs and alcohol, and began addressing the elements of youth development which seemed to underly substance abuse; that is, self-concept, values, social environment, etc. (Schaps et al., 1980). As mentioned previously, this trend grew out of the perceptions that the educational approaches were not effective and that youths were using drugs less out of ignorance and more as a function of deficiencies in personal adjustment. It was reasoned that by clarifying values, shoring up lines of communication, polishing self-concept, and renewing social environments, the youth would not have needs to engage in drug and alcohol abuse. This trend has probably been a good one, but it is not without its flaws, both logical and practical. Just because drug use is associated with (the causal dynamics are still not clear and they are probably complex) a set of personal adjustment problems, it does not necessarily follow that the *most effective* way to prevent drug abuse is to ameliorate those adjustment problems through a school-based program. The most effective prevention method may be, for example, to make it clear that serious sanctions await the user of drugs and alcohol, both at home and at school. Or it may be to get a youth involved in an activity that provides the needed rewards and discipline—basically the alternatives philosophy. The PAY program (and a myriad of other affective education programs like it) takes direct aim at those particular personal adjustment problems and organizes the curriculum units around them. If part of the problem is low self-esteem, sessions are presented in which students and staff discuss self-concept—how it is developed and how it shapes behavior, etc.—and hope that self-esteem rises as a result. If part of the problem is viewed as feelings of social isolation and alienation brought on by poor communications with parents or peers, some sessions are therefore devoted to improving communications skills. This approach rests on two rather questionable implicit assumptions. It assumes that by filling the gaps in the social and psychological makeup of a youth, he or she will no longer need to use drugs (although for PAY staff, the "gapfilling" is an end in itself). Yet the causal dynamics among these elements and drug use are still not very well understood. For example, even if it is true that the causal flow is from some deficiency in personal adjustment to drug use (although in fact it is probably much more interactive than that), what happens when one or two of the critical gaps remain? Do *all* of them have to be filled before a youth is likely to forgo drug involvement—or just a majority of them? This approach further assumes that a frontal assault on each of these elements in the environs of the classroom is the way to restore them to their effective state. Yet all we know about adolescent development tells us that the natural development of interpersonal skills, self-concept, etc., involves a set of dynamics much different and more complex than the experiences comprised in a series of classroom sessions. There are also some very real practical issues here: Even if these personal adjustment elements can be effectively addressed in a classroom, is it realistic to expect that so many of them can be effectively addressed in the course of a single semester? Even if programs choose the affective education route, they would be wise to focus on fewer elements and not spread themselves so thinly over a broad range of affective educational elements.

The virtual omission of curriculum units devoted specifically to drug and alcohol abuse represents a reaction (in rather extreme form, we submit) to the ineffectiveness of past programs which were devoted almost solely to discussion of drugs and alcohol. Moreover, a program like PAY views itself not as a drug abuse prevention program, but as a program designed to promote the general growth and adjustment of adolescents. But why must the topic of drug and alcohol abuse be so assiduously avoided? One suspects that it is mainly because the staff feared that if they talked explicitly at some length about the hazards of drug and alcohol use, the students would perceive them as preachy adults who (like cops and teachers) are really just trying to control them, not understand and help them. But, of course, such discussions need not be simply antidrug in tone but might address the circumstances in which drug and alcohol use is probably not a good idea. (Indeed, this topic was touched upon in the PAY classes but only in the context of coping with stress and negative emotions.) In short, it is difficult to understand why the topic was not given more attention.

The selection and development of the alternative activities are continuing problems. If an activity is to serve as an alternative to drug abuse it must (1) meet needs that are likely to be met through drug or alcohol use, and (2) reflect the preferences of the youths toward whom the program is directed (allowing for individual differences), and not simply the views of program staff. Guidelines for addressing these issues have been developed elsewhere (Cook, Lawrence,

Morse, and Roehl, 1983). These guidelines are designed to maximize the probability that a given activity is attractive to a particular individual, and that it meets needs which might otherwise be met through drug use.

Although the subjects in this study were adolescents, the research results and the alternatives approach have obvious implications for adults as well. For the older general population (ages 20 and above) the alternatives approach may be more appropriately applied to the reduction in use of a variety of licit but unhealthful substances, including smoking, drinking, and misuse of prescription drugs and other medications. More research needs to be conducted on the ways in which adults currently "use" the alternatives approach (without calling it that) to control, reduce, or eliminate their use of hazardous substances; how it can be applied more systematically–individually and collectively–and to what effect.

With respect to the future of the alternatives approach to drug abuse prevention, we submit that the approach continues to hold considerable promise, but that substantial research, both basic and applied, remains to be conducted. We need to examine more closely the relationships between activity, hedonic states, and drug use. Moreover, further systematic research needs to be conducted in a representative school system in which a "true" alternatives program could be launched and tested, making full use of the facilities and staff of a school to engage the large majority (rather than only the talented minority) of youths in healthful activities. As evidence accumulates that physical exercise contributes to the production of the endorphins and enkephalins (Carr et al., 1981), and that it has positive mood effects (Greist et al., 1978)–and as more Americans seem to be recognizing the values of fitness and exercise–the concept of alternatives warrants greater attention from researchers and practitioners alike.

ACKNOWLEDGMENT

This research was supported by grant number R01-DA-02565 from the National Institute on Drug Abuse.

REFERENCES

BARNES, C., and OLSON, F. Usage patterns of nondrug alternatives in adolescence. *J. Drug Educ.* 7(4): 359-368, 1977.

BECKER, H.S. Marijuana: A sociological overview. In D. Solomon (ed.), *The Marijuana Papers.* New York: Signet, 1968.

BRAUCHT, G.N., BRAKARASH, D., FOLLINGSTAD, D., and BERRY, K.L. Deviant drug use in adolescence: A review of psychosocial correlates. *Psychol. Bull.* 79: 92-106, 1983.

CAMPBELL, D.T., and STANLEY, J.C. *Experimental and Quasi-Experimental Designs for Research.* Chicago: Rand McNally, 1966.

CARR, D., BULLEN, B., SKRINAR, G., ARNOLD, M., ROSENBLATT, M., BEITINS, I., MARTIN, J., and MAC ARTHUR, J. Physical conditioning facilitates the exercise induced secretion of beta-endorphin and beta-lipotropin in women. *N. Eng. J. Med.* 304 (10): 560-563, 1981.

CHANIN, A. Understanding adolescence: Alternatives to drug use. *Clin. Pediatr.* 8(1): 6-10, January 1969.

COHEN, A.Y. The journey beyond trips: Alternatives to drugs. *J. Psychedelic Drugs* 3(2): 16-21, 1971.

COHEN, A.Y. *Alternatives to Drug Abuse: Steps Toward Drug Abuse Prevention*. National Clearinghouse for Drug Abuse Information, 1973.

COOK, R.F., HOSTETTER, R.S., and RAMSAY, D.A. Patterns of illicit drug use in the Army. *Am. J. Psychiatry,* 132: 10, October 1975.

COOK, R.F., LAWRENCE, H., MORSE, C., and ROEHL, J. *An evaluation of the alternatives approach to drug abuse prevention.* Report submitted to the National Institute on Drug Abuse (Grant No. R01-DA-02565), 1983.

COOK, R.F., and MORSE, C. *The role of alternative activities in drug abuse prevention: Research results and an emerging model.* Presented at the National Alcohol and Drug Coalition, Washington, DC, September 1980.

COOK, R.F., and MORTON, A. *An assessment of drug education-prevention programs in the U.S. Army.* Army Research Institute for the Behavioral and Social Sciences, 1975.

COOK, R.F., and THEOLOGUS, G. *Development of evaluation instruments for drug abuse prevention programs,* Phase I Final Report. Contract No. 271-75-4017, National Institute on Drug Abuse, July 1976.

COOK, R.F., WALIZER, D., and MACE, D. Illicit drug use in the Army: A social-organizational analysis. *J. Appl. Psychol.* 61(3): 262-272, 1976.

DE ROPP, R.S. *The Master Game: Beyond the Drug Experience.* New York: Delacorte, 1968.

DOHNER, V.A. Alternatives to drugs–A new approach to drug education. *J. Drug Educ.* 2(1): 3-22, 1972.

GOODSTADT, M.S. Myths and methodology in drug education: A critical review of the research evidence. In M.S. Goodstadt (ed.), *Research on Methods and Programs of Drug Education.* Toronto: Addiction Research Foundation, 1974.

GORSUCH, R.L., and BUTLER, M.C. Initial drug abuse: A review of predisposing social psychological factors. *Psychol. Bull.* 83(1): 120-137, 1976.

GREIST, J., KLEIN, M., EISCHENS, R., FARIS, J., GURMAN, A., and MORGAN, W. Running through your mind. *J. Psychosom. Res.* 22: 259-294, 1978.

HANSON, D.J. Drug education: Does it work? In F.R. Scarpitti and S.K. Datesman (eds.), *Drugs and the Youth Culture.* Beverly Hills, Sage Publications, 1980.

HURST, P., COOK, R., and RAMSAY, D. *Assessing the prevalence of illicit drug use in the Army.* Technical Paper 264, Army Research Institute, Alexandria, VA, 1975.

JESSOR, R., and JESSOR, S. *Problem Behavior and Psychosocial Development: A Longitudinal Study of Youth.* New York: Academic Press, 1977.

JOHNSTON, L.D., O'MALLEY, P.M., and EVELAND, L.K. Drugs and delinquency: A search for causal connections. In D. Kandel (ed.), *Longitudinal Research on Drug Use: Empirical Findings and Methodological Issues.* New York: Halstead Press, 1978.

KANDEL, D.B. In D. Kandel (ed.), *Longitudinal Research on Drug Use: Empirical Findings and Methodological Issues.* New York: Halstead Press, 1978.

NIDA Report on Alternative Pursuits for America's 3rd Century. Rockville, MD: National Institute on Drug Abuse, 1974.

PAINE, B. *Getting There Without Drugs.* Esalen Book Series. New York: Viking, 1971.

RICHARDS, L.G. *Evaluation in drug education: Notes on the state of the art.* Presented at National Conference on Research in School Health, Detroit, MI, 1971.

ROSENBERG, M. *Society and the Adolescent Self-Image.* Princeton, NJ: Princeton University Press, 1965.

SCHAPS, E., CHURGIN, S., PALLEY, C., TOKATA, B., and COHEN, A. Primary prevention research: A preliminary review of program outcome studies. *Int. J. Addict.* 15(5): 657-676, 1980.

The International Journal of the Addictions, 19(7), 789–803, 1984

Research Note

Inhalant Abuse and Juvenile Delinquency: A Control Study in Albuquerque, New Mexico

Barbara J. Frost Reed, MA
Philip A. May,* PhD

Department of Sociology
University of New Mexico
Albuquerque, New Mexico 87131

Abstract

This paper examines the relationship between inhalant abuse and delinquency among juveniles in Albuquerque, New Mexico. The arrest records of 100 juvenile delinquents identified as chronic inhalant abusers are compared with two control groups ($N = 100$ each) of other delinquents from Albuquerque. One control group was stratified on age, sex, and ethnicity, and the other was a simple random sample. The demographic characteristics of inhalant abusers indicated an over-representation of young, male Hispanics from large, poor, disrupted families where siblings were involved in both the abuse of inhalants and a variety of other delinquent activities. The inhalant abusers were much more likely to be arrested for virtually every type and category of delinquent activity. Specifically, inhalant abusers are considerably more criminal regarding total offenses committed, status offenses, crimes against property, crimes against persons, and criminal and violent offenses. Therefore, this study has indicated a strong relationship between inhalant abuse and juvenile delinquency.

*To whom correspondence should be addressed.

 0020-773X/84/1907-0789$3.50/0

The growing concern about the various consequences of the use of inhalants is documented by an increasingly large number of recent articles on inhalant abuse (see Novak, 1980; Sharp and Brehm, 1977; and Watson, 1980, for reviews). The study of inhalant abuse encompasses a wide variety of substances (gas, glue, solvents, spray paints, aerosols, etc.) which contain a wide spectrum of chemicals (hydrocarbons, nitrites, ketones, esters, etc.). Therefore, the use of various inhalants will produce a variety of symptoms, reactions, and behaviors. Both acute and chronic use are considered to be an adverse risk to humans in the physiological, psychological, and social aspects of life.

In the United States and other countries, a number of characteristics of inhalant abusers (see Note 1) have appeared in studies with considerable consistency. Most studies have shown inhalant abusers to be young, generally with a mean age between 13 and 15 years (Brozovsky and Winkler, 1965; Press and Done, 1967; Watson, 1980). Some articles, however, have focused on cases of inhalant abuse among adults (Hershey and Miller, 1982; Streicher et al., 1962). Boys are more commonly inhalant abusers than girls, and in some studies the ratio is as high as 10 to 1 (Rubin and Babbs, 1970; Wyse, 1973). Poverty is consistently cited as a factor in inhalant abusers' lives (Rubin and Babbs, 1970; Sharp and Brehm, 1977); however, some more recent findings indicate that some solvent abuse also exists in other socioeconomic settings (Watson, 1980). A number of family variables have been studied which have shown that abusers generally come from large families (e.g., Barker and Adams, 1973; Stybel et al., 1976) which are disorganized or unstable, being characterized by divorce, abandonment, alcoholism, unemployment, etc. (Cohen, 1979; Rubin and Babbs, 1970). School adjustment problems are also common in abusers (Meloff, 1970).

Prevalence literature on inhalant abuse indicates extreme variability by area and over time, but a higher level of use is often found among some minority groups. Spanish-Americans (Note 2) and American Indians who use inhalants consistently outnumber other minorities (Lewis and Patterson, 1974; Sharp and Brehm, 1977). Recent national studies indicate that between 8% and 11% of all youth (12-19 years) have used inhalants (Cohen, 1979; Richards, 1980). Studies on Hispanics and American Indians in the United States have indicated an even higher prevalence of 13-22% (May, 1982; Oetting et al., 1980; Padilla et al., 1979). In the southwestern United States, and New Mexico specifically, Hispanics are the most highly represented in agency files. From 1974 through 1980 Hispanics represented 85.2% of all inhalant abuse cases recorded by New Mexico drug abuse programs even though Hispanics are slightly less than 40% of the state's population (Reed, 1981).

A frequently recorded effect of inhalant use by youth is a tendency toward antisocial behavior. Studies have reported feelings of grandiosity, invulnerability, immense strength, and indifference toward pain as factors contributing to antisocial, negative, self-destructive, and aggressive behaviors of sniffers (Novak,

1980; Wyse, 1973). Also noted is that some inhalant users are characterized by their "unpredictable, bizarre, and impulse-ridden behavior" (Sharp and Brehm, 1977, p. 8). Press and Done (1967, p. 459) stated that sniffing was a "precursor to criminality" in a third of their subjects. Massengale et al. (1963) reported that there is a direct relation, in Denver at least, between glue sniffing and delinquency and antisocial behavior, and that it was an important stimulus to delinquency. Other researchers have reported that delinquency is common among sniffers prior to and independent of their sniffing activities (Ackerley and Gibson, 1964; Chapel and Taylor, 1970). Friedman and Friedman (1973) stated that violence, in obtaining drugs and while under the influence, was common among inhalant abusers. They also found inhalants to be the most frequent type of drug cited in juvenile court and police records (45% of all cases).

In two very recent studies, some relationship was found between delinquency and inhalants, but it was not as significant as those for other drugs. Juvenile assaults in California were found to be most frequently associated with alcohol (Tinklenberg et al., 1981), while inhalants were of relatively little importance. The other study examined the relationship of 13 types of drugs to violent personal crime. Drug experience was higher in juveniles who committed violent personal crimes than in those who committed only property crimes. However, inhalant abuse was not highly correlated with either type of crime. More strongly related to personal offenses were marijuana, alcohol, cocaine, heroin, and LSD (Simonds and Kashani, 1980).

RESEARCH METHODS

In 1981 this study was undertaken as the master's thesis of the first author (Reed, 1981). Data were collected from individual offender files at the Office of Juvenile Probation, City of Albuquerque.

Three groups of juvenile delinquents from Albuquerque were the focus of the study. The experimental group (inhalant abusers) consisted of 100 juvenile delinquents who had been treated by the Inhalant Abuse Program of Albuquerque for chronic inhalant abuse. The experimental group included only individuals who abused volatile solvents (glue, gasoline, aerosols, commercial solvents, and anesthetics) for intoxication, and not those who used narcotic inhalants. The first control group (Control I) consisted of a stratified random sample of 100 juvenile delinquents matched with the experimental group for age, sex, and ethnicity. In view of the overrepresentation of Hispanics found in other studies, ethnicity was the key consideration in this stratified sample. The second control group (Control II) consisted of a simple random sample of 100 juvenile delinquents who had active juvenile probation files.

RESULTS

The most common substance of abuse for inhalant abusers in Albuquerque was found to be spray paint. However, preferences differ from individual to individual, depending in many cases on the availability of products of preference. If an individual cannot afford to buy spray paint, he/she may try to steal it, find a friend to buy it, or turn to the next most accessible product such as glue or gasoline.

Demographic Characteristics

The average age of the abusers in this study was 15.2 years; 84% were male, and 16% were female. Ninety-one percent of the juveniles in the experimental group were Hispanics (mostly Chicanos). Most of the inhalant abusers were living in single-parent homes with their mothers (44%), and over half (57%) of these families had low annual incomes (<$6,000). Half (47%) of the inhalant abusers had siblings who had also been adjudicated as juveniles. The average age of the sniffers at first arrest was 12.7 years, significantly younger than either control group. The most common offense at first arrest was burglary. One-third of the sniffers had dropped out of school, while 14% had been suspended. Also, fewer inhalant abusers were enrolled in school than other delinquents. Regarding the data, it can be said that the demographic variables are consistent with previous inhalant abuse studies. Inhalant abusers in Albuquerque have problems in school, are arrested at a young age, and come from disrupted and disorganized familes of low income. Table 1 summarizes the demographic and social characteristics of the study groups.

Table 1

Demographic and Social Characteristics of Inhalant Abusers and Controls[a]

Characteristics	Inhalant abusers	Control Group I	Control Group II
Sex			
Male	84%	84%	71%
Female	16%	16%	29%
Average age	15.2 yr	15.2 yr	15.0 yr
Ethnicity			
Anglo	4%	4%	49%***
Hispanic	91%	91%	43%***
Black	2%	2%	2%
American Indian	3%	3%	6%
Average age at first arrest	12.7 yr	14.3 yr***	14.1 yr***

(continued)

Table 1 (continued)

Characteristics	Inhalant abusers	Control group I	Control Group II
Living situation			
Natural parents	29%	45%***	51%***
Mother and stepfather	12%	8%	6%
Father and stepmother	2%	2%	2%
Mother alone	44%	37%*	31%*
Other	13%	8%	10%
Average no. of people in household	4.82	4.37*	4.58
Average no. of siblings	3.51	2.78**	2.45***
% with adjudicated siblings	47%	16%***	7%***
Estimated family income			
$6,000/yr	57%	40%**	18%***
$6,000-$15,000/yr	33%	40%**	45%***
$15,000/yr	10%	20%**	37%***
Average no. of grades completed	8.7	9.1*	8.9
Student status			
Enrolled	53%	84%***	85%***
Suspended	14%	3%***	3%***
Dropout	32%	12%***	11%***
Graduate	1%	1%	1%
No. with diagnostic commitment	45.9% (N = 87)	5.6% (N = 88)	2.1% (N = 96)
No. with full commitment	18.4% (N = 87)	1.1% (N = 88)	0% (N = 96)
IQ	80.6 (N = 45)	–	–
Home conditions			
Adequate	67% (N = 39)	–	–
Overcrowded	33% (N = 39)	–	–
Average parental education level			
Fathers	9th grade (N = 39)	–	–
Mothers	9th grade (N = 47)	–	–
Parents with arrest record			
Fathers	69.0% (N = 29)	–	–
Mothers	29.4% (N = 17)	–	–
Employed mothers	53.7% (N = 67)	–	–
Employed juveniles	24.1% (N = 29)	–	–

[a]N = 100 in each category unless otherwise indicated.
*t Test significant at .05 level between experimental group and group where asterisk appears.
**t Test significant at .01 level.
***t Test significant at .001 level.

Arrests and Crime

As a group, the inhalant abusers were arrested for 754 offenses, 2.8 times more frequently than either control group (Control I = 269 offenses, Control II = 216 offenses). The average inhalant-abusing delinquent had been arrested for an average of 7.54 crimes, while the control groups' averages were 2.69 or less (see Table 2). Total career juvenile arrests for these individuals will ultimately be higher due to their young mean age. The largest number of crimes committed by any individual in the inhalant group was 25. Over half of the sniffers had been cited for 1 to 6 crimes. The most common offense committed by the inhalant abuser was burglary, followed by solvent abuse and shoplifting. Therefore, even when the 95 arrests for solvent abuse are eliminated from consideration, the abusers were arrested more frequently. The largest number of arrests for any individual in the matched control group (Control I) was 10. Among Control Group I, 79% had been cited for 1 to 3 crimes, and only 11% had been arrested for 7 or more crimes. The largest number of arrests for any individual in the random sample of delinquents (Control II) was 6. Eighty-six percent had been cited for 1 to 3 crimes, and none had been arrested more than 6 times. The most common offenses committed by controls were shoplifting, burglary, possession of alcohol, and trespassing (see Table 3).

Table 2
Total Number of Arrests for Juveniles in Each Group

	Number of persons		
Number of arrests	Inhalant abusers	Control I	Control II
1 - 3	29	79	86
4 - 6	24	10	14
7 - 9	14	8	0
10 - 12	12	3	0
13 - 15	13	0	0
16 - 18	3	0	0
19 - 21	4	0	0
22 - 25	1	0	0
N	100	100	100
Kendall's $\tau c = -.46, < .001$			
Mean	7.54	2.69	2.16
Mode	3	1	1
Median	6	2	2

Table 3
Specific Criminal Offenses for Each Group

Criminal offenses	Inhalant abusers	Control I	Control II
Arson	2	0	1
Forcible rape	1	0	0
Other sex offenses	0	1	0
Aggravated assault/battery	14	3*	1**
Assault/battery, other	32	10***	4***
Auto theft	12	12	5
Auto burglary	22	3***	2***
Burglary	102	38***	14***
Armed robbery	6	1	0*
Shoplifting	78	41**	55**
Larceny	31	13**	12**
Stolen property	22	12	5**
Forgery	0	2	1
Fraud	0	0	2
Escaping custody	8	1	0*
Resisting arrest	10	2**	2**
Refusing to obey/interfer.	17	10	3**
Possession of marijuana	12	10	10
Selling marijuana	0	2	1
Possession of narcotics	2	0	2
Selling of narcotics	1	0	0
Solvent abuse	95	0***	0***
Vandalism/criminal damage to property	18	12	13
Disorderly conduct	39	16**	7***
Weapons offenses	19	2***	1***
Missiles	5	3	0*
Trespassing	39	14***	17***
Violation of probation	23	1***	1***
Concealing ID	4	2	3
No driver's license	9	6	10
Reckless driving	3	0	1
DWI	13	7	4*
Drinking in a motor vehicle	0	1	0
Leaving the scene of an accident with property damage	1	2	3
Total criminal offenses	640	227***	180***

**t* Test significant at .05 level between experimental group and group where asterisk appears.
***t* Test significant at .01 level.
****t* Test significant at .001 level.

Criminal and Status Offenses

The juveniles in the inhalant group were arrested significantly more often for criminal offenses (N = 640) than those in either control group. Also, the total number of status offenses committed by the inhalant group was much greater than either control group. The detailed distributions of these two categories are shown in Tables 3 and 4, where one can see the major differences between the abusers and the controls. The differences which are highly significant ($p < .001$) include the following: assault and battery, auto burglary, burglary, solvent abuse, disorderly conduct, weapons offenses, trespassing, violation of probation, and curfew violations. Other differences between groups are also significant ($p < .05$) so that in virtually all of the 38 specific offense categories, inhalant abusers had significantly more arrests than controls.

Offense Categories

In this section of analysis and results, and the following one, offenses are grouped into substantive categories for theoretical purposes. In two instances these six offense categories overlap. The violent offense category is composed of the Uniform Crime Reports (Note 3) listing of violent offenses: homicide, rape, robbery, and aggravated assault. Because some crimes against persons (rape, sex offenses, aggravated assault, and armed robbery) are also violent offenses, these categories overlap slightly. In the second instance, Uniform Crime Report (UCR) property offenses (arson, burglary, larceny, and motor vehicle theft) overlap with crimes against property (arson, auto theft, auto burglary, burglary, larceny, shoplifting, vandalism/criminal damage to property, and leaving the scene of an accident). In all other cases the offense categories are mutually exclusive.

Table 4
Types of Status Offenses for Each Group

Status offenses	Inhalant abusers	Control I	Control II
Runaway	26	2**	2**
Truancy	22	6**	6**
Curfew violations	41	13***	8***
Incorrigible	7	2	2
Possession of alcohol	18	19	18
Total status offenses	114	42***	36***

**t Test significant at .05 level between experimental group and group where asterisk appears.
***t Test significant at .01 level.
****t Test significant at .001 level.

Table 5
Mean Number of Offenses in Each Crime Category Per Group

Crime category	Inhalant abusers	Control I	Control II
Average number of arrests/individual	7.54 (N = 754)	2.69*** (N = 269)	2.16*** (N = 216)
UCR violent offenses	0.21	0.04**	0.01**
UCR property offenses	1.47	0.63***	0.32***
Crimes against persons	0.53	0.15***	0.05***
Crimes against property	2.66	1.20***	1.05***
Criminal offenses	6.40	2.27***	1.80***
Status offenses	1.14	0.42***	0.36***

***t* Test significant at .01 level between experimental group and group where asterisk appears.
****t* Test significant at .001 level.

The mean number of arrests per group is shown in Table 5 for each of the six offense categories. As some previous literature indicated, inhalant-abusing delinquents commit more violent and criminal offenses than other delinquents. However, they have also been arrested more for property and status offenses, being significantly higher in arrests for all six categories. Table 6 shows the number of juveniles arrested in each offense category. Thirteen percent of the inhalant abusers committed (UCR) violent crimes; but, because of multiple offenses, these 13 individuals were responsible for a total of 21 violent offenses (1.6 per person). This is a considerably worse record than either control group (1.0 per person). Sixty-three percent of the inhalant abusers committed (UCR) property offenses, compiling a total of 147 property offenses (2.3 per person), considerably more than the control groups. Similar results were also found in crimes against persons. The number of juveniles committing crimes against property did not differ greatly from one group to the next. However, as is shown by mean offenses, the inhalers were more likely to be repeaters in this category. Finally, the inhalant abusers were even more likely to commit status offenses and to do so more frequently. Table 7 also depicts the repetitive nature of abusers arrests. All of the juveniles in the inhalant group committed at least one criminal offense, and the vast majority (87%) were multiple offenders (see Table 7). Even though virtually all of the controls committed at least one criminal offense, they were less likely to be repeaters. Although one might expect criminal offenses to be much lower for the control groups, this may be explained by the fact that shoplifting was the most prevalent crime among

Table 6

Summary of Offenses of Inhalant Abusers and Controls, by Category of Crimes

Offense category[a]	Inhalant abusers (N = 100)		Control I (N = 100)		Control II (N = 100)		Kendall's τ and significance[b]
	N	Offenses per individual	N	Offenses per individual	N	Offenses per individual	
Criminal offenses							
UCR violent offenses	13	(1.6)	4	(1.0)	1	(1.0)	$c = -.08$ $p < .001$
UCR property offenses	63	(2.3)	35	(1.8)	28	(1.1)	$c = -.28$ $p < .001$
Crimes against persons	34	(1.6)	15	(1.0)	5	(1.0)	$c = -.28$ $p < .001$
Crimes agains property	86	(7.4)	73	(3.1)	80	(2.3)	$c = -.30$ $p < .001$
Status offenses	55	(2.1)	29	(1.5)	30	(1.2)	$c = -.21$ $p < .001$

[a]Committed one or more offenses in the category.

[b]Calculated on distribution of total offenses by offender, as in Table 7.

Table 7
Frequency of Juveniles Having Committed Criminal Offenses, by Group

Number of criminal offenses	Inhalant abusers	Control I	Control II
0	0	2	0
1	13	49	50
2	10	23	30
3	13	7	12
4	8	4	7
5 - 9	34	15	1
10 - 14	17	0	0
15 - 20	5	0	0
N	100	100	100

Kendall's $\tau c = -.45, p < .001$.

controls. Shoplifting, while considered by many to be a minor crime, is classified as a criminal offense.

Correlations between Groups

The Pearson correlation coefficients (r) in Table 8 between the experimental group and each control group provide additional information, with the r^2 values indicating the percent of reduction of prediction error. Data indicate an inverse relationship between inhalers and controls for each offense category. The strongest relationships are found in the categories of total offenses and status offenses. These explain the most variance between abusers and both Control Group I ($r^2 = .26$ and $r^2 = .25$ for total and status offenses, respectively) and Control Group II ($r^2 = .33$ and $r^2 = .33$, respectively). Therefore, between 25% and 33% of the criminality for these offenses might be attributed to chronic inhalant abuse. The least amount of variance between groups is explained by the number of violent offenses committed; however, this relationship is significant beyond the .01 level for both groups. In the other five offense categories, all of the correlations are significant beyond the .001 level. Therefore, knowing that a person is an inhalant abuser can significantly aid in the prediction of his/her criminal history.

Table 8
Correlations between Groups on Crime Categories[a]

	Inhalant abusers vs Control I			Inhalant abusers vs Control II		
Crime categories	r	r^2	Significance	r	r^2	Significance
Total offenses	−0.51	.26	$p < .001$	−.057	.33	$p < .001$
Violent offenses	−0.17	.03	$p < .01$	−0.21	.04	$p < .01$
Property offenses	−0.27	.07	$p < .001$	−0.40	.16	$p < .001$
Crimes against persons	−0.26	.07	$p < .001$	−0.34	.12	$p < .001$
Crimes against property	−0.38	.14	$p < .001$	−0.44	.19	$p < .001$
Criminal offenses	−0.28	.08	$p < .001$	−0.31	.10	$p < .001$
Status offenses	−0.50	.25	$p < .001$	−0.57	.33	$p < .001$
N		200			200	

[a]Dummy variables: Abusers = 0; Control = 1.

SUMMARY AND CONCLUSIONS

In investigating the social, demographic, and criminal backgrounds of inhalant abusers and other delinquents in Albuquerque, many findings were both obvious and consistent. Social and demographic variables show the abusers to be young males, who are frequently from large, disrupted, and poor families of Hispanic heritage and low educational attainment. All of the arrest data show chronic inhalant abusers to be more criminal in virtually every way. The strongest categorical relationships between crime and inhalants were found to be in (in descending order): total offenses, status offenses, property crimes, crimes against persons, criminal offenses, and violent offenses.

The demographic data are quite similar to most previous U.S. studies as cited in the literature review of this paper. The criminal data are very consistent with the direction of previous studies but are somewhat more specific regarding the criminal characteristics of inhalant abusers. Past studies have mentioned a wide variety of offenses committed by inhalant abusers, but this study has now provided a specific statistical estimate and prioritizing of their significance. Overall, inhalant abusers in this study are more criminal than controls in all respects, and as much as 33% (r^2 = .33) of this difference can be related to their substance abuse. This is a substantially stronger relationship than was found in two very recent studies (Simonds and Kashani, 1980; Tinklenberg et al., 1981). The reader is reminded that strong correlations are not causal relationships, and some questions remain. Does involvement in habitual sniffing activity cause a juvenile to become delinquent, or do hardcore delinquents engage in the abuse of inhalants simply as another form of deviant behavior? Also, the arrest data used here may only indicate that inhalant abusers allow themselves to be arrested more. Is this because some inhalants anesthetize the individual or disrupt his/her functioning in other ways leading to arrests (see Novak, 1980)? The answers to these questions are illusive. From this study, however, the use of a sample stratified by age, sex, and ethnic status has begun to rule out some variables as other, partial explanations.

It would be beneficial for further research on inhalant abuse and crime to combine statistical data with self-report information (as in Tinklenberg et al., 1981). This would increase information relating to specific causation. Ethnographic research might also prove valuable. Compiling detailed ethnographies or case studies on various agents of abuse used by experimental, social, and habitual inhalant abusers, and on their criminal and behavior patterns would allow for insightful comparisons. Further study of this problem is imperative, for other studies indicate a concern that inhalant abuse may be increasing and affecting new subpopulations (Watson, 1980). It is also of particular importance for Hispanic populations of the southwestern United States and other subpopulations who have been reported as having a higher prevalence of inhalant abuse.

ACKNOWLEDGMENTS

This paper is a summary of the first author's unpublished master's thesis at the University of New Mexico. The research was supported by NIMH grant 5-T01-MH15219. The authors gratefully acknowledge the advice and assistance of the Albuquerque Juvenile Probation Department, Paul Steele, Pedro David, Richard Coughlin, and Cindy Self-Cesarz.

NOTES

1. An inhalant abuser is a person who habitually engages in the intentional smelling, sniffing, or inhaling of fumes or vapors from glues, aerosol spray products, or other chemical substances for the purpose of causing intoxication. "Sniffing" refers to inhalation through the nose, while "huffing" refers to inhalation through the mouth. Both methods can be used simultaneously. In this paper the term "inhalant abuser" is used most frequently, for it is the most generally descriptive. The term "sniffer" is also used occasionally in the paper, for it is a very common term used for inhalant abusers.

2. The terms "Hispanic" and "Spanish-American" are used interchangeably to denote American residents who speak Spanish and trace their ancestry to any country of Spanish culture. The term "Chicano" is a more specific term and is used for U.S. residents of Mexican ancestry.
3. Uniform Crime Reports (UCR) are the annual statistical bulletins of the Federal Bureau of Investigation.

REFERENCES

ACKERLEY, W.C., and GIBSON, G. Lighter fluid sniffing. *Am. J. Psychiatry* 9: 1056-1061, 1964.

BARKER, G.H., and ADAMS, W.T. Glue sniffers. *Sociol. Soc. Res.* 47: 289-310, 1973.

BROZOVSKY, M., and WINKLER, E.G. Glue sniffing in children and adolescents. *NY State J. Med.* 65: 1984-1989, 1965.

CHAPEL, J., and TAYLOR, D. Glue sniffing. *Missouri Med.* 65: 288-296, 1970.

COHEN, S. Inhalants and solvents. In Beschner and Friedman (eds.), *Youth Drug Abuse: Problems, Issues and Treatment.* Lexington, MA: D.C. Heath, 1979.

FRIEDMAN, C.J., and FRIEDMAN, A. Drug abuse and delinquency. *Tech. Pap. 2nd Rep. National Commission on Marijuana and Drug Abuse* 1: 398-484, 1973.

HERSHEY, C.O., and MILLER, S. Solvent abuse: A shift to adults. *Int. J. Addict.* 17(6): 1085-1089, 1982.

LEWIS, P.A., and PATTERSON, D. Acute and chronic effects of the voluntary inhalation of certain commercial volatile solvents by juveniles. *J. Drug Issues* 4: 162-175, 1974.

MASSENGALE, O.N., GLASER, H.H., LE LIEVRE, R.E., DODDS, J.B., and KLOCK, M. Physical and psychological factors in glue sniffing. *N. Engl. J. Med.* 269: 1340-1344, 1963.

MAY, P.A. Substance abuse and American Indians: Prevalence and susceptibility. *Int. J. Addict.* 17(7): 1185-1209, 1982.

MELOFF, W.A. An exploratory study of adolescent glue sniffers. *Diss. Abstr. Int.* 31: 1391-1392, 1970.

NOVAK, A. The deliberate inhalation of volatile substances. *J. Psychedelic Drugs* 12(2): 105-122, 1980.

OETTING, E.R., GOLDSTEIN, G., BEAUVAIS, F., and EDWARDS, R. *Drug Abuse among Indian Children* (NIDA Report). Ft. Collins, CO: Colorado State University, 1980.

PADILLA, E., PADILLA, A., RAMIREZ, R., MORALES, A., and OLMEDO, E. Inhalant, marijuana and alcohol abuse among barrio children and adolescents. Cited in Beschner and Friedman (eds.), *Youth Drug Abuse: Problems, Issues and Treatment.* Lexington, MA: D.C. Heath, 1979.

PRESS, E., and DONE, A.K. Solvent sniffing: Physiologic effects and community control measures for intoxication from the intentional inhalation of organic solvents. I. *Pediatrics* 39: 451-461, 1967.

REED, B.J.F. *Delinquency and inhalant abuse among juveniles in Albuquerque.* Unpublished MA Thesis, The University of New Mexico, 1981.

RICHARDS, L.G. (ed.). Demographic trends and drug abuse 1980-1995. *NIDA Research Monograph*, 35, 1980.

RUBIN, T., and BABBS, J. The glue sniffer. *Fed. Probation* 34: 23-41, 1970.

SHARP, C.W., and BREHM, M.L. (eds.). Review of inhalants: Euphoria to dysfunction. *NIDA Research Monograph*, 15, 1977.

SIMONDS, J.F., and KASHANI, J. Specific drug use and violence in delinquent boys. *Am. J. Drug Alcohol Abuse* 7(3&4): 305-322, 1980.

STREICHER, H.Z., GABOW, P.A., MOSS, A.H., KONO, D., and KAEHNY, W.D. Syndromes of toluene sniffing in adults. *Ann. Int. Med.* 198: 300-303, 1962.

STYBEL, L.J., ALLEN, P., and LEWIS, F. Deliberate hydrocarbon inhalation among low socioeconomic adolescents not necessarily apprehended by police. *Int. J. Addict.* 11(2): 345-361, 1976.

TINKLENBERG, J.R., MURPHY, P., MURPHY, P.L., and PFEFFERBAUM, A. Drugs and criminal assaults by adolescents: A replication study. *J. Psychoactive Drugs* 13(3): 277-287, 1981.

WATSON, J.M. Solvent abuse by children and young adults: A review. *Br. J. Addict.* 75: 27-36, 1980.

WYSE, D.G. Deliberate inhalation of volatile hydrocarbons. *Can. Med. Assoc. J.* 108: 71-74, 1973.

The International Journal of the Addictions, 19(7), 805–818, 1984

Research Note

Self- and Ideal-Self-Perception of Drug Addicts in Therapeutic Communities

Carol A. Preston, BA

Linda L. Viney, PhD

Department of Psychology
The University of Wollongong
Wollongong, NSW, 2500 Australia

Abstract

Ninety-one drug addicts from four residential treatment centers completed a 50-item rating scale for self and ideal self. Factor analysis of their responses revealed two five-factor solutions. As hypothesized, residents who had been in the centers for 10 months or more had higher self-esteem than residents in treatment for shorter periods. They also saw themselves as less pawnlike and were less self-critical. Primary dimensions of the residents' view of ideal self were Pawn and Self-criticism. Implications for program intake procedures, treatment techniques, and goals; criteria for success and failure; and community roles are discussed.

Drug addicts have been described as having a high need for social approval (Scherer, Ettinger, and Mudrick, 1972); as incorporating both self-nurturant and self-destructive feelings about themselves (Boyd, 1971); as exhibiting at the same time passive, dependent behavior and hostile, aggressive tendencies (Chambers, 1972); as experiencing high levels of anxiety (De Leon, Skodal, and Rosenthal, 1971; Koren, 1974); as lacking a sense of identity (Cohen, White, and Schoolar, 1973); and as feeling inferior and powerless to change their behavior (Duster, 1970). There is general agreement among researchers that counseling for social adjustment, academic training, and development of abilities are the most desirable components of treatment for addicts in therapeutic

0020-773X/84/1907-0805$3.50/0

communities (Geis, 1974; Rosenthal, Savoy, Greene and Spillane, 1979; Vaillant, 1973; Westermeyer and Bourne, 1978). However, most researchers report a relapse rate of 80-90% among addicts after treatment. It has been suggested recently (Eiser and Gossop, 1979) that better understanding of addicts' perceptions of themselves, their addiction, and their ability to overcome it, is an important consideration for treatment.

The aims of this research were, then, first to identify some of the views that addicts hold about themselves, and second, to see in what way those views change with treatment. What little research has been done concerning view of self suggests that addicts see themselves as moody, anxious, bored, cynical, impulsive, and rebellious (Robbins, Robbins, Frosch, and Stern, 1970); as easily persuaded, dependent on others, insufficiently intelligent, and suspicious (Alexander and Dibb, 1977). They report feeling morally inferior to nonaddicts (Duster, 1970) and constitutionally incapable of giving up drugs either by their own will or with treatment (Eiser and Gossop, 1979). Researchers who have also investigated addicts' views of their ideal self (Cohen et al., 1973; McKenna-Hartung, Hartung, and Baxter, 1971) have found that addicts report ideals of suspiciousness, passive rebellion, and hostility. These researchers have all concluded that these elements of description of the ideal self argue against the development in the addict of any sense of self-esteem or ego identity. They suggested that addicts' ideals indicate, rather, a rejection of traditional values and an unwillingness to change.

An individual's self-concept has long been considered to be a significant influence on much of his/her behavior and also to be directly related to a general state of mental health (Burns, 1979; Coopersmith, 1967; Fitts, 1965; Lecky, 1945). Generally, individuals who see themselves as worthless or undesirable, and who show a large discrepancy between the way they actually see themselves and the way they would ideally like to be, are said to be less well adjusted than those who are at least moderately satisfied with themselves. Rogers (1951) suggested that an individual develops a self-image early in life which serves to guide and maintain adjustment to the external world. He says that when individuals come to evaluate themselves negatively there is an "omnipresent malaise marked by preoccupation with the self and attention to deficiencies which together reduce the possibility of effective action. Once developed, the self concept resists all efforts at disruption" (p. 507).

Together, the relapse rate, the research into self-perceptions among addicts, and self-concept theory do not present a very optimistic outlook for the treatment of drug addiction. Nevertheless, the present study undertook a systematic investigation of addicts' concepts of self and ideal self in different stages of long-term residential treatment. Such treatment centers emphasize social learning, communication, decision making, self-awareness, and responsibility, and ideally provide a family environment where the resident may make up his/her assumed maturational deficiencies (Geis, 1974). Positive emotional changes over time during residential treatment have been found with psychometric testing (De Leon et al., 1971; Sutker, Allain, and Cohen, 1974; Zuckerman, Sola, Masterson, and Angelone, 1975). They include reduced anxiety and rises in self-confidence and mood evaluation. These findings suggest a movement toward a more positive view of self.

Although the dropout rate from residential centers for drug abusers is very high (about 50%), the abstinence rate among graduates has been reported to be up to 92% (Ogborne and Melotte, 1977). While abstinence is only one measure of successful rehabilitation, it is the one most often associated with reduced crime rate, employment, and social involvement (Levy, 1972; Waldorf, 1970). These improvements may also be associated with positive changes in self-concept and less rejection of social values. It was therefore hypothesized that addicts in later stages of residential treatment would report more positive self-concepts and show less self/ideal-self discrepancy than addicts who had just entered treatment. It was also hypothesized that addicts in treatment retested after a 6-month period would show more positive self-concepts than at first testing.

METHOD

Subjects

Ninety-one residents from four therapeutic community rehabilitation centers for drug abusers participated in the study, during 1980-1981. Interviews with the staff revealed that the programs had in common an emphasis on drug-free living and mutual support among residents. They also all emphasized the development of self-awareness, responsibility, coping skills, self-respect, and the ability to return to the outside community without the aid of drugs. The characteristics of the residents are described in Table 1. The most common drug of abuse was heroin, though most of the residents had also used other drugs including marijuana, barbiturates, amphetamines, and alcohol. The majority of them had been treated in the centers for 5 months or less. These residents were divided into two cohorts, 0-3 months and 3-5 months, in order to distinguish residents who might be expected to have made notable gains. The remaining residents were divided into two approximately equal cohorts, those who had been in treatment 5-10 months and over 10 months.

Procedure

The residents of the rehabilitation centers were asked by the interviewer (C.A.P.) to complete a rating scale under two conditions. They were asked first to rate each of 50 items on a seven-point scale from "not at all like me"

Table 1

Background Characteristics of Residents

Sex (%)		Length of addiction (yr)	
Male	55	$\bar{X}$	7.7
Female	45	SD	3.2
Age (yr)		Range	2-16
$\bar{X}$	24.5	Number of previous treatments	
SD	5.8	$\bar{X}$	3.3
Range	15-52	SD	2.8
Education (yr)		Range	1-12
$\bar{X}$	10.4	Length of residence (wk)	
SD	1.7	$\bar{X}$	21
Range	7-18	SD	5.3
Work experience prior to addiction (%)		Range	1-96
None	26		
Unskilled	47		
Semiskilled	16		
Professional	11		

to "very much like me," according to how they saw themselves at the time (copies of the rating scale are available from the senior author). Then they were asked to rate the items again according to how they would ideally like to be. Six months later the residents were approached a second time and asked to fill in the rating scale again. Forty-three of the 91 residents were still in the centers. Thirty-three had dropped out, five had graduated, seven had been transferred to another center interstate, and three residents were unavailable for retesting. Of those who were retested, 21 were men and 22 were women. Of the 33 who had left, only four completed 5 months of residential treatment before leaving.

Measurement of View of Self and Ideal Self

The items on the rating scale were from the Butler and Haigh Q-Sort (1954), which has become one of the most commonly used instruments in the exploration of self-concept (Burns, 1979). It has been used extensively by Rogers and his associates in studying the self-concept and its change during psychotherapy (Rogers and Dymond, 1954). Test-retest reliability over 6 months has been shown to be .86 (Wylie, 1974). Investigators usually use one of two techniques with the Q-Sort ratings, which result in a "discrepancy" score. However, the discrepancy may not be a satisfactory measure. McCandless (1967) has concluded from research that there is little intersubject variability in ratings of ideal self. The evidence suggests that ideal-self-concepts reflect the cultually desirable;

that is, being intelligent, physically attractive, good, and happy. Also, Wylie (1974) has concluded that discrepancy scores really demonstrate a discrepancy between the subject's concept of him/herself and the cultural norm. She proposed that indices of self-acceptance and possible areas of inadequate adjustment can therefore be reliably inferred from the subject's attitudes toward him/herself as he/she is. However, as has been noted, addicts have been shown to be rejecting of cultural norms and values, and so their ideal-self-ratings may deviate from those ideals obtained from other groups. In order to investigate fully the structure of addicts' views of self and ideal in this study, therefore, factor anayses (Nie, 1975) of self-ratings and ideal-self-ratings were conducted.

RESULTS

Analysis of variance for biographical data revealed no significant difference between residents in different cohorts or in different residential treatment programs on any of the variables. The residents were thereafter considered to be a homogeneous group insofar as age, educational level, length of addiction, and number of attempted treatments were concerned.

Table 2 shows the results of a five-factor principal components solution, after varimax rotation, for self-ratings at first testing. Table 3 shows the solution for ideal ratings. The items clustered together into the same factors for both self and ideal ratings on the first four factors, although the factors emerged in different order according to the amount of variance they accounted for in each solution. These factors consisted of statements of Self-Esteem and Self-Criticism of the kind described by Rogers (1951), Fitts (1965), and Coopersmith (1967); and perceptions of oneself in relation to one's world as Origin and Pawn. De Charms (1968) has proposed that a person who perceives his/her behavior as determined by his/her own choosing be described as an "origin" and a person who perceives his/her behavior as determined by external forces beyond his/her control be described as a "pawn." The concepts are similar to those of internal and external control, as postulated by Rotter (1966), but are independent rather than interrelated (Westbrook and Viney, 1980). The last factor in each solution was the only factor which indicated an essential difference between view of self and view of ideal self. Self-ratings resulted in a factor representing Anger (see Buss, 1961; Gottschalk and Gleser, 1969); and ideal ratings, in one representing Sociality (see Danziger, 1976; Osgood, 1970; Viney and Westbrook, 1979).

Factor scores for each individual were calculated using the factor program (Nie, 1975). ANOVA was then computed on these scales to assess any differences between cohorts on the derived factors. (Means and standard deviations of factor scores are available from the senior author.) There was a significant difference between cohorts for Self-Factors 1 ($F = 2.91, p = .03$), 3 ($F = 5.59$, $p = .001$), 4 ($F = 3.38, p = .02$), and 5 ($F = 3.01, p = .03$). Further analysis using

Table 2

Principal-Component Factor Solution for Initial Self-Ratings

Item	Loading	% of variance accounted for
Factor 1: Self-Esteem		
I feel emotionally mature	.68	
I am satisfied with myself	.63	
I am contented	.59	
I feel adequate	.55	
I understand myself	.54	
I take a positive attitude toward myself	.53	
I am relaxed and nothing really bothers me	.38	46
Factor 2: Origin		
I make strong demands on myself	.68	
I have initiative	.66	
I have an attractive personality	.63	
I am ambitious	.60	
I am a responsible person	.56	
I am assertive	.48	
I can usually make up my mind and stick to it	.43	
I am a good mixer	.43	21
Factor 3: Pawn		
I am really disturbed	.77	
I am disorganized	.66	
All you have to do is insist with me and I give in	.56	
I have a feeling of hopelessness	.48	
I usually feel driven	.47	
My decisions are not my own	.44	
I have to protect myself with excuses and rationalizing	.43	
I am a failure	.43	
I am confused	.42	
I feel insecure within myself	.39	
I feel apathetic	.34	15
Factor 4: Self-Criticism		
I feel hopeless	.67	
I am worthless	.65	
I am unreliable	.57	
I shrink from facing a crisis or difficulty	.46	
I often kick myself for the things I do	.43	
I just don't respect myself	.42	
I am shy	.39	10
Factor 5: Anger		
I am a hostile person	.66	
I tend to be on my guard with people who are more friendly than I expected	.65	
It is difficult to control my aggression	.49	
I usually like people	−.38	8

Table 3

Principal-Component Factor Solution for Initial Ideal-Self-Ratings

Item	Loading	% of variance accounted for
Factor 1: Pawn		
I am really disturbed	.80	
I am confused	.76	
I am a failure	.65	
I have a horror of failing at anything I want to accomplish	.57	
All you have to do is just insist with me and I give in	.41	
I feel insecure within myself	.41	
My decisions are not my own	.30	
Self-control is no problem to me.	–.42	46
Factor 2: Self-Esteem		
I take a positive attitude toward myself	.64	
I am relaxed and nothing really bothers me	.62	
I feel emotionally mature	.56	
I am tolerant	.48	
I feel adequate	.47	
I am contented	.36	
I am a rational person	.30	15
Factor 3: Origin		
I have initiative	.63	
I am a responsible person	.60	
I understand myself	.56	
I am assertive	.54	
I am ambitious	.53	
I am satisfied with myself	.48	
I am a good mixer	.43	
I can usually make up my mind and stick to it	.40	
I make strong demands on myself	.30	
I feel apathetic	–.54	15
Factor 4: Self-Criticism		
I feel worthless	.72	
I just don't respect myself	.71	
I am a hostile person	.68	
I am shy	.55	
I don't trust my emotions	.53	
I feel hopeless	.52	
I am unreliable	.52	
I shrink from facing a crisis or difficulty	.51	
I often kick myself for the things I do	.34	13
Factor 5: Sociality		
I usually like people	.60	
I am liked by most people that know me	.54	
I have warm emotional relationships with others	.45	
I have an attractive personality	.39	11

a priori contrasts (Nie, 1975) indicated that in each case the difference was between Cohort 3 and Cohort 4. Residents in Cohort 4—that is, those who had been over 10 months in residence—were significantly higher than those in Cohort 3 (5-10 months) on Self-Esteem (t = .004), significantly lower on Pawn (t = .010), significantly lower on Self-Criticism (t = .02), and significantly lower on Anger (t = .05). For two factors the contrast between Cohorts 1 and 2 also showed significant differences. Residents in treatment for 3 to 5 months were significantly lower than residents of 0 to 3 months on Pawn (t = .000) and Self-Criticism (t = .019). ANOVA computed in the same way for Ideal-Self Factors showed no significant differences between cohorts. A further ANOVA was computed for all factors with sex as the independent variable to investigate any sex differences. Only two significant differences were found. On the Ideal-Self Factors 4 (Self-Criticism) and 5 (Sociality), women were lower than men ($F = 4.86, p = .03$ and $F = 5.94, p = .01$; respectively).

When factor analyses were computed separately for the "dropouts" and the "stayers" on their first scores, the factors emerged in different orders. For the dropouts it was: Self-Esteem, Pawn, Self-Criticism, and Origin; then a factor representing a mixture of Pawn and Self-Criticism. For the stayers it was Self-Criticism, Pawn, and Origin; followed by Self-Esteem and Anger. The smaller number of residents in the groups may account for the solutions being a little less precise than those reported earlier. However, the self-concepts of those who left the centers and those who stayed contained the same elements, with Self-Criticism accounting for more variance in scores for those who stayed and Self-Esteem accounting for more variance for those who left.

Tables 4 and 5 show the factor analysis solutions on second self- and ideal-self ratings for those who were retested. Again the fifth factor in each solution had only a few items which were not loaded highly on other factors. The smaller number of residents seemed to cloud the solutions so that there was some overlap between Origin and Self-Esteem, and between Pawn and Self-Criticism. Nevertheless, all previous elements are represented in these second solutions. They suggest that the basic structure of the view of self remained constant even though all of the residents had been in treatment for at least 6 months, some up to 2 years. The view of ideal self had altered somewhat, in that Origin accounted for a greater percentage of the variance at second testing. The similarities between these two solutions, too, are more notable than their differences.

DISCUSSION

There are a number of inherent problems in research of this type. A large number of addicts drop out of treatment programs, and many make repeated attempts at rehabilitation. There are also varied influences and motivations which underlie residence in such centers. Such factors make it difficult to

Table 4

Factor Solution for Second Ratings of Self

Item	Loading	% of variance accounted for
Factor 1: Self-Esteem		
I am relaxed and nothing really bothers me	.79	
I feel adequate	.70	
I am contented	.66	
I am satisfied with myself	.65	
I am a responsible person	.58	
I take a positive attitude toward myself	.53	
I understand myself	.46	38
Factor 2: Origin		
I have initiative	.86	
I have an attractive personality	.74	
I am assertive	.68	
I am a good mixer	.66	
I am a rational person	.60	
I am an optimist	.54	
I have a few values and standards of my own	.50	
I make strong demands on myself	.51	
I am ambitious	.48	
I can usually make up my mind and stick to it	.31	23
Factor 3: Self-Criticism		
I am worthless	.79	
I feel hopeless	.78	
I am confused	.66	
I am disorganized	.58	
I have a feeling of hopelessness	.37	
I often feel humiliated	.48	14
Factor 4: Pawn		
I am a failure	.72	
All you have to do is just insist with me and I give in	.71	
I am unreliable	.71	
I have to protect myself with excuses and rationalizing	.65	
I shrink from facing a crisis or difficulty	.62	
I am really disturbed	.58	
I don't trust my emotions	.44	
I just don't respect myself	.43	
I feel insecure within myself	.42	
I usually feel driven	.32	
I have a horror of failing in anything I want to accomplish	.32	14
Factor 5		
My hardest battles are with myself	.56	
My decisions are not my own	.49	
I try not to think about my problems	.40	10

Table 5

Factor Solution for Second Ratings of Ideal Self

Item	Loading	% of variance accounted for
Factor 1: Origin		
I have an attractive personality	.87	
I have initiative	.83	
I am satisfied with myself	.83	
I understand myself	.82	
I am a responsible person	.77	
I am a good mixer	.65	
I am assertive	.62	
I make strong demands on myself	.61	
I can usually make up my mind and stick to it	.56	
Self-control is no problem to me	.39	
I am ambitious	.38	48
Factor 2: Pawn		
I just don't respect myself	.73	
I am a failure	.72	
I have a horror of failing at anything I want to accomplish	.71	
I feel insecure within myself	.68	
I am really disturbed	.66	
I have a feeling of hopelessness	.62	
I have to protect myself with excuses and rationalizing	.61	
I am confused	.60	
It is difficult to control my aggression	.59	
I am disorganized	.49	
All you have to do is just insist with me and I give in	.49	22
Factor 3: Self-Esteem		
I feel adequate	.62	
I usually like people	.61	
I feel emotionally mature	.56	
I am contented	.53	
I have warm emotional relationships with others	.47	
I am tolerant	.46	
I am relaxed and nothing really bothers me	.42	
I am liked by most people who know me	.37	12
Factor 4: Self-Criticism		
I feel hopeless	.91	
I am worthless	.71	
I am unreliable	.32	11
Factor 5		
I feel apathetic	.63	
I usually feel driven	.48	
My decisions are not my own	.39	7

carry out precise assessments of the characteristics of residents or the changes that occur over time. Although the centers included in this study were similar in philosophy and treatment techniques, the implications of this study may not be applicable to other kinds of treatment programs. However, when these limitations are taken into account, the results of the study have some important implications for treatment of drug addiction in residential centers.

The results support the hypothesis that residents in later stages of long-term treatment have a more positive view of self than residents in the early stages. Longer-staying residents had higher self-esteem, saw themselves as less pawnlike, and were less self-critical. The results also show that residents of 3 to 5 months see themselves as less pawnlike and are less self-critical than those who have just entered treatment.

The dropout rate was much greater before 5 months of treatment than after that time. This is consistent with other observations in this area (De Leon et al., 1971). This tendency, and the pattern of scores found, may be interpreted as suggesting that many residents drop out of treatment after approximately 5 months because of a rise in self-esteem and a more positive view of themselves. Those who remain, then, are those who still see themselves as worthless and are more despairing of their ability to take control of their addiction and their lives. The comparison of factor solutions for dropouts and stayers also supports this interpretation. For those who stayed in treatment, self-criticism was of prime importance. For residents who dropped out, self-esteem was paramount.

Numbers left in each cohort at second testing were too small to assess differences between cohorts on factor scores, but for the whole group the structure of drug addicts' view of self is very much the same as at first testing. Overall the view of self obtained suggests that over time in treatment there are significant positive changes in self-concept which could indicate progress toward adequate personal and social adjustment. Drug addicts do not appear to hold ideals consistent with the "culturally desirable," as is found with other groups (McCandless, 1967; Wylie, 1974). Though self-esteem was the primary dimension in their view of self, helplessness was the primary dimension in their view of ideal self. With the "how I am now" instructions, residents were able to see themselves as primarily adequate, satisfied, and in control; but with the "how I would like to be" instructions, residents reported failure and powerlessness in relation to their ideals or goals. Helplessness and self-criticism consistently made up a large part of the addicts' views of their ideal selves, on first and second testing, for those who stayed and for those who dropped out.

This pattern gives some insight into the residents' own perceptions of their future. It suggests that they are ambivalent about their goals and may represent a real fear of returning to the "outside community" where they will be expected to take control of their own lives without the protection and security of the centers. Even though they enter treatment and stay for long periods of time, they seem to be unable to believe that they will eventually be worthwhile, reliable individuals who will be able to take on responsibility and handle difficulties. There was no difference between cohorts in view of ideal self, indicating that even after many months of treatment, thinking about the future evoked self-limiting and self-depreciating concepts.

This unusual view of ideal self may offer some explanation for the low success rates of drug rehabilitation programs. Changes in residents' behavior and self-concepts during treatment may be attributable in part to the addicts feeling protected and secure while away from outside influences, against which they still feel powerless and inadequate. On reentry to society they soon return to familiar and predictable ways of behaving in that situation. Criteria such as abstinence, employment, and social involvement may be valid expectations of a "successfully" rehabilitated addict, but these are only surface indicators of inner changes which in the long run will be necessary for an individual to cope with the stresses, challenges, and disappointments of everyday life, which have been identified as the most common precipitators of return to drug use.

The psychological processes involved in drug addiction, treatment, and reentry to society are complex and variable. An assessment of individuals on entry and periodically through treatment may help both the treatment personnel and the residents to better understand and direct these processes. It would be valuable for staff to be skilled in structuring techniques aimed at enabling the resident to be confident about returning to the community and thinking about the future. Such assessment may also indicate that some residents are ready to live successfully in society much sooner than others. A person who is currently considered a dropout or a failure in treatment may be, in fact, reassessed as someone ready to return to the community.

A further implication involves the role of the community into which the addicts return. Whether or not positive changes in self-concept are maintained by the individuals will be influenced by the attitudes the residents encounter in their communities and families. Rather than being regarded as "cured," they will need acceptance and encouragement to continue to view themselves positively.

The results of this study suggest that while change in self-concept is certainly not the only valid criterion for success in treatment, it can provide valuable information about the progress of addicts toward successful rehabilitation.

REFERENCES

ALEXANDER, B., and DIBB, G. Interpersonal perception in addict families. *Fam. Process*, 1977, pp. 17-28.

BOYD, P. Drug abuse and addiction in adolescents. In J.G. Howells (ed.), *Modern Perspectives in Adolescent Psychiatry*. Edinburg: Oliver and Boyd, 1971.

BURNS, R.B. *The Self Concept.* London: Longman, 1979.

BUSS, A. *The Psychology of Aggression.* New York: Wiley, 1961.

BUTLER, J.M., and HAIGH, G.V. Changes in the relations between self concepts and ideal self concepts consequent upon client-centered counseling. In C.R. Rogers and R.F. Dymond (eds.), *Psychotherapy and Personality Change.* Chicago, 1954.

CHAMBERS, J.L. Need associations of narcotic addicts. *J. Clin. Psychol.* 28(4): 468-469, 1972.

COHEN, C.P., WHITE, E.H., and SCHOOLAR, J.C. Interpersonal patterns of personality for drug abusing patients and their therapeutic implications. *Arch. Gen. Psychiatry* 28: 131-135, 1973.

COOPERSMITH, S. *The Antecedents of Self Esteem.* San Francisco: Freemans, 1967.

DANZIGER, K. *Interpersonal Communication.* New York: Pergamon, 1976.

DE CHARMS, R. *Personal Causation: The Internal Affective Determinants of Behavior.* New York: Academic Press, 1968.

DE LEON, G., SKODAL, A., and ROSENTHAL, M. Phoenix House: Change in psychopathological signs of resident drug addicts. *Arch. Gen. Psychiatry* 24: 353-358, 1971.

DUSTER, T. *The Legislation of Morality: Laws, Drugs and Moral Judgment.* New York: Free Press, 1970.

EISER, R., and GOSSOP, M. Hooked or sick: Addicts' perceptions of their addiction. *Addict. Behav.* 4: 185-191, 1979.

FITTS, W. *Manual: Tennessee Department of Mental Health Self Concept Scale.* Nashville: Counselor Recordings and Tests, 1965.

GEIS, G. A halfway house is not a home: Notes of the failure of a narcotic rehabilitation project. *Drug Forum* 4(1): 7-13, 1974.

GOTTSCHALK, L.A., and GLESER, G.C. *The Measurement of Psychological States from the Content Analysis of Verbal Behavior.* Berkeley: University of California Press, 1969.

KOREN, H. Comparison of psychometric measures in psychiatric patients using heroin and other drugs. *J. Abnorm. Psychol.* 83: 208-212, 1974.

LECKY, P. *Self Consistency.* New York: Island Press, 1945.

LEVY, B.S. Five years after: A follow-up of 50 narcotic addicts. *Am. J. Psychiatry* 128(7): 102-106, 1972.

MC CANDLESS, B. *Children, Behavior and Development.* New York: Holt, 1967.

MC KENNA-HARTUNG, S., HARTUNG, J., and BAXTER, J. Self and ideal self concepts in a drug using subculture. *J. Pers. Assess.* 35: 461-471, 1971.

NIE, N.H. *Statistical Package for the Social Sciences.* New York: McGraw-Hill, 1975.

OGBORNE, A., and MELOTTE, C. An evaluation of a therapeutic community for former drug users. *Br. J. Addict.* 72: 75-82, 1977.

OSGOOD, C.E. Speculation on the structure of interpersonal intentions. *Behav. Sci.* 15: 237-254, 1970.

ROBBINS, E., ROBBINS, L., FROSCH, W., and STERN, M. College students' drug use. *Am. J. Psychiatry* 126: 1743-1751, 1970.

ROGERS, C. *Client Centered Therapy: Its Current Practice, Complications and Theory.* Boston: Houghton Mifflin, 1951.

ROGERS, C.R., and DYMOND, R.F. (eds.). *Psychotherapy and Personality Change.* Chicago: University of Chicago Press, 1954.

ROSENTHAL, B.J., SAVOY, M., GREENE, B.I., and SPILLANE, W.H. Drug treatment outcomes: Is sex a factor. *Int. J. Addict.* 14(1): 45-62, 1979.

ROTTER, J.B. Generalized expectancies for internal versus external control of reinforcement. *Psychol. Monogr.* 80(1): Whole No. 609, 1966.

SCHERER, S.E., ETTINGER, R.F., and MUDRICK, N.J. Need for social approval and drug use. *J. Consult. Clin. Psychol.* 38(1): 118-121, 1972.

SUTKER, B., ALLAIN, A., and COHEN, G.H. MMPI indices of personality change following short term and long term hospitalization of heroin addicts. *Psychol. Rep.* 34: 495-500, 1974.

VAILLANT, C.E. A 20 year follow-up of New York narcotic addicts. *Arch. Gen. Psychiatry* 29: 237-241, 1973.

VINEY, L.L, and WESTBROOK, M.T. Sociality: A content analysis for verbalizations. *Soc. Behav. Pers.* 7: 129-137, 1979.

WALDORF, D. Life without heroin: Some social adjustments during long term periods of voluntary abstention. *Soc. Probl.* 18: 228-243, 1970.

WESTBROOK, M.T., and VINEY, L.L. Scales of origin and pawn perception using content analysis of speech. *J. Pers. Assess.* 44: 157-166, 1980.

WESTERMEYER, J., and BOURNE, P. Treatment outcome and the role of the community in narcotic addiction. *J. Nerv. Ment. Dis.* 166: 51-58, 1978.

WYLIE, R.E. *The Self Concept: A Review of Methodological Consideration and Measuring Instruments.* Lincoln, NB: University of Nebraska Press, 1974.

ZUCKERMAN, M., SOLA, S., MASTERSON, J., and ANGELONE, J. MMPI patterns in drug abusers before and after treatment in therapeutic communities. *J. Consult. Clin. Psychol.* 43(3): 286-296, 1975.

The International Journal of the Addictions, 19(7), 819-825, 1984

Note

Abstinence or Decreasing Consumption among Adolescents: Importance of Reasons

Don W. Reeves,* MS

Department of Community Services
Pitt County Mental Health Center
Greenville, North Carolina 27834

Thomas W. Draper, PhD

Department of Family Sciences
Brigham Young University
Provo, Utah 84601

Abstract

This study determined the pervasiveness of reasons for abstinence or for decreasing alcohol consumption among 196 high school students in eastern North Carolina. Expanding upon prior research, 29 personal, social, and environmental reasons were examined. Generally, the less a student drank, the more important a reason was for abstaining or for a reduction in alcohol intake. Reasons rated important by a majority of all adolescent drinking groups, including heavy drinkers, were related to health, self-esteem/self-control, and parental disapproval/disappointment.

Over the years much research has focused on the reasons why adolescents drink. Recently some investigators have explored the reasons why adolescents do not drink or why they might choose to decrease consumption. Demone (1973) found reasons for abstinence were related to three variables: health, safety, and expense. Rachal, Williams, Brehm, Cavanaugh, Moore, and Eckerman

*To whom requests for reprints should be sent.

 0020-773X/84/1907-0819$3.50/0

(1975) and Barnes (1981) surveyed the degree of importance of each of several reasons related to abstinence or possible cessation of drinking. The Rachal et al. (1975) study found that the drinking levels were inversely related to the perceived importance of those reasons, and the abstainers attached the most importance to the items. Barnes (1981) found more adolescents listed (1) involvement with police, (2) losing one's self-control, and (3) having trouble in getting jobs or getting into school as important reasons for not drinking or for discontinuing to drink.

Previous studies have failed to include many potentially important reasons for abstinence or discontinuance. For example, other personal (to maintain self-esteem), social (better things to do, parents do not approve), and environmental (availability) factors could contribute to the process of building a prevention model. Expanding upon prior research, this study examines the reasons that a sample of rural adolescents gave for ceasing to drink and then seeks to determine the pervasiveness of each reason.

METHOD

The sample consisted of 102 males and 94 females in grades 9 through 12 selected from six high schools located in a relatively rural area of eastern North Carolina. The data were collected in the spring of 1979.

Based upon different quantitative indices, the participants selected the drinking level (abstainer, infrequent, light, moderate, moderate/heavy, heavy) that most reflected his or her own level of consumption. A convenient group of 20 similar students was used to generate 21 additional responses to supplement Rachal et al.'s (1975) eight-item list of reasons that adolescents might give for not drinking or that might influence them to stop or decrease their consumption if they did drink. This technique of using information from one group for the construction of a questionnaire to be given to another group has been described by Anderson, Ball, Murphy, and associates (1975). A Likert scale measured the degree of importance for each of 29 items to the students' decisions to abstain or to drink very infrequently or lightly. For the abstainer, infrequent drinker, and light drinker, each reason was measured as to how important it was in the decision to not drink or to drink very little. The moderate, moderate/heavy, and heavy drinkers were asked to check how important each reason would be to them if they were to stop drinking or decrease their consumption.

RESULTS

The students were divided into three groups on the basis of their reported level of drinking: abstainers, light-to-moderate drinkers, and heavy drinkers. Table 1 provides a breakdown of students' age, sex, and grade, by level of

Table 1

Characteristics of Students, by Drinking Group

	Number of students										
	Age					Sex		Grade			
Drinking group	15	16	17	18	19	M	F	9	10	11	12
Abstainers (N = 85)	7	28	37	11	2	30	55	4	32	42	7
Light to moderate (N = 88)	3	31	40	12	2	56	32	3	16	51	18
Heavy (N = 23)	1	6	10	5	1	16	7	0	3	11	9

drinking. Determinations were made of the percentage of students in each of these three groups that rated each reason for not drinking or ceasing to drink as being either "important" or "very important." A chi-square test of proportionality was administered to determine if the reasons were rated as being of different importance based on the students' alcoholic consumption. For 22 of the 29 reasons, the less students drank, the more important they thought the reason was. Exceptions to this general pattern were Items 2, 5, 11, 18, 20, 27, and 28.

The 29 reasons were arranged into four groups based upon the percentage of students in each drinking group rating the reason as important or very important (Table 2). The four groups were: (1) those reasons that only a minority of students in all three groups thought were important; (2) those reasons that only a majority of the abstainers thought were important; (3) those reasons that only a majority of the abstainers and light-to-moderate drinkers thought were important; and (4) those reasons that a majority of students in all three groups, including heavy drinkers, thought were important.

DISCUSSION

The present study posits that there are many reasons for abstinence or ceasing to drink; however, the reasons are of differing degress of saliency for abstainers, light-to-moderate drinkers, and heavy drinkers. Only those reasons listed in Group D were selected by a majority of students in all three drinking groups, including heavy drinkers, as being important reasons for abstinence or reducing consumption. These reasons were (1) I want to maintain my health, (2) I want to maintain my self-respect, (3) my parents do not approve, (4) I do not want to disappoint my family members, (5) I don't want to lose my self-control, and (6) I want to maintain my positive self-esteem.

Table 2

Importance of Reasons for Not Drinking or Ceasing to Drink

Group A:	A minority of students in all three groups regarded these reasons as important
	Kids I hang around with are against it
	I don't like the smell
	It's too expensive
	It is not readily available to me
	I was raised to use alcohol only on special occasions
	Fear of being excluded from the group I hang around with
	I don't have time to drink
Group B:	Only a majority of the abstainers regarded these reasons as important
	It's against my religion
	It tastes bad to me
	I don't like the effects
	Excessive drinking seems juvenile
	Adolescent drinking is not a sign of becoming an adult
	Drinking often makes you sick to your stomach
	It is just an artificial way of solving your problems or achieving moods
Group C:	A majority of abstainers and light-to-moderate drinkers regarded these reasons as important
	I want to be individual or different
	I have better things to do
	Because of possible negative consequences
	Fear of becoming alcoholic
	I have had little exposure to a drinking environment
	Drinking may lead to unhappiness
	I was raised not to abuse alcohol
	I want to set a good example for others
	I do not need to rebel or seek independence from my family
Group D:	A majority of all three groups, including heavy drinkers, regarded these reasons as important
	I want to maintain my health
	I want to maintain my self-respect
	My parents do not approve
	I do not want to disappoint my family members
	I don't want to lose my self-control
	I want to maintain my positive self-esteem

These data support other research that has found concern over health (Demone, 1973) and fear of losing self-control (Barnes, 1981) to be factors in the adolescent's decision to abstain or potentially reduce consumption. Segal, Rhenberg, and Sterling (1975) have shown that substance-abusing adolescents tend to have poorer self-concept and self-control than non-substance-abusing adolescents. High self-esteem and self-respect do not necessarily assure abstinence or appropriate drinking, but evidently adolescents perceive the loss of such as a salient psychological cost worthy of minimizing or avoiding.

Explanations relative to parental disapproval or disappointment being important are problematic. Roughly 73% of all adolescents surveyed perceived parental disapproval and/or disappointment to be important reasons for abstinence or for decreasing consumption. Burkett and Carrithers (1980) and Rachal, Guess, Hubbard, Maisto, Cavanaugh, Waddell, and Benrud (1980) found, respectively, that 79% and 71.5% of adolescents surveyed expected parental disapproval. Of those students expecting parental disapproval, Burkett and Carrithers found that 44% abstained, and Rachal et al. found only 30% to be abstainers. Rachal et al. found that 15.5% of adolescents expecting parental disapproval were heavy drinkers. If that large a percentage of adolescents expect parental disapproval, and if a majority of adolescents perceive parental disapproval/disappointment to be an important reason for abstinence or for reducing alcohol intake, then why did such a large number of these adolescents drink or drink beyond moderation?

One possibility is that for the adolescent, the cost of not drinking may be greater than the cost he or she experiences by drinking in spite of parental disapproval/disappointment. Adolescent drinking has been referred to as a "rite of passage" into adulthood. Parental disapproval may be a small price to pay for perceived adult status. Another possibility is that developmentally, the adolescent seeks greater independence and autonomy. To disregard or rebel against parental control could be illustrative of their internal determination to procure greater independence. A third possibility is that the most detailed and appropriate set of research questions have not yet been asked. Little is known about how the degree and nature of parental disapproval influence adolescent drinking decisions. Burkett and Carrithers (1980) stated that the effect of parental disapproval seemed to be indirect, such as attempting to influence the selection of their children's friends. Most parents probably realize that their children, sooner or later, will drink, or at least experiment with alcohol. Thus, parental control may be only weakly applied in this area due to the expectations of the parents. As such, parental disapproval toward adolescent drinking may be qualitatively different from parental disapproval in another area, and the form and nature of the control may vary greatly from parent to parent.

Traditional alcohol and drug abuse prevention projects have attempted to modify drinking behavior through increased knowledge or attitudinal change. However, these alcohol/drug education projects have been less than successful (Schaps, Churgin, Palley, Takata, and Cohen, 1980; Staulcup, Kenward, and Frigo, 1979). Contemporary prevention strategies focus upon the development of the individual's interpersonal and intrapersonal skills, self-esteem, and social support systems. That adolescents consider the loss of self-esteem and self-control important lends support to contemporary prevention models in which the enhancement of self-esteem and self-control is an integral component. All aspects of alcohol information curricula may not need to be abandoned; material relative to the effects of substances upon the health of individuals may have salutary results and should be researched further.

Most alcohol prevention programs are directed toward adolescents or young adults, with little attention given to family-oriented strategies. Results from the present study and other correlational data support the importance of the family as a factor, or potential factor, in alcohol and drug use (Schaps et al., 1980). There is a general tendency for adolescents to identify with and imitate parents who are nurturant and involved in their lives in constructive and nonintrusive ways (Douvan and Adelson, 1966). Given this, alcohol abuse prevention programs aimed toward parents could focus upon the development of a strong parent-child relationship, of the family as a support and reference group, and of a greater understanding by parents of child development principles. Further research is needed to delineate specific aspects of the parent-child relationship, or parental qualities, that may contribute to the socialization of appropriate adolescent drinking.

In reviewing the results of this study, the reader needs to be cognizant of the limitations of the present sample. The subjects were from a rural area in a southern state where adherence to traditional family roles and structures is more the rule than the exception. The predominant religious beliefs of people in this area discourage consumption of alcoholic beverages. Since prohibition is more likely to be ascribed by decree than by reason, adolescents who decide to begin drinking may have only limited rationales for ceasing the practice or bringing it under control. Studies with other groups of adolescents are needed to provide a broader understanding of possible precursors of abstinence or decreasing consumption. Since the reasons people give for doing or not doing anything are heavily influenced by their own culture, cross-cultural studies would be particularly fruitful.

REFERENCES

ANDERSON, S.B., BALL, S., MURPHY, R.T., and ASSOCIATES. In *Encyclopedia of Educational Evaluation.* Washington: Jossey-Bass, 1975.

BARNES, G.M. Drinking among adolescents: A subcultural phenomenon or a model of adult behaviors. *Adolescence* 16: 211-299, 1981.

BURKETT, S.R., and CARRITHERS, W.T. Adolescents' drinking and perceptions of legal and informal sanctions. *J. Alcohol Drug Educ.* 41: 839-853, 1980.

DEMONE, H.W. The nonuse and abuse of alcohol by the male adolescent. In *Proceedings of the 2nd Annual Alcoholism Conference.* Rockville, MD: NIAAA, 1973, pp. 24-32.

DOUVAN, E., and ADELSON, J. *The Adolescent Experience.* New York: Wiley, 1966.

RACHAL, J.V., GUESS, L.L., HUBBARD, R.L., MAISTO, S.A., CAVANAUGH, E.R., WADDELL, R., and BENRUD, C.H. The extent and nature of adolescent alcohol and drug use: The 1974 and 1978 national sample studies. In *Adolescent Drinking Behavior*, Vol. 1 (NTS No. PB81 199267). Rockville, MD: National Institute on Alcohol Abuse and Alcoholism, 1980.

RACHAL, J.V., WILLIAMS, J.R., BREHM, M.L., CAVANAUGH, B., MOORE, P.R, and ECKERMAN, W.C. *A National Study of Adolescent Drinking Behavior, Attitudes and Correlates.* Prepared for National Institute on Alcohol Abuse and Alcoholism (Report No. PB-246-002; NIAA/NCALI-75/27). Springfield, VA: U.S. National Technical Information Services, 1975.

SCHAPS, E., CHURGIN, S., PALLEY, C.S., TAKATA, B., and COHEN, A.Y. Primary prevention research: A preliminary review of program outcome studies. *Int. J. Addict.* 15: 657-676, 1980.

SEGAL, B., RHENBURG, G., and STERLING, S. Self-concept and drug and alcohol use in female college students. *J. Alcohol Drug Educ.* 20: 17-21, 1975.

STAULCUP, H., KENWARD, K., and FRIGO, D. A review of federal primary alcoholism prevention projects. *J. Stud. Alcohol* 40: 943-968, 1979.

INFORMATION FOR AUTHORS SUBMITTING MANUSCRIPTS

Send a clear double-spaced typewritten original and one duplicate to Ms. Nancy Reid-Rappolt, Editorial Assistant, *International Journal of the Addictions,* c/o Winch, Smith, Ostermann and Mates, MD's, 4141 Geary, Suite 326, San Francisco, California 94118. Also send one duplicate to the Chief Editor, Dr. Stanley Einstein, Building 113/41, East Talpiot, Jerusalem, Israel. DOUBLE-SPACE the entire manuscript; do not use single spacing anywhere, including references.

Include authors' academic degrees and present affiliation. If applicable, cite auspices under which work being reported was done. Specify address to which requests for reprints should be sent.

Begin your TITLE with a word useful in indexing. A 75- to 100-word ABSTRACT should be provided, which precedes each article. A summary is then not necessary. Major and minor headings may be used in the text; indicate major headings by typing in capitals.

Use METRIC UNITS of measure. If measurements were made in English units, give metric equivalents.

Cite all TABLES and FIGURES in the text. Tables should have titles, and figures should have brief legends. In tables, give each column a heading. Indicate units of measure in parentheses in the heading for each column. Do not use vertical rules. Do not use horizontal rules other than those in the heading and at the bottom. Submit PHOTOGRAPHS as glossy prints, untrimmed and unmounted; identify each with pencil lightly on the back and indicate top.

ARTWORK will not be returned unless specifically requested, and will be disposed of three months after publication.

REFERENCES in the text should be enclosed in parentheses and include the author's surname and the date of the item cited. Keep footnotes to a minimum. Footnotes should be collected at the end of the manuscript in their numerical order of appearance.

The BIBLIOGRAPHY (double-spaced) should be given at the end of the article in alphabetical order. Journal references should include authors, title, name of journal abbreviated according to *Chemical Abstracts List of Periodicals*, inclusive page numbers, and date. Book references should include authors, title, place of publication, publisher, and date.

AUTHOR RESPONSIBILITY: It is the sole responsibility of the author(s) to obtain written permission from the author(s), publisher(s), etc. for figures, tables, or any other information excerpted from previously published works which are used in the manuscript(s) considered for publication. It is understood that the manuscript(s) considered for publication in the *International Journal of the Addictions* have not been previously published nor are they under simultaneous publication consideration elsewhere.

Statements and opinions expressed in the articles and communications herein are those of the author(s) and do not necessarily express those of the Editor or publisher.

THE INTERNATIONAL JOURNAL OF THE ADDICTIONS

Volume 19 Number 7 1984

CONTENTS

Adherence in a Behavioral Alcohol Treatment Program: E. B. Fink, S. Rudden, R. Longabaugh, B. McCrady, and R. Stout 709

Alcohol Education Programs for University Students: A Review of Their Effectiveness: M. S. Goodstadt and A. Caleekal-John 721

Family Mapping: Toward an Understanding of the Interactional Dynamic of the Alcoholic Marital Dyad: K. M. Synol 743

Social Recovery and Therapeutic Mission: L. W. Whorley 753

An Evaluation of the Alternatives Approach to Drug Abuse Prevention: R. Cook, H. Lawrence, C. Morse, and J. Roehl 767

Research Notes

Inhalant Abuse and Juvenile Delinquency: A Control Study in Albuquerque, New Mexico: B. J. F. Reed and P. A. May 789

Self- and Ideal-Self-Perception of Drug Addicts in Therapeutic Communities: C. A. Preston and L. L. Viney 805

Note

Abstinence or Decreasing Consumption among Adolescents: Importance of Reasons: D. W. Reeves and T. W. Draper 819

MARCEL DEKKER, INC., New York and Basel

CODEN: INJABN 19(8) i-ii, 827-962 (1984)
ISSN: 0020-773X

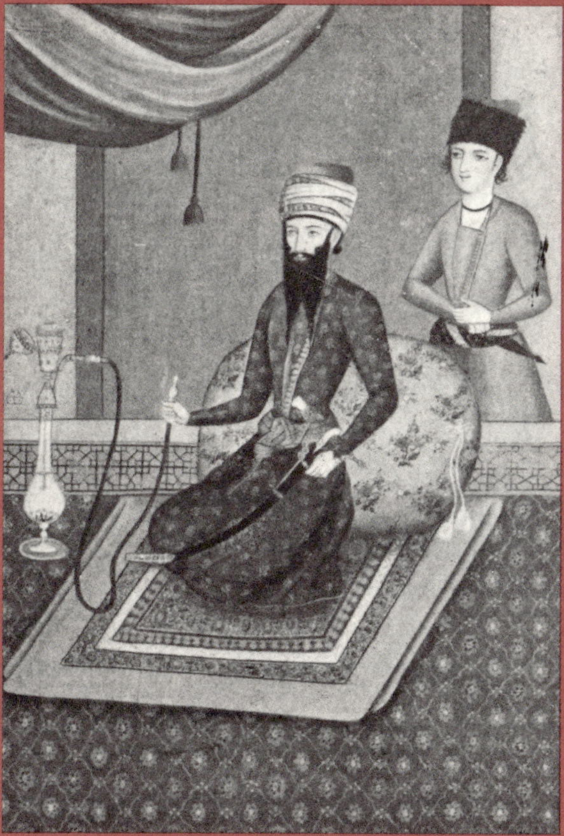

THE INTERNATIONAL JOURNAL OF THE Addictions

Includes Index to Volume 19

Volume 19 Number 8 1984

THE INTERNATIONAL JOURNAL OF THE ADDICTIONS

December 1984

Aims and Scope. This journal is a comprehensive medium for worldwide communication among both concerned laymen and professionals in research, training, and treatment in the field of addiction and substance misuse.

Indexing and Abstracting Services. Articles published in *The International Journal of the Addictions* are selectively indexed or abstracted in:

• Abstracts Journal of the Institute of Scientific Information of the USSR Academy of Sciences • Adolescent Mental Health Abstracts • ASCA • Bibliographic Index of Health Education Periodicals (BIHEP) • BioSciences Information Service of Biological Abstracts (BIOSIS) • Classified Abstracts Archive of the Alcohol Literature • Current Awareness in Biological Sciences • Current Contents/Clinical Practice • Excerpta Medica • Index Medicus • International Pharmaceutical Abstracts • ISI/BIOMED • Psychological Abstracts • Science Citation Index • Selected List of Tables of Contents of Psychiatric Periodicals • Social Sciences Citation Index • State Central Scientific Medical Library/ International Book Exchange—USSR

Articles published in *The International Journal of the Addictions* are listed in Selected List of Tables of Contents of Psychiatric Periodicals.

Manuscript Preparation and Submission. See end of issue.

Subscription Information. *The International Journal of the Addictions* (ISSN: 0020-773X) is published eight times annually in February, April, May, July, August, September, November, and December by Marcel Dekker, Inc., 270 Madison Avenue, New York, New York 10016. The subscription rate for Volume 19 (1984), containing eight numbers, is $225.00 per volume (prepaid). The special discounted rate for individual professionals and students is $112.50 per volume. To secure this special rate, your order must be prepaid by personal check. Add $20.00 for surface postage outside the United States. For airmail to Europe, add $32.48; to Asia, add $40.48.

Mailing Address. *Please mail payment with order to:* Marcel Dekker Journals, P. O. Box 11305, Church Street Station, New York, New York 10249.

Contributions to this journal are published free of charge. Second-class postage paid at New York, New York and additional mailing offices. POSTMASTER: Send address changes to *The International Journal of the Addictions*, P. O. Box 5005, Cimarron Road, Monticello, New York 12701.

Library of Congress Catalog Card Number 66-9896

Portrait of a Persian Prince smoking a hookah, courtesy of the Picture Collection, The Branch Libraries, New York Public Library.

THE INTERNATIONAL JOURNAL OF THE Addictions

The International Journal of the Addictions, 19(8), 827–832, 1984

Nicotine Level as a Predictor of Smoking Frequency: A Case Report

Eric M. Morrell,* PhD

James G. Hollandsworth, Jr., PhD

University of Southern Mississippi
Hattiesburg, Mississippi 39401

Abstract

Laboratory-based evidence is inconsistent regarding the regulation of nicotine intake for habitual smokers. The present case report describes an *in vivo* double-blind alteration of nicotine level for two long-term, heavy smokers. In spite of large changes in nicotine intake, the frequency of smoking remained stable. It was concluded that other variables may play an equal or more important role than nicotine in governing smoking behavior in the natural setting.

The relationship between nicotine content and the number of cigarettes smoked appears to be complex. While a great deal of evidence has been found suggesting that nicotine intake determines smoking frequency (Ashton and Watson, 1970; Frith, 1971; Goldfarb, Gritz, Jarvik, and Stolerman, 1976; Russell, Wilson, Patel, Cole, and Feyerabend, 1973; Turner, Sillett, and Ball, 1974), other studies have failed to support this position (Finnegan, Larson, and Haag, 1945; Goldfarb, Jarvik, and Glick, 1970; Kumar, Cooke, Lader, and Russell, 1977; Mangan and Golding, 1978). All of these studies were planned observations (see Table 1). The present case study describes an unplanned *in vivo* alteration of nicotine level for two long-term, heavy smokers.

*To whom requests for reprints should be sent at his present address: Box 3926, Duke University Medical Center, Durham, North Carolina 27710.

 0020-773X/84/1908-0827$3.50/0

Table 1

Nicotine Manipulations

Author(s)	Year	*Ss*	*N*	Technique	Focus of study	Results
Ashton and Watson	1970	Volunteer smokers	15 females 21 males	High- vs low-retention cigarette filters.	Puffing frequency and nicotine extraction in relation to filter type.	Greater number of puffs for high-retention filters; equivalent extractions of nicotine for both cigarette types.
Finnegan, Larson, and Haag	1945	Volunteer smokers	24	Monthly alterations in cigarette nicotine level.	Smoking rate in relation to nicotine content.	No relationship found.
Frith	1971	Volunteer student smokers	9 males	Varied cigarette nicotine content over 3-day period.	Smoking rate and duration in relation to nicotine content.	Nicotine level: (1) inversely related to smoking rate; (2) positively related to amount of time taken to smoke cigarette.
Goldfarb, Gritz, Jarvik, and Stolerman	1976	Paid smokers	St. 1: 12 males and 8 females St. 2: 12 males and 3 females	Ratings of cigarette strength and satisfaction; recordings of daily numbers of different nicotine level cigarettes; urinalysis for nicotine levels.	(1) Smoker perceptions of nicotine as reinforcing; (2) behavioral and physiological effects of manipulated nicotine levels.	(1) Ratings correlated with nicotine but not tar. (2) Increase in nicotine strength led to slight decrease in cigarette numbers. (3) Urinalysis evidence of altered smoking patterns to maintain nicotine levels.
Goldfarb, Jarvik, and Glick	1970	Paid smokers	15	Simulated (lettuce) cigarettes with	(1) Subject perception of cigarette strength	(1) Accurate perception of strength and qual-

				different nicotine levels.	and quality; (2) smoking rate in relation to nicotine content.	ity; (2) smoking rates independent of nicotine levels.
Kumar, Cooke, Lader, and Russell	1977	Paid smokers	7 males 5 females	Graded ambient tobacco smoke vs intravenous nicotine.	Influence of the two techniques on subsequent cigarette smoking and physiological activity.	Ambient smoke decreased subsequent number of puffs; intravenous nicotine did not. Both produced same physiological effects.
Mangan and Golding	1978	Volunteer smokers	St. 1: 10 males and 11 females St. 2: 5 males and 4 females	Three nicotine alterations over 6 days (Study 1). Two alterations over 8 days (Study 2).	Smoking rate in relation to nicotine content.	No relationship found.
Russell, Wilson, Patel, Cole, and Feyerabend	1973	Sedentary smokers	10	Alteration of cigarette nicotine level at work over 4-day period.	(1) Smoking rate and total weight smoked in relation to nicotine content; (2) influence of altered nicotine content on COHb levels.	(1) Rate and total weight inversely related to nicotine level; (2) change to high or low nicotine from regular brand led to decrease in COHb levels.
Turner, Sillett, and Ball	1974	Volunteer smokers	5 males 5 females	Weekly reduction in cigarette nicotine level.	Effect of nicotine reduction on consumption levels, smoking patterns, and COHb levels.	Increased daily consumption, decreased COHb levels, and altered smoking patterns.

CASE REPORT

The subjects, a married couple, were referred by a physician to the first author in 1981 for a smoking cessation program. The 42-year-old husband had just experienced his second myocardial infarction and had a family history of coronary disease. His father had died of a heart attack when he was 62 years old. Both he and his wife had been smoking for approximately 25 years and had attempted to quit on several previous occasions. Two weeks prior to treatment they were smoking two to three packs a day of a .9 mg nicotine cigarette. At the time of referral, both had switched to a .4 mg nicotine cigarette but were still smoking in excess of two packs a day.

A multicomponent treatment package consisting of brand fading, stimulus control, response substitution, and contingency contracting was implemented. The brand-fading component followed the general procedures outlined by Foxx and Brown (1979). The target nicotine level was reduced by 10% per week. During the first week of the program the subjects were instructed to continue smoking their .4 mg nicotine brand of cigarettes. The target level of nicotine for the second week was set at .34 to .36 mg. Cigarette nicotine levels were determined by referring to the Federal Trade Commission guidelines (Federal Trade Commission, 1979). The subjects were free to smoke as much as they liked, provided they limited their smoking to certain locations (stimulus control). Response substitution consisted of competing behaviors such as chewing gum in nonsmoking areas. A contingency contract involving a $10 weekly forfeiture for noncompliance was also in effect. During the 3 weeks of data collection reported here the treatment conditions in effect were held constant.

During the first week of treatment the subjects smoked a .4 mg nicotine cigarette as instructed. However, due to the poor legibility of a photocopy of the guidelines, a .84 mg nicotine cigarette was mistakenly selected for the second week. Neither the investigator nor the subjects were aware of the error until the end of the second week, at which time the mistake was corrected by choosing a .36 mg nicotine cigarette for Week 3.

The husband smoked an average of 15 cigarettes daily during the first week, 17 during the second, and 17 during the third week. The wife smoked a daily average of 26 cigarettes during Week 1, followed by 24 and 34 cigarettes for Weeks 2 and 3, respectively.

DISCUSSION

Contrary to the literature linking nicotine level to smoking frequency, neither the husband nor the wife decreased the number of cigarettes smoked during the second week, when the nicotine level was unintentionally increased.

In actuality, an approximately 100% increase in nicotine intake for both subjects apparently had no effect on smoking frequency. Additionally, the number of cigarettes smoked by the husband remained stable during the third week. The wife, however, increased her frequency by approximately 50%. This increase would be in keeping with the nicotine regulation hypothesis since the actual level of nicotine intake was cut in half for the third week. What is of interest, though, is the fact that she was aware of this decrease for Week 3 but had been unaware of the increase for Week 2.

Two factors must be considered when discussing these data. First, the data were obtained through self-monitoring, which, of course, is vulnerable to distortion. However, it should be noted that the subjects, both of whom were college professors, were not penalized in any way for increasing or decreasing smoking frequency and that there were no aversive consequences for reporting the data honestly.

Second, there is the possibility that smoking topography differed between weeks. Changes that might have masked data supporting the nicotine regulation hypothesis would include increased puffs (Ashton and Watson, 1970) or increased depth of inhalation (Frith, 1971). While no direct measures of these behaviors were taken, subsequent questioning of the clients did not indicate any awareness of such changes occurring during the 3-week period.

Nicotine regulation has been regarded by many as a major determinant of smoking behavior. The findings of this case report, however, do not support that conclusion. This is particularly surprising given the strong support of this position for long-term, heavy smokers (Schachter, 1977, 1978). While not discounting the possibility that nicotine regulation can be a potentially important factor, the present data would suggest that other variables may be of equal if not greater importance in determining smoking frequency. In designing interventions, therapists would be advised to assess for a multitude of smoking influences and incorporate into treatment all factors that appear contributory.

REFERENCES

ASHTON, H., and WATSON, D.W. Puffing frequency and nicotine intake in cigarette smokers. *Br. Med. J.* 3: 679-681, 1970.

FEDERAL TRADE COMMISSION. *Tar and Nicotine Content of Cigarettes.* Washington, DC: Public Health Service, 1979.

FINNEGAN, J.K., LARSON, P.S., and HAAG, H.B. The role of nicotine in the cigarette habit. *Science* 102: 94-96, 1945.

FOXX, R.M., and BROWN, R.A. Nicotine fading and self-monitoring for cigarette abstinence or controlled smoking. *J. Appl. Behav. Anal.* 12: 111-125, 1979.

FRITH, C.D. The effect of varying nicotine content of cigarettes on human smoking behavior. *Psychopharmacologia* 19: 188-192, 1971.

GOLDFARB, T., GRITZ, E.R., JARVIK, M.E., and STOLERMAN, I.P. Reactions to cigarettes as a function of nicotine and tar. *Clin. Pharmacol. Ther.* 19: 766-772, 1976.

GOLDFARB, T.L., JARVIK, M.E., and GLICK, S.D. Cigarette nicotine content as a determinant of human smoking behavior. *Psychopharmacologia* 17: 89-93, 1970.

KUMAR, R., COOKE, E.C., LADER, M.H., and RUSSELL, M.A.H. Is nicotine important in tobacco smoking? *Clin. Pharmacol. Ther.* 21: 520-529, 1977.

MANGAN, G.L., and GOLDING, J. An "enhancement" model of smoking maintenance? In R.E. Thorton (ed.), *Smoking Behaviour: Physiological and Psychological Influences*. Edinburgh: Churchill Livingstone, 1978.

RUSSELL, M.A.H., WILSON, C., PATEL, U.A., COLE, P.V., and FEYERABEND, C. Comparison of effect on tobacco consumption and carbon monoxide absorption of changing to high and low nicotine cigarettes. *Br. Med. J.* 512-516, 1973.

SCHACHTER, S. Nicotine regulation in heavy and light smokers. *J. Exp. Psychol. (Gen.)* 106: 5-12, 1977.

SCHACHTER, S. Pharmacological and psychological determinants of smoking. *Ann. Intern. Med.* 88: 104-114, 1978.

TURNER, J.A.M., SILLETT, R.W., and BALL, K.P. Some effects of changing to low-tar and low-nicotine cigarettes. *Lancet* 2: 737-739, 1974.

The International Journal of the Addictions, 19(8), 833–848, 1984

Determinants of Relapse among Alcoholics: A Cross-Cultural Replication Study

Christer Sandahl,* MA

Department of Clinical Alcohol and Drug Research
Karolinska Institute
S-104 01 Stockholm, Sweden

Abstract

This study reports on a replication of Marlatt and Gordon's (1980) findings concerning relapse determinants among alcoholics. It was undertaken in a somewhat different drinking culture (Sweden) and with a group of alcoholics also containing patients relapsing after a longer period of abstinence than those in the Marlatt and Gordon study. The difference in drinking culture is reflected in the finding that most subjects in this study took their first drink at home. The group studied by Marlatt and Gordon in Seattle most frequently started to drink in a bar or restaurant. In spite of the differences between the groups, we arrive at a similar picture when it comes to the distribution of relapse determinants according to the model proposed by Marlatt and Gordon. The categories not only have face validity but also construct validity, reflected in meaningful correlations with results on an intelligence test and a personality inventory. A descriptive analysis shows that subjects with poorer results on the intelligence test and having a high tendency to muscle tension and somatized anxiety tended to relapse in intrapersonal situations. Patients who do not readily adjust to other persons' opinions relapsed in interpersonal conflicts, and patients who are more impulsive could not resist social pressure to drink.

*Requests for reprints should be sent to the author at the above address.

 0020-773X/84/1908-0833$3.50/0

The power of general factors to predict recovery or relapse among alcoholics has frequently been studied. Examples of such factors are social stability, family and work situation (Baekeland, 1977; Polich, Armor, and Braiker, 1980; Rönnberg, 1979; Saunders, Phil, and Kershaw, 1979), neuropsychological impairment (Abbot and Gregson, 1981; Gregson and Taylor, 1977; Heilbrun and Tarbox, 1978; O'Leary, Donovan, Chaney, and Walter, 1979), field dependence (Kissin, 1977), self-respect (Heather, Rollnik, and Winton, 1982), and degree of physical dependence (Miller, Pechacek, and Hamburg, 1981; Polich, Armor, and Braiker, 1980). It has not been possible to prove that any given form of treatment modality is more effective when it comes to preventing relapse (Miller and Hester, 1980). However, Ahles, Schlundt, Prue, and Rychtarik (1983) recently found arrangements of aftercare to affect relapse pattern. A few studies have mapped out specific situations preceding a relapse. Tokar, Brunse, Stefflre, Napior, and Södergren (1973) found that alcoholics go to bars, drink, smoke, or take "pills" when they feel helpless or depressed, or are angry or anxious. In another study Ludwig and Stark (1974) found that 80-90% of the alcoholics had a craving experience when they were depressed, nervous, or anxious; felt bad; or were under stress. Only 20-30% used alcohol when they were successful or happy, felt at ease, or were relaxed. Samsonowitz and Sjöberg (1981) found that in most cases relapses were associated with situations of emotional stress. Litman, Eiser, Rawson, and Oppenheim (1979) summarized their findings by categorizing precipitating situations into (1) unpleasant effects, (2) external events and euphoric feelings, (3) social anxiety, and (4) lessened cognitive vigilance. The results from their study suggested that cognitive control and flexibility of coping were more characteristic of those who did not relapse. These earlier studies are summarized in Table 1.

Marlatt and Gordon (1980) interviewed heroin addicts, smokers, and alcoholics regarding the circumstances associated with the last relapse. The answers were arranged in categories based on content analysis with good agreement between two independent raters. Marlatt and Gordon differentiated between determinants of relapse primarily associated with intrapersonal factors and those implying the influence of present or recent interaction with another person. Examples of intrapsychic determinants are: coping with negative emotional states, coping with negative physical/physiological states, enhancement of positive emotional states, testing personal control, and giving in to temptations or urges. Examples of interpersonal determinants are: coping with interpersonal conflict, social pressure, and enhancement of a positive emotional state.

One clinical implication of these findings is that it should be of importance to help alcoholic patients to find ways of coping with these situations in order to prevent relapses. Marlatt and Gordon came to the conclusion that certain situations are more dangerous for some though not for others; that is, every person has his own unique relapse pattern. Marlatt and Gordon have documented empirical support for a scheme to categorize such situations. Their scheme and cognitive-behavioral model of the relapse process are simple and easily defended from a theoretical point of view, and they integrate earlier empirical findings. It also seems reasonable that some individuals should be more sensitive to intrapsychic tensions while others are more sensitive to interpersonal conflicts.

One shortcoming of the Marlatt and Gordon study is that only alcoholics relapsing shortly after treatment were interviewed. All of them were contacted within 90 days, although most relapsed before that.

If every alcoholic has a unique pattern of risk situations, this could partly be influenced by personality factors. Marlatt and Gordon do not discuss such connections, which, however, would appear to be of importance when it comes to predicting relapse situations.

The purpose of this study was to examine the generality of Marlatt and Gordon's means of categorizing relapse precipitants by interviewing alcoholics in a different drinking culture, including also those who successfully abstained from alcohol for longer periods of time. The covariation between relapse determinants and some clinically relevant personality factors was also studied.

METHOD

Subjects

In a clinical research program in Stockholm, KARTAD (Karolinska Project for Research and Treatment of Alcohol Dependence), over 700 alcoholic patients consecutively admitted on medical grounds were examined medically, socially, and psychologically during the period 1976-1980 (Ideström, 1977). The patients were also reinvestigated 6 months and 2 years after discharge. Since the patients belong to the ordinary catchment area of the clinic, some of them return for inpatient detoxification when they have relapsed and had an adverse drinking period.

The subjects in the present study were (1) registered in the KARTAD program and (2) admitted to the clinic for detoxification during a 4-month period in 1980. The patients had had at least one previous stay at the clinic and had therefore, by definition, had a relapse.

Fifty consecutively admitted patients were asked if they would take part in the study. As two refused on the grounds that they did not want to be reminded of their drinking, this report is based on interviews with 48 patients.

In the sample, 17% were women, and the mean age was 44 years. A majority of the patients were either divorced (58%) or had never been married (21%). The educational level was rather low, only 12% having completed schooling comparable to the 12th year of high school. In a male control group from the catchment area, the comparative figure was 36%. Results of neuropsychological

Table 1

Summary of Some Studies of Factors Associated with Relapse

Factor	Author(s)	Subjects	Procedure	Results
Social-economic status and social stability	Baekeland (1977)	Alcoholics	Review of literature on methods for treatment of chronic alcoholism.	Dominant role played by patient rather than treatment factor. Patients with higher social-economic status and social stability had improvement rates varying from 32% to 68% while skid row alcoholics had rates ranging from 0% to 18%.
Family and work situation	Rönnberg (1979)	Alcoholic and problem drinkers	Theoretical discussion of the application of behavioral analysis to alcohol abuse.	Besides the social skill of the consumer, marital support and reinforcing work opportunities seemed to be the most important potentiating variables for alcohol consumption.
Age, dependency symptoms, and marital status	Polich, Armor, and Braiker (1980)	758 alcoholics	Follow-up of subjects 18 months and 4 years after admission to treatment.	Among patients who had high levels of alcohol dependence and who were younger on admission and among older patients with low levels of dependence, those who were married had better prognosis with abstinence as the treatment goal, while the unmarried had a better prognosis with nonproblem drinking.
Life, circumstance changes	Saunders, Phil, and Kershaw (1979)	162 subjects who had experienced alcohol problems in the past	Respondents in a community survey study who had experienced alcohol problems in the past were reinterviewed.	Spontaneous remission occurs most readily in less severe cases and the processes involved in such remission concern significant life circumstance changes such as in marriage and job.
Cognitive control, internal scanning, and self reinforcement	Heilbrun and Tarbox (1978)	60 alcoholics	A battery of tests was administered 2-3 weeks following admission to an	Poorer-outcome alcoholics tended to show a pattern of lower cognitive control and internal scanning, and a higher self-reinforcement.

			outpatient treatment program. The subjects were followed up after 6 months.	
Cognitive impairment	O'Leary, Donovan, Chaney, and Walker (1979)	30 male alcoholics	An index based on a battery of neuropsychological tests was used as the measure which was related to status for 22 subjects located for a 1-year follow-up.	High scores on the index were found to be highly related to fewer relapses, longer abstinence periods, and lower rates of alcohol consumption at the follow-up.
Cognitive impairment	Gregson and Taylor (1977)	90 male alcoholics	A battery of tests was administered during hospitalization. Other data were gathered from records and interviews. Patients were contacted 1, 3, and 6 months after discharge.	Cognitive impairment was the best predictor of relapse.
Cognitive dysfunction	Abbot and Gregson (1981)	106 alcoholics	A battery of tests and an interview were administered during hospitalization. At 3 months and 1 year after discharge, the patients were followed up.	Compared with measures of a wide variety of social demographic and psychological characteristics, indices of cognitive dysfunction were better predictors of treatment outcome.
Social stability, intelligence, and field dependence	Kissin (1977)	450 alcoholics	Subjects were randomly assigned to three different treatment modalities: (1) medical outpatient, (2)	(1) Successes in the medical model tended to be more socially stable, of average intelligence, and field dependent. (2) Successes in the psychological model tended to be more socially stable, above

(continued)

Table 1 (continued)

Factor	Author(s)	Subjects	Procedure	Results
			psychological outpatient, (3) social inpatient. At intake patients were given a social interview and a battery of psychological tests. Only 50% of the original population were successfully contacted after 1 year.	average intelligence, and field independent. (3) Successes in the social model tended to be socially unstable, of average intelligence, and field dependent.
Cognitive control and flexibility of coping	Litman, Eiser, Rawson, and Oppenheim (1979)	120 alcoholics	A questionnaire was administered to a sample of patients chosen with a view to heterogeneity, including patients who had abstained for 6 months or more.	Cognitive control and flexibility of coping seemed to be more characteristic of those who did not relapse.
Self-respect and perceived respectability	Heather, Rollnik, and Winton (1982)	52 alcoholics	Repertory grids were administered to patients shortly after admission to hospital-based ward and just before discharge. 44 subjects were successfully followed up after 6 months.	Measured psychological changes in the variables of self-respect and perceived respectability were significantly related to outcome of treatment.
Severity of problem drinking	Miller, Pechacek, and Hamburg (1981)	35 problem drinkers	28 clients attended three or more sessions of 10 on a once a week basis. A 2-week base-	Indices of severity of problem drinking were found to best predict outcome.

			line was obtained before classes started, and subjects were followed up for 3 months.	
Aftercare arrangements	Ahles, Schlundt, Prue, and Rychtarik (1983)	50 alcoholics	Subjects were assigned to either an intensive aftercare, recruitment procedure or regular clinic aftercare. 36 patients were successfully followed up after 1 year.	Those who received the intensive aftercare procedure showed a delayed relapse.
Dysphoric emotional states	Tokar, Brunse, Stefflre, Napior, Södergren (1973)	56 male alcoholics; 50 male controls	Subjects were asked to relate each of 21 behavioral responses to each of 20 emotional states.	Self-descriptions of behavioral responses in various emotional states by alcoholics and nonalcoholics revealed distinctly different patterns.
Dysphoric emotional states	Ludwig and Stark (1974)	60 male alcoholics	Subjects answered a drinking and craving questionnaire.	Subjects were more likely to experience craving when they felt anxious, worried, depressed, lonesome, or bored, and when they were in situations where alcohol was available.
Emotional stress	Samsonowitz and Sjöberg (1981)	10 socially adjusted alcoholics	Three interviews were carried out with subjects to study their attempts to give up drinking.	Volitional breakdowns occurred mostly under emotional stress and were preceded by various kinds of twisted reasoning to justify giving in to temptation.
Specific situation	Marlatt and Gordon (1980)	70 alcoholics	Subjects were interviewed regarding the circumstances associated with the last relapse.	In each case it was possible to specify a set of specific situations preceding relapse. These relapse episodes were classified to either intrapersonal (61%) or interpersonal (39%) determinants.

examination indicated that as many as 24% showed definite signs of intellectual impairment, particularly with regard to nonverbal and visuospatial functions, though verbal learning and retention were not influenced (Bergman, Borg, Hindmarsh, Idestrom and Mützell, 1980). The mean value for duration of abuse was 10 years. In regard to alcohol-related symptoms, most of the patients had had blackouts (81%), 68% had experienced craving, 90% reported morning drinking, 41% considered themselves as alcoholics, and 26% had experienced delirious episodes. Fifty-seven percent had been treated for alcohol problems before they were admitted to KARTAD, and 40% had been in contact with the local temperance board. As many as 71% had been in hospital treatment at least once during the 5 years preceding the basic examination. Finally, 41% had criminal records. Background characteristics of the sample are summarized in Table 2.

Table 2

Background Characteristics of the Subjects (N = 48)

Social-Anamnestic Data	
Age (yr)	
Mean	44.1
SD	8.5
Range	28-69
Proportion of women	17%
Married	16%
Divorced	58%
Unmarried	21%
Widower/widow	5%
Cohabitation with a partner	32%
Completed secondary modern school	71%
Completed grammar school	12%
Unskilled worker	26%
Permanent employment	63%
Alcohol-Anamnestic Data	
Age started heavy drinking (yr) ($N = 42$)	
Mean	34.0
SD	8.9
Range	18-63
Duration of abuse (yr) ($N = 42$)	
Mean	9.6
SD	6.8
Range	0-24
Reported blackouts	81%
Reported craving	68%
Reported morning drinking	90%

(continued)

Table 2 (continued)

Considered oneself an alcoholic	41%
Reported delirious episodes	26%
Showed signs of intellectual impairment	24%
Treatment Experiences	
Number of times in hospital with diagnosis of alcoholism[a] (*N* = 41)	
Mean	2.6
SD	3.2
Range	0-13
Treated for alcohol problems before admission	57%
No hospital treatment before admission[a]	17%
Somatic care only[a]	12%
Treated on psychiatric and/or somatic and/or alcohol wards[a]	71%
Been in contact with the local Board of Temperance	40%
Legal Status	
Age first time convicted for drunkenness (yr)[a] (*N* = 24)	
Mean	27.6
SD	7.7
Range	17-42
Number of convictions for drunkenness[a] (*N* = 28)	
Mean	3.8
SD	9.0
Range	0-47
Occurring in the criminal records kept by the National Board of Excise[a]	41%

[a]Based on official records and referring to the 5 years preceding the basic examination.

This group was compared to the rest of the patients registered in KARTAD. We found no significant differences between the groups when we compared them with regard to, for example, sex, age, marital status, accommodation, educational level, work situation, intellectual and neuropsychological functioning, results on a personality questionnaire, or alcohol-related symptoms. Thus the sample was representative of patients treated at the clinic during the last years of the 1970s. The clinic has its main catchment area in the northern suburbs of Stockholm City, making the sample fairly representative of the larger Swedish cities.

Procedures

The subjects were interviewed by the author after completing detoxification. The interviews were semistructured, lasted for about three-quarters of an hour, and were tape-recorded. The questions used by Marlatt and Gordon (1980) were translated into Swedish and applied to a Swedish situation. In addition, a few questions were put regarding attitude to Disulfiram and total abstinence, and drinking pattern immediately following the first drink. However, the following were the most central questions:

- In what sort of situation did you take the first drink that led to your losing control over drinking?
- What would you say was the main reason for taking that drink?
- Can you describe any particular circumstances or set of events which triggered your need or desire to take that first drink?
- Do you remember any inner thoughts or emotional feelings that triggered your need or desire to take the first drink at that time?
- What did you think after taking your first drink?
- What sort of feeling did you have after that first drink?

Since not everybody started a drinking bout in connection with the first drink, these questions refer to the first drink that led to loss of control.

Measures

Immediately after the interview a short written summary was made of the most important factors associated with the relapse. The categorizations and assessments of relapse determinants are based on these interview summaries. The elaborate manual described in Marlatt and Gordon (1980) was used in this work.

In a preliminary analysis with four raters receiving minimal information regarding the scoring procedures, the pairwise interrater agreement varied between 58% and 92%. In another context where two other raters received extensive information regarding the categories, the interrater reliability was 87%.

The psychological tests used in KARTAD are well-standardized neuropsychological tests including measures of general intelligence and personality questionnaires assessing, for example, tendency to react with psychic and somatic anxiety to various situations, impulsiveness, socialization, and dependence on other people (Bergman, 1977; Schalling, Edman, and Åsberg, 1983). Questionnaires for social- and alcohol-anamnestic information were also used (Ideström, 1977).

RESULTS

Location of First Drink

There is an interesting cultural difference between the group interviewed in this study (the Stockholm Group) and the group interviewed by Marlatt and Gordon (the Seattle Group). In the Stockholm Group, most people took their

Table 3

Place Where First Drink Was Taken: Comparison between the Groups Studied[a]

Place	Stockholm Study (%)	Seattle Study (%)
At home	56	12
At the home of a friend or relative	23	9
In a bar or restaurant	6	63
Other (a hotel, plane flight, train, sauna, outdoors)	15	16

[a] $p < .001$ in a chi-square test of distribution differences.

first drink in their own homes (56%) or in the homes of friends or relatives (23%), and only 6% in a bar or restaurant. In the Seattle Group, it was quite the opposite—63% started to drink in a bar or restaurant (see Table 3).

Short and Long Relapsers

The median time since discharge from hospital in this study was 5 months, ranging from 1 week to 4 years. The subjects were divided into one group which had managed without hospital care for a longer period than 6 months (44%) and another group which remained outside the hospital for a shorter period than 6 months (56%). The length of time for which the patient had been sober was ascertained, and as expected, a significant difference between the two groups was found. The long relapsers had, on the average, been completely sober for 5 months after treatment. The short relapsers had, on the average, been sober only for 1 month.

When the patients that had remained sober for a longer time were asked what they thought would happen if they took a drink after leaving the clinic this time, we found a significant difference in the attitude toward oneself and toward other patients at the clinic. Of this group, 50% believed that they could have a drink without consequent loss of control, but only 15% believed that the other patients could do the same. In the other group, we could not find this difference; about 30% thought that they could take one drink, and there was no difference in attitude toward oneself as compared to other patients.

If we compare this attitude with what really happened the last time they took a drink after hospitalization, it seems that both groups had a tendency to overestimate their ability to control their drinking. In the group that did not come under care for a longer period, 58% lost control after the first drink; and in the other group, 81% lost control.

It is interesting to look at the drinking pattern after the first drink, and here we can see that very few were satisfied with only one drink (16%) and that a majority took a morning drink the day after (82%). However, that did not lead to uncontrolled drinking for everyone.

Obviously the whole group in this study was somewhat more heterogeneous than the Seattle Group, in which 90% started a drinking bout as a consequence of the first drink, compared to 73% in this study. This difference is significant at the 5% level.

Categorization of Risk Situations

Since this study represents another category of alcoholics, it is interesting to see if it is possible to arrive at a picture similar to the one presented by Marlatt and Gordon. It should be emphasized that the categories have an immediate face validity and that the scorers did not have any trouble in understanding their meaning.

Irrespective of how the material is presented, we get a relative distribution over categories similar to the result obtained by Marlatt and Gordon (see Table 4).

Even the group which stayed sober for a longer period has approximately the same distribution as the others. A few more (49%) relapsed in interpersonal situations, compared to the Seattle Group (39%), but this difference is not statistically significant. Thus, there seems to be a certain amount of universality

Table 4

Distribution of Relapse Situations for the Group Interviewed in Stockholm Compared to the Group Interviewed in Seattle

	Stockholm Study (%)		
Situation	Whole group (N = 48)	Group hospitalized after more than 6 months (N = 21)	Seattle Study (%) (N = 70)
Intrapersonal determinants	50	51	61
Negative emotional states	40	35	38
Negative physical states	2	–	3
Positive emotional states	2	–	–
Testing personal control	2	6	9
Urges and temptations	4	10	11
Interpersonal determinants	50	49	39
Interpersonal conflict	31	19	18
Social pressure	17	30	18
Positive emotional states	2	–	3

regarding risk situations between the American and the Swedish drinking culture, and between those alcoholics who relapse after shorter or longer periods.

The disadvantage of classifying information is that we lose that which is unique and specific for the individual, which is why an accounting of the specific situations that have been classified is perhaps called for. The most commonly reported relapse precipitants in this study were: loneliness, anxiety, friend who drinks, anger, depression, conflicts, holidays, disappointment, and discharge from a treatment institution. Sometimes more than one risk situation obtained at the same time.

Relation between Relapse Determinants and Psychological Characteristics

It was possible to find a few correlations between categories and results on the intelligence test and the personality questionnaire. Those scored on interpersonal relapse determinants had better results on the intelligence test (M_{IQ} = 104) than the others (M_{IQ} = 96). They also scored lower on perceived muscle tension and somatized anxiety. Those who relapsed in interpersonal situations involving conflict scored lower on "social desirability," and those who relapsed because of social pressure scored higher on "impulsivity." All these differences were significant at at least the 5% level.

The poorer results on the intelligence test in the group relapsing in intrapersonal situations were not associated with a longer history of alcohol problems, and there were no age differences between the groups with intra- and interpersonal determinants. Among those who relapsed in intrapersonal situations, there were more who had had contact with the local temperance or social welfare institutions (55% compared to 23%). Also the ward staff more often considered them to be passive (57% compared to 18%) and ambivalent in their attitude to the treatment (67% compared to 28%). All the differences are significant at the 5% level.

DISCUSSION

This study has given strong support to the idea that certain situations are more "dangeorous" than others for alcoholics if they want to remain sober.

Despite the difference in drinking pattern and relapse process, it was possible in the present study to identify and classify relapse determinants. This is of special interest since the study includes a group of alcoholics with a different drinking pattern and a subgroup relapsing after a longer period of time than in the study reported by Marlatt and Gordon (1980).

It does not seem that the different drinking cultures in the United States and Sweden—illustrated here by locations of first drink (bars as opposed to homes)—to any considerable degree affects determinants of relapse. One question not answered by this study, but of importance to alcohol policy, is whether or not the greater accessibility of alcohol in the United States speeds up the relapse process. The results from the present study do not speak in favor of this hypothesis.

The categories proposed by Marlatt and Gordon seem to be psychologically meaningful since there is a connection to results on certain psychological tests and some alcohol-related social variables. Thus, it seems that patients with poorer results on intelligence tests and having a high tendency to muscle tension and somatized anxiety tend to relapse in intrapersonal situations. This group seems more often to make a passive and ambivalent impression on the ward staff. Patients who do not readily adjust to other persons' opinions instead tend to relapse in interpersonal conflicts, and patients who are more impulsive cannot resist social pressure to drink. Covariations of this kind, which have not been reported on before, also give the categories conceptual validity. In future research it should be of interest to elucidate the prognostic value of personality factors in regard to relapse precipitants. This would, of course, not explain the relapse process, but it would add a descriptive dimension valuable in clinical work. It should, however, be emphasized that this kind of analysis is based on group data, and it is not possible to make any reliable predictions in individual cases, based on such simple personality characteristics as those described here.

Since the categories have both face and conceptual validity, there are reasons for using them in future research on the relapse process in alcoholism. In clinical work, however, one should also be careful to map out the specific situations of importance in each single case.

An interesting finding is the tendency toward better prognosis in terms of being sober for a longer period before relapse for those who believed that they could have a drink without losing control and, at the same time, thought that other alcoholics could not. This seems to reflect a certain amount of self-efficacy; that is, a belief in one's capability, which according to Marlatt and Gordon (1980) is another factor of importance for the relapse process.

The high relapse rate seems to be the overwhelming problem in all treatment programs. Based on this study, making prevention of relapse a treatment aim is justified. This can be done by analyzing risk situations and specifying alternative behavior patterns, and by helping the subjects to develop these. The implication would be that staff should be trained to see relapse as a part of the treatment process and should focus on this with a nonjudgmental attitude. The aim would be to reduce relapses with regard to frequency, duration, and intensity. In these terms, criteria for success or failure cannot be dichotomized but should be regarded as a continuum.

Prevention programs should teach the inadvisability of drinking in certain given situations such as when trying to cope with loneliness, depression, pain, anger, etc.

Futher research in this area should focus on preventing relapse, on how to support a realistically self-confident attitude, and on how to teach alcoholics to cope with determinants of relapse.

ACKNOWLEDGMENTS

Preparation of this paper was facilitated by the Swedish Council for Planning and Coordination of Research, grant 82/452 A9-4:1. Thanks to Hans Bergman, Ulf Rydberg, and Sten Rönnberg for valuable comments on the manuscript.

REFERENCES

ABBOT, M.W., and GREGSON, A.M. Cognitive dysfunction in the prediction of relapse in alcoholics. *J. Stud. Alcohol* 42: 1-18, 1981.

AHLES, T.A., SCHLUNDT, D.G., PRUE, D.M., and RYCHTARIK, R.C. Impact of aftercare arrangements on the maintenance of treatment success in abusive drinkers. *Addict. Behav.* 8: 53-58, 1983.

BAEKELAND, F. Evaluation of treatment methods in chronic alcoholism. In B. Kissin and H. Begleiter (eds.), *The Biology of Alcoholism*, Vol. 5. New York: Plenum Press, 1977.

BERGMAN, H. The Karolinska Project for Research and Treatment of Alcohol Dependence: Psychological aspects. In C.-M. Ideström (ed.), *Recent Advances in the Study of Alcoholism*. Amsterdam: Excerpta Medica, Int. Congr. Ser. No. 407, 1977.

BERGMAN, H., BORG, S., HINDMARSH, T., IDESTRÖM, C.-M., and MÜTZELL, S. Computed tomography of the brain and neuropsychological assessment of male alcoholic patients and a random sample from the general male population. In C.-M. Ideström (ed.), *Alcohol and Brain Research.* Copenhagen: Acta Psychiatrica Scandinavica, Suppl. 286, Vol. 62, 1980.

GREGSON, R.A.M., and TAYLOR, G.M. Prediction of relapse in men alcoholics. *J. Stud. Alcohol* 38: 1749-1760, 1977.

HEATHER, N., ROLLNIK, S., and WINTON, M. Psychological change among inpatient alcoholics and its relationship to treatment outcome. *Br. J. Alcohol Alcoholism* 17: 90-97, 1982.

HEILBRUN, A.B., and TARBOX, A.R. Cognitive structure and behavioural regulation in alcoholics: Implications for treatment outcome. *Br. J. Alcohol Alcoholism* 13: 65-73, 1978.

IDESTRÖM, C.-M. (ed.). *Recent Advances in the Study of Alcoholism.* Amsterdam: Excerpta Medica, Int. Congr. Ser. No. 407, 1977.

KISSIN, B. Patient characteristics and treatment specificity in alcoholism. In C.-M. Ideström (ed.), *Recent Advances in the Study of Alcoholism.* Amsterdam: Excerpta Medica, Int. Congr. Ser. No. 407, 1977.

LITMAN, G.K., EISER, R.J., RAWSON, N.S.B., and OPPENHEIM, A.N. Differences in relapse precipitants and coping behavior between alcohol relapsers and survivors. *Behav. Res. Ther.* 17: 89-94, 1979.

LUDWIG, A.M., and STARK, L.H. Alcohol craving: Subjective and situational aspects. *Q. J. Stud. Alcohol* 35: 899-905, 1974.

MARLATT, G.A., and GORDON, F.R. Determinants of relapse: Implications for the maintenance of behavior change. In P. Davidson and S. Davidson (eds.), *Behavioral Medicine: Changing Health Lifestyles*. New York: Brunner-Mazel, 1980.

MILLER, W.R., and HESTER, R.K. Treating the problem drinker: Modern approaches. In W.R. Miller (ed.), *The Addictive Behaviors: Treatment of Alcoholism, Drug Abuse, Smoking and Obesity*. New York: Pergamon Press, 1980.

MILLER, W.R., PECHACEK, T.F., and HAMBURG, S. Group behavior therapy for problem drinkers. *Int. J. Addict.* 16: 829-839, 1981.

O'LEARY, M.R., DONOVAN, D.M., CHANEY, E.F., and WALKER, R.D. Cognitive impairment and treatment outcome with alcoholics: Preliminary findings. *J. Clin. Psychiatry* 40: 397-398, 1979.

POLICH, J.M., ARMOR, D.J., and BRAIKER, H.B. Patterns of alcoholism over four years. *J. Stud. Alcohol* 41: 397-416, 1980.

RÖNNBERG, S. Behavioral analysis of alcohol abuse. In P.O. Sjödén, S. Bates, and W.S. Dockens (eds.), *Trends in Behavior Therapy*. New York: Academic Press, 1979.

SAMSONOWITZ, V., and SJÖBERG, L. Volitional problems of socially adjusted alcoholics. *Addict. Behav.* 6: 385-398, 1981.

SAUNDERS, W.M., PHIL, M., and KERSHAW, P.W. Spontaneous remission from alcoholism–A community study. *Br. J. Addict.* 74: 251-265, 1979.

SCHALLING, D., EDMAN, G., and ÅSBERG, M. Impulsive cognitive style and inability to tolerate boredom: Psychobiological studies of temperamental vulnerability. In M. Zuckerman (ed.), *Biological Bases of Sensation Seeking, Impulsivity and Anxiety*. Hillsdale, NJ: Earlbaum, 1983.

TOKAR, J.T., BRUNSE, A.J., STEFFLRE, V.J., NAPIOR, D.A., and SÖDERGREN, J.A. Emotional states and behavioral patterns in alcoholics and nonalcoholics. *Q. J. Stud. Alcohol* 34: 133-143, 1973.

The International Journal of the Addictions, 19(8), 849-857, 1984

Screening Drug Abuse Clients with the Brief Symptom Inventory

David Royse,* PhD

Research and Evaluation
Greene-Clinton County Mental Health Board
Xenia, Ohio 45385

Kenneth Drude, PhD

School of Professional Psychology
Wright-State University
Dayton, Ohio

Abstract

A sample of 300 new admissions at a rural outpatient drug treatment agency were administered the Brief Symptom Inventory (BSI) during the initial screening. This study sought to determine if the BSI had sufficient discriminative validity to distinguish between groups with various levels of drug abuse, between those having fewer or more life areas affected, and between primary clients and their significant others. The results of the study indicated that the BSI does have usefulness in making such discriminations. Suggestions for its use in clinical care and quality assurance are offered.

Not everyone making a first-time visit to an outpatient drug-counseling agency is an appropriate client. For instance, the nature of the agency may not be intuitively obvious from its name, or it may be confused with a similar-sounding agency providing a completely different service. Even if the person is in the right agency, additional screening is still needed. Families may bring

*To whom requests for reprints should be sent at the Greene County Mental Health Board, 452 West Market Street, Xenia, Ohio 45385.

 0020-773X/84/1908-0849$3.50/0

one member and claim it is *that* person who has the problem. Or, there may be so many problems confronting the client that he or she may not be able to easily distinguish the most important problem. Some clients are in need of immediate hospitalization and are not appropriate for outpatient counseling. Consequently, all clients must be personally screened in some fashion. For most drug abuse agencies it is a necessary but time-consuming process.

Because assessments resulting from the initial screening often vary from counselor to counselor, there has been interest in the identification of an objective instrument which could aid in the determination of appropriateness for treatment and help with other treatment-related decisions. Rather than attempting to develop a new instrument for the assessment of substance abuse clients, this paper reports the results of one rural outpatient counseling agency which implemented the Brief Symptom Inventory (BSI) as a screening instrument for all new admissions.

This study was undertaken to determine if the BSI was effective in distinguishing those persons with "serious" problems from those with "minor" problems. If the BSI could demonstrate such discriminant ability, there would be some potential advantages to its use: (1) Professional time in the intake process could be minimized, (2) the BSI ratings could be compared with diagnoses or impressions determined by staff from clinical interviews, and (3) the instrument would be shown to have the necessary discriminative validity for use as a client outcome measure for program evaluation purposes in drug treatment agencies.

A number of questions were examined in the study. Can the BSI distinguish between people with high (serious) and low (minor) drug abuse frequency? Can the BSI distinguish between drug abuse clients and their significant others? What degree of coincidence exists between BSI ratings and the number of problematic life areas identified by agency staff during the intake interview? However, the primary question explored was: Can an instrument designed to reflect the psychological symptom patterns of psychiatric and medical patients be used advantageously in screening drug abuse clients?

METHOD

Subjects

Subjects were the first 300 clients to be screened and whose cases were closed during the period of January 1981 through March 1982 at an outpatient drug treatment agency in rural southwest Ohio. The agency was a small one (8.5 staff) but had an aggressive outreach program to schools and courts. The sample was composed predominantly of individuals (primarily male adolescents) ordered to the drug agency by local courts (44% of sample) or schools (19%)

because of behavior suspected to be drug related. About 20% were self-referred, and 16% were referred from physicians or other human service agencies. Twenty percent of these subjects were the family members or significant others who received treatment along with the primary client. Ninety-three percent were White, two-thirds were male, and 59% had less than a high school education. The median age was 21 years, and the median family gross income was $15,000 (the latter statistic was reported by only 51% of the subjects).

Thirty-seven percent reported no drug use in the month prior to admission; 10% said that they used drugs less than once a week; 9% reported use once a week; 19%, several times a week; 8%, once daily; 18% reported use greater than once daily. Of those who reported use of drugs, 44% primarily used alcohol and 38% primarily used marijuana.

Procedure

The BSI was given to clients for completion at the time of the first appointment with the agency. This was generally done within 15 to 20 minutes prior to an initial interview with a counselor. During this interview the counselor judged the severity of the drug problem by asking about the frequency of use and type of drug used. Other relevant personal and background information was also obtained at this time.

Instrument

The BSI is a self-report, 53-item instrument providing point-in-time psychological symptom status. It is a condensed version of the Symptom Checklist 90 (SCL-90-R), which was developed from the Hopkins Symptom Checklist. The SCL-90-R was introduced by Derogatis and his associates (Derogatis, Lipman, and Covi, 1973) and later modified and validated in its present form (Derogatis, Rickels, and Rock, 1976). Evaluative reviews of the instrument have identified it as among the best instruments of its type (Edwards, Yarvis, Mueller, Zingale, and Wagman, 1978; Waskow and Parloff, 1975). The instrument has been cited in two different publications prepared to aid community mental health centers in conducting program evaluation (Hagedorn, Beck, Neubert, and Werlin, 1976; Hargreaves, Attkisson, and Sorensen, 1977). The BSI correlates very highly with the SCL-90 across all dimensions (Derogatis, 1977), confirming that the BSI is a valid measure of the SCL-90's symptom constructs. These nine constructs are: Psychoticism, Somatization, Obsessive-Compulsive, Interpersonal Sensitivity, Depression, Anxiety, Hostility, Phobic Anxiety, and Paranoid Ideation. In addition, the BSI has three global indices of distress. The General Severity Index (GSI), as a summary measure of the general level of pathology, is the most important of these and is the only one referred to in this study. More detailed information on the BSI may be obtained in other articles (e.g., Derogatis and Melisaratos, 1983).

FINDINGS

Because there is evidence that the use of drugs is associated with psychiatric symptoms (Gove, Geerken, and Hughes, 1979), it was hypothesized that those clients with low drug use should have lower GSI scores than those with high drug use. Using the categories available from the National Institute on Drug Abuse's Client Oriented Data Acquisition Process (CODAP) Admission Report, the subjects were combined into six groups on the basis of their frequency of use: no use during the month prior to admission, less than once per week, once per week, several times per week, once daily to three times daily, and more than three times daily. As can be seen in Table 1, clients with lower levels of drug use had lower mean GSI scores and clients with higher levels of self-reported drug use had the higher mean GSI scores. Intervening groups had scores between those groups using drugs most and least. The differences among the groups were statistically significant (F [5, 294] = 5.16, $p < .001$) when a one-way analysis of variance was computed.

Since the sample was composed of all those who had terminated the services of the agency, it was possible to examine the relationship between client disposition and initial BSI score. The data lent themselves to five natural divisions: (1) clients who notified the agency that they would no longer be coming for counseling (15%), (2) those clients referred to another agency or practitioner for other services (15%), (3) persons who were terminated because the case manager believed that further care was not indicated (12%), (4) clients who did not notify the agency prior to discontinuing services (41%), and (5) clients who were referred for inpatient hospitalization because of the seriousness of their drug problem (17%).

Table 1

General Severity Index (GSI) and Frequency of Drug Use

Drug use	*N*	Mean	SD
No use	110	0.619	.648
Less than once a week	30	0.611	.571
Once a week	27	0.677	.701
Several times a week	57	0.783	.681
Once daily to 3 times daily	38	0.817	.731
More than 3 times daily	38	1.243	.796
Total	300	0.759	.707

Table 2

General Severity Index (GSI) and Disposition of Case

Case disposition	*N*	Mean	SD
Client withdrew; notified agency	44	0.823	.741
Agency determined no further care needed	35	0.366	.456
Client withdrew; agency not notified	124	0.712	.630
Referral to other agency	45	0.725	.611
Referral for inpatient hospitalization	52	1.110	.896
Total	300	0.759	.707

As can be seen in Table 2, the group with the highest mean GSI score is composed of those persons who were referred for hospitalization. This is what any clinical supervisor would hope would be revealed because it suggests that counselors were perceptive to those with more severe problems. The group with the lowest mean GSI score was composed of those who had been involved in treatment (generally for an extended period) but for whom continued involvement with the agency was no longer believed to be needed.

While there are statistically significant differences among the means of the five disposition groups (F [4, 295] = 6.639, $p < .001$), it is interesting to note that two groups have very similar means. Those who did not notify the agency that they were leaving treatment and those who were referred to another agency (because they still needed additional counseling or because they refused treatment and preferred to take their chances with the court or school) reported comparable levels of symptomatology. The group which notified the agency that they would be terminating services had somewhat higher levels of symptomatology. This group may have offered valid explanations for leaving treatment prematurely (e.g., parents or spouse being transferred out of the area, or the client was transferred to a correctional facility out of the county), but this was certainly not always the case. One might surmise that this group had greater need for treatment but found it too threatening to continue with it, or that the services offered did not meet their needs.

In an effort to better understand the mean scores of the various disposition groups, another one-way analysis of variance was computed for the number of outpatient hours of counseling received. Table 3 indicates that there is not much difference in the number of hours of counseling received by three of the five groups. Those who were referred for hospitalization or to another agency received on the average just about as many hours of counseling as did those who notified the agency that they were withdrawing from treatment. Those who withdrew without notifying the agency had the smallest number of hours, while those for whom no further care was needed received the most hours of

Table 3

Outpatient Counseling Hours Received, by Disposition Group

Client disposition	*N*	Mean	SD
Client withdrew; notified agency	44	6.6	9.5
Agency determined no further care needed	35	21.5	24.6
Client withdrew; agency not notified	124	4.4	5.2
Referral to other agency	45	6.2	5.2
Referral for inpatient hospitalization	51	7.0	16.9
Total	299	7.5	13.1

counseling. The differences among these five disposition groups were once again statistically significant (F [4, 294] = 13.828, $p < .001$). This may suggest that counselors were able to recognize clients who had the greatest potential for response.

One might wonder, with the large percentage of involuntary clients who were screened, if there was a difference in the dispositions between mandated and voluntary clients. A chi-square test was performed to test the hypothesis of no difference, and this was supported ($\chi^2 = 5.98$, $df = 4$, $p > .05$). In other words, voluntary clients were not referred for hospitalization any more often than involuntary clients; nor was the pattern of dispositions remarkably different from that of involuntary clients.

During the intake process, counselors subjectively determined if client problems affected and produced repercussions in one or several of the following areas: (1) legal, (2) marital/family, (3) school/job, and (4) physical health. It was hypothesized that those clients with high GSI scores would have a greater number of life areas affected than those clients with low GSI scores. When the means were examined for each of these four groups, the group with the lowest mean score (.557) was the group judged to have only one life area affected. Those clients determined to have three life areas affected had the highest mean GSI score (.849). Since the means for the groups having two, three, and four life areas affected were fairly similar, a one-way analysis of variance was computed to test for significant differences between those having one or more problematic life areas. There were statistically significant differences between these two groups (F [1, 294] = 8.45, $p < .005$). This would again suggest that the BSI has discriminant validity because those with greater symptomatology also tended to have a greater number of life areas affected by the problem of drug abuse.

Noting that one of the problems with a self-report instrument is that a client may choose not to fill it out accurately (e.g., may distort the number of symptoms or their severity, or completely deny them), we hypothesized that voluntary clients would have significantly higher mean GSI scores than involuntary clients. This hypothesis was supported (t = 4.01, df = 145.4, $p < .001$). Exploring this phenomenon a little more, GSI scores were grouped by the referral source. It was found that the school-referred group had the lowest mean GSI score (.560), followed by the court-referred group (.613). Yet both of these groups of clients had demonstrated behavior which resulted in their referral to the drug-counseling agency. Both of these groups could have an interest in denying symptoms. This is suggested by the fact that referrals from another important group–psychological services and human service agencies–had a higher mean score (.927) than did the court- and school-referred groups. The highest mean score from any of the referral groups was associated with those clients who were self-referred (1.086). This group would have the least amount of interest in distorting their symptoms. The differences among these four groups were statistically significant (F [3, 288] = 9.414, $p < .001$). Obviously, the more the motivation to "fake good," the greater likelihood that low GSI scores will be obtained.

Further evidence that involuntary clients may not have filled out the BSI accuratley is seen when the number of life areas affected by drug abuse was examined by whether the client was voluntary or involuntary. There were no statistically significant differences between voluntary and involuntary clients in the number of life areas staff believed to be affected by drug abuse (χ^2 = 4.27, df = 3, $p > .05$). This demonstrates that counselors at the time of intake did not determine by their own subjective processes that involuntary clients had significantly fewer problem areas than voluntary clients. Since voluntary and involuntary clients have a similar distribution of problematic life areas, one would expect that their GSI scores would also be somewhat similar and would not expect to find statistically significant differences.

Finally, because the agency provided education and treatment to family members as well as to the primary clients, it was possible to compare the GSI scores for these two groups. It was hypothesized that primary clients would have higher mean GSI scores than family members (or significant others). This hypothesis was supported as primary clients had a GSI mean of .831 while the family/significant others had a mean GSI score of .571. These differences were statistically significant (t = 2.88, df = 111.1, $p < .005$). That the mean GSI score for family members was not lower may reflect that primary clients were members of families experiencing more than the usual level of problems. Such clients are often from families revealing high levels of interpersonal problems and social disorganization.

DISCUSSION

The findings presented in this study suggest that the BSI has discriminative validity when administered to a drug-abusing population. This validity was evidenced by the finding that clients who reported using drugs most and least had corresponding highest and lowest average GSI scores. In addition, those clients who were determined to have the most severe problems by their counselors (the group referred for inpatient hospitalization) had the highest GSI scores among the various disposition groupings. Further evidence of the BSI's discriminative validity is seen in that those clients who were determined to have two or more life areas affected by a drug problem had significantly higher BSI scores than those with one life area affected. The last piece of evidence is that primary clients had significantly higher average GSI scores than did their family members or significant others.

It should be noted that while counselors may have taken the opportunity to review the client's BSI form prior to the intake interview, variables such as the counselor's determination of the number of life areas affected, the recommendation for hospitalization, and the reported frequency of drug use were documented without the BSI being scored. In other words, the counselor did not see the client's profile on the nine dimensions of the BSI. All 300 BSIs were scored at the completion of this pilot study by the senior author.

Although the BSI focuses only upon the identified client, other factors such as family and social networks remain important for comprehensive treatment. In spite of its narrow focus on the individual client, the BSI appears to have more than sufficient validity to recommend its use in outpatient substance abuse counseling agencies. It does appear to be sensitive to those in psychological distress associated with drug abuse. Clinicians interested in quality assurance and clinical care studies may find that it can identify, as it did in this study, patient groups most in need of services. Such studies may help clinical and agency directors to target those who may need aggressive outreach or follow-up by the agency. In periods of severe budgetary restrictions, the BSI might be used as an objective way to help prioritize those clients who should be served first. Because of the discriminative validity shown, the BSI would also appear to be an instrument which could be used advantageously in client outcome studies.

Should the BSI be used by drug-counseling agencies for screening all clients? Given the evidence that persons who are mandated to go for screening may not complete the BSI honestly, some agencies may choose not to administer the BSI to involuntary clients. This is not recommended. Even if the client uses the descriptor "not at all" to each of the 53 items on the BSI, there may be some unconscious or at least silent admission that "Hey, I have this problem." This might come out later in the treatment process. The instrument, in these cases, may have a heuristic value. Even the BSIs completed by those clients in this study who indicated having no symptoms provided information to their counselors—usually that they had little interest in seeking help from the agency. Those clients who reported symptoms in certain areas were even more informative. These clients, through use of an impersonal and nonthreatening procedure, facilitated the intake process by identifying problem areas most troublesome for them. The BSI served to bring into focus for the client why he or she had approached the agency. Without this instrument, more time may have been spent in the intake process to identify the client's problem(s).

The BSI provides a standardized means of beginning the problem identification phase of treatment in order to focus attention upon areas to be included in a treatment plan. Data from the BSI inform counselors as to problem areas perceived by clients which can be further explored in a clinical interview. Once these problem areas are identified, specific treatment goals related to these problems can be developed.

A final advantage to using the BSI in an outpatient counseling agency is that it furnishes empirical evidence to funding and allocative bodies that the agency is serving people whose need for services can be objectively documented. It would be possible to show to what extent an agency's clientele surpassed or compared with norms available from samples of outpatient psychiatric patients or nonpatient normals. In this way agencies might show that clients are "deserving" of their services. In this era of great concern for public accountability, directors of outpatient drug-counseling agencies would be wise to explore the use of the BSI with their clientele.

REFERENCES

DEROGATIS, L.R. *The SCL-90 Manual I: Scoring, Administration and Procedures for the SCL-90.* Baltimore: Clinical Psychometric Research, 1977.

DEROGATIS, L.R., LIPMAN, R.S., and COVI, L. The SCL-90: An outpatient psychiatric rating scale–Preliminary report. *Psychopharmacol. Bull.* 9: 13-27, 1973.

DEROGATIS, L.R., and MELISARATOS, N. The Brief Symptom Inventory: An introductory report. *Psychol. Med.* In press, 1983.

DEROGATIS, L.R., RICKELS, K., and ROCK, A.F. The SCL-90 and the MMPI: A step in the validation of a new self-report scale. *Br. J. Psychiatry* 128: 280-289, 1976.

EDWARDS, D.W., YARVIS, R.M., MUELLER, D.P., ZINGALE, H.C., and WAGMAN, W.J. Test-taking and the stability of adjustment scales: Can we assess patient deterioration? *Evaluation Q.* 2(2): 275-291, 1978.

GOVE, W.R., GEERKEN, M., and HUGHES, M. Drug use and mental health among a representative national sample of young adults. *Soc. Forces* 58(2): 572-590, 1979.

HAGEDORN, H.J., BECK, K.J., NEUBERT, S.F., and WERLIN, S.H. *A Working Manual of Simple Program Evaluation Techniques for Community Mental Health Centers.* Rockville, MD: National Institute of Mental Health, 1976.

HARGREAVES, W.A., ATTKISSON, C.C., and SORENSEN, J.E. *Resource Materials for Community Mental Health Program Evaluation.* Rockville, MD: National Institute of Mental Health, 1977.

WASKOW, I., and PARLOFF, M. *Psychotherapy Change Measures.* Rockville, MD: National Institute of Mental Health, 1975.

The International Journal of the Addictions, 19(8), 859–869, 1984

The Drug Addict and the Stigma of Addiction

James C. Dean,* DMin

Office of Chemical Use and Abuse

Faith Rud, MA

Department of Sociology

University of North Dakota
Grand Forks, North Dakota 58202

Abstract

Two hundred and fifty-six respondents from a small, upper-midwestern college town answered a questionnaire designed to assess their first impression images of the term "drug addict." The results indicated that the overwhelming image was of a disoriented, unhealthy, thin, low-class, male "hippie" with behavioral and skin problems who suffered from a disease. Only 11% of the responses described the condition as a crime. This study is compared with a previous, similar study of the first impression of the term "alcoholic," and suggestions are provided to explain the categorization of the conditions as disease states.

BACKGROUND

Scholarly literature on alcohol and other drugs has provided a variety of models to explain the processes of addiction. Bruun (1971), for example,

*To whom requests for reprints should be sent at the Office of Chemical Use and Abuse, P.O. Box 8191, 101 McCannel Hall, University of North Dakota, Grand Forks, North Dakota 58202.

 0020-773X/84/1908-0859$3.50/0

provides eight models of alcohol addiction and seven models or submodels of drug addiction based on the works of Siegler, Osmond, and Newell (Siegler and Osmond, 1968; Siegler, Osmond, and Newell, 1968). The present study was intended to measure the public image of the drug addict and of drug addiction, and to expand a previous study by Dean and Poremba (1983). The present study attempted to answer several questions:

1. What first impression image comes to mind when the term "drug addict" is used?
2. Is drug addiction viewed as a disease, sin, moral weakness, excuse, mental illness, or crime?
3. Do respondents apparently addicted to licit or illicit drugs view the drug addict and addiction in ways similar to or different from respondents who report no personal addictive behavior?

SAMPLE

The 1982 sample was drawn from a small, agricultural, upper-midwestern college town of 40,000. The same population was used in the previous study (Dean and Poremba, 1983) to measure images of the word "alcoholic." The respondents were selected from the telephone book through a systematic probability sample excluding previously called numbers.

The number of potential respondents selected was 450; 246 persons 18 years old or older answered the questionnaire. Of those who responded, 104 (42%) were male, and 141 (58%) were female. Eighty-eight (36%) were single, 127 (52%) married, eight (3%) divorced, 21 (9%) widowed, and two (1%) were separated. Eighty-one (33%) of the respondents were aged 18 to 25, 68 (28%) aged 26 to 35, 29 (12%) aged 36 to 45, 20 (8%) aged 46 to 55, 16 (7%) aged 56 to 65, and 31 (13%) were over 65 years of age.

The respondents included 157 (64%) employed persons and 89 (36%) unemployed. The respondents indicated their present occupational categories:

Occupational category	Number	% of sample
Professional	25	13
Management/administrative	17	9
Sales and skilled	32	17
Clerical/service	65	34
Farmer	2	1
Military	5	3
Housewife	14	7
Student	27	14
Prefer not to answer (PNTA)	4	2

The respondents to this study reported earning the following family unit incomes:

Income category	Number	% of sample
$5,000 or less	18	7
$5,000-$10,000	26	11
$10,000-$15,000	26	11
$15,000-$20,000	20	8
$20,000+	73	30
Not certain	31	13
PNTA	52	21

The reported educational level of respondents was:

Last year (degree) of school	Number	% of sample
Less than junior high	3	1
Junior high	15	6
High school	61	25
College (no degree)	87	35
College degree	58	24
MA	17	7
Doctoral degree	4	2
PNTA	1	0.4

METHOD

The questionnaire was designed to elicit first-impression images by the respondents of individuals labeled "drug addict." The instrument also measured the use of alcohol, tea, coffee, tobacco, Librium, Valium, sleeping pills, marijuana, and cocaine by the respondents. Cross-tabulations were employed to determine whether respondents who used substances at addictive levels had different or similar conceptions of drug addicts compared to those conceptions provided by nonaddicted respondents. Questions designed to elicit first-impression images were the same as in the prior study (see Dean and Poremba, 1983), except "drug addict" was substituted for "alcoholic."

RESULTS

Image of "Hippie+"

The subjects' responses were collected and collapsed into 13 categories (see Table 1). The data, as provided in Table 2, indicated that the image of the drug addict provided by the respondents was that of a "hippie." The term "hippie" was employed although it is no longer in vogue and carries many

Table 1

Subjects' Responses Collected and Collapsed into Categories

Category	Description
1. Hippie	Young, under 30 Unkempt–includes: ragged, sloppy, not well dressed, shabby, a mess, dirty clothes, like a bum, hippie dress, old jacket, disheveled, no belt, not dressed normally, odd appearance, messy Dirty person–includes: not clean, greasy, smells, needs a bath, smoking cigarettes, greasy hair Long hair Bearded–includes: unshaven, moustache Funny eyes–includes: bloodshot eyes, tired eyes, blurry eyes, red eyes, dilated eyes, glasses, dark glasses, shifty eyes, funny expression, funny look, appears not to see well Jeans–includes: jean jacket, T shirt, old brown pants, army greens, old green coat
2. Disoriented	Disoriented–includes: not sure where he is, not sure what he is doing, not alert, out of mind, confused, demented, mixed up, dreamy, weird, mumbling, stupid, dizzy, dazed High–includes: drunk, stoned, doped up, spaced out, out of it, talkative, witty, very exhilarated Staggering–includes: wobbling, stumbling, slow moving, uncoordinated
3. Unhealthy (physically and mentally)	Sad–includes: depressed, sorrowful, unhappy, shaken, troubled, downcast, discouraged, down and out, wretched, downtrodden, alone, pitiful, lonely Scared–includes: afraid, panicked, helpless, hopeless Nervous–includes: twitching, anxious, shaking, jittery, unsteady, hands move, self-conscious, talking to self Desperate–includes: rough looking, bad, terrible, awful, pretty rough, disgruntled, seedy, sleazy, piece of trash, ugly, like they need help, in trouble, in need

(continued)

Table 1 (continued)

Category	Description
	Sick–includes: unhealthy, run down, emaciated, poor health, poor shape, gaunt, undernourished, in a stupor, runny nose, lying on ground
	Tired–includes: weak, half asleep, weary, drowsy, drawn out, dragged out, burnt out, spent, slouched over, not too well, sweating, indifferent, apathetic
4. Thin	Thin–includes: lean, skinny, slender
5. Low class	Low class–includes: poor, selling dope, asking for money, out of work
6. Behavioral problems	Behavioral problems–includes: flirtatious, angry, threatening, uncouth, gets crazy, a goof, uninhibited, obnoxious, suddenly noisy, freaky, no respect, bad manners, uncontrollable, crooked, dangerous, mean, untrustable, sneaky, acts odd, speech problems, can't count money, takes dope
7. Ordinary person	Ordinary person–includes: like anyone else, normal, average, no difference, my son, nice, clean cut, rich, walking, not like a bum, casual dress, medium dress, college student, person, average young person, some act normal
8. Don't know	Don't know–includes: No answer given, never seen one, how do I know?
9. Male	Male
10. Other	Other–includes: Long arms, dark hair, blond hair, brown eyes, short hair, middle part, White, middle aged, old, no glasses, boots, tennis shoes, sandals, leather coat, dark
11. Unclear to researcher	Unclear to researcher–includes: endangered, emancipated, self-cool, animal, surprise, guilt, ice cream parlor, with a group, corner, concern, disgust, drugs, store, needle, magazine, street, I don't want to look, shock
12. Female	Female

Table 2

Descriptive Words by Category for Each Situation

	Descriptive words									
	1		2		3		4		5	
	N	%	*N*	%	*N*	%	*N*	%	*N*	%
First situation										
Hippie+	40	72	34	63	35	79	28	90	18	86
Ordinary person	9	16	8	15	5	11	0	0	1	5
Don't know	5	9	6	11	1	2	1	3	0	0
Other	0	0	4	7	1	2	1	3	0	0
Unclear	2	4	2	4	2	5	1	3	2	10
Second situation										
Hippie+	46	66	54	84	45	79	39	86	25	93
Ordinary person	9	13	6	9	4	7	1	2	0	0
Don't know	10	15	1	2	2	4	2	4	0	0
Other	2	3	1	2	4	7	2	4	0	0
Unclear	2	3	2	3	2	4	1	2	2	7
Third situation										
Hippie+	54	79	51	82	43	81	38	86	26	81
Ordinary person	3	4	6	10	2	4	1	2	1	3
Don't know	7	10	2	3	0	0	1	2	0	0
Other	3	4	3	5	5	9	3	7	4	13
Unclear	1	2	0	0	2	4	1	2	1	3
Fourth situation										
Hippie+	41	78	35	74	31	81	24	86	13	72
Ordinary person	5	9	7	15	3	1	2	7	0	0
Don't know	3	6	1	2	2	5	1	4	0	0
Other	2	4	1	2	0	0	1	4	5	28
Unclear	2	4	3	6	2	1	0	0	0	0

connotations. A specific definition of "hippie" is found in *Webster's New Collegiate Dictionary* (1979, p. 537): "a usually young person who rejects the mores of established society (as by dressing unconventionally or favoring communal living), advocates a nonviolent ethic, and often uses psychedelic drugs or marijuana; broadly: a long haired unconventionally dressed young person." The additional descriptors pictured the drug addict as a disoriented, unhealthy, thin, low-class, male hippie with behavioral and skin problems; this image is identified as "hippie+." The hippie+ image was dominant when all the respondent descriptors were combined from all situations (see Table 3); the hippie+ category included 719 responses, which represented 79% of all the responses.

Table 3

All Descriptive Words; All Situations

Category	*N*	%
Hippie	398	44
Disoriented	78	9
Unhealthy	135	15
Thin	31	3
Low class	11	1
Skin problems	16	2
Behavioral problems	29	3
Male	21	2
Ordinary person	73	8
Don't know	45	5
Other	42	5
Unclear	30	3
Female	1	0.1
	911	100.1[a]

[a]Not all figures equal 100% due to rounding off.

Conceptions of the Condition

Respondents were asked if they considered drug addiction to be a disease, sin, moral weakness, excuse, mental illness, or crime; or preferred not to answer (PNTA). Disease was the dominant category, accounting for 32% (135) of the responses (see Table 4), and 11% (46) of the responses defined drug addiction as a crime.

Table 4

Cognitive Assessment of Drug Addiction

Category	*N*	%
Disease	135	32
Sin	22	5
Moral weakness	87	21
Excuse	78	19
Mental illness	43	10
Crime	46	11
PNTA	8	2
	419	100

Addictive Behavior by Respondent

The image of drug addict in the minds of persons who reported the use of substances at addictive levels was also studied. Sufficient numbers of respondents reported use of coffee or tobacco to allow for analysis. Fifty-one respondents reported drinking 5 or more cups of coffee per day, and 51 reported smoking 20 or more cigarettes per day. For the purposes of this research, 5 or more cups of coffee per day (Ray, 1978, p. 196) or 20 or more cigarettes per day are defined as addictive levels of use (exceeds quantity criteria for tobacco dependence, *DSM III*, 1980, pages 176 and 159). Cross-tabulations were performed on the data, with the results presented in Table 5. These data reveal that all respondents overwhelmingly viewed the drug addict as hippie+ even though 51 of the respondents drank coffee at addictive levels and 51 smoked cigarettes at addictive levels.

A total of 131 respondents who drank coffee also indicated if they believed drug addiction to be a disease, sin, moral weakness, excuse, mental illness, or crime (see Table 6). Of 50 respondents who drank 5 or more cups of coffee per day, 29 viewed drug addiction as a disease (40%), followed by moral weakness (22%), excuse (15%), crime (14%), mental illness (7%), and sin (3%). A total of 79 respondents who smoked also answered the question (see Table 6). Of 49 respondents who smoked 20 or more cigarettes per day, 29 viewed drug addiction as a disease (35%), followed by moral weakness (22%), excuse (15%), crime (15%), mental illness (10%), and sin (4%).

Table 7 provides all responses given by all responders of their image of drug addict cross-tabulated with their categorization of the condition. The data reveal that although 135 respondents believed drug addiction to be a disease, 396 descriptors were provided of the drug addict as hippie+.

Table 5

Coffee and Tobacco Use Compared to Image

	Number of respondents	Hippie+	Ordinary person	Don't know	Other	Unclear	Female
Cups of coffee/day							
1-4	83	232	23	22	11	7	1
5+	51	131	20	10	7	9	0
Cigarettes/day							
1-17	31	87	7	10	7	4	1
20+	51	136	16	7	6	5	0

Table 6

Classification of Drug Addiction by Coffee and Tobacco Users

	Coffee				Cigarettes			
	1-4 cups/ day		5+ cups/ day		1-19/day		20+/day	
	N	%	*N*	%	*N*	%	*N*	%
Disease	38	27	29	40	15	33	29	35
Sin	6	4	2	3	1	2	3	4
Moral weakness	36	26	16	22	9	20	18	22
Excuse	32	23	11	15	12	26	12	15
Mental illness	16	11	5	7	2	4	8	10
Crime	13	9	10	14	7	15	12	15
Total	141	100	73	101	46	100	82	101
No. of respondents	81		50		30		49	

COMPARISON OF THE TWO STUDIES

When all responses were combined in the first study (Dean and Poremba, 1983), 73% (498) of the words conveyed the image of the skid row habitué. In the present study 79% (719) of the words conveyed the image of drug addict as hippie+. In both studies the image of alcoholic and drug addict elicited overwhelming responses of stereotyped skid row habitués and hippies+.

Respondents were also asked if they believed alcoholism or drug addiction to be a disease, sin, moral weakness, excuse, or mental illness, or preferred not to answer. The present study added a category, crime. Fifty-eight percent (164) of the responses categorized alcoholism as a disease, and 32% (135) of the responses categorized drug addiction as a disease.

Table 7

Respondents' Characterization of Addiction Cross-Tabulated with Image of Drug Addict

	Disease	Sin	Moral weakness	Excuse	Mental illness	Crime	PNTA
No. of respondents	135	22	87	78	43	46	8
Hippie+	396	65	261	247	120	126	19
Ordinary person	48	2	18	15	17	8	1
Don't know	20	5	19	16	9	8	3
Other	22	3	11	11	4	9	3
Unclear	12	7	17	8	14	9	0

DISCUSSION

1. The first-impression, nonreflective response to the image of "drug addict" is hippie+. This negative stereotype is similar to the response to "alcoholic," uncovered in the first study.

2. The first study revealed that although 58% of the responses labeled alcoholism a disease, 73% of the responses described the alcoholic as a skid row habitué. In the present study, although 32% of the responses labeled drug addiction a disease, 79% of the responses described the drug addict as hippie+. It may be that the disease label has little impact on the imagery in both cases and that new routes must be pursued to change the public images of alcoholic and drug addict.

3. Only 11% of the responses categorized drug addiction as a crime. Why is the crime response relatively low? Would other populations respond similarly?

4. The categorization of alcoholism and drug addiction as diseases may have resulted from public efforts to shift opinion. It may be, however, that larger, cultural conceptual shifts have taken place which include alcohol and drug issues but go beyond them. Pattison, Bishop, and Linsky (1968) presented data which suggested sources for the change. Their analysis revealed a historical movement from blame of the individual toward blame of societal forces for individual behavior. The authors suggested that these changes were based not on efforts to alter opinion about alcohol and drugs, but on wider societal change which indirectly promoted the disease concept. If this were the case, the alcohol movement can take only partial credit for shifting public opinion.

5. This is not to say that public efforts to change opinion are unimportant. The data reveal that 58% of the responses labeled alcoholism a disease and 32% of the responses labeled drug addiction a disease. The difference between the percentages may be a result of the efforts of the alcohol movement to alter the image of alcoholic and the lack of concentrated effort by similar groups in the drug field.

6. The data reveal that individuals who use coffee and tobacco at addictive levels view drug addicts as hippie+. This may be an example of selective or compartmentalized thinking.

FUTURE RESEARCH

1. This study is limited geographically, and future research should be conducted on other populations in different locations. These studies may reveal cross-cultural differences.

2. Future research should focus on the connection between change in individual concepts of addiction and the impact of that change on behavior. It may be that change in labels does not automatically result in change in personal response to individuals.

3. It is possible that the drug addict label should be abandoned because of its negative stereotypes. If this were done, the impact of the shift should be studied to see if alterations occur in the negative stereotypes.

ACKNOWLEDGMENT

The authors acknowledge the assistance of Ms. Barbara Hills in data collection.

REFERENCES

BRUUN, K.F. The non-medical approach. In L.G. Kiloh and D.S. Bell (eds.), *Alcoholism and Drug Dependencies: Proceedings of the 29th Congress*. Chatswood, Australia: Buttersworth, 1971.

DEAN, J., and POREMBA, G. The alcoholic stigma and the disease concept. *Int. J. Addict.* 18: 739-751, 1983.

Diagnostic and Statistical Manual of Mental Disorders (DSM), 3rd ed. Washington, DC: American Psychiatric Association, 1980.

PATTISON, E., BISHOP, L., and LINSKY, A. Changes in public attitudes on narcotic addiction. *Am. J. Psychiatry* 125: 160-167, 1968.

RAY, O., *Drugs, Society, and Human Behavior.* Saint Louis: Mosby, 1978.

SIEGLER, M., OSMOND, H., and NEWELL, S. Modes of addiction. *Q. J. Stud. Alcohol* 29: 571-591, 1968.

SIEGLER, M., and OSMOND, H. Models of drug addiction. *Int. J. Addict.* 3: 3-24, 1968.

Webster's New Collegiate Dictionary. Springfield, MA: Merriam, 1979.

The International Journal of the Addictions, 19(8), 871–884, 1984

Nonmedical Drug Use Patterns among Medical Students

William Paul Kory,* MD

University of Florida College of Medicine

Lee A. Crandall,† PhD

Department of Community Health and Family Medicine
University of Florida College of Medicine
Gainesville, Florida 32610

Abstract

Interrelationships in the use of nonmedical drug use and tobacco use are explored based on self-reports by 165 medical students at an average-sized southeastern medical school. Lifetime and current use of drugs among these students appears consistent with earlier studies. Several background and demographic characteristics are correlated with drug use; higher rates of use are found among males, older students, and students who frequently miss classes. No correlation is observed between drug use and class standing, sibling position, social relationships, or family drug use patterns. Tobacco use was found to be low among these medical students but was highly correlated with nonmedical drug use. Drug use patterns appear to have developed in high school and college, and to persist, albeit at a diminished rate, during medical school. The findings provide little support for the belief that marijuana or cocaine use substitutes for alcohol use; higher consumption of virtually any recreational drug is predictive of higher use of other recreational drugs.

*Present address: Department of Pathology, University of Miami, Miami, Florida.
†To whom all correspondence should be sent at Box J-222, JHMHC, Gainesville, Florida 32610.

 0020-773X/84/1908-0871$3.50/0

Over the past two decades a substantial number of researchers have examined nonmedical drug use among American medical students. The majority of these studies, which are summarized in Table 1, have focused on description of lifetime and/or current drug use and have demonstrated great variability in definition, research design, response rate, and types of drugs studied. Few of these studies dealt comprehensively with the issue of medical student drug use. For example, of the 12 studies of drug use reviewed, only three dealt with alcohol use. Nine provided information on marijuana use while six dealt with hallucinogens, six studied amphetamines or other stimulants, and only one reported data on use of cocaine. Furthermore, the interrelationships among use patterns of the various drugs have not been well documented, and only a few of these studies have attempted to obtain information on life problems associated with recreational use (Mechanick et al., 1973; Thomas, Luber, and Smith, 1977).

Early recognition of drug problems may help to prevent the morbidity and mortality associated with physician impairment. Thus, one purpose of the present study was to gather information on patterns of drug use and drug problems which may be precursors of impairment during later stages of the physician's career. While only a longitudinal study can provide definitive data on future impairment, the present study does examine the relationship between students' background and the type and number of substances used, and in addition provides an update on drug use by medical students which may reflect the changing popularity of recreational drugs.

METHODS

Data were collected by mailing an anonymous questionnaire to all medical students in an average-sized southeastern medical school during spring 1980. Two follow-up mailings were used to increase the response rate. While mailed surveys notoriously produce lower response rates than face-to-face interviews, the issue of recreational drug use is one which is highly sensitive and where a lack of absolute anonymity may produce misleading findings, especially with regard to current use (Leutgert and Armstrong, 1973; Smith and Nacer, 1977). Surveys presented to captive populations such as students in classroom settings often must forego collection of demographic data in order to avoid inadvertent identification of respondents based on age, sex, race, etc. Furthermore, the present study raised questions about acts which were illegal (e.g., cocaine use) and/or might invoke administrative sanctions (e.g., working on the wards while under the influence of drugs). As a consequence, the authors employed a mailed survey in order to allow full treatment of items dealing with behaviors and demographic data without compromising the study's validity or the students' anonymity. Nevertheless, underreporting of controversial and illegal acts seems likely in social research. The estimates reported here thus seem more likely to underestimate drug use by medical students than to overestimate this behavior.

Table 1

Drug Use among Medical Students: Published Reports

Authors (publication year)	Study year	Technique	Sample population	Recreational drugs studied[a]	Major findings	Limitations of study
Smith and Blachly (1966)	1964	Anonymous questionnaire–mailed return	All students in one medical school (70%) response	AMP	Greatest initial use during freshman year 44% lifetime use	Failed to distinguish recreational from medically prescribed use Single institution
Blaine, Lieberman, and Hirsh (1968)	1966	Anonymous questionnaire–mixed mailed return and on-site completion	All students in one medical school (response rate varied from 34% to 100% by class year)	AMP ETOH TRANQ BARB MAR HAL OPIAT	Frequent recourse to drugs to alleviate somatic complaints Amphetamines used as adjunct to studying Trend to increased marijuana use among younger students No evidence of dependence on opiates, codeine, barbiturates, amphetamines	Single institution
Solursh, Weinstock, Saunders, and Ungerleider (1971)	?	Anonymous questionnaire–distributed and completed on site	All students in one U.S. (Calif.) and one Canadian (Ont.) medical school	MAR ETOH TOB	U.S. students more familiar with cannabis U.S. students more permissive than Canadian students regarding use by patients and legalization	Single institution in each country

(continued)

Table 1 (continued)

Authors (publication year)	Study year	Technique	Sample population	Recreational drugs studied[a]	Major findings	Limitations of study
Lipp, Benson, and Taintor (1971); also Lipp, Tinklenberg, Benson, Melges, Taintor, and Peterson (1972)	1970	Anonymous questionnaire–mailed	All students in four "widely separated" U.S. medical schools	MAR	Slightly over half of respondents reported lifetime use Geographic differences exceeded those due to age, sex, or marital status Current use ranged from 6% to 44% (average of 4 schools was 30%)	Study purposes were descriptive; thus, no correlations with respondents' characteristics are reported
Slaby, Lieb, and Schwartz (1972)	1970	Confidential questionnaire–mailed	All medical and law students attending Yale University	MAR HAL AMP	Medical student use: MAR, 68%; HAL (LSD), 9.5%; AMP, 7.0% Inverse relationship of religiousity to drug use	Low response rates raise issues of representativeness Single institution
Polakoff and Lowinger (1972)	1969	Mixture of questionnaires distributed at national conferences and at a large urban medical school	Mixture: volunteers at convention and freshman/sophomores at one medical school	MAR HAL COC OPIAT	47% "had exposure to drugs not intended for medical uses" Of 325 respondents, number using drugs was: MAR, 81%; AMP, 31%; HAL, 16%; "hard drugs" (cocaine, opium, heroin), 6%	Convenience sample combined with institutional sample

Grotheer (1973)	?	Questionnaire–distributed to first- and second-year students for on-site completion; mailed to other students	All medical students in one midwestern medical school	MAR	Higher lifetime use among underclassmen Current use highest among junior class Of 81 current MAR smokers, 62 did not currently smoke (tobacco) cigarettes	Single institution Questionnaire limited to 15 questions
Mechanick, Mintz, Gallagher, Lapid, Rubin, and Good (1973)	1970, 1972	Anonymous questionnaire–mailed with stamped return envelope	All medical students at the University of Pennsylvania	MAR HAL AMP BARB	Lifetime drug use increased between 1970 and 1972 1972 lifetime MAR use 70% Current MAR use declined slightly from 1970 to 1972 Cannabis use and positive attitudes toward it are fading	Single institution Short time period for meaningful longitudinal research
Thomas, Luber and Smith (1977)	?	Anonymous questionnaire–distributed in classroom situations	Students from all classes in a midwestern medical school	ETOH MAR AMP HAL TRANQ BARB TOB	40% of seniors were TOB smokers 95% of respondents drank ETOH 10% drank "in a concerning manner" 53% lifetime MAR 14% lifetime AMP Significant relationship between TOB use and use of ETOH, TRANQ	Single institution Population and sampling methods not clearly described Relatively low response rate (35%)

(continued)

Table 1 (continued)

Authors (publication year)	Study year	Technique	Sample population	Recreational drugs studied[a]	Major findings	Limitations of study
					Significant relationship between familial use of ETOH and student use ETOH use positively related to use of other substances Higher familial income correlated with higher use of most drugs	
Rochford, Grant, and LaVigne (1977)	?	Administered questionnaire	134 freshman medical students	MAR HAL AMP	No significant differences between MAR users and nonusers on any of six neuropsychological tests	Representativeness of students not specified Apparently single institution

					Lifetime use: ETOH, 94%; MAR, 72%; HAL or AMP, 24%; NARC, 7%; TOB, 37% MAR users consume significantly more ETOH on a weekly basis than naive subjects Positive correlation of family income and use of MAR	
Rosenberg, Orkin, and Springstead (1979)	?	Distributed anonymous questionnaire	"Medical and dental students at a nearby university"	ANES (N_2O)	"Depending on class year, N_2O has been used in a social setting by 8.5% to as many as 20% of students" No significant difference in use of rates between medical and dental students	Response rate unspecified ("high") Single institution

[a] AMP, amphetamines; ANES, nitrous oxide (N_2O), other anesthetics; BARB, barbiturates; COC, cocaine; ETOH, ethyl alcohol; HAL, LSD, mescaline, other hallucinogens; MAR, marijuana, hashish, other cannibinoids; NARC, narcotics; OPIAT, heroin, opium, other opiates; TOB, cigarettes, other tobacco products; TRANQ, tranquilizers.

Of the approximately 450 students registered at the time of the survey, 165 (37%) completed and returned our questionnaire. No significant differences were found among responses from each of the three mailings. While the rate of response was relatively low, demographic data suggest that the respondents are representative of the student body with two exceptions. Females, who represented approximately 24% of the student body at the time of the study, comprised 28.6% of respondents. Respondents also were likely to report that they were in the middle third (40%) or upper third (53%) of their class rather than the lower third. It is unclear whether this second finding represents a skew of respondents toward better students or simply an overestimation of class standing by respondents. When findings from our study were compared with a study conducted in a classroom setting in the same medical school, results were amazingly similar despite that study's participation rate of 77% (Gravenstein, Kory, and Marks, 1983). Our study showed a lifetime use rate of marijuana of 76% versus 75% for the classroom study and a lifetime use rate of 31% for cocaine versus 38% for the classroom study. Thus, comparisons with demographic characteristics of the student body and comparisons with a classroom study (for which demographic data were unknown) suggest that data from our study represent the students and their drug use quite accurately.

FINDINGS

Table 2 shows the educational level at which medical students first used each of 10 drugs recreationally and the lifetime prevalence of use of each drug. Alcohol appeared to be widely used and to have been used first while students

Table 2

Educational Level at Time of Initial Recreational Use and Lifetime Prevalence of Use of 10 Recreational Drugs

	Percent, by educational level at time of first use			Lifetime prevalence (%)
	High school	College	Medical school	
Alcohol	73.9	20.6	0.6	95.1
Marijuana	37.6	29.7	8.5	75.8
Cocaine	4.2	17.6	9.1	30.9
Tranquilizers	7.3	6.7	6.1	20.1
Hypnotics	6.1	9.7	4.8	20.6
Amphetamines	7.3	15.8	1.8	24.9
Hallucinogens	11.5	7.3	0.0	18.8
Barbiturates	6.1	3.0	0.6	9.7
Opiates	2.4	4.8	1.2	8.4
Anesthetics	1.8	6.7	0.6	9.1

were in high school. Similarly over 75% of respondents had sampled marijuana, and 37.6% reported initial use as high school students. Other types of drugs used recreationally at some time by more than 10% of respondents included hallucinogens, cocaine, amphetamines, tranquilizers, and hypnotics. Most drugs appeared to have been initially used prior to entry into medical school, if at all. Only marijuana, cocaine, tranquilizers, and hypnotics were reported by a substantial number of students as being first used for recreational purposes in medical school.

Table 3 provides a clearer picture of the current use of drugs (i.e., monthly or more frequent use) among these medical students. Only two substances were reported to be used on a daily basis (marijuana and alcohol), and this frequency of current use was reported by only a few students. Nearly 90% of respondents reported current use of alcohol, and a majority reported use on at least a weekly basis. The only drug currently used recreationally by a large portion of students was marijuana. However, over half of respondents reported that they were not current users; this included 40% who reported that they never used it.

Cocaine use was reported by nearly one fourth of respondents, but its frequency of use appeared low as only 10% of respondents reported use on a monthly or more frequent basis. Tranquilizers were the only other drug class which was reported by any substantial number of students as the subject of weekly or monthly recreational use. This drug is subject to more confusion

Table 3

Annual Use and Current Use of 10 Recreational Drugs While in Medical School

	Percent reporting various frequencies of use					
			Current use[a]			
	No use	Annual use	Monthly use	Weekly use	Daily use	Total current use (%)
Alcohol	5.5	6.7	31.1	52.4	4.3	87.8
Marijuana	40.0	16.4	21.8	13.4	8.5	43.6
Cocaine	76.4	13.9	9.1	0.6	0.0	9.7
Tranquilizers	79.9	7.3	6.7	6.1	0.0	12.8
Hypnotics	90.3	6.1	3.6	0.0	0.0	3.6
Amphetamines	92.7	5.5	0.6	1.2	0.0	1.8
Hallucinogens	93.3	6.1	0.6	0.0	0.0	0.6
Barbiturates	97.6	1.2	1.2	0.0	0.0	1.2
Opiates	97.6	1.8	0.6	0.0	0.0	0.6
Anesthetics	98.2	1.2	0.6	0.0	0.0	0.6

[a]Current use as defined by the *National Survey on Drug Abuse* (Fishburne, Abelson, and Cisin, 1980).

regarding self-treatment and medically appropriate use versus recreational use than is the case for alcohol, marijuana, or cocaine. Thus its frequency may have been overreported.

These findings appear consistent with a number of other studies of recreational drug use by college students and health professions students cited earlier in this paper. The major purpose of the present research, however, is not to describe medical student drug use, but to investigate relationships between background characteristics of medical students and their recreational drug use and abuse, and to examine the interrelationships among use patterns of these drugs.

Table 4 shows that several background and demographic characteristics of medical students were correlated with an overall index of their drug use. These included: sex, with males reporting substantially more drug use; age, with older students reporting somewhat greater drug use; and class, with juniors and seniors reporting greater drug use than freshmen and sophomores. Drug use was also associated with a decrease in class standing and decreased class attendance. In contrast to a number of other studies, we found few significant correlations (only one of eight examined) between students' current use of drugs and measures of family drug use (i.e., mother's, father's, or sibling's abuse of drugs

Table 4

Correlation between Background and Demographic Characteristics of Medical Students and Overall Index of Drug Use

Characteristic	Correlation coefficient	p[a]
Sex	.23[b]	<.01
Age	.16[c]	<.05
Sibling position	–.01[b]	NS
Class year	.14[b]	<.05
Class standing	–.05[b]	NS
Frequency of class attendance	–.16[b]	<.05
Number of social relationships	.05[b]	NS
Mother's function impaired by drugs	–.01[b]	NS
Father's function impaired by drugs	–.02[b]	NS
Older sibling's function impaired by drugs	–.05[b]	NS
Younger sibling's function impaired by drugs	–.07[b]	NS
Mother has sought help for drug problem	.03[b]	NS
Father has sought help for drug problem	.03[b]	NS
Older sibling has sought help for drug problem	.11[b]	<.05
Younger sibling has sought help for drug problem	.05[b]	NS

[a]NS, not statistically significant.
[b]Kendall's tau B.
[c]Pearson's *R*.

or seeking help for drug use). However, the number of students reporting substantial parental or sibling impairment was quite small.

Drug use during medical school clearly is not a phenomenon which is isolated from earlier behavior. Those medical students who reported early initial use of virtually any of the drugs surveyed also reported a greater variety and frequency of drug use in medical school. Similarly, a high frequency of use during college of most of the drugs surveyed was correlated with more frequent current drug use as medical students. Most students reported that their drug use had not increased during medical school. One-third (32.9%) of students reported that their level of drug use had decreased during medical school, while over half (51.6%) reported no change in their use of drugs during medical school. Most of those who did report an increase during medical school were very low users of drugs during their undergraduate years.

Drug use may have had some adverse impact on medical students' performance. One of every eight respondents (12.1%) reported that he/she was under the influence of a recreational drug at some time while present on the wards. Similarly, 15.3% of medical students reported that they believed that drugs had caused some level of impairment of their function at some time. The types of impairment reported included damaged social relations, missed classes, and lowered grades. Approximately half of those who perceived impairment reported that this had occurred during medical school with alcohol or marijuana, the most frequent causal agents.

The issue of polydrug use, which has been widely discussed in the literature, was addressed by correlating the students' current frequency of use of each of the 10 drugs with a numerical index which summarized use of the other nine

Table 5

Medical Students' Use of 10 Common Drugs by Index of Use of Nine Other Drugs

	Kendall's tau B	p
Alcohol by Index 1[a]	.43	< .0001
Cocaine by Index 2	.49	< .0001
Marijuana by Index 3	.61	< .0001
Hallucinogens by Index 4	.29	< .0001
Amphetamines by Index 5	.29	< .0001
Barbiturates by Index 6	.21	< .001
Tranquilizers by Index 7	.34	< .0001
Opiates by Index 8	.20	< .01
Hypnotics by Index 9	.33	< .0001
Anesthetics by Index 10	.17	< .01

[a]Index 1 = use of all drugs in Table 4 except alcohol; Index 2 = use of all drugs in Table 4 except cocaine; etc.

drugs. Each of the 10 drugs was strongly positively related to the index score for use of the other drugs (Table 5). In addition, an examination of all possible intercorrelations among measures of use of these 10 drugs showed that 38 of the 46 possible correlation coefficients were statistically significant. These findings suggest that the 10 drugs were not used as substitutes for one another, but rather that use of any of these substances was part of a larger pattern of substance use which was consistent and appeared to encompass most recreational drugs. The use of alcohol, marijuana, and cocaine appeared to be particularly strongly associated with the use of other drugs. This no doubt reflects the fact that use of all three of these recreational drugs may be simultaneously discouraged or encouraged by one's peer group, depending on the nature of that group, and the likelihood that social settings in which one of these drugs is used will also encompass use of other drugs.

This paper has so far ignored the issue of tobacco use. This drug was used by some of the medical students, although its use was surprisingly low. Only 23 (13.9%) of the respondents reported any tobacco use; and of these only six reported daily use, while five reported weekly use, six reported monthly use, and six reported having used tobacco only on a yearly basis while medical students. National data for 1979 show that 37.1% of males and 33.5% of females in the 20-24 age group were current smokers (Fishburne, Abelson, and Cisin, 1980). Those medical students who reported more frequent use of tobacco, and those who began smoking earlier, appeared to use a wider variety and higher frequency of recreational drugs and reported more problems associated with drug use. For example, 78% of respondents reporting any tobacco use also reported use of alcohol or marijuana on at least a monthly basis. Among nonsmokers only 19% reported such use. Table 6 shows the results when a trichotomous index of recreational drug use (which excludes tobacco use) is cross-tabulated with current use of tobacco. Nearly two-thirds of current tobacco users are in the highest category of recreational drug use, while only one-fourth of nonusers of tobacco fall in this category. The lowest category of recreational drug use, which represents an extremely conservative use of drugs, includes only 12% of current tobacco users but 30% of nonusers.

Table 6

Trichotomous Index of Current Recreational Drug Use by Current Tobacco Use

	Index of current recreational drug use		
Current tobacco use	Extremely low	Low	Moderate or more
No	30%	44%	26%
Yes	12%	23%	65%

Kendall's tau B = .22; $p < .01$

DISCUSSION

The lifetime use of drugs, except for tobacco, by medical students responding to this survey was very similar to the pattern seen in the National Survey on Drug Use for young adults collected in 1979 (Fishburne, Abelson, and Cisin, 1980). Current use, defined in the National Survey as use of a drug in the month prior to information collection, was also remarkably similar.

One of the major purposes of this study was to examine the interrelationships among use patterns of recreational drugs. The findings provide little support for beliefs that marijuana and cocaine serve as substitutes for alcohol. Indeed, higher frequency of consumption of virtually any recreational drug appears to be predictive of higher consumption of other recreational drugs.

The use of tobacco and its relationship to other drugs was especially striking. Daily use of tobacco among medical students was markedly lower than use among age peers. It appears that medical students, who regularly observe patients suffering from smoking-related illnesses, refrain from habitual use of this substance. Moreover, those medical students who were regular tobacco users were much more likely to be substantial users of recreational drugs. This suggests that tobacco use may reflect a general pattern of hedonism in drug use or may indicate the existence of certain physicians with a predisposing personality more susceptible to drug dependency, especially in this population where the dangers of tobacco are widely appreciated.

From the intercorrelations of drug use seen in this study, one may postulate that a changing pattern may emerge for drug abuse. The availability of marijuana, cocaine, and other illicit agents may not significantly increase the total population of physician drug abusers. Rather the broader spectrum of drugs used suggests that polydrug abuse, already a common pattern seen in physician addicts, may become a greater segment of the problem. Still, the predominant drug of use and abuse remains alcohol.

Conversely, one may infer that the reported polydrug use by medical students is not a serious problem since our research suggests that: (1) The number at risk remains relatively constant throughout medical school, (2) these medical students report relatively little impairment at present, and (3) drug use appears to be largely recreational and sporadic rather than habitual. Nevertheless, the recreational drug use patterns of these students appear to include a substantially broader array of drugs than was believed to be the case among their predecessors of two decades ago. The reported incidence of illicit drug use among medical students may not portend a serious problem ahead with physician drug abuse when the present group of medical students enters the medical profession. Nevertheless, the long-range impact of these new drug patterns on physician impairment and on physicians' understanding and treatment of drug abuse merits further attention.

REFERENCES

BLAINE, J.D., LIEBERMAN, C.M., and HIRSH, J. Preliminary observations on patterns of drug consumption among medical students. *Int. J. Addict.* 3: 389-398, 1968.

FISHBURNE, P.M., ABELSON, H.I., and CISIN, I. *National Survey on Drug Abuse: Main Findings: 1979.* Rockville, MD: National Institute on Drug Abuse, 1980.

GRAVENSTEIN, J.S., KORY, W.P., and MARKS, R.G. Drug use by anesthesia personnel. *Anesth. Analg.* 62: 467-472, 1983.

GROTHEER, M.H. The use of marijuana by medical students. *J. Kansas Med. Soc.* 74: 142-144, 1973.

LEUTGERT, M.J., and ARMSTRONG, A.H. Methodological issues in drug usage surveys: Anonymity, recency, and frequency. *Int. J. Addict.* 8: 683-689, 1973.

LIPP, M.R., BENSON, S.G., and TAINTOR, Z. Marijuana use by medical students. *Am. J. Psychiatry* 128: 207-212, 1971.

LIPP, M., TINKLENBERG, J., BENSON, S., MELGES, F., TAINTOR, Z., and PETERSON, M. Medical students' use of marijuana, alcohol and cigarettes: A study of four schools. *Int. J. Addict.* 7: 141-152, 1972.

MECHANICK, P., MINTZ, J., GALLAGHER, J., LAPID, G., RUBIN, R., and GOOD, J. Nonmedical drug use among medical students. *Arch. Gen. Psychiatry* 29: 48-50, 1973.

POLAKOFF, P.L., and LOWINGER, P. Do medical students "turn on?" *Compr. Psychiatry* 13: 185-188, 1972.

ROCHFORD, J., GRANT, I., and LA VIGNE, G. Medical students and drugs: Further neuropsychological and use pattern considerations. *Int. J. Addict.* 12: 1057-1065, 1977.

ROSENBERG, H., ORKIN, F., and SPRINGSTEAD, J. Abuse of nitrous oxide. *Anesth. Analg.* 58: 104-106, 1979.

SLABY, A.E., LIEB, J., and SCHWARTZ, A.H. Comparative study of the psychosocial correlate of drug use among medical and law students. *J. Med. Educ.* 47: 717-723, 1972.

SMITH, B., and NACER, Y. Drug usage as determined under conditons of anonymity and high questionnaire return rate. *Int. J. Addict.* 12: 1057-1065, 1977.

SMITH, S.N., and BLACHLY, P.H. Amphetamine usage by medical students. *J. Med. Educ.* 41: 167-170, 1966.

SOLURSH, L.P., WEINSTOCK, S.J., SAUNDERS, C.S., and UNGERLEIDER, J.T. Attitudes of medical students toward cannabis. *J. Am. Med. Assoc.* 217: 1371-1372, 1971.

THOMAS, R.B., LUBER, S.A., and SMITH, J.A. A survey of alcohol and drug use in medical students. *Dis. Nerv. Syst.* 38: 41-43, 1977.

The International Journal of the Addictions, 19(8), 885-902, 1984

Follow-Up Difficulty with Substance Abusers: Predictors of Time to Locate and Relationship to Outcome

Richard N. Bale,* PhD

Department of Psychiatry and Behavioral Sciences
Stanford University School of Medicine

Veterans Administration Medical Center
Palo Alto, California

Barbara H. Arnoldussen, RN

Alexandra M. Quittner, MA

Veterans Administration Medical Center
Palo Alto, California

Abstract

A sample of 76 alcoholics and 31 drug abusers who had been inpatients at a Veterans Administration Medical Center were followed up 6 months after termination of treatment. Of this population, 100 (93.5%) were located, and additional data were recorded as to both the length of time required for location and the sources which proved useful in the process. Two-thirds of the sample were located within 1 month and most before the fourth month. Multivariate analyses revealed that criminal history, longer time in treatment, and previous treatment each were independent predictors of difficulty in location. Personal addresses provided by the subjects at intake were crucial in the tracking

*To whom requests for reprints should be sent at the Department of Psychiatry and Behavioral Sciences, Stanford University School of Medicine, Stanford, California 94305.

 0020-773X/84/1908-0885$3.50/0

process, as well as female relatives named by addicts. The time to locate a subject was not generally related to outcome. Employed subjects were somewhat harder to find, and those drinking daily—or not at all—were easier to locate.

Useful, valid evaluative research on treatment outcome depends on an adequate sampling of the treated population. Many well-conceived and well-executed studies of drug and alcohol abuse treatment have failed to locate more than 50-70% of their subjects and been unable to draw generalizable conclusions from limited samples (Bale, 1979b). Locating treated subjects is difficult in all outcome studies but is perhaps more difficult with substance abusers, regarded as characterologically manipulative and untrustworthy, and often leading nomadic, criminal, and/or clandestine lives (Bale, 1979a). Often they are also being pursued by criminal justice authorities, probation officers, collection agencies, street business acquaintances, family members, and others who may have other than scientific motivations. The follow-up researcher must often achieve both adequate trust and creative location strategies to overcome obstacles set up to thwart these other inquiries.

Achieving a sample of located subjects adequate to make valid generalizations about treatment outcome depends on (1) the ability of the researcher to achieve a high location rate and (2) some information from studies of similar subjects to allow speculation on the functioning of those subjects who were not located. These issues are interdependent: A sufficiently high completion rate makes information about nonrespondents less important. Alternatively, data indicating no differences between responding and nonresponding subjects make high location rates unnecessary. Previous reports of follow-up methodology have focused on both techniques producing high location rates and differences between responding and nonresponding subjects.

PREVIOUS REPORTS OF LOCATION TECHNIQUES

While many studies have reported on the progress of substance abusers after discharge from treatment (Bale, 1979b), only a few have described tracking, location, and interview techniques; or have quantitatively studied the relationship of difficulty in location to posttreatment social functioning. No studies have systematically investigated the relative effectiveness of different follow-up strategies.

In an early archival study, Nurco and Lerner (1971) examined the feasibility of locating drug addicts in a large metropolitan community using information from police files, social services, and neighborhood residents. Some 70% of the subjects were located through these community sources.

In another field study, Goldstein, Abbott, Paige, Sobel, and Soto (1977) distinguished between three types of information sources or "networks" for locating drug abusers in the community. The authors suggested that initial field contacts begin with family and friends, followed by more formal, institutional sources. However, they did not provide data on the actual number of subjects contacted or the follow-up completion rates. In contrast to the use of institutional sources, the field methodology employed in this study is rarely employed because of its prohibitive cost.

In a third study of addicts, Bale, Cabrera, and Brown (1977) provided a detailed description of their follow-up location techniques, including suggestions for information to be gathered at admission for tracking (public records including DMV [Department of Motor Vehicles] and criminal justice systems), the use of certified mail, and ways of establishing contacts with employers and social service agencies. Also emphasized were effective methods of staff teamwork and supervision. Follow-up completion rates using these strategies were above 96%.

An anecdotal report by Craig (1979) reiterated the Bale et al. (1977) study's emphasis on information gathering at admission as vital to the tracking process and reported the particular usefulness of mothers, other drug programs, and the DMV in locating some 80% of 62 addicts who had dropped out of VA treatment. The general usefulness of DMV information in both tracking subjects and validating self-reported data was reviewed by the Sobells (1978).

The various studies of follow-up strategies are summarized in Table 1. No study to date has investigated the predictors of location difficulty and examined the relative effectiveness of various sources in the tracking process. In the present report we determine those demographic variables which are associated with difficulty in location and assess the relative usefulness of various information given by the subject.

PREVIOUS STUDIES OF LOCATION DIFFICULTY VERSUS OUTCOME

Several reports of substance abusers have reported an apparent correspondence between poor outcome and difficulty of location. Three of these studies systematically quantified location efforts. Moos and Bliss (1978) achieved a 94% follow-up rate combining mail and telephone procedures to locate 505 alcoholics 6 months after treatment. Once the subject's location was obtained, a questionnaire was mailed, followed by a 2-week waiting period. If there was no response, then telephone and mail contact urged the subject's cooperation. Approximately one-fifth of the alcoholic subjects required three or four contacts with community agencies (e.g., social service, police, public and private treatment programs) for both location and completion of the questionnaire.

Table 1

Follow-Up Strategies

Author	Year	After treatment?	Method	Location results: *N*	%	Difficulties
Nurco and Lerner	1971	No	Field workers	28 out of 41 addicts	68	Access to files *S*s dead Geographic location Uncooperative *S*s
Sobell and Sobell	1978	Yes	Mailed requests	452 of 500 records of alcoholics	90	Out-of-state *S*s Record fees Special forms *S* data needed
Goldstein et al.	1977	No	Field workers	NA (addicts)	NA	Trust Confidentiality *S*s transience

						Uncooperative *S*s Timing of attempts *S*s privacy
Bale et al.	1978	Yes	Mail and phone	545 of 585 addicts	93	Trust Confidentiality Phone disconnected *S*s moved Record fees Access to files
Craig	1979	Yes	Mail and phone	50 of 62 addicts	80	Trust Mobility of *S*s Language barriers Confidentiality Bureaucracies

(No attempt, however, was made to determine which of the family or community sources was most useful in providing information or actual leads to the subject.)

The study found that subjects who required a greater number of follow-up activities to locate and interview tended to have the poorest treatment outcomes, a finding consistent with two other less systematic studies (Edwards, Chandler, and Hensman, 1972a; Edwards, Chandler, Hensman, and Peto, 1972b; Wolff and Holland, 1964). However, those differences in outcome were accounted for by sociodemographics and functioning at intake. A further analysis revealed that among a subgroup of subjects who were relatively uncooperative in providing information, the differences were not attributable to characteristics at intake.

Similar initial results showing an association between poor outcome and difficulty of location were described by Polich, Armor, and Braiker (1980), who also reported that the differences were accounted for by characteristics assessed at intake. In a study of 922 male alcoholics, Polich et al. recorded the time elapsed to locate, the number of persons or agencies contacted, and the number of hours spent in locating a case. All measures of effort were moderately related to poorer outcome until a 60-70% response rate was reached, at which point there was essentially no relationship between effort and outcome. The authors concluded that additional data from the expensive process of locating the final 20-30% of a subject population may not be worth the effort, and that follow-up studies are probably not affected by nonresponse, given at least a 60-70% completion rate.

Another study of substance abusers showed no significant relationship between locatability and posttreatment functioning. LaPorte, McLellan, Erdlen, and Parente (1981) located 96% of 150 consecutive male alcoholic and drug abuse admissions to a VA hospital. Most were located through telephone contacts with friends, relatives, and agencies; and the number of required contacts before location was noted. No relationship between the number of contacts and outcome was found for either addicts or alcoholics, and further analyses revealed that the results were also not related to time in or since treatment.

The relationship of location difficulty to outcome remains unclear for substance abusers. The only study (LaPorte et al., 1981) which included both addicts and alcoholics found differences in locatability between the two groups; however, those differences were not examined in a multivariate analysis including other related demographics. Further, two of three systematic studies (LaPorte et al., 1981; Moos and Bliss, 1978) gave equal weight to each follow-up contact regardless of the amount of effort actually spent, perhaps limiting the variability of the effort score. The effect of this procedure may have been to reduce the correlation between location effort and outcome. In the only study which assessed effort in terms of time (Polich et al., 1980), a negative correlation was found between location difficulty and outcome, until a 60-70% return rate was achieved. The several reports of location difficulty versus outcome are summarized in Table 2.

In the present report the relationship of actual time to locate with outcome is assessed for both addicts and alcoholics. Drug diagnosis is anlayzed in multivariate analyses including a variety of other variables.

METHOD

Treatment Settings

Subjects in the study spent a 2-week period undergoing withdrawal from alcohol and/or heroin or other drugs in a residential program at the Menlo Park Division of the Veterans Administration Medical Center in Palo Alto. Following this withdrawal period, the veterans could opt for continuation of treatment in one of five therapeutic communities. These treatment residences incorporated aspects of Synanon-style confrontation as well as the professionally staffed structure of Maxwell Jones, and ranged in length from 45 days to 6 months. The relative characteristics (Bale and Potter, 1976; Van Stone, 1974; Van Stone and Gilbert, 1972; Van Stone, Engelsing, Bale, and Zarcone, 1976; Zarcone, 1975, 1982) and outcome (Bale, 1982; Bale, Van Stone, Kuldau, Engelsing, Elashoff, and Zarcone, 1980) of several of these programs have been reported elsewhere, as well as the validity of self-reports from their former patients (Bale, 1979a; Bale et al., 1981).

Subjects

One hundred and seven veterans who left treatment (from March '79 to September '80) comprised the original study population. Ninety-seven completed a follow-up questionnaire by mail or phone, and three subjects who had returned to treatment were interviewed in person. Another six subjects who had also left treatment during this period were not located, and one subject was located but refused to provide information (yielding a completion rate of 100/107 = 93.5%, typical for this ongoing study during the last 10 years). Seventy-two of the 100 subjects located were addicted to alcohol, whereas the remaining 28 were using heroin and/or other drugs prior to admission. Other demographic characteristics of the located subjects are outlined in Table 3.

Of these 100 subjects, 87 had spent some time in one of the longer-term residential treatment programs following their withdrawal period. The remaining 13 subjects were chosen randomly from a larger group of veterans who underwent withdrawal but did not continue in longer-term treatment (an ongoing evaluation protocol involves sampling this withdrawal-only group).

Table 2

Author	Year	Treatment		Subjects	Location results
		Type	Length		
Wolff and Holland	1964	Inpatient	3 weeks (av)	364 alcoholics	94 interviewed 17 dead 41 no contact 135 collateral 1 refused 76 not sought
Edwards et al.	1972a, 1972b	None	NA	1,039 adults from general population	918 interviewed
Moos and Bliss	1978	5 residential programs	Not stated	505 alcoholics	429 interviewed 11 dead 35 refused
Polich et al.	1980	Inpatient and outpatient	Contact (min) Average not stated	922 alcoholics	668 interviewed 113 dead
La Porte et al.	1981	Inpatient	5 days (min) 56 days (av)	150 addicts	142 interviewed 2 dead

Studies of Location Difficulty Versus Outcome

% found at follow-up time	Field study?	Location difficulties	Rating of difficulty	Outcome criteria
39%, ranging 0 to 30 months after discharge	No	Time since discharge Unmarried subjects Non-home owners No field workers Time available Uncooperative subjects (especially women)	Response to questionnaire	Drinking and employment
89%	Yes	Subjects not at home	Residential instability	Drinking problems
94%, at 5 months after discharge	No	Uncooperative subjects Subject transience	Numbers and type of contacts or attempts	Drinking behavior and consequences, employment, social and psychological functioning
85%, at 4 years after admission	Yes	Undetermined deaths Population mobility Geographical distance Incapacitated subjects	Time in study, no. of contacts, location time	Drinking behavior, symptoms and consequences
96%, at 6 months after admission	No	Unlisted phones Incarceration Lack of phones Uncooperative subjects	Grouped nos. of contact attempts	Alcohol use, drug use, employment, family/social and psychological problems

Table 3

Demographics of the Population at Admission (N = 100)

Variable	%	Variable	%
Drug diagnosis		On probation/parole	21
Alcohol	72	Married currently	32
Drugs	28	Married ever	68
Age over 33 yr (median)	51	Employed during past year	48
Some college	48	Living arrangement	
Ethnic background		Alone	46
White	74	Wife or girlfriend	17
Black	16	Parents	17
Chicano	10	Friends	17
Arrested in past 2 yr	54	No stable arrangement	3

The Follow-Up Staff

Trained follow-up personnel (at the time of this study, two RNs) were involved in the initial interview, location, and follow-up of subjects. Neither follow-up worker was involved in significant counseling or other psychotherapeutic contact with the subjects after admission, and both were administratively and physically separate from the longer-term programs and their staff.

Procedure

On or shortly after his day of admission, each subject was interviewed by a staff member, who gathered data on a wide variety of background information, including patterns of substance abuse, past treatment, employment, and arrests and convictions, as well as standard demographic information.

Additionally, the follow-up worker explained the nature and purpose of the follow-up project, and explained that the information provided would be confidential and restricted to the program staff. She then showed the questionnaire to the subject and told him that he would be receiving the same questionnaire in 6 months. The subject was free to decline participation at this point. If he did consent, he was asked to provide the following information to assist in the location procedure:

1. His present address and phone number
2. The address and phone number at which he expected to reside following treatment
3. The names, addresses, and phone numbers of two people that he expected might know his whereabouts after he left the hospital.

He understood that should all sources fail to locate him, institutional sources would be utilized (e.g., VA hospital records, criminal indices, etc.). However, he was assured that the research worker would always identify herself as inquiring regarding "Veterans Administration business" and not for hospital or treatment concerns.

Two weeks prior to the 6-month point, the location process began. First, a questionnaire was mailed to the predicted future residence of the subject, if it detailed a street address. If it did not, the form was mailed to the subject's admission address. If no response was received in 2 weeks, the staff member called the corresponding phone number. If that produced no results, the staff person contacted the two additional information sources given by the subject. If all sources provided by the subject proved unsuccessful, the staff member turned to institutional sources.

For the period reported in this methodology study, the researcher recorded the following key data on the tracking process:

1. The length of time in months until the questionnaire was completed
2. Whether the original addresses given by the subject himself contained street addresses and/or phone numbers
3. The nature of sources given by the subject (e.g., mother, sibling, employer, friend, etc.)
4. Whether each source given by the subject (if needed) was "useful," meaning that a solid lead was provided or the person or place proved to be a liaison; or "not useful," meaning unable to contact by telephone or receive a mailed response, incorrect addresses, no helpful information provided, etc.
5. The type of institutional source(s), if any, utilized in tracking that was not provided by the subject (e.g., criminal justice systems, treatment programs, etc.)

RESULTS

Time to Locate

During the 6 months allowed for follow-up, 100 (93.5%) of the original group of 107 subjects were located. After 1 month, almost two-thirds of the group of 100 had been located and completed the questionnaire (Table 4). This return rate, characteristic of many follow-up studies, reflects rather straightforward use of personal address information gathered at intake.

As the follow-up team began to employ additional leads given by the subject and their own institutional leads, an additional 16% were found in the second month. Further efforts produced diminishing returns, and only one additional subject was located in each of the fourth, fifth, and sixth months, when follow-up efforts ceased (at 100, 93.5% of the original group of 107).

Table 4

Time to Locate

Time (months)	Located, of 107 subjects N	%
1	70	65.4
2	87	81.3
3	94	87.9
4	98	91.6
5	99	92.5
6	100	93.5

Usefulness of Personal Addresses

We obtained personal addresses at admission from 79 of the 100 subjects who were located (Table 5). The remaining 21 subjects had no stable address or a P.O. box only. These subjects were much more difficult to locate within 1 month ($\chi^2 = 11.03$, $p < .01$). The locatability of subjects was less clearly related to the availability of an anticipated "future" address at admission.

Interestingly, a phone number was not crucial (even though the follow-up process relied heavily on the use of a phone). All 10 subjects who provided a street address without a telephone number were readily located. The usefulness of the present address was related to recent moving; if a veteran had more than two addresses in the past year, the address was useful only 43% of the time, compared to 69% for two moves or less ($\chi^2 = 4.75, p < .05$). The usefulness of address information was not related to drug diagnosis or marital or employment status.

Table 5

Personal Addresses

Description	Admission address N	Admission address % found < 1 month	Future address N	Future address % found < 1 month
Street address and phone no.	69	75.4	46	78.3
Street address	10	100.0	1	100.0
P.O. box	5	16.7	1	100.0
No information	16	43.8	52	61.5
	100		100	

Usefulness of Additional Sources Provided by the Subject

The subject was asked at admission to provide two additional names and addresses of people who would know his whereabouts. The pattern was striking and consistent with previous anecdotal reports (Bale et al., 1977; Craig, 1979); female relatives were by far the most often named (Table 6). Again, the mother was not only the most often named source (52%), but she was useful in more than half of those instances (28% of the total). Other female relatives were both less often named and less useful. On the whole relatives were useful in 52% of cases.

Some sources were rarely named (e.g., business colleague–12%) but were very useful in location (6% of total). Conversely, some sources were often named (e.g., male friends–24%) but rarely useful (3% of total). Friends–both male and female–were useful in only 10% of all cases.

This pattern of sources named was unrelated to drug diagnosis except in the case of the mother. Half of the alcoholics (45.8%) compared with two-thirds (67.9%) of the addicts named the mother as an additional source ($\chi^2 = 3.09$, $p < .01$).

Table 6

Additional Sources from Subject

Source	% of subjects naming source	% useful
Mother	52	28
Wife	29	6
Sister	29	10
Male friend	24	3
Father	24	6
Brother	23	3
Other male relative	22	5
Female friend	16	3
Other female relative	14	3
Business colleague	12	6
Employer	12	2
Female cohabitor	8	2
Son	7	1
Parole/probation officer	5	3
Daughter	2	1

Usefulness of Institutional Sources

The follow-up workers employed a variety of information sources when leads given by the subject were not successful. Only three sources were useful (Table 7): (1) the subjects' own treatment program (useful in 10% of the cases), (2) other VA hospital departments (7%), and (3) parole officers not listed by the subject but accessed through public records (4%).

Other Factors Related to Time to Locate

In summary, those subjects giving a personal street address at admission were more quickly located, and certain sources given (e.g., mother) were generally useful in location. These are factors over which the follow-up worker may have some control; that is, she may press for detailed information and/or concentrate follow-up efforts on these sources. How important were other factors, such as demographic characteristics, drug diagnosis, and length of stay in treatment, etc., to the ease of location after 6 months?

In order to examine the relative contribution of these variables, a linear discriminant function analysis was completed which accounted for the interaction between the variables and rank ordered them in order of their separate contribution to time to locate. (A two-group analysis was performed: those located in less than 1 month vs those located in more than 1 month.) The results (Table 8) confirm that while adequate address information was indeed crucial, other factors were independently important ($\chi^2 = 28.96$, $p < .01$).

Criminality (any jail time previous to admission) was the first factor inhibiting location. Those with a criminal past required more time to locate, when all other variables were held constant. A person with a history of previous withdrawal treatment was also harder to locate. The experience over time of the follow-up workers was also important, as those subjects followed up later in the project were completed more quickly. Those subjects living alone or with friends were more difficult to locate. Finally, those subjects who stayed in treatment longer were more difficult to follow up.

Table 7

Institutional Sources

Source	% of subjects for which source useful
VA treatment program	10
Other hospital departments	7
Probation/parole officers	4

Table 8

Contributing Factors to Time to Locate

Variable	Rank of importance[a]
Any jail time[b]	1
Repeat admission to withdrawal program	2
Earlier follow-up	3
Adequate address	4
Living alone or with friends	5
Longer treatment program	6

[a]In a linear discriminant function ($\chi^2 = 28.96$, $df = 8$, $p < .001$).
[b]Polarity is related to longer time to locate; e.g., if a subject had spent some time in jail, he was harder to locate.

Interestingly, while univariate analyses revealed that alcoholics as a group were easier to follow up (consistent with an earlier report by LaPorte et al., 1981), drug diagnosis was not a factor when all variables were considered together in the multivariate analysis (linear discriminant function). Similarly, age and ethnic background, while having univariate significance, were not independent contributors. All other demographics were not related to time to locate, including marital status, education, employment, number of recent moves, and legal status.

Difficulty of Location Versus Posttreatment Functioning

Generally, the time to locate a subject was not related to how well he was functioning at follow-up. Chi-square analyses revealed no significant differences between time to locate and criminality, legal status, drug use, living arrangements, relationships with significant other, subsequent treatment, or plans for further treatment. Employed subjects were somewhat less likely to be found in the first month (62%) than those not employed (80%)—a comparison just short of significance at the .05 level. Alcohol use was a significant predictor, but not in a linear fashion. Those subjects drinking daily—or not at all—were significantly more likely to be reached in 1 month (84%) than those who were drinking moderately (55%) ($\chi^2 = 5.72$, $p < .05$).

DISCUSSION

The results of this study shed additional light on both the factors related to effective location of substance abusers and the relationship between difficulty of location and outcome.

Unlike some previous studies (Edwards et al., 1972a, 1972b; Wolff and Holland, 1964), we did not find that those subjects who were harder to locate were doing more poorly at follow-up. Further, our finding that alcoholics were easier to locate than addicts corresponds with LaPorte et al.'s results (1981), but multivariate analyses revealed that this difference was accounted for by variables associated with drug diagnosis: criminality, previous treatment, and longer time in treatment. Our unprecedented results showing an association between location and good outcome, combined with earlier reports showing no association (Moos and Bliss, 1978; Polich et al., 1980), leave an unclear picture for researchers to generalize from limited samples. Certainly it remains important to generate high location rates from which to draw valid conclusions.

Our data on predictors of location difficulty suggest several ways to improve follow-up rates. First, the follow-up worker should be very careful to solicit both complete information about present address and information about female relatives. This becomes especially crucial when the subjects have criminal backgrounds, are repeat admissions, or are living alone or with friends. Address and location information should be updated if the subject is in treatment for some time, as the address information as well as the relationship with the named sources may change over time. Finally, if initial location efforts are less than successful, there is a redeeming result: Our data show that follow-up workers do get better over time.

Most of our former patients and their families were very cooperative during the location process. It is important, however, for follow-up workers to be sensitive to the various kinds of resistance they may experience from non-respondents. Sometimes a distrustful patient with a poor treatment experience will simply not believe a researcher's word that his future treatment will not be affected by disclosures at follow-up, and in these cases cooperation will only follow reentry into treatment. For many other patients, including those who are functioning well, the follow-up assessment is a painful reminder of unpleasant memories, and the resistance to the interview/questionnaire is not too different from that experienced by the therapist in treatment. We have found, in fact, that the routine assessment is an extremely stressful situation for many respondents, something useful for the interviewer to remember.

Similarly, participating program staff often have considerable anxiety, distrust, and resistance to the assessment effort, for a variety of reasons including concern about how the data will be interpreted and used. (Staff resistance to follow-up studies is discussed in detail in a previous article in this journal: Bale, 1979b.) A useful suggestion for the researcher is to frame the project as just what it really is—intended to raise questions rather than to answer them. This process can be facilitated by a gamelike presentation of results, in which there is considerable give and take (described in detail in Bale, 1982), rather than the traditional (and often unread) written report. When properly approached, treatment personnel are often hungry for a lively debate on clinical implications of the follow-up data.

The conclusions of this study are limited by several important factors. Our population was composed of male veterans, all with sufficient premorbid history to qualify for military service, and our conclusions can be strictly generalized only to that group. We have made some crucial simplifications in our approach to the data; for example, we assume that difficulty of location is highly related to time to locate. A more precise study needs to be done where amount of effort is systematically quantified and assessed as a separate variable.

Finally, the usefulness of empirically derived follow-up strategies awaits a field test. Can the results of our assessment, in turn, improve our own location rates? In an efficient ongoing follow-up evaluation, results such as these would be fed back to alter, modify, and improve the assessment and location protocols, and then tested for their effectiveness.

ACKNOWLEDGMENTS

This study was supported by the staff and residents of the Drug and Alcohol Rehabilitation Unit of the Menlo Park Division of the Veterans Administration Medical Center, Palo Alto. We especially wish to thank William Orr, Arline Thomas, and Dr. Tom Engelsing for their continued support of evaluative efforts in our unit. A special thanks to the unit's former residents who participated in this study, who collaborated with us during a difficult and challenging time in their lives.

REFERENCES

BALE, R. Outcome evaluation of therapeutic communities. In R. Craig and S. Baker (eds.), *Drug Dependent Patients: Treatment and Research.* Springfield, IL: C.C. Thomas, 1982, pp. 309-348.

BALE, R. The validity and reliability of self-reported data from heroin addicts: Mailed questionnaires compared with face-to-face interviews. *Int. J. Addict.* 14: 993-1000, 1979(a).

BALE, R. Outcome research in therapeutic communities for drug abusers: A critical review: 1963-1975. *Int. J. Addict.* 14: 1053-1074, 1979(b).

BALE, R., CABRERA, S., and BROWN, J. Follow-up evaluation of drug abuse treatment. *Am. J. Drug Alcohol Abuse* 4: 233-249, 1977.

BALE, R., and POTTER, B. Treating drug abuse by treating its causes. In J. Krumboltz and C. Thoresen (eds.), *Behavioral Counseling Methods.* New York: Holt, Rinehart and Winston, 1976, pp. 150-157.

BALE, R., VAN STONE, W., KULDAU, J., ENGELSING, T., ELASHOFF, R., and ZARCONE, V. Therapeutic communities vs. methadone maintenance. *Arch. Gen. Psychiatry* 37: 179-193, 1980.

BALE, R., VAN STONE, W., KULDAU, J., ENGELSING, T., and ZARCONE, V. The validity of self-reported heroin use. *Int. J. Addict.* 16(8): 1387-1398, 1981.

CRAIG, R. Locating drug addicts who have dropped out of treatment. *Hosp. Commun. Psychiatry* 30(6): 402-404, 1979.

EDWARDS, G., CHANDLER, J., and HENSMAN, C. Drinking in a London suburb. I: Correlates of normal drinking. *Q. J. Stud. Alcohol* Suppl. No. 6: 69-93, 1972(a).

EDWARDS, G., CHANDLER, J., HENSMAN, C., and PETO, J. Drinking in a London suburb. II: Correlates of trouble with drinking. *Q. J. Stud. Alcohol* Suppl. No. 6: 94-119, 1972(b).

GOLDSTEIN, P., ABBOTT, W., PAIGE, W., SOBEL, I., and SOTO, F. Tracking procedures in follow-up studies of drug abusers. *Am. J. Drug Alcohol Abuse* 4(1); 21-30, 1977.

LA PORTE, D., MC LELLAN, A., ERDLEN, F., and PARENTE, R. Treatment outcomes as a function of follow-up difficulty in drug abusers. *J. Consult. Clin. Psychol.* 49(1): 112-119, 1981.

MOOS, R., and BLISS, F. Difficulty of follow-up and outcome of alcoholism treatment. *J. Stud. Alcohol* 39: 473-490, 1978.

NURCO, D., and LERNER, M. The feasibility of locating addicts in the community. *Int. J. Addict.* 6: 52, 1971.

POLICH, J., ARMOR, D., and BRAIKER, H. *The Course of Alcoholism: Four Years after Treatment.* New York: Wiley, 1980.

SOBELL, L., and SOBELL, M. Driver records: An aid in follow-up tracking and verification of self-reports of alcoholics. *Int. J. Addict.* 12(4): 429-438, 1978.

VAN STONE, W. Treating the drug dependent veteran–Perspective from a Veteran's Administration Hospital. *Int. J. Addict.* 9(4): 593-604, 1974.

VAN STONE, W., ENGELSING, T., BALE, R., and ZARCONE, V. Treating the drug dependent veteran. In J. Masserman (ed.), *Current Psychiatric Therapies*, Vol. 16. New York: Grune and Stratton, 1976, pp. 215-222.

VAN STONE, W., and GILBERT, R. Peer confrontation groups: What, why and whether? *Am. J. Psychiatry* 129: 583-589, 1972.

WOLFF, S., and HOLLAND, L. A questionnaire follow-up of alcoholic patients. *Q. J. Stud. Alcohol* 25: 108-118, 1964.

ZARCONE, V. *Drug Addicts in a Therapeutic Community: The Satori Approach.* Baltimore: York Press, 1975.

ZARCONE, V. Residential treatment for drug dependence. In R. Craig and S. Baker (eds.), *Drug Dependent Patients: Treatment and Research.* Springfield, IL: C.C. Thomas, 1982, pp. 67-89.

The International Journal of the Addictions, 19(8), 903–917, 1984

The Social Networks of Opioid Abusers

Mark W. Fraser, PhD

Social Research Institute, Graduate School of Social Work
University of Utah, Salt Lake City, Utah 84112

J. David Hawkins, PhD

Center for Social Welfare Research, School of Social Work
University of Washington, Seattle, Washington 98195

Abstract

Using social network analysis, the pretreatment social networks of 106 street drug abusers are examined. While no significant sociodemographic differences are found between opioid and nonopioid abusers, eight significant univariate differences in the characteristics of their social networks are reported. Four of these differences account for 32% of the variation between the two groups of abusers. The social networks of opioid abusers appear significantly less conventional than those of nonopioid abusers; however, opioid abusers appear less committed to the values and behaviors displayed by their network members. Network reconstruction is discussed as an explicit, empirically supportable rehabilitation strategy.

The misuse of psychoactive drugs is a widespread phenomenon (Drug Abuse Council, 1980, p. 4). For over a decade the misuse of opioid drugs in particular has been a major focus of multimillion dollar federal and state drug policy, enforcement, and treatment efforts. Across the United States, close to 60% of all federally subsidized drug treatment slots have been specifically designated for opioid abusers (National Institute on Drug Abuse, 1978). Nonmedical use of opioids appears to be generally less socially acceptable in this society than the use or misuse of other psychoactive drugs, at least as gauged by federal and state policies.

Concerns over opioid drug abuse have generated extensive research regarding its etiology. This research is remarkable in its diversity, focusing upon socio-

 0020-773X/84/1908-0903$3.50/0

demographic, biomedical, psychological, and pharmacological aspects of opioid addiction. Taken as a whole, it presents a broad range of competing hypotheses about the causes of abuse, including: poor family relations (Cloe Madanes, Dukes, and Harbin, 1980), low self-esteem (Pittel, 1971), biogenetic predisposition (Rasor, 1958), peer influence (Kandel, 1973), weak attachments to conventional others (Hirschi, 1969), impaired impulse and mood regulation (Treece and Nicoholson, 1980), metabolic need (Dole and Nyswander, 1967), depression or hypophoria (Cowan, Kay, Neidert, Ross, and Belmore, 1980), lack of assertiveness (Williams, Scott, Stout, and Hertzel, 1981), and external locus of control (Manganiello, 1978). Most of these hypotheses attempt to define personal life experiences and social interactions that lead to opioid use.

Some researchers have used ethnographic methods to distinguish "social worlds" or "drug subcultures" that are nested within the larger society (see Becker, 1963). These subcultures are described as separate systems with culturally distinct roles and norms that prescribe behavior (Lindesmith, 1938; Preble and Casey, 1969). Heroin abusers, for example, are thought to develop life-styles that are organized around the procurement of illicit drugs. An addict's personal style and self-concept are shaped by the associations that he must maintain in order to secure a consistent supply of drugs (Fiddle, 1976). Rich in detail, ethnographic studies describe a web of social relationships that provide little support for conventional behavior. These studies suggest that the most serious forms of drug abuse, particularly opioid abuse, are maintained and reinforced by the social context in which they are embedded.

To date, the research which supports this perspective has been largely anecdotal and impressionistic. There has been little effort to compare the social support for opioid abuse with competing forces in the social environment of the user. Nor have there been systematic comparisons of the social contexts of opioid abuse and the abuse of other drugs. There is, however, growing evidence that the use of heroin and other opioids is associated with greater interpersonal disruption than is the use of nonopioid drugs (Kandel, 1974; Kandel, Treiman, Faust, and Single, 1976).

The dearth of such comparative research may have resulted from the paucity of methods for systematically comparing personal social environments. While the interactional environment of a drug user is likely to be complex, consisting of influences from family, friends, school, work, criminal connections, gangs or social organizations, neighbors, and the like, standard sociometric investigations have typically confined attention to family and peer influences. In this study, using the method of social network analysis, the standard sociometric approach was expanded in order to compare the interactional systems of addicts who use illegal opioids including heroin, morphine, illegally obtained methadone, and Darvon with those of abusers of other illegal drugs. The investigation proceeds from the assumption that the rewards accrued in daily social interaction provide strong incentives to engage in or abstain from the use of drugs. Personal social networks provide opportunities for patterned interactions which may inhibit or induce drug use or misuse.

In the last decade, social network analysis has emerged as a tool for measuring the structural and interactional aspects of people's social environments. As defined by Mitchell (1969), a social network is a

> . . . specific set of linkages among a defined set of persons, with the additional property that the characteristics of these linkages as a whole may be used to interpret the social behavior of the persons involved. (p. 2)

Social support and social networks appear to be somewhat different. Networks are patterns of connections between people; they may be supportive, intrusive, binding, freeing, or neutral. Connections have been found to support conforming, conventional behavior (Phillips, 1981, p. 121), and they have also been reported to support deviant behavior like delinquency (Cohen, 1955) and drug abuse (Fraser, 1981; Hawkins and Catalano, 1980; Hawkins and Fraser, 1981). Networks can be described in both structural and interactional terms. In this study, we identify structural and interactional aspects of social networks that appear to support opioid abuse.

THE SAMPLE

The subjects for this investigation were residents in four drug treatment centers (therapeutic communities) between November 1979 and June 1980. They included both those who had used illegal opiates prior to treatment and those who had used other psychoactive substances. To guard against local geographic effects, two treatment programs in a northwestern city and two in a western city were purposely selected. The overall research effort studied the community reintegration of treated clients from therapeutic communities; however, this paper reports only on pretreatment social networks, as described by respondents in retrospective client history interviews conducted by the research team. The pretreatment networks of opioid users are compared with those of respondents who used other drugs including amphetamines, barbiturates, cocaine, and hallucinogens prior to treatment.

Eligibility for the original sample was defined as residence in treatment for 3 or more months. All eligible clients in two small therapeutic communities were sampled, and a systematic random sample of eligible clients at the two larger programs was constituted. All sampled residents elected to participate in the research, producing a sample of 106 respondents (Program 1 = 21; Program 2 = 16; Program 3 = 29; Program 4 = 40).

As shown in Table 1, respondents have long histories of life-styles associated with drug addiction, selling and using heroin, other opiates, and amphetamines, as well as barbiturates, cocaine, and hallucinogens. Seventy-four clients (69.8%) reported regular use of heroin at some time in their life, and 50 (47.2%) reported regular use of other opiates like morphine, codeine, or Darvon. Clearly, the residents sampled are not incidental users. Many have engaged in criminal behaviors more serious than the sale of illegal drugs. These include crimes against persons (murder, assault, rape), crimes of profit (robbery, burglary, shoplifting), and crimes against property (vandalism). Only a small percentage (4.7%) have never committed a crime.

Subjects range in age from 16 to 48, and the average age is 28.3 years. As shown in Table 2, 76% are male. Ten percent are Chicano; 20%, Black; 5%, Native American, Asian, or other; and the remaining 65% are White. Table 2 compares statistics describing the subjects of this study with statistics describing the Drug Abuse Report Program (DARP) national sample of 20,630 opiate users referred to drug treatment from 1969 to 1974 (Bale et al., 1980). The DARP study oversampled methadone maintenance programs, which were not sampled in this study. Nonetheless, the two samples are remarkably similar in sex distribution and various measures of deviance. The present sample has a significantly lower proportion of Black respondents and is slightly older. Few residents are currently married. Respondents appear to have experienced more family disruption during childhood and more previous involvement with drug treatment programs.

Table 1

Drug Use and Crime Participation Characteristics of the Sample (N = 106)

Drug use: regular use	
Heroin	69.8%
Morphine, codeine, Darvon	47.2%
Amphetamines	66.2%
Age at first regular use	
Heroin	14.3
Amphetamines	11.7
Crime: ever	
Drug related	95.3%
Burglary, robbery, theft	29.2%
None	4.7%
Arrests	
Ever	96.2%
Average number	11.0
Average age at first arrest	15.9
Currently on probation	67.0%
Committed illegal act in 30 days prior to treatment	74.5%

Table 2

Comparative Demographic Data

Variable	Study sample (%) (N = 106)	DARP study (%) (N = 20,630)
Male	76	77
White	65	54
Black	20[a]	43
Chicano	10	10
Never married	56	48
Currently married	14[b]	28
Age, older than 25	64[a]	43
Parents' marriage intact until subject aged 12 years	51	64
Previous drug abuse treatment	62	51
Age at first arrest, younger than 18 years	38	41
Currently on parole or probation	21	24
Cost of drug habit, more than $50/day	44	34

[a] χ^2, $df = 1$, $p < .001$.
[b] χ^2, $df = 1$, $p < .05$.

Overall, the current data, when compared with DARP data, are not inconsistent. The observed differences may be due to time of test or cohort effects. For example, inflation has affected the cost of most drugs on the street. The current respondents cannot be said to be more serious drug abusers on the basis of a cost-of-habit variable, because the purchasing power of $50 decreased between 1974 and 1980. Similarly, differences in marital status may be due to changes in the social institution of marriage and may not reflect greater deviance within the current sample. The distribution within the race/ethnicity variable appears to corroborate others' observations that therapeutic communities tend to serve more Whites, while methadone maintenance programs serve more minority clients (Bale et al., 1980). On the other hand, this may represent a regional or geographic effect. Finally, the fact that the 1969-1974 DARP population is younger suggests a cohort effect. It is possible that fewer young people are becoming involved in street-level addict life-styles, and that the drug addict population as a whole is getting older. Such speculation leads to questions which are beyond the domain of the current investigation. Returning to the current sample, no great departures from the expected characteristics of drug abusers in 1980 are noted. Where departures from DARP data are observed, plausible alternative explanations exist. In general, if sampling bias exists in the original sample, it does not pose a serious threat to the external validity of results from this study.

ASSESSING SOCIAL NETWORKS AND DRUG ABUSE

The operational measures used in this study to classify respondents as abusers of opioid or nonopioid drugs, to describe their background characteristics, and to describe their social networks are defined as follows:

- *Opioid abuse*: Interviewers asked respondents to indicate the average number of times they had used heroin or other opioids in the month preceding admission to treatment. For each type of opioid drug, responses were coded in eight categories (not at all = 0; used as an addiction substitute when drug of choice was not available = 1; less than once a month = 2; less than once a week = 3; weekly = 4; several times a week, but only on weekends = 5; several times a week = 6; and daily = 7). Inspection of the frequencies revealed a distinct dichotomous underlying variable of opioid abuse or abstention. Only 19 respondents reported moderate opioid use in Categories 2, 3, 4, or 5. Therefore, the frequency of use categories were collapsed into a two-point scale of abuse and abstinence. Respondents were categorized as opioid abusers if they reported use of either heroin or other opiates daily (7), several times a week (6), or as an addiction substitute (1). Respondents who reported no use of any opioids (0) were defined as abstainers. The 19 respondents whose opioid use was moderate (2, 3, 4, or 5) were dropped from this analysis. It is important to note that abstinence from opioid abuse, as operationalized here, does not imply abstinence from all drug abuse. All respondents had been referred to drug treatment, and thus it can be assumed that abstainers from opioids were users of other nonopioid drugs: amphetamines, barbiturates, nonprescribed tranquilizers, cocaine, hallucinogens, marijuana, hashish, or alcohol.
- *Proportion of "alters" (network members) classified by domain*: Social interaction can be classified by the social context in which it occurs. For this study, eight contexts or domains were defined: work/school, social organizations, friends, "informal business" (largely street crime), business, neighbors, residence, and family. Respondents identified network members by the domain in which the relationship usually occurred. From these data, it was possible to compute the proportion of alters in each domain of each respondent's social network.
- *Length of acquaintance*: The reported duration of each relationship in respondents' social networks was obtained and averaged.
- *Use of hard drugs by alters*: The average degree (4 = daily user; 3 = use 2-3 times a week; 2 = use 2-3 times a month; 1 = use less than once a month) to which network members are reported to use heroin, other opiates, barbiturates, amphetamines, cocaine, nonprescribed tranquilizers, and hallucinogens.

- *Use of any drugs by alters*: The average degree (5 = daily use of hard drugs; 4 = use of hard drugs 2-3 times a week; 3 = use of hard drugs 2-3 times a month; 2 = exclusive use of marijuana or alcohol; 1 = use of a hard drug less than once a month) to which network members are reported to use any drug.
- *Use of alcohol only by alters*: The proportion of network members who use alcohol exclusively.
- *Use of alcohol, marijuana, or hashish only by alters*: The proportion of network members who use alcohol, marijuana, or hashish exclusively.
- *Attitude toward use of hard drugs*: The degree (average) to which network members support the use of hard drugs (as defined in Item 4).
- *"Be kind of"*: The degree (average) to which respondents "want to be the kind of" people others in their social networks are.
- *Closeness*: The degree (average) to which respondents feel close to network members.
- *Share thoughts*: The degree (average) to which respondents share thoughts and feelings with network members.
- *Network size*: The number of people in each social network, not counting the respondent. (A natural log transformation was used to normalize this variable.)
- *Network density*: The proportion of alters who know one another. (A natural log transformation was used to normalize this variable.)
- *Equal status*: The proportion of alters who are reported to be of equal status with the respondent.
- *Share special days*: The proportion of alters with whom the respondent is reciprocally and intimately involved, defined in terms of recognizing one another's birthdays and sharing holidays and special occasions.
- *Mutual lending*: The proportion of network members with whom the respondent is reciprocally and instrumentally involved, defined in terms of lending one another money or "things."

Each of the network variables satisfies the requirements for interval scales. They are proportions or average scores characterizing respondents' social networks. For example, if a respondent reported 15 alters and 3 of these alters were from his/her family, the domain score for "% alters from family" would be .20. Similarly, five-point scaled items describing dyadic relations between the respondent and each network member were summed and divided by the network size to produce an average score which characterizes a person's total social network but is independent of its size.

DATA COLLECTION METHOD

To gather these data, confidential structured interviews were used because the information sought was detailed and sensitive. The method is reported as reliable and valid when reports of drug use and criminal behavior are desired (Bale, 1979; Bale et al., 1980; Whitehead and Smart, 1972). Recall is a potential source of bias in network-focused interviewing, since respondents are asked to identify interactions that occurred in the past. The reliability and validity of these self-reports continue to be controversial (Bernard and Killworth, 1977; Killworth and Bernard, 1976, 1979).

We attempted to reduce this bias by using a modified Q-sort interview technique (Kerlinger, 1973). Respondents were asked to list on cards the first names of people with whom they had significant contact in the 4 weeks prior to incarceration, hospitalization, or admission to treatment; that is, during their most recent month on the street. Interviewers were trained to use frequent prompts to enhance the recall of participants, who were asked about specific events and activities related to their own residence, employment, schooling, organizational affiliations, social contacts, receipt of services, illegal activities, quality of relationships, and drug use. After each set of questions, respondents were instructed to add additional network members with whom they interacted in that activity area. Sixteen clients added a total of 18 names to the original card sorts as a result of this probe procedure. While these data should be interpreted with some caution, our focus upon major social relationships and the use of systematic prompts should reduce biases due to recall (Hammer, 1980a, 1980b, 1980c; Hammer, Polgar, and Salzinger, 1969).

RESULTS

Demographic Differences

No significant differences between the 54 opioid abusers and the 33 non-opioid abusers were found on any of the sociodemographic background indices: age, sex, ethnicity, years of schooling, number of arrests ever, and longest continuous period of employment.

Social Network Differences

As shown in Table 3, eight differences at the .05 level of significance were found in the pretreatment social networks of opioid abusers and abusers of non-opioid drugs using a one-way analysis of variance procedure. Only one of these could be expected on the basis of chance. Three trends with p values between .05 and .10 were also observed.

Table 3

Comparison of Social Network Characteristics of Opioid Abusers and Abusers of Nonopioid Drugs Using One-Way Analyses of Variance (N = 87)[a]

Variable	Opioid abusers (*N* = 54)		Abusers of nonopioids (*N* = 33)			
	Mean	SD	Mean	SD	*F* ratio	*p* value
1-8. Alters (proportion from):						
1. Work/school	0.034	0.085	0.109	0.139	7.524	.007
2. Organizations	0.009	0.051	0.073	0.166	7.034	.010
3. Friends	0.242	0.187	0.271	0.216	0.464	.498
4. Street crime	0.293	0.247	0.099	0.111	18.180	.001
5. Business	0.061	0.114	0.076	0.109	0.345	.558
6. Neighbors	0.011	0.033	0.029	0.064	2.914	.092
7. Residence	0.150	0.124	0.097	0.146	3.285	.073
8. Family	0.194	0.167	0.249	0.181	2.099	.151
9. Length	4.118	0.643	4.089	0.795	0.035	.852
10. Use hard drugs[b]	2.131	0.969	1.253	0.914	17.570	.001
11. Use any drugs	3.102	1.017	2.414	0.949	9.844	.002
12. Use only alcohol (prop.)	0.146	0.207	0.238	0.190	4.327	.041
13. Use alcohol and marijuana only (prop.)	0.200	0.214	0.396	0.262	14.430	.001
14. Feel hard drugs ok	3.297	0.950	2.406	0.972	17.690	.001
15. "Be kind of"	2.322	0.904	2.632	0.869	2.477	.119
16. Close	3.829	0.619	3.838	0.745	0.004	.950
17. Share thoughts	2.756	0.957	2.988	1.008	1.159	.284
18. Network size (ln)	2.496	0.542	2.593	0.653	0.558	.457
19. Network density (ln)	3.862	0.562	3.719	0.856	0.885	.350
20. Prop. of equal status	0.371	0.275	0.408	0.316	0.323	.571
21. Share special days	0.381	0.264	0.495	0.282	3.679	.059
22. Mutual lending	0.401	0.319	0.307	0.317	1.766	.188

[a]Univariate *F* ratio with 1 and 87 degrees of freedom.

[b]Expressed as percentages, 52.1% of opioid abusers' network members are regular users of hard drugs and 30.0% of nonopioid abusers' network members are regular users of hard drugs.

On the average, opioid abusers named 12.7 people in their social networks, while 15.3 were named by drug program clients who had abstained from opioid use in the month prior to treatment. Though these average network sizes are not significantly different statistically, they may have clinical importance. Pattison, De Francisco, Wood, Frazier, and Crowder (1979) reported network sizes of 22.4 members for normal respondents (i.e., no reported disabilities), of 14.6 members for heroin addicts, of 16.4 members for alcoholics, and of 13.3 members for persons with psychotic thought disorders. Similarly, Sokolovsky, Cohen, Berger, and Geiger (1978) reported smaller networks of 10.2 members for schizophrenics with active symptoms. Street-level drug abusers of both types appear to lack the network resources of normal adults. Their networks appear to be close in size to those of other drug abusers and persons with serious mental illness. From a rehabilitation perspective, further differentiation is important. It may be useful, for example, to describe the composition of these small networks, the nature of interactions within them, or the support for rehabilitation rendered by network members.

In this regard, the members of opioid abusers' networks appear less involved in conventional activities than do the members of nonopioid abusers' networks. The networks of opioid abusers have significantly fewer members who are involved in work or school and social organizations, and significantly more members who are involved in street crime. The density analysis, though not significant, shows opioid abusers to have networks in which a higher proportion of alters know one another. These patterns suggest that opioid abusers may be embedded in more tightly knit and more deviant interaction networks than are abusers of other drugs.

This suggestion, that the networks of opioid abusers are particularly deviant, is supported by the results of the tests of interactional measures. Significantly more of the network members of opioid abusers use and approve of the use of hard drugs. The networks of abusers of nonopioid drugs appear to contain significantly more members who use only "conventional" drugs like alcohol and marijuana.

Discriminant Analysis of Drug Abuse Categories

To find a more concise combination of social network variables that distinguish opioid abusers from abusers of other drugs, discriminant analysis was used (Harris, 1975). As shown in Table 4, a four-variable discriminant function accounts for close to 32% ($r_c^2 = .563^2$) of the variance between groups. The results confirm that opioid abusers' network members are less involved in conventional activities and more involved in hard drug use and street crime.

A smaller proportion of the network members of opioid addicts in this population sustain organizational connections and use only conventional drugs

Table 4

Discriminant Analysis: Social Network Characteristics That Distinguish Opioid Abusers from Abusers of Nonopioid Drugs (N = 87)

Variables	Standardized discriminant function	
	Coefficient	*p* value
1. Proportion of network members in social organizations	–.449	.023
2. Proportion of network members involved in street crimes	.561	.005
3. Proportion of network members using only alcohol or marijuana	–.521	.009
4. Proportion of network members from place of residence	.393	.046
Canonical correlation	0.563	
Wilks lambda	0.683	
Chi square	31.605	
Degrees of freedom	4	
Significance of function	< 0.001	
Correctly classified (%)	78.16	
Classification gain (%)	16.09	

like alcohol and marijuana. The standardized coefficients suggest that the most important factor distinguishing the networks of opioid abusers from those of nonopioid abusers is participation in street crime. In this regard, the network members of opioid addicts appear to be involved in significantly more sales of illegal drugs and nonviolent crimes of profit. Finally, suggesting significant life-style differences, opioid addicts reported networks in which a higher proportion of members were from their own place of residence. When all four measures were used to classify the 87 respondents, 78.16% were correctly classified, and this represents a gain of 16.09% over simply classifying all respondents as opioid abusers. (In such a case, 54/87 [or 62.07%] would be correctly classified.)

This network depiction of opioid abuse is clarified by inspection of the structure loadings or zero-order correlations between network variables and the discriminant function. As shown in Table 5, the most important single variable is alters' involvement in street crime. Use of hard drugs by network members appears as the converse of exclusive use of soft drugs. The social networks of opioid abusers appear more likely than those of abusers of other drugs to encourage participation in street crime and to discourage abstinence from hard drug use.

Table 5

Structure Loadings: Zero-Order Correlations between Social Network Variables and Discriminant Function[a]

Variable	Loading/correlation
1. Alters (%) in street crime	.679
2. Use of only marijuana/alcohol by alters	–.605
3. Use of hard drugs by alters	.589
4. Use of only alcohol by alters	–.538
5. Use of any drug by alters	.427
6. Alters (%) in social organization	–.423
7. Alters (%) from family	–.333
8. "Want to be kind of person"	–.305
9. Network density	.295
10. Alters (%) from residence	.289
11. Alters (%) who are friends	–.216
12. Alters (%) from work or school	–.178
13, Network size	–.168

[a]Only loadings greater than $r = \pm.150$ are reported.

The networks also appear less capable of providing opportunities for conventional activities. The opioid addicts in our sample have fewer contacts with network members from social clubs, churches, and athletic groups (–.423); with family members (–.333); with friends (–.216); and with work or school associates (–.178) than do users of other drugs. In slightly smaller (–.168) and more dense networks (.295), they sustain proportionately more relationships in their place of residence than abusers of other drugs (.289). In sum, the networks of opioid addicts appear unlikely to provide opportunities or rewards for conventional behavior.

There is, however, a faintly encouraging note in these data. When asked whether they wanted to be the kind of people members of their networks were, opioid addicts tended to reply more negatively (–.305) than did abusers of other drugs. Thus, while their networks appear less conventional than the networks of other drug abusers, opioid abusers appear less committed to the values and behaviors modeled by their friends and associates. Opioid addicts who enter treatment do not emulate many of those with whom they interacted prior to treatment. This is an important finding, for it indicates that the subculture of opioid abuse may not be characterized by deep commitments to deviant values.

DISCUSSION

This study has important implications for drug treatment. As long as opioid abusers remain embedded in their pretreatment social networks, they are likely to experience strong pressures to use "hard drugs." Drug treatment programs which seek to assist clients in avoiding relapse should explicitly focus on the composition of clients' social networks in order to reduce the influence of members who are supportive of drug abuse. So long as treated former addicts continue to have routine contact with their old network members, they will experience compelling social support for opioid abuse. This support is not likely to decrease without intentional establishment of new relationships with others who support more conventional living patterns. In their exploratory study of natural recovery from opioid addiction, Waldorf and Biernacki (1981) have described several cases in which severing connections with drug users and establishing associations with more conventional others appear linked to the successful cessation of opioid use.

If former opioid abusers are to decrease interactions with network members who are drug abusers and who participate in street crime, they will need help. While residential treatment removes street addicts from these influences, creating a closed network of social support for conventional behavior, the construction of a network supportive of rehabilitation is not likely to occur spontaneously upon reentry to the community. Nor does development of such a network appear particularly likely for clients treated in nonresidential programs. Ex-addicts may seek out and be sought out by former friends if they do not develop supportive relationships with new people in the community. Treatment, then, should seek to connect former abusers with people involved in conventional activities. Specifically, it might set treatment goals to develop bonds of attachment to people in the network domains of social organizations, work or school, family, neighborhood, and business.

We know of no single proven network construction strategy, but a key to this approach is found in the structure loadings. Recall that opioid abusers appear less likely to admire or emulate their network members. The data suggest that opioid abusers are likely to have few network members after whom they wish to pattern their lives. If treatment is to assist opioid abusers in the development of new networks supportive of rehabilitation, it is likely to be most successful when it links formers addicts with conventional others who are respected as potential role models.

ACKNOWLEDGMENT

The research reported in this paper was supported by grant number H81 DA02071-01S1 from the Treatment Research Branch, National Institute on Drug Abuse.

REFERENCES

BALE, R. The validity and reliability of self-reported data from heroin addicts: Mailed questionnaires compared with face-to-face interviews. *Int. J. Addict.* 14(7): 993-1000, 1979.

BALE, R.N., VAN STONE, W.W., KULDAN, J.M., ENGELSING, T.M.J., ELASHOFF, R.M., and ZARCONE, V.P. Therapeutic communities versus methadone maintenance. *Arch. Gen. Psychiatry* 37: 179-193, 1980.

BECKER, H.S. *Outsiders: Studies in the Sociology of Deviance.* New York: Free Press, 1963.

BERNARD, H.R., and KILLWORTH, P.D. Informant accuracy in social network data. II. *Human Commun. Res.* 4(1): 3-18, 1977.

CLOE MADANES, L., DUKES, J., and HARBIN, H. Family ties of heroin addicts. *Arch. Gen. Psychiatry* 37: 889-894, 1980.

COHEN, A.K. *Delinquent Boys: The Culture of the Gang.* Glencoe, IL: Free Press, 1955.

COWAN, J.D., KAY, D.C., NEIDERT, G.L., ROSS, F.E., and BELMORE, S.M. Defeated and joyless: Potential measures of change in drug abuse characteristics. *J. Nerv. Ment. Dis.* 168(7): 391-399, 1980.

DOLE, V., and NYSWANDER, M. Heroin addiction: A metabolic disease. *Arch. Int. Med.* 120: 19-24, 1967.

DRUG ABUSE COUNCIL. *The Facts about "Drug Abuse."* New York: Free Press, 1980.

FIDDLE, S. Sequences in addiction. *Addict. Dis.* 2(4); 553-567, 1976.

FRASER, M.W. *The social support networks of street drug abusers.* Unpublished doctoral dissertation, University of Washington, 1981.

HAMMER, M. Predictability of social connections over time. *Soc. Networks* 2: 165-180, 1980a.

HAMMER, M. Reply to Killworth and Bernard. *Connections* 3(3): 14-15, 1980b.

HAMMER, M. Some comments on the validity of network data. *Connections* 3(1): 13-15, 1980c.

HAMMER, M., POLGAR, S.K., and SALZINGER, K. Speech predictability and social contact patterns in an informal group. *Human Org.* 28: 235-242, 1969.

HARRIS, R.J. *A Primer of Multivariate Statistics.* New York: Academic Press, 1975.

HAWKINS, J.D., and CATALANO, R.F. *Reversing drug abuse: A theory of rehabilitation.* Paper presented at the Pacific Sociological Association Meeting, San Francisco, CA, 1980.

HAWKINS, J.D., and FRASER, M.W. *The social networks of drug abusers before and after treatment: Implications for drug abuse treatment.* Paper presented at the International Congress on Drugs and Alcohol, Jerusalem, Israel, 1981.

HIRSCHI, T. *Causes of Delinquency.* Berkeley, CA: University of California Press, 1969.

KANDEL, D.B. Adolescent marihuana use: Role of parents and peers. *Science* 181: 1067-1069, 1973.

KANDEL, D.B. Interpersonal influence on adolescent illegal drug use. In E. Josephson and Eleanor E. Carroll (eds.), *Drug Use: Epidemiological and Sociological Approaches.* Washington, DC: Wiley, 1974.

KANDEL, D.B., TREIMAN, D., FAUST, R., and SINGLE, E. Adolescent involvement in legal and illegal drug use: A multiple classification analysis. *Soc. Forces* 55(2): 438-458, 1976.

KERLINGER, F.N. *Foundations of Behavioral Research.* New York: Holt, Rinehart, and Winston, 1973.

KILLWORTH, P.D., and BERNARD, H.R. Informant accuracy in social network data. *Human Org.* 35(3): 269-286, 1976.

KILLWORTH, P.D., and BERNARD, H.R. Informant accuracy in social network data. III. *Soc. Networks* 2(1): 19-46, 1979.

LINDESMITH, A. A sociological theory of drug addiction. *Am. J. Sociol.* 43: 593-613, 1938.

MANGANIELLO, J.A. Opiate addiction: A study identifying three systematically related psychological correlates. *Int. J. Addict.* 13(5): 839-847, 1978.

MITCHELL, J.C. *Social Networks in Urban Situations.* Manchester, England: Manchester University Press, 1969.

NATIONAL INSTITUTE ON DRUG ABUSE. *Nonresidential Self-Help Organizations and the Drug Abuse Problem: An Exploratory Conference.* Washington, DC: U.S. Government Printing Office, 1978.

PATTISON, E.M., DE FRANCISCO, D., WOOD, P., FRAZIER, H., and CROWDER, J.A. A psychosocial kinship model for family therapy. *Am. J. Psychiatry* 132(12): 1246-1251, 1979.

PHILLIPS, S.L. Network characteristics related to the wellbeing of normals: A comparative base. *Schizophrenia Bull.* 7(1): 117-123, 1981.

PITTEL, S.M Psychosocial aspects of heroin and other drug dependence. *J. Psychedelic Drugs* 4: 40-45, 1971.

PREBLE, E., and CASEY, J.J. Taking care of business: The heroin user's life on the streets. *Int. J. Addict.* 4(1): 1-24, 1969.

RASOR, R. Narcotics addicts: Personality characteristics and hospital treatment. In P. Hock and J. Zubin (eds.), *Problems of Addiction and Habituation.* New York: Grune and Stratton, 1958.

SOKOLOVSKY, J., COHEN, C., BERGER, D., and GEIGER, J. Personal networks of ex-mental patients in a Manhattan SRO hotel. *Human Org.* 37(1): 5-15, 1978.

TREECE, C., and NICOHOLSON, B. DSM-III personality type and dose level in methadone maintenance patients. *J. Nerv. Ment. Dis.* 168(10): 621-628, 1980.

WALDORF, D. *Rock Bottom: Careers in Dope.* Englewood Cliffs, NJ: Prentice-Hall, 1973.

WALDORF, D., and BIERNACKI, P.F. The natural recovery from opiate addiction: Some preliminary findings. *J. Drug Issues* 11(1): 61-74, 1981.

WHITEHEAD, P.C., and SMART, R.G. Validity and reliability of self-reported drug use. *Can. J. Criminol. Correction* 14: 1-7, 1972.

WILLIAMS, J.H., SCOTT, A., STOUT, J., and HERTZEL, R. The relationship between assertiveness, conformity, and drug use. *J. Drug Educ.* 11(1): 47-51, 1981.

The International Journal of the Addictions, 19(8), 919–923, 1984

Note

A Communication Approach to Drug Use Intervention

Stanley Einstein,* PhD

Middle Eastern Summer Institute on Drug Use

Abstract

A schema has been designed to enable intervention planners to more functionally select, and to more effectively utilize a communication model for drug use/misuse intervention which is suitable for the focus of their efforts and which meets the necessary demands of *prevention, education, training,* and *information dissemination.*

Drug education is a communication approach to drug use intervention. It is a general heading which includes a variety of types of programs. These programs can be categorized in the following ways: *prevention, education, training,* and *information dissemination.*

The programs or approaches of each type are suited to particular goals and target populations, are associated with the use of certain techniques which are most effective in particular places, demand specific staff who are knowledgeable in certain skills, must be carried out for specific periods of time, need the help and cooperation of certain types of agency and community support systems, and are associated with varied criteria for judging success and failure over time.

For example, *education* is a process by which a heterogeneous or homogeneous group becomes the focus of certain goals and techniques applied by educators, and terminates this process as a heterogeneous group. *Training*, on the other hand, is a process by which a group (heterogeneous or homogeneous) is aided by skilled trainers-technicians in becoming a homogeneous one for

*Address correspondence to the author at 113/41 East Talpiot, Jerusalem, Israel.

 0020-773X/84/1908-0919$3.50/0

specific behaviors, skills, abilities, attitudes, values, etc. *Information dissemination* is an event or process in which specific information is communicated by a "media" specialist. Whether this information is understood, integrated, and/or used is often not known or even evaluatable. *Prevention* may be an ideology, a goal, technique, or process, designed to affect drugs and/or their effects, drug use or abstinence, behavior, or life-styles.

These distinctions are not minor ones nor semantic ones when one considers that current programs are designed to:

1. Reinforce certain patterns of drug use (healthy use of medicines)
2. Inhibit other patterns and types of drug use (unacceptable use of medicines and the use of "drugs")
3. Facilitate non-drug-use-related values, behaviors, and life-styles

To date the various approaches which have been developed under the general heading of *drug education* can be categorized into the various "models" listed in Table 1. Although these "models" have mainly been used with youth, and mostly in Western cultures, they are not unique to specific ages, sexes, or countries/cultures. They are "models" in the sense that each of them is based upon particular assumptions regarding the etiology of drug use and its prevention. These "models" in no way encompass the variety of programs which we

Table 1

Categorizing the Primary Prevention Process by Focus[a]

Individual focus	Interpersonal focus	Systemic focus
Self-esteem	Communication skills	Racism
Values clarification	Peer influence	Sexism
Norm setting	Role delineation	Power
Decision making	Interpersonal/group rituals	Economic
Problem solving	Simulation	Policy making
Counseling	Status enhancement	Culture
Coping skills	Empathy training	Media
Adaptation skills		Institutions
Functioning skills		Social structures
Attitude confrontation		Environments
Affective education		Communities
Self-evaluation		
Scare techniques		
Factual drug information dissemination		
Natural high(s)		
Life-styles		

[a]Preventing drug use and its various consequences (primary prevention) is a multifocus process and effort. We may choose to focus upon the individual, interpersonal factors, or upon systems. Each focus brings with it its own traditions, goals, strategies, techniques, staff, sites for intervention, and policies, as well as desirable and undesirable outcomes.

can develop. They are simply examples of what others have done to date. Their primary effect upon us is twofold: They permit us to discover how we can become involved in a program suitable to our needs and roles, and they act as conceptual catalysts for developing other types of programs.

Table 2 summarizes a selected number of independent factors which affect communication-based/related program effectiveness. Table 3 is designed as a conceptual tool to permit us to analyze what minimal program factors must be considered when using a specific communication model. Our task is to define and to select the needed program factors, to understand their meaning(s), utility, and limitations within a usable communication program which is evaluatable. Since communication—verbal as well as nonverbal—is an integral part of healthy human adaptation, as well as being a significant factor in maladaptation, we should permit ourselves to develop needed effective models and programs for drug use intervention.

Table 2

Independent Factors Affecting Drug Education Program Effectiveness

Source factors:	• Expertness (knowledge, status, values, interests, ethnicity, age, drug use/misuse experience and status) • Reliability • Intentions • Activeness • Personal attractiveness • The majority opinion of the listener's associates • Non-status threatening • Control of information sources and dissemination (total control → no control)
Message factors:	• Content (one sided, two sided, multifaceted, fear arousing, neutral)
Channel factors:	• Medium impact • Exposure time
Receiver factors:	• Age • Sex • Intelligence • Education level • Anxiety • Active versus passive participation • Level(s) of suggestibility • Drug use/misuse status and experience
Destination factors:	• Longevity of effect and rate(s) of decay • Sleeper effects • Behavior commitment • Behavior change orientation • Attitude change orientation

Table 3

A Communication Approach to Drug Use Intervention

Types of models	Type of strategy: ______	Time to initiate	Target population	Goals	Policies	Needed knowledge	Techniques	Site	Temporal aspects	Staff	Needed support system	Ongoing evaluation	Outcome criteria: success/ failure
Self-esteem													
Values clarification													
Norm setting													
Decision making													
Problem solving													
Coping skills													
Adaptation skills													
Attitude confrontation													
Affective education													
Self-examination													
Roles and status development/ reinforcement													
Role playing													
Creation of new cognitive structures													

Logical arguments	
Appeal to authority (individual, group, institution, tradition, experience)	
Negative reinforcement (scare techniques)	
Simulation (drama, art, etc.)	
Role playing	
Life-style evaluation and confrontation	
Empathy training	
Communication skills	
Factual drug information	
Other: specify ________ ________ ________	

The International Journal of the Addictions, 19(8), 925–929, 1984

Note

Drug Use Community Intervention: Issues and Options

Stanley Einstein,* PhD

Middle Eastern Summer Institute on Drug Use

Abstract

A schema has been designed for intervention planners to facilitate their effective use of the concept/entity of *community*, in its variety of types, meanings, and implications, for drug use/misuse intervention.

THE BACKGROUND

During the 1950s *the community*, as a concept, process, and entity, was rediscovered as a factor leading to mental, physical, and social problems as well as being recognized as a critical factor for effective intervention. The terms used were *community mental health* and *community health*. These terms, and the world view underlying them, resulted in the creation of treatment sites/programs called "community mental health centers," "crisis intervention centers," and "community health centers." Both drug use and alcoholism were viewed as legitimate concerns for community intervention.

From this perspective effective drug use/medication misuse community intervention is possible if we come to terms with the following critical factors:

1. Definitions of *drugs and their consequences*
2. Definitions of *drug use and misuse*
3. Definitions of *sickness, pathology, and health*
4. Definitions of *community*
5. Selection and definition of reasonable *criteria for success and failure*

*Address correspondence to the author at 113/41 East Talpiot, Jerusalem, Israel.

 0020-773X/84/1908-0925$3.50/0

6. Acknowledgment of (a) the *multiplicity of factors* which may reinforce, inhibit, or be irrelevant for any of man's chemical appetites; and (b) the state of political, economic, and social affairs at any given point in time

The major consequence of the four classical sources of drug definitions (religious-social, medical, legal, and scientific) is that the condemning or condoning of specific types of drugs or types of drug use is related not to their actual dangers but rather to social-political-economic decision making. The major consequence of analyzing definitions of drug use and misuse, sickness, pathology, and health, and the community, is the finding that none of these concepts is homogeneous even though they continue to be thought of in such a manner. The major challenge to community drug intervention program planners and to citizens engaged in community intervention is to develop the necessary frameworks which will permit them to choose roles that are consonant with their abilities as well as their interests.

There is no such entity as "The Community Drug Intervention Program." The sooner we recognize this—and go on to develop programs which are meaningful, achievable, acceptable, and flexible as well as necessary—the sooner we can divest ourselves of the sham which all too often continues to pass for community intervention.

THE COMMUNITY: CONCEPTS, ENTITIES, AND OPTIONS

Many of us, when we hear or read the term *community* know what it is. But if we really are to develop useful and effective community drug use/misuse intervention programs, we should be aware of the many meanings which have been and continue to be associated with *community*, as well as the actual and potential implications of these meanings. Table 1 briefly summarizes 12 types of communities. You the reader can no doubt add other definitive types of communities which could serve as a reasonable and needed basis for developing some type of community-based/related intervention program. What is at stake is that once we understand the broad variety of actual as well as potential communities, we should be able to better select and develop appropriate programs.

Table 2 is designed to help the reader think about, analyze, and then to determine the type of drug use/misuse community intervention program which seems to be most reasonable and suitable. Drug use community intervention is more than just another type of option. It clearly and dramatically reminds us that drug use does not exist in a vacuum, away from us. Nor is it simply the interaction between the users (whoever and whatever they are) and the drugs that they choose (prefer, or which are available). Drugs, drug use, and the drug users (as well as the abstainers) are developed, exist, continue, and disappear in

Table 1

Types of Communities

1. Territorial, geographical communities (building, street, region)	Crucial factor: Individuals identifying with a physical area for attitudinal and behavioral activity (e.g., neighborhood, town, city, nation, etc.)
2. Functional communities	Crucial factor: Various functions which people perform (e.g., artists, drivers, policy planners, law enforcement agents, MDs, therapists, etc.)
3. Organizational communities	Crucial factor: Membership in or identification with various organizations (e.g., unions, professional organizations, service groups, etc.)
4. Belief system communities	Commitment to or identification with particular belief systems (e.g., politicalisms, religious systems, drug use belief systems, abstinence belief systems, etc.)
5. Familial communities	Crucial factor: Membership in a blood-related family structure (e.g., primary family, extended family, etc.)
6. Legal communities	Crucial factor: The legal status and functions (e.g., profit and nonprofit corporations, law enforcement, etc.)
7. Political communities	Adherence to or identification with various political theories, organizations, and aspirations (e.g., political parties, philosophies, etc.)
8. Economic communities	Practice of or identification with economic theories or types of delivery systems (e.g., capitalism, communism, socialism, EEC, centrally directed delivery of services systems, laissez-faire delivery of services systems, etc.)
9. Mutual interdependence systems	Crucial factor: Going beyond the usual agreed upon community concepts to achieve a greater goal of mutual aid (e.g., EEC, ecumenical councils, UNESCO, WHO, etc.)
10. Common destiny communities	Crucial factor: Belief in and a sense of common destiny (e.g., age delineations such as under 30, retirees, Grey Panthers; counterculture; religious sects; visible street drug users; racism groups; etc.)
11. Symbolic communities	Crucial factor: Symbolic structuring of communities (e.g., humankind, youth culture, deviants, etc.)
12. Self-perception communities	Crucial factor: The person's view of him/herself (e.g., patriots, go-getters, passives, doers, recipients, abstainers, etc.)
13. Semantic-imputed communities	Crucial factor: The imputation, by self and/or others, of a "community" status, structure, function (e.g., "the community," "them," "the neighborhood," etc.)

Table 2

Drug Use Community Intervention

Type of community model	Area for intervention	Type of strategy	Time to initiate	Goals	Policies	Needed knowledge	Techniques/ materials	Sites	Temporal aspects	Staff	Needed support systems	Ongoing evaluation	Criteria for success/ failure
Territorial													
Functional													
Organizational													
Belief system													
Familial													
Legal													
Political													
Economic													
Mutual interdependence													
Common destiny													
Symbolic													
Self-perception													
Semantic imputed													
Other: specify ________ ________ ________													

many communities which are part of our own life-styles. Therefore effective intervention *demands of us* a willingness to consider *community* as an integral part of what we plan and do. In doing so we have responsibility to determine and to select our own roles, responsibilities, obligations, and rights. We cannot live without communities. Obviously, without us there are no communities—neither as concepts nor entities. Equally obvious is that drug use, drug misuse, or abstinence does not, cannot exist outside of the various communities that have been defined in this note—and not without our active or passive involvement.

The International Journal of the Addictions, 19(8), 931–936, 1984

Note

Drug Use Intervention with and for Special Populations

Stanley Einstein,* PhD

Middle Eastern Summer Institute on Drug Use

Abstract

A schema has been designed to enable intervention planners to more reasonably and effectively integrate the concept of *special populations*, its varied meanings and their implications, and to better meet the special/unique needs of individuals and systems in drug use/misuse intervention programs.

In the good old days, when it was clear *who* the drug user was, as well as *what* he was using and *why*, one didn't have to worry or even think about "them." Someone, generally not us, reacted to *them* for us. We just footed the bill. But times have changed—perhaps even forever. Now instead of *the drug user* we are made aware, almost constantly, of young ones including newborn "addicts"; old ones; black ones, white ones, and red ones; poor ones, middle-class and rich ones; educated ones; illiterates; males, females, heterosexuals, and homosexuals; etc.—in simple terms: different populations. And different populations, just like different individuals, may have (or do have) special/unique needs. Such needs, whatever they are, cannot be met, at least not adequately, by continuing to use a single homogenizing concept such as *the drug user.* Under such circumstances it becomes useful to introduce the idea of drug use intervention with and for special populations. It should be obvious to the reader that the groups we include under *special populations* and the criteria which we use to determine them are totally our own choice. The examples given may not satisfy the reader. If this is so, simply add to, delete from, or change what is listed in Table 1.

*Address correspondence to the author at 113/41 East Talpiot, Jerusalem, Israel.

 0020-773X/84/1908-0931$3.50/0

Table 1

Intervening with Special Populations: 16 Selected Program Factors, by Selected Typologies of Special Populations

	A: Program factors 1-8							
Selected criteria for categorizing special populations	Why intervene?	Who intervenes?	Budget	Target population	Policies	Strategies	Assessment process	Intervention site(s)
Responsivity to intervention: compliant/noncompliant								
Potential for change								
Intellectual status: abilities/ functioning								
Motivational status								
Geographical status: close/ distant								
Parenting status								
Health status								

Economic status: self-support/ public-other support	
Race/ethnicity	
Sex role	
Statistical proportions	
Power/powerlessness	
Stigma/discrimination	
Cultural differences	
Status: alienation/integration	
Beliefs: religious/secular	
Status: legal	
Theoretical concepts ("at risk")	

Table 1 (continued)

Selected criteria for categorizing special populations	B: Program factors 9-16							
	Goals	Techniques	Intervention agent(s)	Roles	Needed support system(s)	Ongoing evaluation	Follow-up/ outcome	Outreach/early case finding
Responsivity to intervention: compliant/noncompliant								
Potential for change								
Intellectual status: abilities/ functioning								
Motivational status								
Geographical status: close/ distant								
Parenting status								
Health status								

Economic status: self-support/
public-other support

Race/ethnicity

Sex role

Statistical proportions

Power/powerlessness

Stigma/discrimination

Cultural differences

Status: alienation/integration

Beliefs: religious/secular

Status: legal

Theoretical concepts ("at risk")

Table 1 (parts A and B) schematizes a selected number of types of special populations by a selected number of types of intervention factors. What is critical for intervention planning is to learn whether the basic factors differ greatly, little, or not at all, when we focus on the special attributes as well as needs of different types of populations.

If indeed *special populations* is not simply a didactic concept, but a dynamic series of structures and systems which may or may not be related, we will be challenged to develop specific intervention models which are suitable for a specific population. If, on the other hand, there is a basic formulation for intervention, and if the uniqueness of the population is a secondary or minor issue, fewer types of models will be needed.

The reader is asked to "play" with Table 1. The "game" is worthwhile. In the West the increasing uniqueness of special populations has been acknowledged. Their unique needs are being researched. Articles and books are being published. Lectures, workshops, and conferences are being held with greater frequency. And yet there appears to be little evidence that the quality of intervention has been improved or that the outcome is any better than it was when we were unaware of special groups and their needs.

Whatever the truth is regarding the *role* and actual as well as potential *meaning(s)* of *special populations* as a concept, tool, or factor in drug use intervention planning and programs, we certainly owe it to ourselves to be aware of it and its various implications. In the process of doing this we should raise the issue of how important it is that we continue to separate the drug user from the rest of the population—from us.

The International Journal of the Addictions, 19(8), 937–956, 1984

Cumulative Index
International Journal of the Addictions
Volume 19

SECTION 1, AUTHOR-TITLE LIST

Issue No.	Page	Author	Title
19:1	iii	S. Einstein	Editorial: Coping and Drug Misuse Intervention
	1	N. Ben-Yehuda S. Einstein	Human Garbage and Physical Garbage: A Sociological Case Example of Institutional Violence
	25	N. R. Mann V. C. Charuvastra V. K. Murthy	A Diagnostic Tool with Important Implications for Treatment of Addiction: Identification of Factors Underlying Relapse and Remission Time Distributions
	45	R. M. Costello K. A. Wicoff	Impression Management and Testing for Control Locus in an Alcoholic Sample
	57	J. D. Swisher T.-W. Hu	A Review of the Reliability and Validity of the Drug Abuse Warning Network
	79	J. Sexter A. P. Sullivan S. F. Wepner R. Denmark	Substance Abuse: Assessment of the Outcomes of Activities and Activity Clusters in School-Based Prevention
	93	J. A. Woodward R. L. Retka L. Ng	Construct Validity of Heroin Abuse Estimators
19:2	iii	S. Einstein	Editorial: Considering the Risks of "Populations at Risk"

Issue No.	Page	Author	Title
19:2	119	J. V. Spotts F. C. Shontz	Drug-Induced Ego States. I. Cocaine: Phenomenology and Implications
	153	L. S. Aiken L. A. LoSciuto M. A. Ausetts B. S. Brown	Paraprofessional Versus Professional Drug Counselors: Diverse Routes to the Same Role
	175	W. R. Blount R. Dembo	The Effect of Perceived Neighborhood Setting on Self-Reported Tobacco, Alcohol, and Marijuana Use among Inner-City Minority Junior High School Youth
	199	F. Suffet R. Brotman	A Comprehensive Care Program for Pregnant Addicts: Obstetrical, Neonatal, and Child Development Outcomes
	221	R. R. Blanck N. W. Ream J. S. Deleese	Infectious Complications of Illicit Drug Use
19:3	iii	S. Einstein	Editorial: Drug Use Intervention and Control Mechanisms
	233	L. LoSciuto L. S. Aiken M. A. Ausetts B. S. Brown	Paraprofessional Versus Professional Drug Abuse Counselors: Attitudes and Expectations of the Counselors and Their Clients
	253	O. E. Achalu D. F. Duncan	Drug Taking by Nigerian Students in American Universities: Prevalences for Four Commonly Used Drugs
	265	R. T. Dull	An Empirical Examination of the Social Bond Theory of Drug Use
	287	L. Eriksen K. G. Götestam	Conditioned Abstinence in Alcoholics: A Controlled Experiment
	295	J. V. Spotts F. C. Shontz	The Phenomenological Structure of Drug-Induced Ego States. II. Barbiturates and Sedative-Hypnotics: Phenomenology and Implications
	327	H. H. Dawley, Jr. B. J. Fleischer L. T. Dawley	Smoking Cessation with Hospital Employees: An Example of Worksite Smoking Cessation

Issue No.	Page	Author	Title
19:3	335	A. Cohen	The "Urge to Classify" the Narcotic Addict: A Review of Psychiatric Classification. II.
	355	S. Einstein	Drug Misuse/Abuse Intervention: A Schematic Tool for Decision Making and Planning
19:4	iii	S. Einstein	Editorial: Preventing Change through Current Substance Use Intervention: A Role Analysis
	367	R. Larson M. Csikszentmihalyi M. Freeman	Alcohol and Marijuana Use in Adolescents' Daily Lives: A Random Sample of Experiences
	383	L. S. Aiken L. A. LoSciuto M. A. Ausetts B. S. Brown	Paraprofessional Versus Professional Drug Counselors: The Progress of Clients in Treatment
	403	E. J. Futch S. A. Lisman M. I. Geller	An Analysis of Alcohol Portrayal on Prime-Time Television
	411	M. T. Malcolm	Alcohol and Drug Use in the Elderly Visited at Home
	419	J. M. Moskowitz E. Schaps G. A. Schaeffer J. H. Malvin	Evaluation of a Substance Abuse Prevention Program for Junior High School Students
	431	P. M. Moody	Human Smoking Patterns and Smoke Deliveries
	441	D. N. Nurco J. W. Shaffer I. H. Cisin	An Ecological Analysis of the Interrelationships among Drug Abuse and Other Indices of Social Pathology
	453	W. M. Allison D. W. A. Jerrom	Glue Sniffing: A Pilot Study of the Cognitive Effects of Long-Term Use
	459	P. M. Flynn R. C. McMahon	An Examination of the Drug Abuse Scale of the Millon Clinical Multiaxial Inventory
	469	S. Einstein	Drug Use Intervention and Individual/Group Adaptation: Facilitation of Coping in Potential Worlds of Adaptation
	475	S. Einstein	An Experiential Model for Drug Use Intervention

Issue No.	Page	Author	Title
19:5	479	M. S. Goldstein M. Surber D. M. Wilner	Outcome Evaluations in Substance Abuse: A Comparison of Alcoholism, Drug Abuse, and Other Mental Health Interventions
	503	C. C. Presson L. Chassin S. J. Sherman R. Olshavsky M. Bensenberg E. Corty	Predictors of Adolescents' Intentions to Smoke: Age, Sex, Race, and Regional Differences
	521	C. J. Rogalski	Professional Psychotherapy and Its Relationship to Compliance in Treatment
	541	B. Segal S. S. Hobfoll F. Cromer	Alcohol Use by Juvenile Offenders
	551	I. Vogt	Defining Alcohol Problems as a Repressive Mechanism: Its Formative Phase in Imperial Germany and Its Strength Today
	571	K. E. Friend P. A. Koushki	Student Substance Use: Stability and Change across College Years
	577	M. R. Haack T. C. Harford	Drinking Patterns among Student Nurses
	585	R. A. Holland R. C. Evenson	Prediction of Readmission in a Cohort of Alcoholics: A 2-Year Follow-Up
	591	S. Einstein	A Task Approach to Drug Use Intervention
	595	S. Einstein	A Functional Approach to Drug Use Intervention
19:6	601	S. D. Robinson	Women and Alcohol Abuse—Factors Involved in Successful Interventions
	613	S. M. Hall	The Abstinence Phobias: Links between Substance Abuse and Anxiety
	633	H. L. Voss R. R. Clayton	"Turning on" Other Persons to Drugs
	653	M. L. Waring G. Petraglia L. Cohen E. Busby	Alcohol Use among Graduate Business Administration Students

Issue No.	Page	Author	Title
19:6	665	R. J. Craig	Can Personality Tests Predict Treatment Dropouts?
	675	R. J. Battjes	Symbolic Interaction Theory: A Perspective on Drug Abuse and Its Treatment
	689	R. O. Pihl M. Smith B. Farrell	Individual Characteristics of Aggressive Beer and Distilled Beverage Drinkers
	697	S. Einstein	Considering Motivation and Ability for Drug Use Intervention: Some Implications
	701	S. Einstein	Outcome of Drug User Treatment: A Selection of Additional Needed Factors
19:7	709	E. B. Fink S. Rudden R. Longabaugh B. McCrady R. Stout	Adherence in a Behavioral Alcohol Treatment Program
	721	M. S. Goodstadt A. Caleekal-John	Alcohol Education Programs for University Students: A Review of Their Effectiveness
	743	K. M. Synol	Family Mapping: Toward an Understanding of the Interactional Dynamic of the Alcoholic Marital Dyad
	753	L. W. Whorley	Social Recovery and Therapeutic Mission
	767	R. Cook H. Lawrence C. Morse J. Roehl	An Evaluation of the Alternatives Approach to Drug Abuse Prevention
	789	B. J. F. Reed P. A. May	Inhalant Abuse and Juvenile Delinquency: A Control Study in Albuquerque, New Mexico
	805	C. A. Preston L. L. Viney	Self- and Ideal-Self-Perception of Drug Addicts in Therapeutic Communities
	819	D. W. Reeves T. W. Draper	Abstinence or Decreasing Consumption among Adolescents: Importance of Reasons
19:8	827	E. M. Morrell J. G. Hollandsworth, Jr.	Nicotine Level as a Predictor of Smoking Frequency: A Case Report

Issue No.	Page	Author	Title
19:8	833	C. Sandahl	Determinants of Relapse among Alcoholics: A Cross-Cultural Replication Study
	849	D. Royse K. Drude	Screening Drug Abuse Clients with the Brief Symptom Inventory
	859	J. C. Dean F. Rud	The Drug Addict and the Stigma of Addiction
	871	W. P. Kory L. A. Crandall	Nonmedical Drug Use Patterns among Medical Students
	885	R. N. Bale B. H. Arnoldussen A. M. Quittner	Follow-Up Difficulty with Substance Abusers: Predictors of Time to Locate and Relationship to Outcome
	903	M. W. Fraser J. D. Hawkins	The Social Networks of Opioid Abusers
	919	S. Einstein	A Communication Approach to Drug Use Intervention
	925	S. Einstein	Drug Use Community Intervention: Issues and Options
	931	S. Einstein	Drug Use Intervention with and for Special Populations

SECTION 2, SUBJECT INDEX

This subject index follows the format of the National Library of Medicine's *Index Medicus.* Headings have been added.

Entries take this form: volume and number, senior author, first page of article. For example, 19:6 Einstein (697) refers to the article "Considering Motivation and Ability for Drug Use Intervention: Some Implications," by S. Einstein, found in issue 6 of this volume, beginning on page 697. From this section of the index, reference can be made to Section 1 for the full title and authors of a particular article.

All original contributions to *The International Journal of the Addictions*, Volume 19, are indexed. Book reviews and communications are not included.

Ability for drug use intervention
19:6 Einstein (697)
Abstinence–Conditioned abstinence in alcoholics
19:3 Eriksen (287)
Abstinence–Time distributions
19:1 Mann (25)
Abstinence from alcohol–Reasons in adolescents
19:7 Reeves (819)
Abstinence phobias in substance abuse
19:6 Hall (613)
Adaptation–Intervention goals
19:4 Einstein (469)
Adherence
See also Compliance; Dropout
Adherence–Behavioral alcohol treatment
19:7 Fink (709)
Adolescent daily life–Alcohol and marijuana use
19:4 Larson (367)
Adolescents–Inhalant abuse and delinquency
19:7 Reed (789)
Adolescents–Reasons for abstinence from alcohol
19:7 Reeves (819)
Adolescents–Reasons for alcohol use
19:5 Segal (541)
Adolescent smoking intentions–Predictors
19:5 Presson (503)
Adults
See also Elderly medical patients; Graduate business administration students
Adults–Social bonds and drug use
19:3 Dull (265)
Africa
See Nigerian students in the U.S.
Age
See also Elderly medical patients
Age differences in adolescent smoking intentions
19:5 Presson (503)
Aggression in social drinkers
19:6 Pihl (689)
Albuquerque, NM–Inhalant abuse
19:7 Reed (789)
Alcohol abstinence–Reasons in adolescents
19:7 Reeves (819)
Alcohol abuse–Anxiety relationship
19:6 Hall (613)
Alcohol abusers–Women
19:6 Robinson (601)
Alcohol education–University students
19:7 Goodstadt (721)
Alcoholic marital dyads–Interactional dynamics
19:7 Synol (743)
Alcoholics–Conditioned abstinence
19:3 Eriksen (287)
Alcoholics–Follow-up difficulties
19:8 Bale (885)
Alcoholics–Impression management and control locus
19:1 Costello (45)
Alcoholics–Prediction of recidivism
19:5 Holland (585)
Alcoholics–Relapse determinants
19:8 Sandahl (833)
Alcoholism outcome evaluation–Methodology
19:5 Goldstein (479)

Alcohol portrayal on TV
19:4 Futch (403)
Alcohol problems–Definitions as repressive mechanisms
19:5 Vogt (551)
Alcohol treatment–Adherence
19:7 Fink (709)
Alcohol use–Adolescent daily life
19:4 Larson (367)
Alcohol use–Aggression in social drinkers
19:6 Pihl (689)
Alcohol use–Elderly medical patients
19:4 Malcolm (411)
Alcohol use–Graduate business administration students
19:6 Waring (653)
Alcohol use–Neighborhood perception effects
19:2 Blount (175)
Alcohol use–Nigerian students
19:3 Achalu (253)
Alcohol use–Self-reported reasons in juvenile offenders
19:5 Segal (541)
Alcohol use–Social bond effects
19:3 Dull (265)
Alcohol use–Stability across college years
19:5 Friend (571)
Alcohol use–Student nurses
19:5 Haack (577)
Alternatives approach–Alcohol education
19:7 Goodstadt (721)
Alternatives approach–Drug abuse prevention
19:7 Cook (767)
Amphetamine use–Nigerian students
19:3 Achalu (253)
Amphetamine use–Social bond effects
19:3 Dull (265)
Antecedents
See also Determinants
Antecedents to alcohol use–TV portrayal
19:4 Futch (403)
Assessment
See also Diagnostic instruments; Screening
Assessment–Alcoholic dyads
19:7 Synol (743)
Assessment–Elderly medical patients
19:4 Malcolm (411)
Attention in long-term glue sniffers
19:4 Allison (453)
Attitudes–Alcohol education effects
19:7 Goodstadt (721)
Attitudes–Alternatives prevention program effects
19:7 Cook (767)
Attitudes–Counselors and clients
19:3 LoSciuto (233)

Baltimore–Drug abuse and social pathology
19:4 Nurco (441)
Barbiturate-induced ego states
19:3 Spotts (295)
Barbiturate use–Social bond effects
19:3 Dull (265)
Beer drinkers–Aggression scores
19:6 Pihl (689)
Behavior–Alcohol education effects
19:7 Goodstadt (721)
Behavior–Alternatives prevention program effects
19:7 Cook (767)
Behavioral alcohol treatment–Adherence
19:7 Fink (709)
Behavioral consequences of alcohol use–TV portrayal
19:4 Futch (403)
Behavioral correlates in drug use transmission
19:6 Voss (633)
Behavioral responses to alcohol-related stimuli
19:3 Eriksen (287)
Behavior of drug abusers–Symbolic interaction analysis
19:6 Battjes (675)
Black youth–Neighborhood perceptions and substance use
19:2 Blount (175)
Bonding
See Social bond theory
Brief Symptom Inventory in drug abuser screening
19:8 Royse (849)
Business administration students–Drinking patterns
19:6 Waring (653)

Capture-recapture estimation of heroin abuse
19:1 Woodward (93)
Care program for pregnant addicts
19:2 Suffet (199)
Case studies
See Representative Case Method
Causality–Barbiturate and sedative-hypnotic users
19:3 Spotts (295)
Causality–Cocaine effects
19:2 Spotts (119)
Census tract analysis of drug abuse and social pathology
19:4 Nurco (441)
Change prevention in intervention (editorial)
19:4 Einstein (iii)
Change in self-concept–Addicts in treatment
19:7 Preston (805)
Change in substance use across college years
19:5 Friend (571)
Characteristics of aggressive drinkers
19:6 Pihl (689)
Characteristics of drug abusers–Symbolic interaction analysis
19:6 Battjes (675)
Characteristics of drug use transmitters
19:6 Voss (633)
Child development outcome in pregnant addict care
19:2 Suffet (199)
Civic functioning as measure of social recovery
19:7 Whorley (753)
Classification of narcotic addicts
19:3 Cohen (335)
Classroom program
See Effective Classroom Management
Client attitudes and expectations
19:3 LoSciuto (233)
Client progress–Counselor effects
19:4 Aiken (383)
Clinical assessment
See also Diagnostic instruments
Clinical assessment–Dropout prediction
19:6 Craig (665)
Clinical characteristics and adherence in treatment
19:7 Fink (709)
Cocaine-induced ego states
19:2 Spotts (119)
Cocaine use transmission
19:6 Voss (633)
Cognitive effects–Glue sniffing
19:4 Allison (453)
Cognitive functioning–Barbiturate and sedative-hypnotic users
19:3 Spotts (295)
Cognitive functioning–Cocaine effects
19:2 Spotts (119)
College student drug use–Nigerians in the U.S.
19:3 Achalu (253)
College students
See also Graduate business administration students; Medical students; Nursing students
College students–Alcohol education
19:7 Goodstadt (721)
College students–Stability of substance use
19:5 Friend (571)
Communication approach to drug use intervention
19:8 Einstein (919)
Community intervention for drug use
19:8 Einstein (925)
Community-treatment program relations–Israel
19:1 Ben-Yehuda (1)
Competing-risk distribution of relapse and remission
19:1 Mann (25)
Compliance
See also Adherence
Compliance in treatment–Psychotherapy effects
19:5 Rogalski (521)
Concepts of alcohol problems as repressive mechanisms
19:5 Vogt (551)
Concepts of community
19:8 Einstein (925)
Concepts of drug addiction–General population
19:8 Dean (859)

Conditioned abstinence–Alcoholics
19:3 Eriksen (287)
Consistency–Millon Inventory Drug Abuse Scale scoring
19:4 Flynn (459)
Construct validity–Heroin abuse estimators
19:1 Woodward (93)
Control groups in outcome evaluation
19:5 Goldstein (479)
Control mechanisms in intervention (editorial)
19:3 Einstein (iii)
Control theory
See Social bond theory
Coping–Individual and institutional (editorial)
19:1 Einstein (iii)
Coping–Intervention goals
19:4 Einstein (469)
Coping as reason for alcohol use
19:5 Segal (541)
Corporate administrators–Drinking patterns
19:6 Waring (653)
Correlates of early treatment termination
19:7 Fink (709)
Counselors–Paraprofessional vs professional
19:2 Aiken (153)
19:3 LoSciuto (233)
19:4 Aiken (383)
Criminal activity–Adolescent inhalant abusers
19:7 Reed (789)
Cross-cultural study of alcoholic relapse
19:8 Sandahl (833)

Daily adolescent life–Alcohol and marijuana use
19:4 Larson (367)
Data-gathering procedures–DAWN
19:1 Swisher (57)
Decision making for intervention
19:3 Einstein (355)
Definitions of alcohol problems as repressive mechanisms
19:5 Vogt (551)
Delinquency
See Juvenile delinquency
Demographic characteristics – Inhalant abusers
19:7 Reed (789)
Demographic variables–Adolescent smoking intentions
19:5 Presson (503)
Demographic variables and social bonds–Adults
19:3 Dull (265)
Design problems
See Research design problems
Determinants
See also Antecedents
Determinants of relapse–Alcoholics
19:8 Sandahl (833)
Development
See Child development
Deviance in drug abuse etiology
19:6 Battjes (675)
Deviance label and institutional violence
19:1 Ben-Yehuda (1)
Diagnostic instruments–Brief Symptom Inventory
19:8 Royse (849)
Diagnostic instruments–Drug Abuse Scale of Millon Inventory
19:4 Flynn (459)
Disease concept in public images of drug addicts
19:8 Dean (859)
Distilled beverage drinkers–Aggression scores
19:6 Pihl (689)
Dropout
See also Adherence; Outcome
Dropout–Personality test prediction
19:6 Craig (665)
Drug abuse–Alternatives approach to prevention
19:7 Cook (767)
Drug abuse–Social pathology relationship
19:4 Nurco (441)
Drug abuse etiology–Symbolic interaction analysis
19:6 Battjes (675)
Drug abuse outcome evaluation–Methodology
19:5 Goldstein (479)
Drug abusers–Follow-up difficulties
19:8 Bale (885)

Drug abusers–Psychotherapy effect on compliance
19:5 Rogalski (521)
Drug abusers–Screening
19:8 Royse (849)
Drug abusers–Social networks
19:8 Fraser (903)
Drug Abuse Scale–Millon Clinical Multiaxial Inventory
19:4 Flynn (459)
Drug Abuse Warning Network–Data reliability and validity
19:1 Swisher (57)
Drug addicts–Dehumanization in treatment
19:1 Ben-Yehuda (1)
Drug addicts–Opiate
19:1 Mann (25)
Drug addicts–Public images
19:8 Dean (859)
Drug addicts–Self-perception changes in treatment
19:7 Preston (805)
Drug education for abuse prevention–Junior high school
19:4 Moskowitz (419)
Drug education models
19:8 Einstein (919)
Drug use–Adolescent daily life
19:4 Larson (367)
Drug use–Elderly medical patients
19:4 Malcolm (411)
Drug use–General adult population
19:3 Dull (265)
Drug use–Inner-city minority youth
19:2 Blount (175)
Drug use–Medical complications
19:2 Blanck (221)
Drug use–Medical students
19:8 Kory (871)
Drug use–Nigerian students in the U.S.
19:3 Achalu (253)
Drug use–Stability across college years
19:5 Friend (571)
Drug use intervention
See Intervention
Drug use transmission
19:6 Voss (633)
Dyads
See Alcoholic marital dyads
Dysfunction as factor in relapse
19:1 Mann (25)

Ecological analysis–Drug abuse and social pathology
19:4 Nurco (441)
Editorial–Control mechanisms
19:3 Einstein (iii)
Editorial–Coping by individuals and institutions
19:1 Einstein (iii)
Editorial–Intervention as obstacle to change
19:4 Einstein (iii)
Editorial–Risk/susceptibility
19:2 Einstein (iii)
Education
See Alcohol education; Drug education
Effective Classroom Management program for substance abuse prevention
19:4 Moskowitz (419)
Ego states–Barbiturate and sedative-hypnotic induced
19:3 Spotts (295)
Ego states–Cocaine induced
19:2 Spotts (119)
Elderly medical patients–Alcohol and drug use
19:4 Malcolm (411)
Emotionality–Barbiturate and sedative-hypnotic users
19:3 Spotts (295)
Emotionality–Cocaine effects
19:2 Spotts (119)
Endocarditis in drug users
19:2 Blanck (221)
Environment
See Ecological analysis; Perceived neighborhood setting
Epidemiology–Transmission of drug use
19:6 Voss (633)
Estimation of heroin abuse
19:1 Woodward (93)
Etiology of drug abuse–Symbolic interaction analysis
19:6 Battjes (675)
Europe
See Germany; Sweden

Evaluation
See Assessment; Treatment evaluation
Ex-addict counselors
19:2 Aiken (153)
19:3 LoSciuto (233)
19:4 Aiken (383)
Expectations–Counselors and clients
19:3 LoSciuto (233)
Expectations in treatment outcome
19:6 Einstein (701)
Experience Sampling Method study of adolescent drug use
19:4 Larson (367)
Experiential model for intervention
19:4 Einstein (475)
Externality
See Internal-external control locus

Factor analytic estimation of heroin abuse
19:1 Woodward (93)
Failure
See "Planned failure"
Familial functioning as measure of social recovery
19:7 Whorley (753)
Family mapping–Alcoholic dyads
19:7 Synol (743)
Family in treatment seeking by women
19:6 Robinson (601)
Follow-up difficulties–Substance abusers
19:8 Bale (885)
Follow-up in outcome evaluation
19:5 Goldstein (479)
Functional approach to drug use intervention
19:5 Einstein (595)

General population images of drug addicts
19:8 Dean (859)
Germany–Alcohol problem definitions and repression
19:5 Vogt (551)
Glue sniffing
See also Inhalant abuse
Glue sniffing–Cognitive effects
19:4 Allison (453)
Government data–DAWN
19:1 Swisher (57)
Government role in methadone distribution–Israel
19:1 Ben-Yehuda (1)
Graduate business administration students–Drinking patterns
19:6 Waring (653)
Group adaptation–Intervention goals
19:4 Einstein (469)

Health as motive for decreased alcohol use
19:7 Reeves (819)
Health professionals
See also Staff
Health professionals–Medical student drug use
19:8 Kory (871)
Health professionals–Nursing student drinking patterns
19:5 Haack (577)
Health professionals in treatment seeking by women
19:6 Robinson (601)
Hepatitis
See Viral hepatitis
Heroin abuse estimation
19:1 Woodward (93)
Heroin use transmission
19:6 Voss (633)
High school students–Alcohol and marijuana use
19:4 Larson (367)
History–Alcohol problem definitions
19:5 Vogt (551)
Home visits–Elderly medical patients
19:4 Malcolm (411)
Hospital employees–Smoking cessation program
19:3 Dawley (327)
Hypnotics
See Sedative-hypnotic induced ego states

Ideal-self-perceptions–Drug addicts in treatment
19:7 Preston (805)
Images of drug addicts
19:8 Dean (859)

Impression management and control locus–Alcoholics
19:1 Costello (45)
Individual adaptation–Intervention goals
19:4 Einstein (469)
Infectious complications of drug use
19:2 Blanck (221)
Inhalant abuse
See also Glue sniffing
Inhalant abuse and juvenile delinquency
19:7 Reed (789)
Inner-city minority youth–Neighborhood perceptions and substance use
19:2 Blount (175)
Institutional violence in methadone distribution
19:1 Ben-Yehuda (1)
Intelligence in long-term glue sniffers
19:4 Allison (453)
Intentions to smoke–Adolescents
19:5 Presson (503)
Interaction
See Symbolic interaction analysis
Interactional dynamics–Alcoholic marital dyads
19:7 Synol (743)
Interactional systems–Opioid abusers
19:8 Fraser (903)
Internal-external control locus–Alcoholics
19:1 Costello (45)
Interpersonal relations as therapeutic goals
19:7 Whorley (753)
Intervention
See also Treatment programs
Intervention–Change prevention factors (editorial)
19:4 Einstein (iii)
Intervention–Communication approach
19:8 Einstein (919)
Intervention–Community approach
19:8 Einstein (925)
Intervention–Control mechanisms (editorial)
19:3 Einstein (iii)
Intervention–Coping and adaptation goals
19:4 Einstein (469)
Intervention–Coping options (editorial)
19:1 Einstein (iii)
Intervention–Experiential model
19:4 Einstein (475)
Intervention–Functional approach
19:5 Einstein (595)
Intervention–Motivation and ability factors
19:6 Einstein (697)
Intervention–Potential areas and foci
19:3 Einstein (355)
Intervention–Special populations
19:8 Einstein (931)
Intervention–Task approach
19:5 Einstein (591)
Intervention–Women alcohol abusers
19:6 Robinson (601)
Israel–Methadone distribution
19:1 Ben-Yehuda (1)

Junior high school students–Neighborhood perceptions and substance use
19:2 Blount (175)
Junior high school students–Substance abuse prevention
19:4 Moskowitz (419)
Juvenile delinquency and inhalant abuse
19:7 Reed (789)
Juvenile offenders–Reasons for alcohol use
19:5 Segal (541)

Knowledge–Alcohol education effects
19:7 Goodstadt (721)

Location difficulty at follow-up
19:8 Bale (885)
Long-term glue sniffing–Cognitive effects
19:4 Allison (453)

Marijuana use–Adolescent daily life
19:4 Larson (367)
Marijuana use–Neighborhood perception effects
19:2 Blount (175)
Marijuana use–Nigerian students
19:3 Achalu (253)
Marijuana use–Social bond effects
19:3 Dull (265)

Marijuana use transmission
19:6 Voss (633)
Marital dyads–Alcoholics
19:7 Synol (743)
Materiality–Barbiturate and sedative-hypnotic users
19:3 Spotts (295)
Materiality–Cocaine effects
19:2 Spotts (119)
Measurement in outcome evaluation
19:5 Goldstien (479)
Media portrayal of alcohol use–TV
19:4 Futch (403)
Medical complications in drug use
19:2 Blanck (221)
Medical factors in treatment seeking by women
19:6 Robinson (601)
Medical students
See also Nursing students
Medical students–Drug use patterns
19:8 Kory (871)
Medication use by elderly patients
19:4 Malcolm (411)
Memory in long-term glue sniffers
19:4 Allison (453)
Men–Aggression in social drinkers
19:6 Pihl (689)
Mental health outcome evaluation–Methodology
19:5 Goldstein (479)
Methadone–Child development effects
19:2 Suffet (199)
Methadone distribution in Israel
19:1 Ben-Yehuda (1)
Methodology–DAWN data utilization
19:1 Swisher (57)
Methodology–Experience Sampling Method
19:4 Larson (367)
Methodology–Functional approach to intervention
19:5 Einstein (595)
Methodology–Heroin abuse estimation
19:1 Woodward (93)
Methodology–Intervention for coping and adaptation
19:4 Einstein (469)
Methodology–Intervention planning
19:3 Einstein (355)
Methodology–Location for follow-up
19:8 Bale (885)
Methodology–Outcome analysis
19:6 Einstein (701)
Methodology–Outcome evaluation
19:5 Goldstein (479)
Methodology–Task approach to intervention
19:5 Einstein (591)
Methodology–Testing alcoholics' locus of control
19:1 Costello (45)
Middle East
See Israel
Millon Clinical Multiaxial Inventory–Dropout prediction
19:6 Craig (665)
Millon Clinical Multiaxial Inventory–Drug Abuse Scale consistency
19:4 Flynn (459)
MMPI diagnosis of narcotic addicts
19:3 Cohen (335)
Models–Abstinence phobias
19:6 Hall (613)
Models–Drug education
19:8 Eisntein (919)
Models–Experiential intervention
19:4 Einstein (475)
Models–Prevention programs
19:1 Sexter (79)
Models–Structural equations for heroin abuse estimation
19:1 Woodward (93)
Mood alteration as reason for alcohol use
19:5 Segal (541)
Motivation for drug use intervention
19:6 Einstein (697)
Motivation as factor in abstinence and relapse
19:1 Mann (25)
Motivation for treatment seeking–Women alcohol abusers
19:6 Robinson (601)
Motives–Adolescent alcohol use
19:5 Segal (541)
Motives–Alcohol abstinence in adolescents
19:7 Reeves (819)

Narcotic abuse–Census tract analysis
19:4 Nurco (441)
Narcotic addicts–Psychiatric classification
19:3 Cohen (335)
Needle use role in medical complications
19:2 Blanck (221)
Neighborhood perception relationship to substance use
19:2 Blount (175)
Neonatal outcome in pregnant addict care
19:2 Suffet (199)
Networks
See Social networks
Neurosis in narcotic addicts
19:3 Cohen (335)
Nicotine delivery–Smoking pattern effects
19:4 Moody (431)
Nicotine level and smoking frequency
19:8 Morrell (827)
Nigerian students in the U.S.–Drug use prevalences
19:3 Achalu (253)
Nonmedical drug use–Medical students
19:8 Kory (871)
Nursing students
See also Medical students
Nursing students–Drinking patterns
19:5 Haack (577)

Obesity–Anxiety relationship
19:6 Hall (613)
Obstetrical outcome in pregnant addict care
19:2 Suffet (199)
Occupational functioning as measure of social recovery
19:7 Whorley (753)
Opiate abuse–Anxiety relationship
19:6 Hall (613)
Opiate addicts–Relapse and remission time distributions
19:1 Mann (25)
Opiate use transmission
19:6 Voss (633)
Opioid abusers–Social networks
19:8 Fraser (903)
Outcome
See also Dropout; Recidivism; Relapse
Outcome–Alcohol education
19:7 Goodstadt (721)
Outcome–Counselor effects
19:4 Aiken (383)
Outcome–Follow-up difficulty relationship
19:8 Bale (885)
Outcome–"Planned failure" (editorial)
19:4 Einstein (iii)
Outcome–Pregnant addict care
19:2 Suffet (199)
Outcome–School-based prevention
19:1 Sexter (79)
Outcome analysis–Methodology
19:6 Einstein (701)
Outcome evaluation–Methodology and rigor
19:5 Goldstein (479)

Paraprofessional vs professional counselors–Attitudes and expectations
19:3 LoSciuto (233)
Paraprofessional vs professional counselors–Client progress
19:4 Aiken (383)
Paraprofessional vs professional counselors–Roles
19:2 Aiken (153)
Parental disapproval as motive for decreased alcohol use
19:7 Reeves (819)
Parental factors–Alcoholic dyads
19:7 Synol (743)
Patterns of drinking–Business administration students
19:6 Waring (653)
Patterns of drinking–Student nurses
19:5 Haack (577)
Patterns of drug use–Medical students
19:8 Kory (871)
Patterns of smoking and smoke delivery
19:4 Moody (431)
Perceived nieghborhood setting effects on substance abuse
19:2 Blount (175)
Personality disorder in narcotic addicts
19:3 Cohen (335)
Personality tests in dropout prediction
19:6 Craig (665)

Phenomenology–Barbiturate and sedative-hypnotic use
19:3 Spotts (295)
Phenomenology–Cocaine ego state
19:2 Spotts (119)
Phobias
See Abstinence phobias
Physiological responses to alcohol-related stimuli
19:3 Eriksen (287)
"Planned failure" (editorial)
19:4 Einstein (iii)
Planning intervention programs
19:3 Einstein (355)
Planning intervention programs–Communication approach
19:8 Einstein (919)
Planning intervention programs–Community approach
19:8 Einstein (925)
Planning intervention programs–Coping and adaptation goals
19:4 Einstein (469)
Planning intervention programs–Experiential model
19:4 Einstein (475)
Planning intervention programs–Functional approach
19:5 Einstein (595)
Planning intervention programs–Special populations
19:8 Einstein (931)
Planning intervention programs–Task approach
19:5 Einstein (591)
Populations
See also General population images of drug addicts; Special population drug use intervention
Populations at risk (editorial)
19:2 Einstein (iii)
Positive Alternatives for Youth prevention program
19:7 Cook (767)
Prediction of alcoholic recidivism
19:5 Holland (585)
Prediction of dropout–Personality test effectiveness
19:6 Craig (665)
Prediction of relapse and remission
19:1 Mann (25)
Prediction of smoking frequency from nicotine level
19:8 Morrell (827)
Prediction of substance use–Neighborhood perception factors
19:2 Blount (175)
Predictors of adolescent intentions to smoke
19:5 Presson (503)
Predictors of time to locate at follow-up
19:8 Bale (885)
Pregnant addict care program
19:2 Suffett (199)
Prevalence of heroin abuse–Estimation
19:1 Woodward (93)
Prevention activities–Substance abuse effects
19:1 Sexter (79)
Prevention programs – Alternatives approach to drug abuse
19:7 Cook (767)
Prevention programs–Junior high school
19:4 Moskowitz (419)
Prime-time TV portrayal of alcohol
19:4 Futch (403)
Professional counselors
See Paraprofessional vs professional counselors
Professional psychotherapy–Compliance effects
19:5 Rogalski (521)
Progress of clients–Counselor effects
19:4 Aiken (383)
Prospective research design in outcome evaluation
19:5 Goldstein (479)
Psychedelic use transmission
19:6 Voss (633)
Psychiatric classification–Narcotic addicts
19:3 Cohen (335)
Psychological characteristics in alcoholic relapse
19:8 Sandahl (833)
Psychological symptom screening of drug abusers
19:8 Royse (849)

Psychosis in narcotic addicts
19:3 Cohen (335)
Psychotherapy–Compliance effects
19:5 Rogalski (521)
Psychotherapy for barbiturate and sedative-hypnotic users
19:3 Spotts (295)
Psychotherapy for cocaine users
19:2 Spotts (119)
Puerto Rican youth–Neighborhood perceptions and substance use
19:2 Blount (175)
Puff characteristics in cigarette smoking
19:4 Moody (431)
Pulmonary infections in drug users
19:2 Blanck (221)

Questionnaires–Drinking pattern survey
19:6 Waring (653)

Race differences in adolescent smoking intentions
19:5 Presson (503)
Recidivism
See also Outcome; Relapse
Recidivism in alcoholics–Prediction
19:5 Holland (585)
Reference groups in drug abuse etiology
19:6 Battjes (675)
Regional differences in adolescent smoking intentions
19:5 Presson (503)
Relapse
See also Recidivism
Relapse in alcoholics–Determinants
19:8 Sandahl (833)
Relapse and remission time distributions
19:1 Mann (25)
Reliability–Drug Abuse Warning Network data
19:1 Swisher (57)
Representative Case Method study–Barbiturate and sedative-hypnotic users
19:3 Spotts (295)
Representative Case Method study–Cocaine users
19:2 Spotts (119)
Repression through alcohol problem definitions
19:5 Vogt (551)
Research design problems in outcome evaluation
19:5 Goldstein (479)
Research instruments–Brief Symptom Inventory
19:8 Royse (849)
Research instruments–Drug Abuse Scale of Millon Inventory
19:4 Flynn (459)
Research instruments–Millon Clinical Multiaxial Inventory
19:6 Craig (665)
Research instruments – Social Recovery Inventory
19:7 Whorley (753)
Risk
See also Competing-risk distribution of relapse and remission
Risk factors–Cocaine abuse
19:2 Spotts (119)
Risk situations–Alcoholic relapse
19:8 Sandahl (833)
Risk/susceptibility (editorial)
19:2 Einstein (iii)
Roles–Intervention program (editorial)
19:4 Einstein (iii)
Roles–Paraprofessional and professional counselors
19:2 Aiken (153)
Roles–Professional psychotherapists in drug abuse treatment
19:5 Rogalski (521)
Roles in treatment outcome
19:6 Einstein (701)
Rural adolescents–Abstinence from alcohol
19:7 Reeves (819)

Scales and tests
See Research instruments
School-based prevention–Substance abuse effects
19:1 Sexter (79)
Screening
See also Assessment

Screening drug abusers–Brief Symptom Inventory
19:8 Royse (849)
Sedative-hypnotic induced ego states
19:3 Spotts (295)
Sedative use transmission
19:6 Voss (633)
Self-esteem as motive for decreased alcohol use
19:7 Reeves (819)
Self-perceptions–Drug addicts in treatment
19:7 Preston (805)
Self-reported drug use–Medical students
19:8 Kory (871)
Self-reported reasons for adolescent alcohol use
19:5 Segal (541)
Sensorimotor functioning–Barbiturate and sedative-hypnotic users
19:3 Spotts (295)
Sensorimotor functioning–Cocaine users
19:2 Spotts (119)
Sepsis in drug users
19:2 Blanck (221)
Setting
See also Ecological analysis; Perceived neighborhood setting
Setting and alcoholic relapse
19:8 Sandahl (833)
Sex differences in adolescent smoking intentions
19:5 Presson (503)
Sex differences in drinking patterns–Business administration students
19:6 Waring (653)
Smoking
See also Tobacco
Smoking cessation program–Hospital employees
19:3 Dawley (327)
Smoking frequency–Nicotine level effects
19:8 Morrell (827)
Smoking intentions–Adolescents
19:5 Presson (503)
Smoking patterns and smoke deliveries
19:4 Moody (431)
Sniffing
See Glue sniffing; Inhalant abuse
Social bond theory of drug use
19:3 Dull (265)
Social characteristics–Inhalant abusers
19:7 Reed (789)
Socialization in drug abuse etiology
19:6 Battjes (675)
Social networks–Opioid abusers
19:8 Fraser (903)
Social pathology–Drug abuse relationship
19:4 Nurco (441)
Social recovery and therapeutic goals
19:7 Whorley (753)
Sociological example of institutional violence
19:1 Ben-Yehuda (1)
Sociopathy in narcotic addicts
19:3 Cohen (335)
Spatiality–Barbiturate and sedative-hypnotic users
19:3 Spotts (295)
Spatiality–Cocaine users
19:2 Spotts (119)
Special population drug use intervention
19:8 Einstein (931)
Stability of substance use across college years
19:5 Friend (571)
Staff–Attitudes and expectations
19:3 LoSciuto (233)
Staff–Client progress effects
19:4 Aiken (383)
Staff–Early treatment termination effects
19:7 Fink (709)
Staff–Paraprofessional vs professional roles
19:2 Aiken (153)
Staff–Professional psychotherapists
19:5 Rogalski (521)
Staff–Smoking cessation program
19:3 Dawley (327)
Stereotypes of drug addicts
19:8 Dean (859)
Stigma of addiction
19:8 Dean (859)
Stimulant use–Nigerian students
19:3 Achalu (253)
Stimulant use transmission
19:6 Voss (633)
Structure of opioid abuser social networks
19:8 Fraser (903)

Students
See also College students; High school students; Junior high school students
Student substance abuse–Prevention activity effects
19:1 Sexter (79)
Styles in treatment outcome
19:6 Einstein (701)
Subjective responses to alcohol-related stimuli
19:3 Eriksen (287)
Substance abuse–Anxiety relationship
19:6 Hall (613)
Substance abuse–Prevention activity effects
19:1 Sexter (79)
Substance abuse–Prevention in junior high school
19:4 Moskowitz (419)
Substance abusers–Follow-up difficulties
19:8 Bale (885)
Substance use–Stability and change in college
19:5 Friend (571)
Susceptibility/risk (editorial)
19:2 Einstein (iii)
Sweden–Relapse in alcoholics
19:8 Sandahl (833)
Symbolic interaction analysis of drug abuse etiology
19:6 Battjes (675)
System variables and adherence in treatment
19:7 Fink (709)

Tar delivery–Smoking pattern effects
19:4 Moody (431)
Task approach to drug use intervention
19:5 Einstein (591)
Tasks in treatment outcome
19:6 Einstein (701)
Television
See Prime-time TV
Temporal analysis–Alcoholic relapse
19:8 Sandhal (833)
Temporal analysis–Changes in self-perception in treatment
19:7 Preston (805)
Temporal analysis–Drug abuse prevention program
19:7 Cook (767)
Temporal analysis–Drug use transmission
19:6 Voss (633)
Temporal analysis–Relapse and remission
19:1 Mann (25)
Temporality–Barbiturate and sedative-hypnotic users
19:3 Spotts (295)
Temporality–Cocaine effects
19:2 Spotts (119)
Tests and scales
See Research instruments
Thematic Locus of Control results in alcoholics
19:1 Costello (45)
Therapeutic communities–Client self-perception changes
19:7 Preston (805)
Time to locate at follow-up
19:8 Bale (885)
Tobacco
See also Smoking
Tobacco dependence–Anxiety relationship
19:6 Hall (613)
Tobacco use–Medical students
19:8 Kory (871)
Tobacco use–Neighborhood perception effects
19:2 Blount (175)
Tobacco use–Nigerian students
19:3 Achalu (253)
Tobacco use–Social bond effects
19:3 Dull (265)
Treatment evaluation–Substance abuse prevention in junior high school
19:4 Moskowitz (419)
Treatment program development
See Planning intervention programs
Treatment programs
See also Intervention; Methadone; Staff
Treatment programs–Client self-perception changes
19:7 Preston (805)
Treatment programs–Pregnant addict care
19:2 Suffet (199)

Treatment programs – Psychotherapy effects on compliance
19:5 Rogalski (521)
Treatment programs–Screening
19:8 Royse (849)
Treatment programs–Smoking cessation
19:3 Dawley (327)
Treatment programs–Social recovery goals
19:7 Whorley (753)
Treatment programs–Supports and barriers for women
19:6 Robinson (601)
Treatment programs–System variables and adherence
19:7 Fink (709)
"Turning on" other persons to drugs
19:6 Voss (633)
Typologies–Communities
19:8 Einstein (925)
Typologies–Drug abuse
19:3 Einstein (355)
Typologies–Special populations
19:8 Einstein (931)

University students
See College students
Urban drug abuse–Social pathology relationship
19:4 Nurco (441)
Urban substance abuse
19:2 Blount (175)

Validity
See also Construct validity
Validity–Brief Sympton Inventory
19:8 Royse (849)
Validity–Drug Abuse Warning Network data
19:1 Swisher (57)
Validity–Millon Clinical Multiaxial Inventory Drug Abuse Scale
19:4 Flynn (459)
Violence
See Aggression; Institutional violence
Viral hepatitis in drug users
19:2 Blanck (221)

Wear-out as factor in relapse
19:1 Mann (25)
Women–Alcohol abuse intervention factors
19:6 Robinson (601)
Women–Drinking habits in West Germany
19:5 Vogt (551)
Women–Nursing student drinking patterns
19:5 Haack (557)
Women–Pregnant addict care
19:2 Suffet (199)
Women–Prevention program effects in junior high school
19:4 Moskowitz (419)
Working class repression through alcohol problem definitions
19:5 Vogt (551)
Worksite smoking cessation program
19:3 Dawley (327)

The International Journal of the Addictions, 19(8), 957-962, (1984)

COLLECTIVE CONTENTS TO VOLUME 19

Volume 19 **Number 1** **1984**

Editorial: Coping and Drug Misuse Intervention: S. Einstein iii

Human Garbage and Physical Garbage: A Sociological Case Example of Institutional Violence: N. Ben-Yehuda and S. Einstein 1

A Diagnostic Tool with Important Implications for Treatment of Addiction: Identification of Factors Underlying Relapse and Remission Time Distributions: N. R. Mann, V. C. Charuvastra, and V. K. Murthy 25

Impression Management and Testing for Control Locus in an Alcoholic Sample: R. M. Costello and K. A. Wicoff 45

A Review of the Reliability and Validity of the Drug Abuse Warning Network: J. D. Swisher and T.-W. Hu 57

Substance Abuse: Assessment of the Outcomes of Activities and Activity Clusters in School-Based Prevention: J. Sexter, A. P. Sullivan, S. F. Wepner, and R. Denmark 79

Construct Validity of Heroin Abuse Estimators: J. A. Woodward, R. L. Retka, and L. Ng 93

Volume 19 **Number 2** **1984**

Editorial: Considering the Risks of "Populations at Risk": S. Einstein . . iii

Drug-Induced Ego States. I. Cocaine: Phenomenology and Implications: J. V. Spotts and F. C. Shontz 119

Paraprofessional Versus Professional Drug Counselors: Diverse Routes to the Same Role: L. S. Aiken, L. A. LoSciuto, M. A. Ausetts, and B. S. Brown 153

The Effect of Perceived Neighborhood Setting on Self-Reported Tobacco, Alcohol, and Marijuana Use among Inner-City Minority Junior High School Youth: W. R. Blount and R. Dembo 175

A Comprehensive Care Program for Pregnant Addicts: Obstetrical, Neonatal, and Child Development Outcomes: F. Suffet and R. Brotman 199

Note

Infectious Complications of Illicit Drug Use: R. R. Blanck, N. W. Ream, and J. S. Deleese 221

Volume 19 Number 3 1984

Editorial: Drug Use Intervention and Control Mechanisms: S. Einstein . . . iii

Paraprofessional Versus Professional Drug Abuse Counselors: Attitudes and Expectations of the Counselors and Their Clients: L. LoSciuto, L. S. Aiken, M. A. Ausetts, and B. S. Brown 233

Drug Taking by Nigerian Students in American Universities: Prevalences for Four Commonly Used Drugs: O. E. Achalu and D. F. Duncan . . . 253

An Empirical Examination of the Social Bond Theory of Drug Use: R. T. Dull 265

Conditioned Abstinence in Alcoholics: A Controlled Experiment: L. Eriksen and K. G. Götestam 287

The Phenomenological Structure of Drug-Induced Ego States. II. Barbiturates and Sedative-Hypnotics: Phenomenology and Implications: J. V. Spotts and F. C. Shontz 295

Smoking Cessation with Hospital Employees: An Example of Worksite Smoking Cessation: H. H. Dawley, Jr., B. J. Fleischer, and L. T. Dawley 327

The "Urge to Classify" the Narcotic Addict: A Review of Psychiatric Classification. II: A. Cohen 335

Note

Drug Misuse/Abuse Intervention: A Schematic Tool for Decision Making and Planning: S. Einstein 355

Volume 19 **Number 4** **1984**

Editorial: Preventing Change through Current Substance Use Intervention: A Role Analysis: S. Einstein iii

Alcohol and Marijuana Use in Adolescents' Daily Lives: A Random Sample of Experiences: R. Larson, M. Csikszentmihalyi, and M. Freeman 367

Paraprofessional Versus Professional Drug Counselors: The Progress of Clients in Treatment: L. S. Aiken, L. A. LoSciuto, M. A. Ausetts, and B. S. Brown 383

An Analysis of Alcohol Portrayal on Prime-Time Television: E. J. Futch, S. A. Lisman, and M. I. Geller 403

Alcohol and Drug Use in the Elderly Visited at Home: M. T. Malcolm 411

Evaluation of a Substance Abuse Prevention Program for Junior High School Students: J. M. Moskowitz, E. Schaps, G. A. Schaeffer, and J. H. Malvin 419

Human Smoking Patterns and Smoke Deliveries: P. M. Moody 431

An Ecological Analysis of the Interrelationships among Drug Abuse and Other Indices of Social Pathology: D. N. Nurco, J. W. Shaffer, and I. H. Cisin 441

Research Note

Glue Sniffing: A Pilot Study of the Cognitive Effects of Long-Term Use: W. M. Allison and D. W. A. Jerrom 453

Notes

An Examination of the Drug Abuse Scale of the Millon Clinical Multiaxial Inventory: P. M. Flynn and R. C. McMahon 459

Drug Use Intervention and Individual/Group Adaptation: Facilitation of Coping in Potential Worlds of Adaptation: S. Einstein 469

An Experiential Model for Drug Use Intervention: S. Einstein 475

Volume 19 **Number 5** **1984**

Outcome Evaluations in Substance Abuse: A Comparison of Alcoholism, Drug Abuse, and Other Mental Health Interventions: M. S. Goldstein, M. Surber, and D. M. Wilner 479

Predictors of Adolescents' Intentions to Smoke: Age, Sex, Race, and Regional Differences: C. C. Presson, L. Chassin, S. J. Sherman, R. Olshavsky, M. Bensenberg, and E. Corty 503

Professional Psychotherapy and Its Relationship to Compliance in Treatment: C. J. Rogalski 521

Alcohol Use by Juvenile Offenders: B. Segal, S. S. Hobfoll, and F. Cromer 541

Defining Alcohol Problems as a Repressive Mechanism: Its Formative Phase in Imperial Germany and Its Strength Today: I. Vogt 551

Research Notes

Student Substance Use: Stability and Change across College Years: K. E. Friend and P. A. Koushki 571

Drinking Patterns among Student Nurses: M. R. Haack and T. C. Harford 577

Notes

Prediction of Readmission in a Cohort of Alcoholics: A 2-Year Follow-Up: R. A. Holland and R. C. Evenson 585

A Task Approach to Drug Use Intervention: S. Einstein 591

A Functional Approach to Drug Use Intervention: S. Einstein 595

Volume 19 **Number 6** **1984**

Women and Alcohol Abuse—Factors Involved in Successful Interventions: S. D. Robinson 601

The Abstinence Phobias: Links between Substance Abuse and Anxiety: S. M. Hall 613

"Turning on" Other Persons to Drugs: H. L. Voss and R. R. Clayton 633

Alcohol Use among Graduate Business Administration Students: M. L. Waring, G. Petraglia, L. Cohen, and E. Busby 653

Can Personality Tests Predict Treatment Dropouts?: R. J. Craig 665

Symbolic Interaction Theory: A Perspective on Drug Abuse and Its Treatment: R. J. Battjes 675

Research Note

Individual Characteristics of Aggressive Beer and Distilled Beverage Drinkers: R. O. Pihl, M. Smith, and B. Farrell 689

Notes

Considering Motivation and Ability for Drug Use Intervention: Some Implications: S. Einstein 697

Outcome of Drug User Treatment: A Selection of Additional Needed Factors: S. Einstein 701

Volume 19 Number 7 1984

Adherence in a Behavioral Alcohol Treatment Program: E. B. Fink, S. Rudden, R. Longabaugh, B. McCrady, and R. Stout 709

Alcohol Education Programs for University Students: A Review of Their Effectiveness: M. S. Goodstadt and A. Caleekal-John 721

Family Mapping: Toward an Understanding of the Interactional Dynamic of the Alcoholic Marital Dyad: K. M. Synol 743

Social Recovery and Therapeutic Mission: L. W. Whorley 753

An Evaluation of the Alternatives Approach to Drug Abuse Prevention: R. Cook, H. Lawrence, C. Morse, and J. Roehl 767

Research Notes

Inhalant Abuse and Juvenile Delinquency: A Control Study in Albuquerque, New Mexico: B. J. F. Reed and P. A. May 789

Self- and Ideal-Self-Perception of Drug Addicts in Therapeutic Communities: C. A. Preston and L. L. Viney 805

Note

Abstinence or Decreasing Consumption among Adolescents: Importance of Reasons: D. W. Reeves and T. W. Draper 819

Volume 19 **Number 8** **1984**

Nicotine Level as a Predictor of Smoking Frequency: A Case Report: E. M. Morrell and J. G. Hollandsworth, Jr 827

Determinants of Relapse among Alcoholics: A Cross-Cultural Replication Study: C. Sandahl 833

Screening Drug Abuse Clients with the Brief Symptom Inventory: D. Royse and K. Drude 849

The Drug Addict and the Stigma of Addiction: J. C. Dean and F. Rud 859

Nonmedical Drug Use Patterns among Medical Students: W. P. Kory and L. A. Crandall 871

Follow-Up Difficulty with Substance Abusers: Predictors of Time to Locate and Relationship to Outcome: R. N. Bale, B. H. Arnoldussen, and A. M. Quittner 885

The Social Networks of Opioid Abusers: M. W. Fraser and J. D. Hawkins 903

Notes

A Communication Approach to Drug Use Intervention: S. Einstein 919

Drug Use Community Intervention: Issues and Options: S. Einstein 925

Drug Use Intervention with and for Special Populations: S. Einstein 931

Index to Volume 19 937

THE AMERICAN JOURNAL OF DRUG AND ALCOHOL ABUSE

Volume 10, Number 2, 1984

CONTENTS

A Longitudinal Study of Offspring Born to Methadone-Maintained Women. I. Design, Methodology, and Description of Women's Resources for Functioning 135
J. Marcus, S. L. Hans, C. B. Patterson, and A. J. Morris

A Longitudinal Study of Offspring Born to Methadone-Maintained Women. II. Dyadic Interaction and Infant Behavior at 4 Months 161
V. Bernstein, R. Jeruchimowicz Jeremy, S. L. Hans, and J. Marcus

A Longitudinal Study of Offspring Born to Methadone-Maintained Women. III. Effects of Multiple Risk Factors on Development at 4,8, and 12 Months 195
J. Marcus, S. L. Hans, and R. Jeruchimowicz Jeremy

The Index of Choice: Indications of Methadone Patients' Selection of Naltrexone Treatment 209
E. G. Singleton, M. F. Sherman, and G. E. Bigelow

Teacher Training in Affective Education for the Primary Prevention of Adolescent Drug Abuse 223
J. H. Malvin, J. M. Moskowitz, G. A. Schaeffer, and E. Schaps

Heroin Addicts and Nonaddicted Brothers 237
J. F. Maddux and D. P. Desmond

Strategies to Improve Compliance with Narcotic Antagonists 249
T. R. Kosten and H. D. Kleber

Therapeutic Communities: What Are the Retention Rates? 267
G. De Leon and S. Schwartz

Frequency of Heroin Use and Drug Users' Life-Style 285
E. W. Flaherty, L. Kotranski, and E. Fox

Books Received 315

MARCEL DEKKER, INC.

270 MADISON AVENUE, NEW YORK, N.Y. 10016

(212) 696-9000

INFORMATION FOR AUTHORS SUBMITTING MANUSCRIPTS

Send a clear double-spaced typewritten original and one duplicate to Ms. Nancy Reid-Rappolt, Editorial Assistant, *International Journal of the Addictions,* c/o Winch, Smith, Ostermann and Mates, MD's, 4141 Geary, Suite 326, San Francisco, California 94118. Also send one duplicate to the Chief Editor, Dr. Stanley Einstein, Building 113/41, East Talpiot, Jerusalem, Israel. DOUBLE-SPACE the entire manuscript; do not use single spacing anywhere, including references.

Include authors' academic degrees and present affiliation. If applicable, cite auspices under which work being reported was done. Specify address to which requests for reprints should be sent.

Begin your TITLE with a word useful in indexing. A 75- to 100-word ABSTRACT should be provided, which precedes each article. A summary is then not necessary. Major and minor headings may be used in the text; indicate major headings by typing in capitals.

Use METRIC UNITS of measure. If measurements were made in English units, give metric equivalents.

Cite all TABLES and FIGURES in the text. Tables should have titles, and figures should have brief legends. In tables, give each column a heading. Indicate units of measure in parentheses in the heading for each column. Do not use vertical rules. Do not use horizontal rules other than those in the heading and at the bottom. Submit PHOTOGRAPHS as glossy prints, untrimmed and unmounted; identify each with pencil lightly on the back and indicate top.

ARTWORK will not be returned unless specifically requested, and will be disposed of three months after publication.

REFERENCES in the text should be enclosed in parentheses and include the author's surname and the date of the item cited. Keep footnotes to a minimum. Footnotes should be collected at the end of the manuscript in their numerical order of appearance.

The BIBLIOGRAPHY (double-spaced) should be given at the end of the article in alphabetical order. Journal references should include authors, title, name of journal abbreviated according to *Chemical Abstracts List of Periodicals*, inclusive page numbers, and date. Book references should include authors, title, place of publication, publisher, and date.

AUTHOR RESPONSIBILITY: It is the sole responsibility of the author(s) to obtain written permission from the author(s), publisher(s), etc. for figures, tables, or any other information excerpted from previously published works which are used in the manuscript(s) considered for publication. It is understood that the manuscript(s) considered for publication in the *International Journal of the Addictions* have not been previously published nor are they under simultaneous publication consideration elsewhere.

Statements and opinions expressed in the articles and communications herein are those of the author(s) and do not necessarily express those of the Editor or publisher.

THE INTERNATIONAL JOURNAL OF THE ADDICTIONS

Volume 19 Number 8 1984

CONTENTS

Nicotine Level as a Predictor of Smoking Frequency: A Case Report: E. M. Morrell and J. G. Hollandsworth, Jr 827

Determinants of Relapse among Alcoholics: A Cross-Cultural Replication Study: C. Sandahl 833

Screening Drug Abuse Clients with the Brief Symptom Inventory: D. Royse and K. Drude 849

The Drug Addict and the Stigma of Addiction: J. C. Dean and F. Rud 859

Nonmedical Drug Use Patterns among Medical Students: W. P. Kory and L. A. Crandall 871

Follow-Up Difficulty with Substance Abusers: Predictors of Time to Locate and Relationship to Outcome: R. N. Bale, B. H. Arnoldussen, and A. M. Quittner 885

The Social Networks of Opioid Abusers: M. W. Fraser and J. D. Hawkins 903

Notes

A Communication Approach to Drug Use Intervention: S. Einstein 919

Drug Use Community Intervention: Issues and Options: S. Einstein 925

Drug Use Intervention with and for Special Populations: S. Einstein 931

Index to Volume 19 937

Collective Contents to Volume 19 957

MARCEL DEKKER, INC., New York and Basel